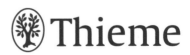

Current Concepts of Sleep Apnea Surgery

Thomas Verse, MD
Professor of Otorhinolaryngology
Director of Department of Otorhinolaryngology–Head and Neck Surgery
Asklepios Clinic Harburg
Asklepios Campus Hamburg of Semmelweis University
Hamburg, Germany

Nico de Vries, MD, PhD
Professor of Otolaryngology
Department of Otorhinolaryngology–Head and Neck Surgery
OLVG Hospital
Department of Oral Kinesiology
ACTA Amsterdam
Amsterdam, The Netherlands
Department of Otorhinolaryngology–Head and Neck Surgery
University of Antwerp
Antwerp, Belgium

281 illustrations

Thieme
Stuttgart • New York • Delhi • Rio de Janeiro

Library of Congress Cataloging-in-Publication Data is available from the publisher.

© 2019 by Georg Thieme Verlag KG

Thieme Publishers Stuttgart
Rüdigerstrasse 14, 70469 Stuttgart, Germany
+49 [0]711 8931 421, customerservice@thieme.de

Thieme Publishers New York
333 Seventh Avenue, New York, NY 10001, USA
+1-800-782-3488, customerservice@thieme.com

Thieme Publishers Delhi
A-12, Second Floor, Sector-2, Noida-201301
Uttar Pradesh, India
+91 120 45 566 00, customerservice@thieme.in

Thieme Publishers Rio de Janeiro,
Thieme Publicações Ltda.
Edifício Rodolpho de Paoli, 25º andar
Av. Nilo Peçanha, 50 – Sala 2508
Rio de Janeiro 20020-906 Brasil
+55 21 3172 2297 / +55 21 3172 1896

Cover design: Thieme Publishing Group
Typesetting by DiTech Process Solutions Pvt. Ltd., India

Printed in Germany by CPI Books   5 4 3 2 1

ISBN 978-3-13-240119-8

Also available as an e-book:
eISBN 978-3-13-240263-8

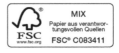

Contents

Videos

Video 6.1: Argon plasma coagulation technique for tonsillotomy.

Video 8.1: Z-palatopharyngoplasty (Z-PPP) technique.

Video 8.2: Relocation—uvulopalatopharyngoplasty (UPPP) in obstructive sleep apnea (OSA).

Video 8.3: Expansion sphincter pharyngoplasty (ESP) evolutive technique.

Video 8.4: Implantation of selective upper airway stimulation.

Video 8.5: Primary collapse of the epiglottis in an adult male.

Video 8.6: Three-dimensional planning of maxillomandibular advancement surgery in an OSA patient.

Video 8.7: Operative procedure of maxillomandibular advancement surgery in an OSA patient.

Video 8.8: Distraction osteogenesis maxillary expansion (DOME).

Preface

Obstructive sleep apnea (OSA) is one of the most frequent and common diseases all over the globe. In 1981, both continuous positive airway pressure (CPAP) and uvulopalatopharyngoplasty (UPPP) were introduced in the treatment of OSA. That year marked the birth of modern sleep medicine. We have since learnt a lot about the pathophysiology of OSA. Today, there is a variety of treatment modalities for OSA, snoring and related disturbances including conservative (i.e., diet, behavior therapy, positional treatments), medical device treatment (i.e., oral devices, CPAP), and operative treatments. After a period that was characterized by the search for the optimal single treatment, we today know that often a combination of different treatment modalities provides the best results.

Sleep apnea surgery is a relatively young discipline that is developing rapidly. Surgical procedures aimed to treat sleep apnea need to be selected in awareness of the individual underlying pathology, pathophysiology and anatomy, and severity of the disease, and comorbidities must also be taken into account. The first part of the book is designed to provide the reader with fundamental knowledge about the pathophysiology and diagnosis of OSA and to give a practical approach on how to choose the best treatment(s) for every individual case.

The second part concentrates on surgical approaches to treat OSA. Both of us have performed sleep apnea surgery for decades and witnessed, and to a certain extent influenced, the development of sleep apnea surgery for many years. Today, there are too many surgeries or modifications to include in one book. Therefore, we have discussed those techniques that work best in our hands. Leading experts in the field of surgery from all over the world have contributed as coauthors for specific topics and surgical techniques. Of course, there are other modifications of sleep surgeries that might work well or come up in future. However, we are convinced that this book provides a variety of effective surgical treatments that will help successfully treat the biggest part of the clinical cases. The easy-to-read text is accompanied by figures and videos of best quality, and the readers are provided with a variety of solutions for their sleep surgery cases. We very much hope that this book will become a helpful tool in sleep apnea surgery.

Thomas Verse, MD
Nico de Vries, MD, PhD

Contributors

José Enrique Barrera, MD, FACS
Associate Professor
Uniformed Services University
Bethesda, Maryland, USA
Clinical Associate Professor
University of Texas Health Sciences Center
Medical Director
Texas Facial Plastic Surgery and ENT
San Antonio, Texas, USA

Annemieke Beelen, MD
Department of Otorhinolaryngology–Head and Neck
  Surgery
OLVG Hospital
Amsterdam, The Netherlands

Chiara Bellini, MD
Department of Otolaryngology–Head and Neck Surgery
Head-Neck and Oral Surgery Unit
G.B. Morgagni-L. Pierantoni Hospital
Forli, Italy

Linda B. L. Benoist, MD
Department of Otorhinolaryngology and Head and Neck
  Surgery
Erasmus University Medical Center
Rotterdam, The Netherlands

Jolien Beyers, MD
Faculty of Medicine and Health Sciences
University of Antwerp
Antwerp, Belgium
Department of ENT, Head and Neck Surgery
Antwerp University Hospital UZA
Edegem, Belgium

Marc Blumen, MD
Head, Department of Otolaryngology/Sleep and Breathing
Centre Medical Veille-Sommeil
Paris, France

Marina Carrasco-Llatas, Md, PhD
ENT Consultant
Hospital Universitario Dr. Peset
Valencia, Spain

Alessandra Castrogiovanni, MD
Clinic for Pneumology and Allergology
Center of Sleep Medicine and Respiratory Care
Bethanien Hospital
Solingen, Germany

Khai Beng Chong, MD
Department of Otorhinolaryngology
Tan Tock Seng Hospital
Tan Tock Seng, Singapore

Marijke Dieltjens, MBS, PhD
Department of ENT, Head and Neck Surgery
Antwerp University Hospital UZA
Edegem, Belgium

Mohamed Salah El-Rashwan, MD
Department of Otolaryngology
Suez Canal University Teaching Hospitals
Ismailia, Egypt

Michael Friedman, MD, FACS
Department of Otolaryngology–Head and Neck Surgery
Division of Sleep Surgery
Rush University Medical Center
Department of Otolaryngology
Advanced Center for Specialty Care
Advocate Illinois Masonic Medical Center
Chicago, Illinois, USA

Christian Guilleminault, DM, MD, DBIOL
Professor
Department of Psychiatry and Behavioral Sciences
Stanford University School of Medicine
Stanford, California, USA

Evert Hamans, MD, PhD
ENT surgeon
Department of Otorhinolaryngology
Hospital Network Antwerp
Antwerp, Belgium

Clemens Heiser, MD, Prof.
Provisional Medical Director
Head of Sleep Laboratory
Department of Otorhinolaryngology, Head and Neck
 Surgery
Klinikum Rechts der Isar
Technical University of Munich
Munich, Germany

Simon Herkenrath, MD
Clinic for Pneumology and Allergology
Center of Sleep Medicine and Respiratory Care
Bethanien Hospital
Solingen, Germany

PD Dr. med. habil. Michael Herzog
Chief Doctor
Clinic for ENT diseases, Head and Neck Surgery
Carl-Thiem-Klinikum Cottbus gGmbH
Cottbus, Germany

Aarnoud Hoekema, MD, DMD, PhD
Oral and Maxillofacial Surgeon
Department of Oral and Maxillofacial Surgery
Tjongerschans Hospital
Heerenveen, The Netherlands
Department of Oral Kinesiology
Academic Centre for Dentistry Amsterdam (ACTA)
MOVE Research Institute Amsterdam
University of Amsterdam and VU University Amsterdam
Amsterdam, The Netherlands
Department of Oral and Maxillofacial Surgery
Academic Medical Center (AMC)
Amsterdam, The Netherlands
Department of Oral and Maxillofacial Surgery
University Medical Center Groningen
Groningen, The Netherlands

Jan de Lange, MD
Maxillofacial Surgeon
Chairman, Department of Maxillofacial Surgery
University of Amsterdam
Amsterdam, The Netherlands

Hsin-Ching Lin, MD, FACS, FICS
Professor and Chairman
Department of Otolaryngology
Sleep Center and Robotic Surgery Center
College of Medicine, Chang Gung University
Kaohsiung Chang Gung Memorial Hospital
Kaohsiung City, Taiwan

Stanley Yung-Chuan Liu, MD, DDS
Assistant Professor of Otolaryngology
Co-Director, Sleep Surgery Fellowship Stanford University
 School of Medicine
Stanford, California, USA

Peter van Maanen, MD, PhD
Department of Otorhinolaryngology–Head and Neck Surgery
OLVG Hospital
Amsterdam, The Netherlands

Andrea Marzetti, MD
Department of Otolaryngology
San Carlo di Nancy Hospital
Rome, Italy

OA Dr. med. Joachim T. Maurer
Deputy Hospital Director
University ENT Clinic Mannheim
Head of Sleep Medical Center
Mannheim, Germany

Giuseppe Meccariello, MD
Department of Otolaryngology–Head and Neck Surgery
Head-Neck and Oral Surgery Unit
G.B. Morgagni-L. Pierantoni Hospital
Forli, Italy

Carla Miltz, MD
Clinic for Pneumology and Allergology
Center of Sleep Medicine and Respiratory Care
Bethanien Hospital
Solingen, Germany

Filippo Montevecchi, MD
Department of Otolaryngology–Head and Neck Surgery
Head-Neck and Oral Surgery Unit
G.B. Morgagni-L. Pierantoni Hospital
Forli, Italy

Edward B. Pang
Student, Otolaryngology
Asia Sleep Centre
Paragon, Singapore

Kathleen A. Pang
Student, Otolaryngology
Asia Sleep Centre
Paragon, Singapore

Kenny P. Pang, FRCSEd, FRCSI(OTO)
Consultant, Otolaryngology
Asia Sleep Centre
Paragon, Singapore

Dirk Pevernagie, MD, PhD
Director
Center for Sleep Medicine
Kempenhaeghe Foundation
Heeze, The Netherlands
Department of Internal Medicine
Faculty of Medicine and Health Sciences
Ghent University
Ghent, Belgium

Prof. Dr. med. Wolfgang Pirsig
Professor Emeritus for Otorhinolaryngology
University of Ulm
Ulm, Germany

Anne-Lise Poirrier, MD
Rhinology and Facial Plastic Surgery
University Hospital of Liege
Liège, Belgium

Robert Poirrier, MD
Sleep Center, Department of Neurology
University Hospital of Liege
Liège, Belgium

Christel de Raaff, MD
Department of Surgery
Albert Schweitzer Hospital
Dordrecht, The Netherlands

Winfried J. Randerath, MD
Clinic for Pneumology and Allergology
Center of Sleep Medicine and Respiratory Care
Bethanien Hospital
Solingen, Germany

Madeline Ravesloot, MD, PhD, MSc
Department of Otorhinolaryngology–Head and Neck
    Surgery
OLVG Hospital
Amsterdam, The Netherlands

Martin Roesslein, MD
Department of Anesthesiology and Critical Care Medicine
University Medical Center
Freiburg, Germany

Kerstin Rohde†, MD
Private Practice
Hamburg, Germany

Jim Smithuis, MD, PhD
Department of Otorhinolaryngology–Head and Neck
    Surgery
OLVG Hospital
Amsterdam, The Netherlands

Ullrich Sommer, MD
Clinic for ENT Diseases
Helios University Clinic Wuppertal
Wuppertal, Germany

PD Dr. med. Armin Steffen
Managing Senior Physician
Department of Otolaryngology
University Hospital Schleswig-Holstein
Lübeck, Germany

Boris A. Stuck, MD
Clinic for ENT Diseases
Philipps-Universität Marburg
Marburg, Germany

Olivier M. Vanderveken, MD, PhD
Faculty of Medicine and Health Sciences
University of Antwerp
Antwerp, Belgium
Department of ENT, Head and Neck Surgery
Antwerp University Hospital UZA
Edegem, Belgium

Johan Verbraecken, MD, PhD
Pulmonologist and Medical Coordinator
Department of Pulmonary Medicine
Multidisciplinary Sleep Disorders Centre
Antwerp University Hospital UZA
Edegem, Belgium

Thomas Verse, MD
Professor of Otorhinolaryngology
Director of Department of Otorhinolaryngology–Head and
    Neck Surgery
Asklepios Clinic Harburg
Asklepios Campus Hamburg of Semmelweis University
Hamburg, Germany

Claudio Vicini, MD
Department of Otolaryngology–Head and Neck Surgery
Head-Neck and Oral Surgery Unit
G.B. Morgagni-L. Pierantoni Hospital
Forli, Italy

Nico de Vries, MD, PhD
Professor of Otolaryngology
Department of Otorhinolaryngology–Head and Neck Surgery
OLVG Hospital
Department of Oral Kinesiology
ACTA Amsterdam
Amsterdam, The Netherlands
Department of Otorhinolaryngology–Head and Neck Surgery
University of Antwerp
Antwerp, Belgium

Anneclaire Vroegop, MD
Faculty of Medicine and Health Sciences
University of Antwerp
Antwerp, Belgium
Department of ENT, Head and Neck Surgery
Antwerp University Hospital UZA
Edegem, Belgium

Bart van Wagensveld, MD
Department of Bariatric Surgery
Quro Obesity Center
Dubai, United Arab Emirates

David White, MD
Professor of Medicine, Part Time
Harvard Medical School
Boston, Massachusetts

Audrey Jung-Sun Yoon, MD
Orthodontist
Stanford, California, USA
Clinical Faculty, Lecturer
Section of Pediatric Dentistry
University of California Los Angeles
Los Angeles, California, USA
Honorary Assistant Professor
Orthodontics, Faculty of Dentistry
The University of Hong Kong
Sai Wan, Hong Kong

1 Introduction and History of Sleep Apnea Surgery

Abstract

Symptoms and surgical procedures for snoring and obstructive sleep apnea (OSA) are known from antiquity especially from Greece, where uvulas were crushed, nasal polyps removed, and fine needles thrust into the belly of Dionysius to stop his OSA-originated sleep. In the Renaissance, caustic methods were introduced by Arabian physicians of the Middle Ages and snares were installed to reduce obstructive tissues of the upper airways. In addition, guillotine-like devices for uvulectomy and tonsillotomy were developed and used until the 20th century. In 1878, Meyer added the effective adenoidectomy to the procedures for sleep-disordered breathing, while in 1969 Kuhl et al proved tracheostomy to be an effective therapy to heal even severe OSA. With the development of modern sleep medicine in the 1970s, palatal surgery, tongue base techniques, maxillofacial procedures, and multilevel surgery enabled a tailored treatment of the patients which for the moment is culminating in the successful hypoglossal nerve stimulation procedure.

Keywords: sleep surgery, history, obstructive sleep apnea, snoring

1.1 Introduction

David White

This book has been written to describe which patients with obstructive sleep apnea (OSA) can be identified as appropriate candidates for upper airway surgery, to describe in detail the various procedures available, and to discuss how a particular surgery can be selected for a given patient. Upper airway surgery, in general, assumes that the primary cause of OSA is an anatomically small pharyngeal airway and that the surgical procedure can adequately correct this anatomical abnormality to allow for unobstructed breathing during sleep. It has been known for years that abnormal pharyngeal anatomy is an important part of OSA pathophysiology and this will be discussed further. However, the success or failure of upper airway surgery to reduce or eliminate disordered breathing is likely dependent on a number of variables only some of which relate to anatomy. These include:

- The severity of the anatomical abnormality.
- The site or sites, severity, and configuration of collapse and their proper identification.
- The role and importance of nonanatomical traits in the pathogenesis of OSA in a particular patient.

The role of abnormal anatomy in the pathogenesis of OSA has been well described over the years. Haponik et al[1] were the first to suggest this possibility when they demonstrated a smaller pharyngeal airway lumen in OSA patients compared with a control group using CT scanning in 1982. This led to numerous assessments of pharyngeal anatomy in OSA patients using a variety of imaging techniques including cephalometry, acoustic reflection, CT scanning, and MRI. The work of Richard Schwab[2,3] using MRI for the past 10 to 15 years has convincingly demonstrated that the upper airway lumen is smaller and that certain tissue structures are larger in OSA patients compared with various control groups. These enlarged structures include the tongue, the lateral pharyngeal walls, the parapharyngeal fat pads, and the soft palate/uvula among others. However, virtually all such imaging has been conducted during wakefulness when pharyngeal muscles are active, making pure assessment of anatomy difficult. Ultimately Isono et al[4] studied patients during neuromuscular blockade and found the pressure-area plots of patients with OSA to be quite different from controls, indicating a clear anatomic deficiency in the apnea patients.

In addition to studies directly assessing pharyngeal anatomy, metrics of pharyngeal collapsibility obtained during sleep have been used for the past 30 years to quantify the severity of the anatomic abnormality. Alan Schwartz and colleagues[5,6] at Johns Hopkins developed the methods to quantify the critical closing pressure (Pcrt) that can be measured with and without pharyngeal muscle activity (active versus passive Pcrt). This metric has proved quite valuable as a physiologic measure of the severity of the anatomic abnormality and has been used widely. However, no measure of anatomy whether quantified awake or asleep, with or without muscle activity, or using imaging or physiologic techniques has correlated well with the severity of OSA.[7] Indeed some patients without OSA have a similar or more collapsible airway than many OSA patients.[8] Patients with a very high passive Pcrt (above 2–3 cm H_2O) generally have more severe OSA than those with a lower Pcrt (−2 to 0 cm H_2O). However, there remains huge variability in the apnea–hypopnea index (AHI) at any measured level of pharyngeal collapsibility.[7,8] This failure to predict apnea severity can be interpreted in a number of ways. First, AHI may be a poor measure of OSA severity. Second, Pcrt may be a less quantitative assessment of the pure anatomy than originally thought. However, third, and most likely, is the fact that anatomy is not the entire explanation for the presence or severity of OSA. Other physiologic traits are likely important as well and these will be addressed later. That being said, anatomy is the most important trait in the majority of OSA patients, and OSA is likely to resolve if surgery can completely correct the anatomic deficiency yielding a minimally collapsible airway (Pcrt below −6 or −7 cm H_2O).[8] However, this is often difficult.

Recognizing that anatomy is not often the entire explanation for the presence of OSA, it is not surprising that the techniques described earlier for quantifying pharyngeal anatomy/collapsibility have not proved very useful in predicting who will and will not respond to upper airway surgery. Again, this may reflect our inability to adequately quantify collapsibility or the importance of nonanatomic traits. However, considerable effort has been put into at least identifying the site(s) of collapse as clearly as possible and directing the surgery at the appropriate site(s). Not surprisingly, assessing the site of collapse during sleep, generally using drug-induced sleep endoscopy (DISE), has proved the most fruitful.[9] However, in the author's opinion, no study has combined DISE and measurement of Pcrt to predict surgical outcomes, and such a study is needed as both the site of collapse and the severity of collapsibility seem likely to dictate surgical success.

It has become evident over the past 10 to 15 years that nonanatomical traits are important in OSA pathogenesis.[10,11,12] Most evidence suggests that there are four phenotypic traits that dictate who will and will not develop OSA. As outlined earlier, anatomy is one such trait. The others include:

- **The upper airway response:** This is the ability of the pharyngeal dilator muscles to respond to standard stimuli (airway negative pressure and rising PCO_2) during sleep. Conceptually, virtually all patients with OSA breathe normally while awake with little difficulty maintaining a patent upper airway. Thus pharyngeal dilator muscles can compensate for even the most anatomically deficient airway during wakefulness.[13] It is the failure of this compensatory muscle activation during sleep that leads to airway collapse in most patients. However, there is considerable variability in the responsiveness of these muscles during sleep. In some patients these muscles can activate quickly during sleep yielding stable respiration despite considerable airway collapsibility. In other patients with a minimally abnormal airway, the muscles cannot compensate during sleep and airway collapse occurs rapidly. Thus, variability in upper airway muscle responsiveness importantly dictates who does and who does not develop sleep apnea.
- **Arousal threshold to respiratory stimulation:** Based on what has been said earlier, when there is deficient pharyngeal anatomy, upper airway muscles must respond during sleep to open the airway if apneas or hypopneas are to be prevented. However, the stimuli to the upper airway muscles (increasingly negative airway pressure and rising PCO_2) develop slowly after the onset of airway obstruction.[14] Thus the individual must stay asleep long enough for these stimuli to reach adequate levels to activate the dilator muscles and restore airway patency. If the individual awakens from sleep before the required level of muscle activation has been reached, stable breathing during sustained periods of sleep will become difficult to achieve. Thus a high respiratory arousal threshold may help prevent disordered breathing by allowing pharyngeal dilator muscles adequate time to activate. On the other hand, individuals with a low respiratory arousal threshold will readily awaken shortly after each episode of airflow obstruction and therefore cycle between sleep and wake.
- **Loop gain (ventilatory control instability):** *Loop gain* is an engineering term used to describe the gain of any system controlled by feedback loops.

Respiratory control is very much a feedback-controlled system designed primarily to control arterial PCO_2. Loop gain is most easily understood as the respiratory response to a disturbance divided by that disturbance, i.e., response/disturbance. A high loop gain is characterized by a large respiratory response to a small disturbance. In such a case, a small increase in PCO_2 leads to a large increase in ventilation to correct it. When this occurs, ventilation can become unstable with waxing and waning between hyperpnea and hypopnea/apnea. Thus individuals with a high loop gain have a tendency toward unstable respiratory control.[15] If that same individual has a collapsible upper airway, then small airway obstructions can lead to large ventilatory overshoots, which leads to the next obstructive event.

Thus, although upper airway anatomy is fundamentally important in the pathogenesis of OSA, it is far from the entire cause of this disorder.

The fact that sleep apnea has a multifactorial cause should not deter efforts focused primarily on improving pharyngeal anatomy such as upper airway surgery. As stated previously, if the anatomy can be adequately addressed, the other traits generally become unimportant. It is when surgery is unsuccessful or only partially successful that the other contributors to OSA need to be considered. Currently if surgery does not lead to an adequate reduction in AHI, doctors revert to standard approaches to apnea management, i.e., continuous positive airway pressure (CPAP), mandibular advancing devices, or further surgery; all approaches again focus on correcting the anatomy. An alternative approach would be to recognize that improving anatomy increases the potential role of the nonanatomic traits described before and makes therapies focused on these other traits more likely to be successful. As an example, two recently completed but unpublished studies (oral communication from Dr. Scott Sands in September 2017) indicate that the single most important trait distinguishing OSA patients who failed pharyngeal surgical procedures versus being cured was a particularly high loop gain, not badly abnormal anatomy. This would suggest, although the studies have not been performed, that treating this high loop gain in the surgical failures with acetazolamide or nocturnal oxygen might well turn failures into successes.

In conclusion, upper airway surgery in appropriately selected OSA patients is a viable therapy focused on correcting deficient pharyngeal anatomy, the primary cause of sleep apnea. Thus, if the anatomic defect is not too great, the site and type of surgery are correct, and the other nonanatomic traits are not terribly abnormal, surgery should be successful. However, when surgery is not successful, continuing to address only anatomy may not be in the best interest of the patient and efforts to improve the other traits may yield surprisingly good results. Such an approach, however, will require further research before it is broadly accepted.

1.2 A Short History of Surgery for Sleep-Disordered Breathing: From the Uvula Crusher to the Stimulation of the Hypoglossus Nerve

Wolfgang Pirsig

1.2.1 Antiquity

Observations about symptoms and surgical procedures to influence snoring and OSA are transmitted from antiquity. Let us start with the so-called "Sleeping Lady of Malta," a 5,000-year-old terracotta sculpture from the Stone Age in the Hypogeum of Malta. She looks like a snoring woman suffering from obesity and hypersomnia.

In Greek mythology, the family of the Gods of the Underworld is associated with sleep in a fascinating interrelationship: Nyx (night) is the mother of the twins Hypnos (sleep) and Thanatos (death), and Morpheus (dreams) is the son of Hypnos. Detailed observations on the multiple facets of sleep-disordered breathing (SDB) were documented by the ancient Greeks and Romans, not only as to medical aspects but also in the Greco–Roman literature. Albert Esser (1885–1972) gave us an inspiring insight into these ancient sources about SDB.[16] Snoring may be caused by exogenous factors such as excessive eating and drinking, supine position, dropping of the lower jaw, or an epidemic disease of the nose. Esser also cites endogenous or constitutional factors that induce snoring such as age, small children and old people, or the pyknic or plethoric sleeper with a well-fed neck. In the ancient literature there are some detailed observations of the characteristics of the snoring sounds, including the extremely loud and interrupted snoring and the apneic snoring combined with a stop of breath. The main inspiratory type of snoring was recognized, as were the respiratory effort and body movements associated with snoring.

Comparable body dimensions as "The Sleeping Lady of Malta" can be supposed for Dionysius (360–305 BC), tyrant of Heraclea on the Euxine (Black Sea). He loved eating and Athenaeus ("Deipnosophistae" ca. 200 AD) transmitted Dionysius' wish on how to die: "One thing for my own self I desire - and this seems to me the only death that is a happy dying - to lie on my back with its many rolls of fat, scarce uttering a word, gasping for breath, while I eat and say 'I am rotting away in pleasure.'"[17] Athenaeus also reported that the physicians prescribed that he should get some fine needles, exceedingly long, which they thrust through his ribs and belly whenever he happened to fall into a very deep sleep. Now up to a certain point under the flesh, completely calloused as it was by fat, the needle caused no sensation; but if the needle went through so far as to touch the region which was free of fat, then he would be thoroughly aroused. At last Dionysius was choked by his own fat.[18]

In the 1980s, 2,300 years later, a modern form of bariatric surgery was applied in the United States to successfully treat obesity-related OSA.[19] A study about 330 patients who were successfully treated by bariatric surgery was published by Kleinhans and Verse.[20]

Hippocrates (460–359 BC), clearly described how a nasal polyp causes snoring 2,400 years ago: "When the polyp comes from the nose, hanging down the middle cartilages like a uvula, softly expanding with expiration outside the nose, retracting with inspiration, it causes a croaky voice and snoring during sleep."[21] Hippocrates surgically treated the polyps with loops or using the sponge method which was nicely depicted by Baldewein[22] (▶ Fig. 1.1).

In the past, uvula pathology appears to have been a common cause of different symptoms among them those associated with SDB. As the access to the uvula is easy, no wonder it became the scapegoat being sacrificed for all types of diseases for thousands of years as first documented in the Indian Sushruta 3,000 years ago. Hippocrates clearly recommended when to crush the uvula (Prognostic XXII): "It is dangerous to cut away or lance the uvula while it is red and enlarged, … Where, however, … forming what is called 'the grape,' that is when the front of the uvula is enlarged and vivid, while the upper part is thinner, it is safe to operate."

Early instruments to amputate the uvula were excavated in Roman tombs. Usually they were manufactured

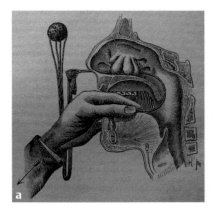
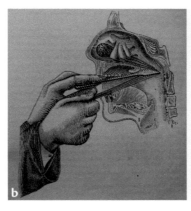

Fig. 1.1 (a, b) Baldewein's drawing of Hippocrates' technique for removal of nasal polyps in snorers.[22]

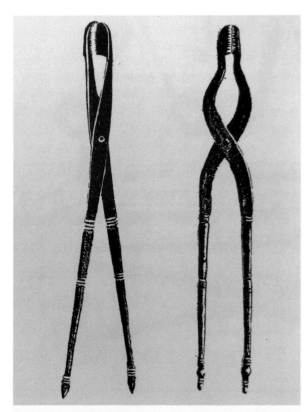

Fig. 1.2 Staphylagra for crushing the uvula, bronze, Roman period (Milne, 1907; ► Table 32.3)

from bronze. The forceps for crushing the uvula, termed *staphylagra*, is shown in ► Fig. 1.2. It was buried in about 275 AD and found in a physician's tomb in Paris.[23]

1.2.2 Renaissance

In his book, *Wund Artzney oder Artzneyspiegell*, Ambroise Paré (1510–1590) mentioned that the swollen uvula causes prevention of sleep, coughing, and fear of being choked.[24] This can be stopped by cauterizing it using nitric acid or a snare. The snare is depicted on a woodcut on page 267 of the book. In 1608, the same type of snare like that of Paré and a ligature carried on the outside of the ring was applied by Wilhelm Fabry von Hilden (1560–1634) to amputate the extremely long uvula disturbing respiration and eating in a noble man. The resected uvula and the snare in action are naturally shown in ► Fig. 1.3.[25]

Thomas Bartholin (1616–1680) reported about a guillotine-knife type of uvulotome, but indicated that it was originally devised by a Norwegian peasant, Canute de Thorbern. This instrument is described and depicted by Johann Scultetus (1595–1645) from Ulm in his German book edition of 1666 (Scultetus 1666 p. 19–22 and Tabula IX Fig. I and Fig. II).[26] Canute de Thorbern's uvulotome (► Fig. 1.4) later became the precursor of the tonsil guillotine for the rapid excision of the tonsils.

1.2.3 19th Century

In the 19th century several milestones were set in the field of medicine. César Jean Legallois (1812) described the neuronal influence on breathing and the heart. John Cheyne (1818) and William Stokes (1854) found connections between heart disorders and irregular breathing with central apneas.[27,28] The poet Charles Dickens (1812–1870) gave excellent symptomatic descriptions of OSA in the character of Joe, (the little fat boy), and in the obese Samuel Pickwick in his continuing booklet papers (The Posthumes Papers of the Pickwick Club).[29,30] In 1877, Sir Henry Broadbent (1835–1907), less poetically but meticulously, described an OSA: "When a person, especially advanced in years, is lying on his back in heavy sleep and snoring loudly, it very commonly happens that every now and then the inspiration fails to overcome the resistance of the pharynx, of which stridor or snoring is the audible sign, and there will be perfect silence through two, three or four respiratory periods, in which there are ineffectual chest movements; finally air enters with a loud snort, after which there are several compensatory deep inspirations …".[31]

Concepts and instruments for sleep surgery relating to adenotomy, uvulectomy, tonsillotomy, tracheostomy, and nasal surgery were published in the second half of 19th century.

Hans Wilhelm Meyer (1824–1895) from Copenhagen, scholarly studied the adenoids and their symptoms, especially their impact on children during sleep.[32] His descriptions of the symptoms (hearing problems, mouth breathing, sleep disturbance, snoring, floppy features, and sleepiness in children) are still valid today, and also his experience about the positive outcome after adenotomy as to snoring, sleep quality, and daytime sleepiness.

Thorbern's uvular guillotine was modified for the use as tonsillotome in the 19th century by Philip Syng Physick (1828), William B. Fahnestock (1832), Morrel Mackenzie (1880), and Albert Mathieu (1883) (► Fig. 1.5a, b). The Fahnestock-type tonsil guillotine still remained in use until the 1950s for tonsillotomy. Several casuistics about tonsillotomy for snoring children can be found in the 19th century. One example is the case report of Dr. Friedrich Betz about a 3-year-old boy: "… as sometimes snoring is caused by hypertrophic tonsils … In such a case, snoring can be reduced by amputation of the tonsils, or according to the circumstances can radically be healed."[33] However, the polysomnographic evidence that hypertrophic tonsils cause OSA in children who can be healed by adenotonsillectomy was shown not before 1965 when several centers in France, United States, and Canada published their results.[34,35]

In the just founded *Lancet* of 1848, tracheostomy for snoring in patients with epilepsy, severe drunkenness, and apoplexy was published by Marshall Hall (1790–1857).[36] But it took more than 120 years before Wolfgang

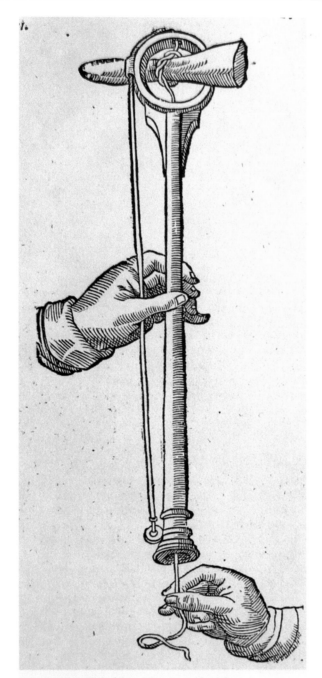

Fig. 1.3 Woodcut of the uvula resected (p. 93); snare resecting the uvula (p. 98).[25]

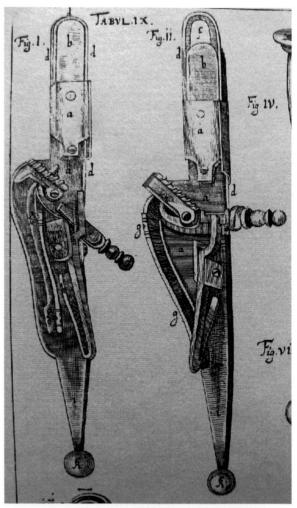

Fig. 1.4 Canute de Thorbern's uvulotome in Scultetus 1666, Table IX.[26]

Cline published a case study of the relief of excessive daytime sleepiness following nasal surgery, and Wells reported an increase of daytime vigilance in 8 of 40[10] patients after nasal surgery.[39,40]

1.2.4 20th Century

In the 19th century, insomnia, sleep apnea, and narcolepsy had been described; however, any type of documentation of sleep phenomena was lacking. In 1928, Hans Berger (1873–1941), a psychiatrist from Jena, registered the electrical activity of the human brain at the surface of the head and named the method *electroencephalography*.[41] Thus, some sleep phenomena could be monitored continuously. However, sleep research was not actively pursued until the early 1950s when Nathaniel Kleitmann (1895–1999) and Eugene Aserinsky (1921–1998) first registered rapid eye movements (REMs) during sleep

Kuhlo and colleagues from Freiburg im Breisgau polysomnographically proved that SDB due to a Pickwickian syndrome could be healed (▶ Fig. 1.6).[37]

By the end of the 19th century, nasal surgery was also indicated in children and adults to improve their sleep quality and reduce snoring. Krieg successfully performed a submucous septal resection in a girl with obstructed nose, snoring, and attacks of suffocation during sleep.[38]

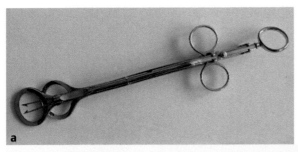
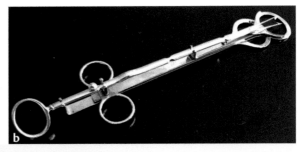

Fig. 1.5 (a, b) Mathieu-type tonsil guillotine, steel plated, designed in 1883, collection Pirsig.

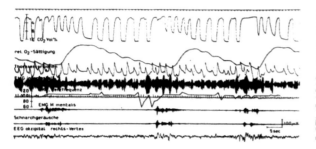
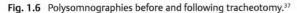
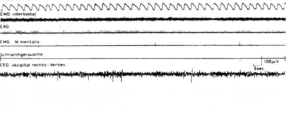

Fig. 1.6 Polysomnographies before and following tracheotomy.[37]

by means of electro-oculography in 1953.[42] The pattern of sleep was differentiated in non–rapid eye movement (non-REM) and REM phases with regular cyclical periods. In 1973, sleep apnea as a syndrome was first described by Guilleminault et al.[43] This group also established a sleep clinic at Stanford University. Until the late 1970s, mostly physiologists, neurologic and psychiatric specialists in their sleep laboratories diagnosed SDB using electroencephalographic (EEG) recordings, while pulmonary and intern departments investigated cardiopulmonary parameters. In the late 1970s, the diagnostics and treatments of SDB were taken over by interdisciplinary university sleep centers such as at Stanford, Detroit, Cleveland in the United States, Bologna in Italy, and Freiburg im Breisgau, Munich, and Marburg in Germany. In the 1980s, surgical disciplines were also integrated in these sleep centers.

The 1980s paved the way for new methods to treat SDB with device options, namely CPAP, oral appliances, and electrostimulation. Colin E. Sullivan, pneumologist from Sidney, has been an outstanding pioneer. In 1981, he published with his group the reversal of OSA by nasal CPAP.[44]

In 1982, German psychiatrist Karlheinz Meier-Ewert proved in a self-experiment over 9 months that an oral appliance functioning according to the principle of the Esmarch movement of the mandible could keep the upper airway open during sleep (1984 Munich Poster).[45]

The 1980s also saw otorhinolaryngologists and maxillofacial surgeons being inventive in developing new approaches for sleep surgery with varying degrees of success according to the level of the obstruction of the upper airway.

1.2.5 Palatal Surgery

Palatoplasty with a partial uvulectomy for loud snoring was first performed in 1964 by Takenosuke Ikematsu in Japan. He published his results in 152 patients in 1964.[46]

In 1977, Quesada et al from Barcelona proved by polysomnography that they could delete or reduce obstructive apneas by partial resection of the soft palate, uvulectomy, and tonsillectomy in patients with Pickwickian syndrome.[47] In 1981, Shiro Fujita's publication of uvulopalatopharyngoplasty (UPPP) spurred a new era in the surgical treatment of SDB.[48] This rather invasive technique with several side effects was modified in many countries until the end of the century. The enthusiasm about UPPP decreased after Sher's meta-analysis about UPPP showing that its overall positive efficacy was only 40%.[49] Furthermore, Sher recognized that the success rate of sleep surgery also depends on the level of pharyngeal obstruction during sleep. In 1978, Hill et al had already studied the complex pattern of collapse of the pharyngeal walls during OSAs using fiberoptic and electromyographic (EMG) studies.[50] During 1980s, the diagnostic tools of acoustic information in snoring noises, such as flexible nasopharyngoscopy, pharyngeal pressure measurements, and Müller maneuver during wakefulness, did not deliver the expected results to predict the levels of pharyngeal obstruction during sleep. Croft and

Pringle (1991) introduced DISE to improve the detection of the proper levels for upper airway surgery in the daily work.[51]

Several modifications of the "standard UPPP" tried to improve the outcome of the palatal surgery, starting with Powell's uvulopalatal flap (1996). In chronological order the following modifications were published: extended uvulopalatal flap (EUPF 2003), lateral pharyngoplasty (LP 2003), Z-palatoplasty (ZPP 2004), Han-UPPP (2005), expansion sphincter pharyngoplasty (ESP 2007), microdebrider-assisted extended uvulopalatoplasty (MEUP 2008), relocation pharyngoplasty (rPP 2009), Z-palato-pharyngoplasty (Z-PPP 2010), and soft palate webbing flap (SPWF 2015). Details about the improvements, side effects, and references of these modifications, published after a mean follow-up of 10 months have recently been reported.[52]

1.2.6 Lower Pharyngeal Airway Procedures

Many invasive and less invasive procedures to achieve an enlargement of the pharyngeal tube at the tongue base level have been published. One principle was to reduce the amount of tongue base tissue and other procedures aimed to shift the tongue and/or surrounding tissues toward anteriorly. The first transoral tongue base resection was described by Djupesland et al in 1987.[53] By 1992, Djupesland published the technique of palatopharyngoglossoplasty.[54] In 1991, Fujita et al reported about the midline glossectomy using the laser.[55] Chabolle performed the most extended tongue base reduction via an external approach and presented the results in 1999.[56] In the same year, the feasibility of interstitial radiofrequency (RFQ) surgery of the tongue base as minimally invasive surgical therapy was first investigated in 15 OSA patients by Powell et al.[57]

Surgery on the hyoid bone to widen the upper airway for OSA was described by Kaya in 1984.[58] Two years later Riley et al combined hyoid myotomy-suspension with inferior sagittal osteotomy of the mandible to treat OSA.[59] This last technique has been modified by the Stanford group in 1994 under the term *hyoid suspension*, although it is a hyoidthyroidpexia.[60] A less invasive modification, also applicable under local anesthesia, was introduced by Hörmann et al in 2001.[61]

1.2.7 Devices for the Tongue Base Suspension

By 1992, Faye-Lund et al verified the idea of tongue suspension by fixing the tongue base at the chin with homologous fascia lata, but this technique proved to involve great expense.[62] The idea of tongue base suspension regained actuality in the 21st

century in the form of some minimally invasive systems: the first invention of the Influ-ENT Repose system was published by DeRowe et al.[63] Other existing medical devices for tongue suspension are lateral hyoid expansion (Aspire), Tongue anchor (Aspire), Advance system (Aspire), Flour-of-mouth Attracting System (Apneon), Pavad, and ReVent.

1.2.8 Laryngeal Obstructive Sleep Apnea

Laryngeal structures relatively rarely cause OSA in comparison to soft palate, tonsils, and tongue. In 1981, Olsen et al reported a case of OSA due to a laryngeal cyst in an infant, which was healed after removal of the cyst.[64] In 1987, Zalzal et al described that newborns, especially preterm, with laryngeal abnormalities and presenting laryngomalacia needed procedures such as epiglottoplasty.[65] In adults, a floppy epiglottis is the most common reason for laryngeal OSA and can be treated by laser surgery.[66]

1.2.9 Multilevel Surgery

The pathophysiological concept of a two level–pharyngeal collapse (retropalatal and retrolingual) proved to be too simplified and was replaced by a dynamic multiple level collapse concept, reflecting the complex pattern of collapsibility of the whole upper airway during sleep. This concept was especially successful in treating patients with SDB intolerant of nasal CPAP. Multilevel surgery for OSA was first performed in 1985 in Chicago by Caldarelli et al.[67] They showed an increased positive outcome by adding a tongue retaining device and palatopharyngoplasty to nasal surgery in comparison to the success rate of the three methods alone. The step of treating OSA by surgical procedures of the nose, soft palate, tongue, mandible, and maxilla was published by Waite et al in 1989.[68] Following Fujita's division of the pharynx into three levels, Riley et al in 1993 termed this type of treatment as *multilevel surgery*, which is now achieved in all combinations of the single procedures.[69,70]

1.2.10 Hypoglossal Stimulation

In 1988, Miki et al found significant reduction in OSA in six patients who were electrically stimulated with surface electrodes in the submental region.[71] This observation triggered a new effective treatment modality for patients with OSA rejecting CPAP or other therapies. The enormous progress and the efficacy of this new nerve stimulation method was recently published in the prospective cohort study—the STAR trial of 2017, reporting the successful stimulation of the hypoglossal nerve at follow-up after 48 months[72] (see ▶ Fig. 1.7).

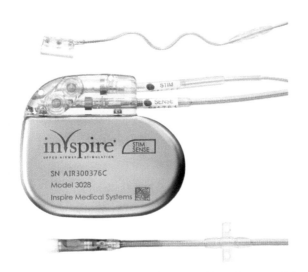

Fig. 1.7 Tools for hypoglossal nerve stimulation with Inspire.

1.2.11 Maxillofacial Surgery

Since the 1980s, maxillomandibular advancement (MMA) has proved to be the most successful surgical option after tracheotomy in the treatment of OSA and was especially performed in patients with craniofacial deformities. This procedure was either performed on the mandible or maxilla or on both facial bones, and also in combination with above-mentioned procedures. By 1972, Cosman and Crikelair reported two cases of respiratory difficulty associated with micrognathia that responded to mandibular advancement, respectively, with hyoid advancement.[73]

Kuo et al performed mandibular advancement in three patients with OSA in 1979.[74] In 1989, Waite et al published their results of maxillomandibular advancement surgery in 23 patients with OSA. In 1992, McCarthy et al introduced osteogenesis especially in infants with grossly retropositioned mandible or midface distraction.[75] The enthusiasm about the initially good results had been dampened because follow-up showed partial recurrence of the malformation during growth.

1.2.12 Final Remark

The years of the 1980s were the "golden decade of therapy for SDB," sleep surgery included. In the meantime, SDB had increasingly been recognized as a widespread disease with multidisciplinary aspects. Its many symptomatic facets in children and adults probably are the reason why patients with SDB often were not adequately diagnosed and treated in the past. Some surgical procedures started rather radical and turned into less invasive versions, while others disappeared. Since the beginning of the 21st century new devices have been integrated

into sleep surgery. The enormous progress as to research, diagnostics, and treatment modalities in sleep medicine in the past 30 years is not only the result of technical improvements, but also of the increasingly interdisciplinary cooperation worldwide, the exchange of knowledge, and the growing World Wide Web. To be a witness of this development was an inspiring experience for the author as an otorhinolaryngologist who had performed adenotonsillectomies and tracheotomies in the 1970s without knowing that some of these patients suffered from OSA. In 1985, the author joined the group of sleep medicine to understand more of this fascinating specialty.

References

[1] Haponik EF, Smith PL, Bohlman ME, Allen RP, Goldman SM, Bleecker ER. Computerized tomography in obstructive sleep apnea. Correlation of airway size with physiology during sleep and wakefulness. Am Rev Respir Dis. 1983; 127(2):221–226

[2] Schwab RJ, Gupta KB, Gefter WB, Metzger LJ, Hoffman EA, Pack AI. Upper airway and soft tissue anatomy in normal subjects and patients with sleep-disordered breathing. Significance of the lateral pharyngeal walls. Am J Respir Crit Care Med. 1995; 152(5 Pt 1):1673–1689

[3] Schwab RJ, Pasirstein M, Pierson R, et al. Identification of upper airway anatomic risk factors for obstructive sleep apnea with volumetric magnetic resonance imaging. Am J Respir Crit Care Med. 2003; 168(5):522–530

[4] Isono S, Remmers JE, Tanaka A, Sho Y, Sato J, Nishino T. Anatomy of pharynx in patients with obstructive sleep apnea and in normal subjects. J Appl Physiol (1985). 1997; 82(4):1319–1326

[5] Schwartz AR, Smith PL, Wise RA, Gold AR, Permutt S. Induction of upper airway occlusion in sleeping individuals with subatmospheric nasal pressure. J Appl Physiol (1985). 1988; 64(2):535–542

[6] Kirkness JP, Peterson LA, Squier SB, et al. Performance characteristics of upper airway critical collapsing pressure measurements during sleep. Sleep. 2011; 34(4):459–467

[7] Sforza E, Petiau C, Weiss T, Thibault A, Krieger J. Pharyngeal critical pressure in patients with obstructive sleep apnea syndrome. Clinical implications. Am J Respir Crit Care Med. 1999; 159(1):149–157

[8] Eckert DJ, White DP, Jordan AS, Malhotra A, Wellman A. Defining phenotypic causes of obstructive sleep apnea. Identification of novel therapeutic targets. Am J Respir Crit Care Med. 2013; 188(8):996–1004

[9] Kezirian EJ. Nonresponders to pharyngeal surgery for obstructive sleep apnea: insights from drug-induced sleep endoscopy. Laryngoscope. 2011; 121(6):1320–1326

[10] White DP. Pathogenesis of obstructive and central sleep apnea. Am J Respir Crit Care Med. 2005; 172(11):1363–1370

[11] Wellman A, Eckert DJ, Jordan AS, et al. A method for measuring and modeling the physiological traits causing obstructive sleep apnea. J Appl Physiol (1985). 2011; 110(6):1627–1637

[12] Wellman A, Edwards BA, Sands SA, et al. A simplified method for determining phenotypic traits in patients with obstructive sleep apnea. J Appl Physiol (1985). 2013; 114(7):911–922

[13] Mezzanotte WS, Tangel DJ, White DP. Waking genioglossal electromyogram in sleep apnea patients versus normal controls (a neuromuscular compensatory mechanism). J Clin Invest. 1992; 89(5):1571–1579

[14] Wiegand L, Zwillich CW, White DP. Collapsibility of the human upper airway during normal sleep. J Appl Physiol (1985). 1989; 66(4):1800–1808

[15] Wellman A, Jordan AS, Malhotra A, et al. Ventilatory control and airway anatomy in obstructive sleep apnea. Am J Respir Crit Care Med. 2004; 170(11):1225–1232

[16] Esser AM. Snoring in the ancient world. Sleep Breath. 2002; 6(1):29–39

[17] Gulick CP. Athenaeus: The Deipnosophists. (trans). Cambridge, MA: Harvard University Press; 1863:491

[18] Kryger MH. Sleep apnea. From the needles of Dionysius to continuous positive airway pressure. Arch Intern Med. 1983; 143(12):2301–2303

[19] Peiser J, Lavie P, Ovnat A, Charuzi I. Sleep apnea syndrome in the morbidly obese as an indication for weight reduction surgery. Ann Surg. 1984; 199(1):112–115

[20] Kleinhans H, Verse T. Bariatric Surgery. In: Hörmann K, Verse T. Surgery for Sleep Disordered Breathing. 2nd ed. Springer, Heidelberg. 2010:221–230

[21] Littré E. Oevres Complètes d'Hippocrate, Paris: Baillière; 1853

[22] Baldewein R. Die Rhinologie des Hippokrates. Zschr Ohrenheilk. 1896; 28:101–118

[23] Milne JS. Surgical Instruments in Greek and Roman Times. Oxford: Clarendon Press; 1907

[24] Paré A. Wund Artzney oder Artzneyspiegell. Edition J. Guillemeau in the Teutsche Sprach. Franckfurt, Caspar Rötell für Fischers Erben, 1635:266–267

[25] Fabry W. [Guilhelm Fabritius Hildanus] Observationum et curationum chirurgicarum centuriae. 6 vols. Basle, Frankfort, & Lyons, 1606–1641 Centuria I, Observatio XIX p. 93

[26] Scultetus J. Wund-Arneyisches Zeug-Hauß. Johann Gerlin, Franckfurt. 1666, Table IX (Faksimile-Druck Kohlhammer, Stuttgart. 1974)

[27] Cheyne J. A case of apoplexy in which the fleshy part of the heart was converted into fat. Dublin Hosp Rep. 1818; 2:216–223

[28] Stokes W. The diseases of the heart and aorta. Dublin, Ireland: Hodges & Smith; 1854

[29] Dickens C. The Posthumes Papers of the Pickwickian Club. London: Chapman & Hall; 1836

[30] Dickens C. The Posthumous Papers of the Pickwickian Club. Reprint: London: Penguin Books; 1994:5–81

[31] Broadbent WH. On Cheyne-Stokes' respiration in cerebral haemorrhage. Lancet. 1877; 109(2792):307–309

[32] Meyer W. On adenoid vegetations in the nasopharyngeal cavity, their pathology, diagnosis and treatment. Hospitalstidende, Copenhagen. 1868; 11:177–178

[33] Betz F. Ueber das Schnarchen ganz kleiner Kinder (About the snoring of infants). Memorabilien, Heilbronn. 1858; 3:73–77

[34] Menashe VD, Farrehi C, Miller M. Hypoventilation and cor pulmonale due to chronic upper airway obstruction. J Pediatr. 1965; 67:198–203

[35] Noonan JA. Reversible cor pulmonale due to hypertrophied tonsils and adenoids: studies in two cases. Circulation. 1965; 31/32:164

[36] Hall M. The instrument for tracheotomy. Lancet. 1848; 2:530

[37] Kuhl W, Doll E, Franck MC. [Successful management of Pickwickian syndrome using long-term tracheostomy] Dtsch Med Wochenschr. 1969; 94(24):1286–1290. [The correct name of Kuhlo is Kuhl.]

[38] Krieg R. Resection der Cartilago quadangularis septi narium zur Heilung der Scoliosis septi. Medizinisches Correspondenz-Blatt württembergischer ärztlicher Vereinigung, Stuttgart. 1886; 56:209–213

[39] Cline CL. The effects of intra-nasal obstruction on the general health. Med Surgical Rep. 1892; 67:259–260

[40] Wells WA. Some nervous and mental manifestations occurring in connection with nasal disease. Am J Med Sci. 1898; 116:677–692

[41] Berger H. Über das Elektroenkephalogramm des Menschen. Arch Psychiatr Nervenkr. 1929; 87:527–575

[42] Aserinsky E, Kleitman N. Regularly occurring periods of eye motility, and concomitant phenomena, during sleep. Science. 1953; 118(3062):273–274

[43] Guilleminault C, Eldridge FL, Dement WC. Insomnia with sleep apnea: a new syndrome. Science. 1973; 181(4102):856–858

[44] Sullivan CE, Issa FG, Berthon-Jones M, Eves L. Reversal of obstructive sleep apnoea by continuous positive airway pressure applied through the nares. Lancet. 1981; 1(8225):862–865

[45] Meier-Ewert KH, Schäfer H, Kloß W. Treatment of sleep apnea by a mandibular protracting device. 7th Sleep Res Soc Congress, Munich, Sept. 3–7, 1984, Abstract

[46] Ikematsu T. Study of snoring: therapy [in Japanese] J Jpn Otol Rhinol Laryngol Soc. 1964; 64:434–435

[47] Quesada P, Botet J, Fuentes E, Perelló E. Resección parcial del paladar blando como tratamiento del sindrome de hipersomnia y respiración de los obesos. ORL Dips. 1977; 5:81–88

[48] Fujita S, Conway W, Zorick F, Roth T. Surgical correction of anatomic azbnormalities in obstructive sleep apnea syndrome: uvulopalatopharyngoplasty. Otolaryngol Head Neck Surg. 1981; 89(6):923–934

[49] Sher AE, Schechtman KB, Piccirillo JF. The efficacy of surgical modifications of the upper airway in adults with obstructive sleep apnea syndrome. Sleep. 1996; 19(2):156–177

[50] Hill MW, Guilleminault C, Simmons FB. Fiberoptic and EMG Studies in Hypersomnia-Sleep Apnea Syndrome. Sleep Apnea Syndromes. New York, NY: Allen R. Riss; 1978

[51] Croft CB, Pringle M. Sleep nasendoscopy: a technique of assessment in snoring and obstructive sleep apnoea. Clin Otolaryngol Allied Sci. 1991; 16(5):504–509

[52] Verse T, Stuck BA. [Modern modifications of uvulopalatopharyngoplasty] HNO 2017; 65(2):90–98

[53] Djupesland G, Lyberg T, Krogstad O. Cephalometric analysis and surgical treatment of patients with obstructive sleep apnea syndrome. A preliminary report. Acta Otolaryngol. 1987; 103(5–6):551–557

[54] Djupesland G, Schrader H, Lyberg T, Refsum H, Lilleås F, Godtlibsen OB. Palatopharyngoglossoplasty in the treatment of patients with obstructive sleep apnea syndrome. Acta Otolaryngol Suppl. 1992; 492(Suppl 492):50–54

[55] Fujita S, Woodson BT, Clark JL, Wittig R. Laser midline glossectomy as a treatment for obstructive sleep apnea. Laryngoscope. 1991; 101(8):805–809

[56] Chabolle F, Wagner I, Blumen MB, Séquert C, Fleury B, De Dieuleveult T. Tongue base reduction with hyoepiglottoplasty: a treatment for severe obstructive sleep apnea. Laryngoscope. 1999; 109(8):1273–1280

[57] Powell NB, Riley RW, Guilleminault C. Radiofrequency tongue base reduction in sleep-disordered breathing: A pilot study. Otolaryngol Head Neck Surg. 1999; 120(5):656–664

[58] Kaya N. Sectioning the hyoid bone as a therapeutic approach for obstructive sleep apnea. Sleep. 1984; 7(1):77–78

[59] Riley RW, Powell NB, Guilleminault C. Inferior sagittal osteotomy of the mandible with hyoid myotomy-suspension: a new procedure for obstructive sleep apnea. Otolaryngol Head Neck Surg. 1986; 94(5):589–593

[60] Riley RW, Powell NB, Guilleminault C. Obstructive sleep apnea and the hyoid: a revised surgical procedure. Otolaryngol Head Neck Surg. 1994; 111(6):717–721

[61] Hörmann K, Hirth K, Erhardt T, Maurer JT, Verse T. [Modified hyoid suspension for therapy of sleep related breathing disorders. operative technique and complications] Laryngorhinootologie. 2001; 80(9):517–521

[62] Faye-Lund H, Djupesland G, Lyberg T. Glossopexia–evaluation of a new surgical method for treating obstructive sleep apnea syndrome. Acta Otolaryngol Suppl. 1992; 492(Suppl 492):46–49

[63] DeRowe A, Günther E, Fibbi A, et al. Tongue-base suspension with a soft tissue-to-bone anchor for obstructive sleep apnea: preliminary clinical results of a new minimally invasive technique. Otolaryngol Head Neck Surg. 2000; 122(1):100–103

[64] Olsen KD, Suh KW, Staats BA. Surgically correctable causes of sleep apnea syndrome. Otolaryngol Head Neck Surg. 1981; 89(5):726–731

[65] Zalzal GH, Anon JB, Cotton RT. Epiglottoplasty for the treatment of laryngomalacia. Ann Otol Rhinol Laryngol. 1987; 96(1 Pt 1):72–76

[66] Andersen APD, Alving J, Lildholdt T, Wulff CH. Obstructive sleep apnea initiated by a lax epiglottis. A contraindication for continuous positive airway pressure. Chest. 1987; 91(4):621–623

[67] Caldarelli DD, Cartwright RD, Lilie JK. Obstructive sleep apnea: variations in surgical management. Laryngoscope. 1985; 95(9 Pt 1):1070–1073

[68] Waite PD, Wooten V, Lachner J, Guyette RF. Maxillomandibular advancement surgery in 23 patients with obstructive sleep apnea syndrome. J Oral Maxillofac Surg. 1989; 47(12):1256–1261, discussion 1262

[69] Fujita S. Obstructive sleep apnea syndrome: pathophysiology, upper airway evaluation and surgical treatment. Ear Nose Throat J. 1993; 72(1):67–72, 75–76

[70] Riley RW, Powell NB, Guilleminault C. Obstructive sleep apnea syndrome: a review of 306 consecutively treated surgical patients. Otolaryngol Head Neck Surg. 1993; 108(2):117–125

[71] Miki H, Hida W, Inoue H, Takishima T. A new treatment for obstructive sleep apnea syndrome by electrical stimulation of submental region. Tohoku J Exp Med. 1988; 154(1):91–92

[72] Gillespie MB, Soose RJ, Woodson BT, et al; STAR Trial Investigators. Upper airway stimulation for obstructive sleep apnea: patient-reported outcomes after 48 months of follow-up. Otolaryngol Head Neck Surg. 2017; 156(4):765–771

[73] Cosman B, Crikelair GF. Mandibular hypoplasia and the late development of glossopharyngeal airway obstruction. Plast Reconstr Surg. 1972; 50(6):573–579

[74] Kuo PC, West RA, Bloomquist DS, McNeil RW. The effect of mandibular osteotomy in three patients with hypersomnia sleep apnea. Oral Surg Oral Med Oral Pathol. 1979; 48(5):385–392

[75] McCarthy JG, Schreiber J, Karp N, Thorne CH, Grayson BH. Lengthening the human mandible by gradual distraction. Plast Reconstr Surg. 1992; 89(1):1–8, discussion 9–10

2 Pathophysiology

Abstract

Obstructive sleep apnea (OSA) is diagnosed more frequently now than in the past. The characteristics of this potentially life-threatening disorder are (socially) disturbing snoring, excessive daytime sleepiness, disturbed concentration and memory, personality changes as well as cardiovascular, metabolic, and cognitive morbidities. Snoring is usually the cardinal symptom, but is aspecific, while the disorder can be suspected based on a thorough history taking (and physical-technical examination). In high-risk populations, OSA can contribute to the course of the underlying disorder, and influence its outcome. Due to its high prevalence and multiple interactions with most organ systems, OSA is a huge burden for the healthcare systems worldwide which deserves explicit attention.

Keywords: epidemiology, prevalence, apnea, fatigue, sleepiness, nocturia, prediction, consequences, comorbidities, hypertension, stroke, arrhythmias, coronary artery disease, metabolic, cognitive, obesity, chronic heart failure

mellitus,[9,10,11] metabolic syndrome,[12] and endocrinopathies.[9,13] Often patients with SDB suffer from excessive daytime sleepiness, though other symptoms can be present as well, while some others remain asymptomatic. In some cases, patients express fatigue, tiredness, or lack of energy rather than sleepiness itself, which can be related to a comorbid medical disorder, but can also be the cardinal symptom of OSA.[14,15,16,17] However, these symptoms are aspecific and can be caused by many different sleep disorders, and hence adequate workup is mandatory. If patients suffering from OSA also suffer from other medical disorders then the negative effects are more common, rapid, and intensive. If OSA is present with other disorders then their consequences will be increased mutually.[18]

The objective of this chapter is to describe the most common signs and symptoms of OSA, which can be helpful in identifying these patients. Emphasis will be on OSA, which is the most common type of SDB associated with pathological sleepiness. At the same time, cardiovascular, metabolic, cognitive, and economic consequences will be highlighted.

2.1 Epidemiology

Johan Verbraecken

2.1.1 Introduction

Epidemiological studies provide strong evidence that sleep-disordered breathing (SDB), especially OSA, is highly prevalent not only in the general population (▶Table 2.1), but also in specific patient categories with obesity,[1,2] systemic hypertension,[3,4] cardiovascular disease,[5,6,7,8] diabetes

2.1.2 Definitions

Obstructive sleep apnea syndrome (OSAS) is part of a spectrum of sleep-related breathing disorders, described with a widely used term SDB.[17] The International Classification of Sleep Disorders (ICSD-3) has defined four major categories of SDB: OSA disorders, central sleep apnea (CSA) disorders, sleep-related hypoventilation disorders, and sleep-related hypoxemia disorders.[30] The fundamental difference between the first two major categories is the pathophysiological mechanism that

▶ **Table 2.1** Prevalence of OSA based on community-based population studies

First author, reference	Country of study	Age range (years)	AHI ≥ 5	AHI ≥ 10	AHI ≥ 15	AHI ≥ 5 + symptoms	AHI ≥ 15 + symptoms
Young et al[19]	U.S.	30–60	24/9	15/5	9/4	4/2	
Bixler et al[20]	U.S.	20–100			7.2/2.2	3.9/1.2	
Duran et al[21]	Spain	30–70	26/28	19/15	14/7		
Young et al[22]	U.S.	39–99	33/26		25/11		
Hrubos-Strøm et al[23]	Norway	30–65	21/13		11/6		
Franklin et al[24]	Sweden	20–70	/50		/20	/17	
Ip et al[25]	Hong-Kong	30–60				4.1/0	
Ip et al[26]	Hong-Kong	30–60				0/2.1	
Kim[27]	Korea	40–69				4.5/3.2	
Reddy et al[28]	India	30–65				4/1.5	
Heinzer et al[29]	Switzerland	40–85					49.7/23.4

Abbreviations: AHI, apnea-hypopnea index; OSA, obstructive sleep apnea; U.S., United States.

exerts the respiratory disturbance.[31] In OSA, the upper airway occlusion is usually caused by abnormal anatomy and/or abnormal control of the muscles that maintain the patency of the upper airway. In CSA, dysfunctional ventilatory control in the central breathing center is involved, finally resulting in loss of ventilatory effort. Many patients have a combination of obstructive and central sleep apnea, which suggests that the mechanisms responsible for different types of apnea must overlap. An obstructive apnea/hypopnea can be defined as a respiratory event that lasts for at least 10 seconds and is characterized by a transient partial (hypopnea) or complete (apnea) upper airway obstruction during sleep.[17] Based on the American Academy of Sleep Medicine (AASM) criteria from 2012, a hypopnea can be defined as a decrease from baseline in the amplitude of flow, based on a peak signal excursion drop by more than or equal to 30% of pre-event baseline using nasal canula, with a duration of more than or equal to 10 seconds, and more than or equal to 3% oxygen desaturation from pre-event baseline or the event is associated with an arousal,[32] which is a simplification of previous definitions.

CSA refers to a reduction or cessation of airflow due to reduced or absent respiratory effort, lasting for at least 10 seconds (in adults), due to transient loss of neural output to the respiratory muscles.[17] Its severity is based on the number of apneas and hypopneas occurring during 1 hour of sleep (apnea–hypopnea index or AHI) and the degree of daytime symptoms. According to ICSD-3, the criteria for the diagnosis of a clinically significant obstructive sleep apnea-hypopnea syndrome are: presence of criterion (A and B) or C satisfy the criteria.[30] The different levels of severity in OSA can be defined as "mild" for an AHI above or equal to 5 and below 15, "moderate" for an AHI above or equal to 15 and below or equal to 30, and "severe" for an AHI above 30.[33] Based on these criteria, "sleep apnea" occurs in 4% of men and 2% of women who are between 30 and 60 years of age.[19] The current definition of OSA takes into considreration two components: (1) breathing pattern abnormalities during sleep and (2) daytime symptoms. This definition indicates that there are also asymptomatic subjects. Nowadays, asymptomatic cases can be referred to as OSA, and the symptomatic ones as OSAS, although this subclassification and use of these terms is not performed systematically. It is possible that nonsleepy OSA patients may have an innate increased sleep threshold or greater level of activations.[34] In one study, only 15% of males and 22% of females with OSA reported sleepiness on the three subjective measures used.[19] Interestingly, patients with OSA who deny the occurrence of sleepiness report other daytime complaints, such as a lack of energy or short memory, which can be the subjective perception of unrecognized sleepiness.[35,36,37]

OSA can be subdivided into adult type and pediatric type, since the diagnostic criteria and clinical presentation for abnormal breathing during sleep are different for pediatric cases and adult ones.[32] Obstructive events may include apneas, hypopneas, and also respiratory effort–related arousals (RERAs).[38] A RERA can be defined as a sequence of breaths characterized by increasing respiratory effort leading to arousal from sleep, but not fulfilling the precise criteria for apnea or hypopnea.[32,38] Moreover, these events are characterized by a pattern of progressively more negative esophageal pressures, terminated by an abrupt change in pressure to a less negative level and finally an arousal. Esophageal pressure measurement is still recommended as gold standard,[32,39] but the flattening of the flow curve obtained by nasal pressure is explicitly mentioned, together with induction plethysmography, as acceptable alternatives.[32] In routine care, nasal pressure is the method of choice for most sleep laboratories. These events also last at least 10 seconds. Upper airway resistance syndrome (UARS) is characterized by increased upper airway resistance, followed by repetitive arousals, finally resulting in (excessive) daytime sleepiness.[40,41] The essential polysomnographic (PSG) features are absence of OSAs, an AHI below 5, and a lack of significant oxygen desaturations, which differ from the laboratory findings of OSAS.[32] The term UARS is no longer used as an independent disease, but is incorporated under the diagnosis OSA(S) because the pathophysiology does not significantly differ from that of OSA(S).

The diagnosis of CSA is made by criteria recommended by ICSD-3.[30] Patients are diagnosed with primary CSA if they present with the following:

- Sleepiness or difficulty initiating or maintaining sleep, frequent awakenings, or nonrestorative sleep or awakening, short of breath or snoring, or witnessed apneas.
- PSG demonstrates five or more central apneas and/or hypopneas per hour of sleep. The number of central apneas and/or central hypopneas is more than 50% of the total number of apneas and hypopneas, with absence of Cheyne-Stokes breathing (CSB).
- There is no evidence of daytime or nocturnal hypoventilation.
- The disorder is not better explained by another current sleep disorder, medical or neurological disorder, medication use, or substance-use disorder.

All these criteria must be met. Usually, patients with CSA have mild hypocapnia or normocapnia, but rarely, hypoventilation and hypercapnia are also observed. A periodic pattern of waxing and waning of ventilation with episodes of hyperventilation alternating with central apnea/hypopnea is defined as CSB. According to ICSD-3, CSB can be considered if:

- There is presence of one or more of the following: (1) sleepiness, (2) difficulty initiating or maintaining sleep, frequent awakenings, or nonrestorative sleep, (3) awakening short of breath, (4) snoring, or (5) witnessed apneas.
- There is presence of atrial fibrillation/flutter, congestive heart failure (CHF), or a neurological disorder.

- PSG (during diagnostic or positive airway pressure titration) shows all of the following: (1) Five or more central apneas and/or central hypopneas per hour of sleep; (2) the total number of cenral apneas and/or hypopneas is above 50% of the total number of apneas and hypopneas; and (3) the pattern of ventilation meets criteria for CSB.
- The disorder is not better explained by another current sleep disorder, medication use, or substance-use disorder.

Although symptoms are not mandatory to make the final diagnosis, patients often suffer from daytime sleepiness, repetitive arousals and awakenings during sleep, insomnia, or awakening because of shortness of breath.[30]

A last patient group in the spectrum of SDB is termed sleep-related hypoventilation/hypoxemic syndrome. Sleep-induced hypoventilation is characterized by elevated levels of arterial carbon dioxide tension ($PaCO_2$) of more than 45 mm Hg while asleep or disproportionately increased relative to levels during wakefulness.[17] This group includes obesity hypoventilation syndrome (OHS), congenital central alveolar hypoventilation syndrome, late onset central hypoventilation with hypothalamic dysfunction, idiopathic central alveolar hypoventilation, sleep-related hypoventilation due to a medication or substance use, and sleep-related hypoventilation due to a medical disorder.[30] Among these categories, OHS is the most prevalent clinical presentation of this syndrome. OHS is primarily defined as the association of obesity (body mass index [BMI] > 30 kg/m²) and hypercapnia ($PaCO_2$ > 45 mm Hg) that is not due to lung parenchymal or airway disease, pulmonary vascular pathology, chest wall disorder (other than mass loading from obesity), medication use, neurologic disorder, muscle weakness, or a known congenital or idiopathic central alveolar hypoventilation syndrome.[42,43,44,45,46] However, there is not a commonly accepted definition for OHS. Finally, sleep-related hypoxemia is characterized by significant hypoxemia during sleep. This group is believed to be secondary to a medical or neurological disorder. PSG, polygraphy (PG), or nocturnal oximetry show the arterial oxygen saturation (SaO_2) during sleep of less than or equal to 88% in adults for more than or equal to 5 minutes. Sleep hypoventilation has been excluded.

Over time, different definitions have been proposed by the AASM for the different entities of SDB (ICSD-3 vs Scoring manual), which may complicate the understanding of the problem.[30,32,39]

2.1.3 Signs and Symptoms Suggestive of Obstructive Sleep Apnea

The symptoms of OSA can be classified as symptoms experienced by the patient and symptoms recognized by the bed partner.[47,48] Individuals with symptoms suggestive of OSA, especially excessive daytime sleepiness, are candidates for a formal overnight sleep study as patients with such a history have more than 70% probability of having sleep apnea.[33,44] Nocturnal symptoms in OSA are more specific than those appearing during daytime. Since symptoms progress gradually, many patients do not become fully aware of their problems until their daytime function and performance are severely affected. Relevant symptoms are summarized in ▶ Table 2.2.

Snoring and Witnessed Apneas

OSA is clinically characterized by heavy snoring. Snoring may be defined as a vibratory, sonorous noise made during inspiration.[49] It is associated with a vibration of the soft pharyngeal tissues producing a fluttering noise. Often, snoring is more cumbersome for the bed partner than for the patient and it mostly exists for a long time. Four or five loud snores, followed by a silence (apnea) and another series of loud snores is a highly suggestive description of a subject with OSA. Resumption of respiration can be associated with loud stridorous breathing ("gasping" or "snorting"). Typically, these symptoms are most prominent in the supine position or after alcohol intake. However, in rare conditions, snoring may not be so prominent, even in the presence of severe OSA.[50] There is also convincing evidence that snoring might cause daytime sleepiness in the absence of OSA.[19] This might occur due to UARS or by upper airway inflammation due to snoring induced vibrations within the pharynx.[38,51] In the general population, 25% of men and 15% of women are habitual snorers (snore almost every night) but the prevalence of snoring increases progressively with age: 60% of men and 40% of women between the ages 41 and 65 years snore habitually.[52] The prevalence of heavy snoring in the general population ranges from 15 to 47% in men and from 6 to 33% in women.[53,54,55] Snoring can be quantified either by frequency (how many nights per week) or by intensity, or by directly asking the patient how often they snore loudly or about vibratory qualities; but this information is only modestly helpful for making a clinical decision.[56] In a large PSG study in 1,040 patients

▶ Table 2.2 Common symptoms in obstructive sleep apnea

Night-time symptoms	Daytime symptoms
Heavy snoring	Not waking up fresh in the morning
Restless sleep, awakenings, insomnia, nightmares	Matinal headache
Witnessed apneas	Dry mouth on arising
Nocturnal choking or gasping	Excessive sleepiness
Dyspnea	Fatigue
Nocturia	Mood disturbance
Excessive sweating	Irritability
Impotence/sexual dysfunction/ decreased libido	Memory and concentration problems
Gastroesophageal reflux	Decreased performance

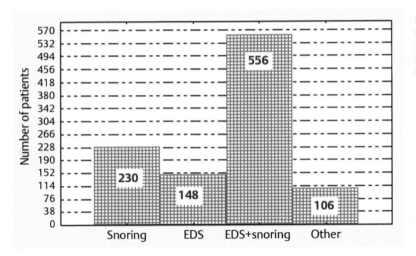

Fig. 2.1 Distribution of cardinal symptoms in a series of 1,040 referred patients with suspicion of obstructive sleep apnea (OSA). EDS, excessive daytime sleepiness.

referred with suspicion of OSA, socially disturbing snoring was associated with OSA (AHI ≥ 10) in 37% of the patients referred to exclude sleep apnea (▶Fig. 2.1). The combination of heavy snoring with excessive daytime sleepiness revealed OSA in 56% of the referred patients.[57] In the absence of snoring, the diagnosis of OSA becomes less likely but cannot be excluded (e.g., in patients after uvulopalatopharyngoplasty [UPPP]). Often, snoring is underestimated or denied by the snorers themselves and is reported by their bed partners and environment. Of the patients who deny snoring, 75% are proven to be snorers when measured objectively.[58] Usually, patients develop strategies to cope with heavy snoring. Nevertheless, snoring is a cause of poor sleep quality for the patient's bed partner, affecting the partner's quality of life.[59] Often alcohol intake and sleep deprivation aggravate snoring and sleep apneas. Symptoms of dry mouth during sleep or in the morning together with a globus sensation in the pharynx may also be suspected for heavy snoring.

Witnessed apneas and choking at night are related to apneic events and are reported by bed partners or roommates. Inquiring about the frequency of apneas observed by the partner has about the same (low) diagnostic utility as asking about snoring frequency. Bed partners seldom give accurate information about frequency of repetitive hypopneas. It is more useful to ask patients whether the bed partner reports to them choking or gasping during the night than it is to simply ask the patients if they wake up experiencing these symptoms. Attacks of choking or dyspnea that wake them from sleep may result in referral for a sleep study. Patients usually report it as being wakened by snoring, and are able to register events only after the airway has opened and they are in the middle of the postapneic snore. In conjunction with an arousal, patients often feel a sensation of tachycardia. Episodes of choking have to be differentiated from sleep choking (typically at initiating sleep) and sleep-related laryngospasm (typically in the middle of the night).[60] In such conditions, patients describe dramatic episodes where they wake up

during the night gasping because of complete airway closure, despite violent efforts to reopen the airway. After some time the airway suddenly opens and patients feel fine. Patients are usually extremely frightened, often feel they are going to die, and are unable to breathe properly for much longer than patients with OSA (often several minutes versus a fraction of < 15–30 seconds).

Pathological Daytime Sleepiness

Pathological or excessive daytime sleepiness is the second key symptom in the diagnosis of sleep apnea.[47,61,62] According to the AASM, excessive daytime sleepiness can be defined as "sleepiness that occurs in a situation when an individual would usually be expected to be awake and alert."[63] It is caused by increased respiratory effort and hypoxemia, which finally results in the so-called "arousal," with sleep fragmentation and loss of rapid eye movement (REM) sleep and slow-wave sleep as a consequence. Extreme daytime sleepiness is characterized by falling asleep during motor activity (talking, eating). Unequivocal sleepiness is characterized by falling asleep in quiet conditions (under boring situations or during periods of physical inactivity) or while driving. Extension of physiological diurnal sleepiness is considered mild sleepiness.

Sleepiness casued by inadequate sleep is very common in the general population; therefore it is hard to distinghuish from sleepiness due to an underlying sleep disorder or a medical disease.

In general, patient and environment will not give too much attention toward this symptom, as far as it does not lead to repetitive traffic accidents or occupational accidents. Tasks arising at regular intervals can be performed at decreased levels of vigilance, but this is not the case for unexpected tasks and (traffic) events. Therefore, up to 9% of all traffic accidents are attributed to sleepiness and falling asleep, 13% of the accidents with physical harm, and 17% of the accidents with fatality.[64] In car accidents where sleepiness was the obvious cause, the rate of deaths was three times as high as in other accidents. According to a French study, falling asleep while driving seemed to be the cause of 3% of the accidents causing material damage, 20% of the accidents causing injuries, and 50% of the accidents causing death.[65] As a consequence, a recent accident can give occasion to consult a physician. On the other hand, sleepiness is often underestimated or denied by patients with OSA, since they get adapted to this condition over time.[66]

Different rating scales have been developed to assess sleepiness, such as visual analogue scales,[67] the Karolinska Sleepiness Scale,[68] the Stanford Sleepiness Scale (SSS),[69] and the Epworth Sleepiness Scale (ESS).[70] These tools have different indications and are useful to assess patient's perception of current sleepiness and the feelings and symptoms associated with drowsiness.[67,68,69] These tools are fast, simple, easy to understand, cheap to administer, and reflect the patient's own opinion on the severity of his/her sleepiness. Usually, these scales are used to supplement the history and to follow the effects of treatment. The SSS was one of the first self-rating scales introduced in 1972 to quantify sleepiness.[69] This scale asks subjects to rate their degree of sleepiness at a single moment of time from seven descriptions, ranging from "feeling active and vital; alert wide awake" to "almost in reverie; sleep onset soon; lost struggle to remain awake." The SSS is fast and easy to administer. However, there are no reference values and it has not been validated with other physiologic measures.[34] The ESS is a measure to assess the tendency to nod off[70] and enables the quantification of excessive daytime sleepiness. The ESS was developed in 1991 as a trait to measure the tendency to fall asleep in several specific situations. It is a subjective tool to measure how sleepiness interferes with an individual's daily activities in eight situations. Although very popular in daily clinical practice, the test is limited by the situations assessed that patients may actually experience rarely or never (e.g., driving). Many sleepy subjects may also score in the normal range, since they do not actually fall asleep, despite being drowsy, either because of lack of opportunity or because of effective compensatory measures.[34] Its reliability and validity have also been questioned because of its weak or absent correlation with objective measures of sleep, but it is still the most widely used instrument. These scales can only be used well if subjects have insight into their symptoms and the capacity to dissociate sleepiness from other symptoms, such as fatigue.

Specific tests have been developed to measure sleepiness more objectively,[36,71] such as the multiple sleep latency test (MSLT), maintenance of wakefulness test (MWT), and vigilance tests such as Oxford Sleep Resistance Test (OSLER) test or Psychomotor Vigilance Task (PVT).[63,72,73] MSLT and MWT are considered the gold standard measures of objective sleepiness. The MSLT is an objective measure of the tendency to fall asleep under standardized conditions and in the absence of alertness stimulating factors. The MWT is an objective measure of the ability to stay awake for a defined period of time.[63,73]

According to the AASM, the MSLT is not routinely indicated in the initial evaluation and diagnosis of OSA or in the assessment of change following treatment; however, it is strictly indicated when a patient with OSA is suspected of having narcolepsy. Patients with OSA frequently underestimate the severity of sleepiness. Objectifying sleepiness may be important for the evaluation of OSA severity and its consequences on the individual level.[74] In daily practice, MSLT, MWT, and vigilance testing are restricted to patients with persistent hypersomnolence despite adequate continuous positive airway pressure (CPAP) therapy or surgical or oral device therapy. On the other hand, routine use of these tests can be recommended for medicolegal reasons, but is not routinely feasible.[65,73] Unfortunately, in MWT, completely normal values do not necessarily ensure absolute safety. Therefore, clinical judgement should always prevail in a context of ability to drive.

As with ESS, the AHI also poorly correlates with quantified measures of sleepiness, which could indicate that some individuals cope better with sleep fragmentation than others, while brain susceptibility and subjective perception of the consequences of hypoxemia could also be involved.[75] Using a cutoff value of 18 respiratory events per hour, a sensitivity of 71% and a specificity of 60% for identifying subjects with excessive daytime sleepiness was obtained. When subtle flow limitations are not taken into account, the sensitivity/specificity is even worse.[76] Hence, for clinical purposes, it is obvious that the respiratory disturbance index is a more reliable parameter, but even then, its correlation with daytime symptoms remains suboptimal. In the Sleep Heart Health Study (SHHS) a poor correlation between the AHI and sleepiness was reported: the ESS only rose from 7.2 to 9.3 when the AHI changed from less than 5 to more than 30.[77] However, in clinical decision making, it is important to identify patients in whom CPAP therapy should be instituted to treat daytime sleepiness.

In severe cases of OSA it is difficult to identify excessive daytime sleepiness resulting from other causes than sleep apnea. Depression, disturbed mood, diabetes mellitus, and cardiovascular diseases are among the most important confounding factors,[78,79,80] as well as sleep disorders other than OSA or side effects due to medical treatment.[81,82,83] In a large epidemiological study (n = 16,583 subjects), depression was the most significant risk factor for excessive daytime sleepiness, followed by age, BMI, sleep duration, diabetes mellitus, smoking, and finally sleep apnea.[81] Obesity alone may interfere through systemic inflammation (adipokines and chemokines) being activated even in the absence of OSA. In OSA, stress activation involving both the sympathetic system and the hypothalamic pituitary adrenal (HPA) axis may also be involved. Some patients have persistent symptoms while on adequate treatment. Whether residual sleepiness (ESS ≥11) is related to residual apneas is an unanswered question. Some extrapolations could be made. In a series of adequately treated OSA (baseline ESS >10, 6 months CPAP, compliance ≥4 h/d),[84] Koutsourelakis et al found that 55% of their patients had an abnormal ESS score (>10) (16 ± 3) at follow-up, which was related to a history of depression, diabetes, heart disease, and a higher ESS score (16 ± 3 vs 14 ± 3) and lower AHI (44 ± 28 vs 59 ± 34) at baseline conditions. Unfortunately, their study group was blurred by patients with mild OSA (AHI > 5). Stradling et al studied 572 patients on CPAP and compared them with a control group of 525 individuals from a community survey.[85] There was no difference in the percentage of patients with an ESS above 10 in the CPAP group compared with the controls (16 vs 14%). In the study of Pépin et al, 12% remained sleepy on CPAP, or 6% after exclusion of associated major depression, restless legs syndrome, and narcolepsy.[86] This again emphasizes that mood disturbance is often involved in (residual) sleepiness. However, a link between residual sleepiness and residual apneas in selective patients is not ruled out. Maybe more insight will be obtained when pathophysiology of (obstructive) sleep apnea identified on CPAP or oral devices is disentangled. Verbruggen et al reported residual excessive sleepiness in 27 out of 84 patients (32%) on oral appliance therapy, despite normalization of AHI in patients with mild to moderately severe OSA. These patients had a significantly higher baseline ESS (15 ± 4 vs 9 ± 4; P < 0.001) and were younger (43 ± 9 vs 47 ± 9; P = 0.028) compared with patients without residual sleepiness.[87]

Fatigue

Fatigue can be defined as an overwhelming sense of tiredness, lack of energy, and a feeling of exhaustion, associated with impaired physical and/or cognitive functioning.[88] Exhaustion could potentially reflect changes in mood, known to be common in chronic illness, but can also be the symptom of unknown or neglected OSA.[14] Fatigue is frequently reported as the main symptom in patients with OSA, in up to 50% of referred cases, and is more common and more distressing to OSA patients than excessive daytime sleepiness.[89,90] Increased fatigue has also been closely related to increased levels of depressive symptoms in OSA patients.[91,92] Fatigue is also a common and distressing complaint in the general population and a major problem in a wide range of diseases in internal and sleep medicine. Previous studies have demonstrated that self-reported sleep quality is independently associated with fatigue, even after taking into account demographic, comorbid conditions, OSA severity, sleepiness, and depressive symptoms. Hence, patients complaining about fatigue have a worst perception of sleep quality.[93] It has important implications for clinical practice, where lack of energy, fatigue, and tiredness may lead to investigations, including sleep studies, and differential diagnosis that do not address the

medical problem. The fatigue of the various disorders is not disease-specific, and is likely caused from interplay of physiological, psychological, and lifestyle-related factors. However, typical symptoms of OSA are less predictive in the presence of comorbid conditions, or might be attributed to these medical disorders, while consideration for OSA may be missed. Instruments to assess fatigue are the Fatigue Severity Scale,[94] visual analogue scales,[95] and specific questionnaires such as the fatigue-inertia subscale of the Profile of Mood States[96] and the vitality subscale of the SF-36 quality-of-life questionnaire.[97]

Fatigue or Sleepiness?

Excessive daytime sleepiness is a cardinal feature of OSA, which is frequently used interchangeably with fatigue, likely because patients often complain of both types of symptoms. Daytime sleepiness, reflecting a physiological need for sleep, can be objectively quantified with tests, while fatigue is more elusive and relies almost exclusively on self-report.[98] Nevertheless, symptoms compatible with OSA may be caused by OSA itself, or by comorbid medical disorders that can predispose a patient to sleep disturbance. Clinicians must be aware that absence of complaints of fatigue, tiredness, sleepiness, or lack of energy does not rule out the possibility of OSA.[15]

Other Daytime Symptoms

Thorough anamnesis of patient and bed partner can make clear the association between the main symptoms and sleep apnea syndrome by bringing to light complaints related to poor sleep quality. These complaints include profuse body sweating, matinal headache (due to nocturnal carbon dioxide [CO_2] accumulation, usually dull and generalized), not feeling fresh in the morning, nasal obstruction, behavioral alterations, memory and concentration problems, decreased cognitive performance, depressed mood, anxiety, automatic behavior, social problems, marital problems, decreased libido, unexplained muscle pain, all resulting in a decreased quality of life. Also, symptoms of reflux have been more frequently reported; however, these symptoms improve with OSA treatment.

These symptoms can be explained by pronounced intrathoracic pressure changes induced by vigorous breathing attempts against an occluded airway along with regurgitation of gastric fluid.

There is also evidence of an association between erectile dysfunction and OSA, based on self-report and small case series,[99] but underreporting can be estimated. CPAP therapy has shown to reverse this problem.

Disturbed Sleep, Insomnia, Nocturnal Sweating

Most patients with OSA have little difficulty initiating sleep and have short sleep latencies during sleep studies.[100] On the other hand, problems of maintaining sleep, early morning awakenings, nightmares, abnormal motor activity, nocturnal dyspnea, nocturnal asphyxia, and nocturia are frequently reported. OSA patients also often have a restless sleep. Apneas can be associated with body movements or movements limited to mild limb movements. Occasionally, abrupt arm and limb movements with involuntary hitting of the bed partner occur.[101] Due to this increased motor activity at night, patients with OSA often suffer from nocturnal sweating. It is striking that, despite these typical symptoms, the interval between the first symptoms and the final diagnosis can often take some years. Nevertheless, OSA patients are usually convinced that they are sleeping well and are unaware of the breathing stops. Infrequently, patients may have insomnia as their major symptom. Moreover, a significant proportion of insomniacs have sleep apnea (25–50%), which is most likely to reflect recurrent sleep fragmentation and increased wakefulness during the night. This manifestation is described as occult sleep apnea, provoked by an increased number of arousals and sleep/wake transitions, which per se may induce unstable breathing. Women may report more insomnia and less witnessed apneas. Rarely, arousal triggered by obstructive events may induce nonrapid eye movement (NREM) parasomnias, such as nocturnal eating syndrome. In case of increased nocturnal sweating, a number of medical reasons have to be checked, such as infections, endocrinological alterations (hypoglycaemia, thyroid dysfunction), cardiovascular disorders with increased sympathetic activity, malignancy, chronic pain, stress disorders, and substance abuse or withdrawal (benzodiazepines, opioids, ethanol).

Nocturia

Nocturia can be defined as waking up more than once during the night to urinate (each void is preceded by and followed by sleep).[102] The prevalence of nocturia is high and increases suddenly with age. About 20% of elderly males and 25% of elderly women report regular nocturia (NYHANES III study).[103] It has been reported to be up to 50% in patients with OSA, and the number of voids at nights seems to correlate with the severity of OSA.[104,105,106] Nocturia can be attributed to increased levels of atrial natriuretic peptide (ANP) levels, related to the generation of negative intrathoracic pressures in OSA. These pressure swings cause false signals of volume overload to the endocardium, with resulting increase in ANP secretion and increased urine production. Umlauf et al found increased nocturia and elevated urinary ANP only when the AHI was more than or equal to 15 per hour.[106] Fitzgerald et al demonstrated that CPAP could decrease nocturia in OSA patients.[107] Although less well supported, nocturia in OSA could also develop due to an increased awareness of bladder fullness secondary to arousal and/or transmission to the bladder of

positive intra-abdominal pressure provoked by repetitive obstructive events.[108,109] Thorough medical history taking with respect to hypertrophic benign prostate, diabetes mellitus, chronic heart failure, renal disease, and use of diuretics is mandatory. Increased intake or late consumption of liquids is also one potential explanation to be excluded.

2.1.4 Age and Gender Bias

Most of the studies have been performed in middle-aged subjects (range 40–60 years), overweight male subjects with moderate to severe OSA. As a consequence, the features and neurobehavioral as well as cardiometabolic sequellae in OSA mainly apply to this specific cohort. Nevertheless, OSA can also have a substantial impact on daytime vigilance and quality of life in the elderly (>70 years old). Remarkably, anamnesis and daytime symptoms can be less specific in advanced ages.[110] A gender bias also takes place in the OSA population, as discussed earlier. In general, men and women report many of the same typical symptoms. However, women may report insomnia, and are more likely to complain of depression, morning headache, and fatigue.[111]

2.1.5 Symptoms of OSA in Older Subjects

The symptoms of OSA in aged people are similar to and could be confused with some of the functional deteriorations in elderly. Both OSA and ageing lead to disturbed sleep, cognitive dysfunction, and increased cardiometabolic alterations. With age, sleep becomes more fragmented, independent of OSA, and there is a well-documented age-related decline in sleep quality.[112,113,114,115,116] These features of sleep in aged people have led to the suggestion that older OSA patients may be habituated to the added disease-related sleep disruption of OSA, and hence, do not suffer from symptoms of daytime sleepiness compared with young OSA patients. In the SHHS, it has been shown that age is associated with a reduction in subjective sleepiness measured with the ESS in females, but not in males.[117] However, in another study comparing older people with and without OSA, patients with OSA were more sleepy than those without OSA.[118] In older OSA patients from clinical cohorts, subjective daytime sleepiness was found to be similar to that experienced by younger patients matched for BMI and disease severity[119] and less in another.[120] Altogether, the current information on the symptoms of sleepiness in older people with OSA is controversial.

Estimates of the prevalence of OSA suggest that it is higher in the geriatric population than in the general population, and the clinical consequences may be different.[121]

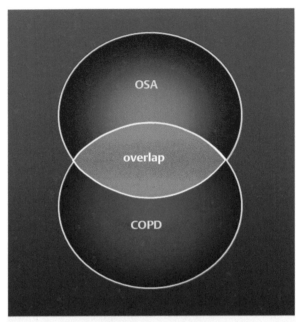

Fig. 2.2 The two components of the overlap syndrome.

2.1.6 Symptoms in Overlap Syndrome

Based on established prevalence figures, OSA and chronic obstructive pulmonary disorder (COPD) should coexist in about 1% of the adult general population, with even higher figures likely depending on the definitions employed for diagnosis (▶ Fig. 2.2).[122] Sleep quality is typically poor in COPD, with diminished amounts of REM and slow-wave sleep, which may contribute to the daytime fatigue frequently reported by these patients.[123] Patients with overlap syndrome present with the clinical features of each disorder to a greater or lesser extent, depending on the balance between the OSA and COPD components. However, there are likely to be additional clinical features that reflect the higher prevalence of hypoxemia, hypercapnia, and pulmonary hypertension. Specifically, morning headache reflecting hypercapnia, cyanosis reflecting hypoxemia, and peripheral edema reflecting cor pulmonale are likely to be common in overlap patients. Such finding should facilitate the selection of COPD patients for further assessment regarding the likelihood of OSA.

2.1.7 Focused History

Referral of patients to sleep facilities is mandatory, but risk stratification and triage of patients is highly desirable, given the diagnostic capacity of sleep centers is limited and waiting lists tend to grow.[124] Relevant clinical information (symptoms, past medical history, family history) should be obtained from the patient, supplemented by collateral history from a bed partner, relatives, friends,

or caregivers. Details of patient's typical night sleep time and sleep-wake schedule are always required, along with the observation of other symptoms. The degree and relevance of sleepiness should always be evaluated clinically, and special emphasis should be paid to driving performance. Patients with suspected OSA should undergo careful physical examination. Overall, it may be hard to produce objective, reproducible findings because of observer and reporter bias. Persistent efforts have been made to increase standardization. Use of questionnaires allows for both the identification of individuals with a high likelihood of OSA and for triage according to their symptomatology. Questionnaires that make use of isolated symptoms have a limited effectiveness. For instance, loud snoring is a primary symptom in OSA that has a sensitivity of almost 100% but lacks specificity. As a result, snoring has a low positive predictive value.[125] On the other hand, the report of "breath holding" has a low sensitivity, but a high specificity for OSA.[125] Furthermore, the diagnostic performance of the ESS score above 10 to predict AHI more than 5 per hour has a sensitivity of 54% and a specificity of 63%.[126] Also, subjective clinical impressions of OSA tend to have inadequate sensitivity (60%) and specificity (63%). Therefore, attempts were made to develop novel clinical prediction models with optimized sensitivity and specificity, however, without beneficial outcome.[127]

2.1.8 Screening Questionnaires and Clinical Prediction Models

Several screening questionnaires that incorporate risk factors, clinical symptoms, and physical examination parameters have been developed to facilitate the diagnosis of OSA. Some of these have been validated for perioperative screening[128]: the Berlin questionnaire,[129,130] the American Society of Anesthesiologists (ASA) checklist,[131] the STOP-Bang questionnaire (acronym for snoring, tiredness, observed apneas, hypertension, BMI, age, neck circumference, and male gender),[132] and the Flemons Index (Sleep Apnea Clinical Score [SACS]).[133] Attempts to establish a reliable diagnosis based on a clinical prediction model without a simultaneous objective sleep test have failed.[134] The oldest of these tests is the Flemons Index, which combines neck circumference, presence or absence of arterial hypertension, and historical features (habitual snoring, partner report of gasping, choking). The test provides an SACS and it has been shown that a score of more than or equal to 15 has been associated with a high likelihood to find OSA (odds ratio [OR] of 5.17 and a positive predictive value of 81%).[133] Furthermore, the SACS has been associated with postanesthesia care complications.[135] Takegami et al developed a four-variable screening tool based on gender, BMI, blood pressure, and snoring.[136] This tool was highly discriminative, but mathematical corrections were needed to calculate an end score.

The Berlin questionnaire was the outcome of Conference on Sleep in Primary Care in Berlin, Germany (April 1996).[137] The questionnaire has a high specificity for identifying subjects with moderate to severe OSA, while rather low specificity. It classifies subjects as low or high risk for OSA based on responses in three different categories: (1) snoring history, (2) daytime sleepiness, and (3) history of obesity or arterial hypertension. If a patient responds positively in two of the categories assessed, he/she can be considered at a high risk for OSA. The Apnea Risk Evaluation System (ARES) questionnaire is an attractive tool that combines features of the Berlin questionnaire, the Flemons' Index, and the ESS and classifies the patients as "no apparent risk," "low risk," or "high risk," with a sensitivity of 94% and a specificity of 79% for an AHI above 5. In 2,877 patients screened with the ARES questionnaire in a preoperative setting, 23.7% had high risk for OSA (661) and among these 82% had OSA.[138] An increased sensitivity (90.4%) at the expense of a lower specificity (43.2%) to find an AHI above or equal to 15 compared to the Berlin questionnaire was reported.[139] The ASA scoring checklist combines history of apparent airway obstruction, somnolence, and physical characteristics. Its sensitivity is good (72–87%), while its specificity is low (36–38%). The STOP and STOP-Bang questionnaires are self-administered questionnaires developed by Chung et al.[132] STOP is the acronym for four questions addressing the presence of snoring, tiredness (daytime fatigue), observed apneas, and arterial hypertension. The STOP-Bang questionnaire is a refinement of the STOP questionnaire and incorporates questions on BMI (>35 kg/m^2), age (>50 years), neck circumference (>40 cm), and gender (male) with improved sensitivity at the cost of a little lower specificity. Both questionnaires have a high sensitivity for identifying subjects with OSA, but, on the other hand, relatively low specificity. The STOP-questionnaire labels a patient with a high risk for SDB if at least two positive answers are present, while the STOP-Bang questionnaire uses a cut-off value of more than or equal to three positive answers. Due to its simplicity, the STOP-Bang tool is often used to predict severity of underlying OSA and to facilitate triage of patients. In a recent study comparing STOP, the Berlin questionnaire, and the ASA scoring checklist, the last one showed the highest sensitivity but the lowest specificity.[140,141] Overall, the potential usefulness of these tools for prioritization of an objective diagnostic test is limited. The best model so far is the OSA50 questionnaire, which combines a simple questionnaire with oximetry. For clarity, OSA50 is the acronym for obesity (waist circumference: males >102 cm; females >88 cm), snoring (Has your snoring ever bothered other people?), apnea (Has anyone noticed that you stop breathing during your sleep?), and 50 (Are you aged 50 years or over?). If yes, a score of 3, 3, 2, and 2 points, respectively, is assigned. If a cutoff is above or equal to 5/10 and an oxygen desaturation index (ODI) above or equal to 16 per hour is applied for OSA, a sensitivity of 97%, a specificity

of 87%, and a diagnostic accuracy of 83% is obtained.[142] The authors preferred oximetry over nasal pressure for their two-stage model, because the failure rate for the oximetry signal (3%) was one-third of that observed for the nasal pressure signal (9%). Recently, Perioperative Sleep Apnea Prediction (P-SAP) score was introduced. This score incorporates six out of eight elements of the STOP-BANG questionnaire and some other elements used in the standard perioperative assessment (Mallampati score, presence of diabetes, thyromental distance <6 cm).[143] For each of the nine risk factors, 1 point is assigned (unweighted scale) and scores are summed up. This results in a very high sensitivity and a very low specificity in the lower range, but a very low sensitivity and very high specificity in the higher range. Anyway, it was concluded that the score requires further refinement.

2.1.9 Consequences

Most compelling evidence described here (▶Fig. 2.3 and ▶Fig. 2.4) is based on cross-sectional population-based investigations, looking for associations between the prevalence of a cardiovascular consequence (e.g., diabetes mellitus) at a given time with the severity of OSA, based on various levels of AHI. Others follow a population over a time period and determine the amount of new cases (called "incidence"). Such approach enables to determine the risk of developing consequences at various disease levels. It is worth remembering that conclusions from investigations in clinical cohorts could be different from those in population-based asymptomatic individuals, and these clinical cohorts are subject to referral bias.

Cardiovascular Morbidities

OSA is increasingly recognized as an independent risk factor for systemic hypertension, stroke, cardiac arrhythmias, and coronary artery disease (CAD).[144,145,146]

Systemic Hypertension

Elevated blood pressure values can be present during sleep as a consequence of OSA.[147] Moreover, systemic hypertension during wakefulness may be related to OSA. At least 45% of patients with OSA have systemic hypertension. In OSA, hypoxia increases sympathetic tone via chemo- and baroreflex activation, which finally results in increasing blood pressure.[147,148] Increased negative intrathoracic pressures (promoting venous return) and arousal from sleep, both in association with apneic events, also contribute to the rise in blood pressure seen in OSA.[149,150,151] Lack of a normal decrease in blood pressure during sleep, often described as "non-dipping," may be the earliest sign of OSA-induced hypertension and an independent risk factor for developing CAD,[152,153] as well as heart failure, especially heart failure with preserved ejection fraction (HFpEF) and a strong risk factor for stroke.

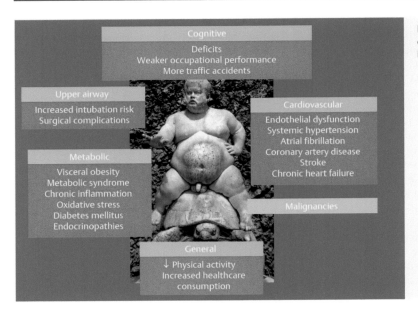

Fig. 2.3 Major consequences of untreated obstructive sleep apnea (OSA). (Statue of Bachus in Boboli Gardens, Firenze, Italy)

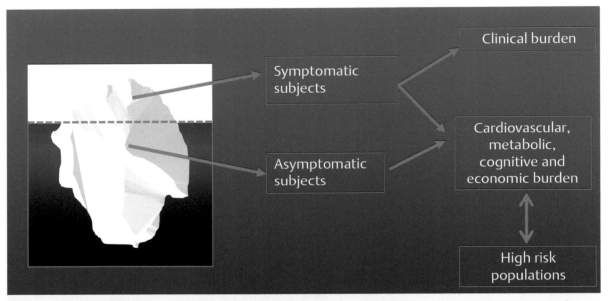

Fig. 2.4 Most of the patients with obstructive sleep apnea (OSA) in the general population are asymptomatic, but are prone to the consequences of the disorder.

The Wisconsin Sleep Cohort Study, one of the largest population-based studies (n = 1,060), reported a close dose-response relationship between OSA and hypertension. After correction for established risk factors for hypertension, this relationship was still present.[154] Moreover, the Sleep Heart Health Study (SHHS) (n = 6,424) identified OSA as an independent risk factor for systemic hypertension.[155] In the following 4 years, the OR of developing systemic hypertension increased gradually and linearly with increasing AHI.[156] In the European Sleep Apnea Database (ESADA), it was shown in a multiple regression analysis (with both ODI and AHI in the model) that ODI was independently associated with prevalent hypertension, whereas AHI was not: OR (95% CI) for ODI was 2.01 (1.61–2.51) and regarding AHI 0.92 (0.74–1.15) ($P < 0.0001$ and $P = 0.3054$, respectively).[157]

Stroke

Evidence from a broad variety of studies has suggested an increased risk of stroke in OSA patients,[158,159,160] with the 10-year predicted occurrence of stroke being 14%.[161]

At the same time, a high prevalence of OSA was also demonstrated in patients with stroke.[162,163,164,165] Central apneas and Cheyne-Stokes respiration have been shown to occur rather commonly in the acute phase of stroke, but spontaneously resolve with time and its clinical impact is not proven. Intermittent hypoxemia is probably the most critical factor in the cerebrovascular abnormalities predisposing OSA patients to stroke. Moreover, impaired cerebrovascular response to hypoxemia has been reported in OSA patients, which is consistent with underlying endothelial alterations. Overall, fluctuations in blood pressure, reduction in cerebral blood flow, altered cerebral autoregulation, endothelial dysfunction, accelerated atherogenesis, and prothrombotic and proinflammatory states are mechanisms involved in the increased risk for stroke in OSA.[166] Studies have found a direct relationship between nocturnal oxygen dipping, intima media thickness, and atherosclerotic plaques in the carotid arteries, independent of the presence of systemic hypertension, and thereby support a direct relation between OSA, atherosclerosis, and subsequent stroke.[167,168] Another correlation was found between increased severity of OSA and incidence of stroke and death in a cohort of OSA patients after a follow-up period of 3.4 years.[158] Consequently, increased mortality was found in patients with severe OSA (AHI > 30) after stroke[163,169] and cross-sectional data from the SHHS have shown greater risks for stroke in the highest quartile (AHI > 11) (OR 1.58 [95% CI 1.02–2.46]) than in the lower quartile (AHI 4.4–11) (OR 1.42 [75% CI 0.91–2.21]).[160] Another group showed an OR of 4.33 (95% CI 1.32–14.24) for prevalent stroke in moderate-to-severe OSA (AHI ≥ 20), after correction for other risk factors, compared to patients without OSA. After 4 years of follow-up, an AHI of more than or equal to 20 at baseline was associated with an increased incidence for stroke, after adjustment for age and sex, but not for BMI (OR 4.48 [95% CI 1.31–5.33]). However, after correction for age, sex, and BMI, the OR was still elevated, but without statistical significance (OR 3.08 [95% CI 0.74–12.81]).[159] Nevertheless, OSA in patients with stroke often results in worse functional outcomes and higher mortality.[170,171]

Cardiac Arrhythmias

The whole spectrum of cardiac arrhythmias has been observed and associated with OSA. The most common among them are nonsustained tachycardia, sinus arrest, second-degree atrioventricular conduction block, and premature ventricular contractions. Their prevalence and complexity increases with the severity of the OSA and following hypoxemia.[172,173,174] In the SHHS, it was suggested that patients with OSA have increased likelihoods of atrial fibrillation (OR 4.02 [95% CI 1.03–15.74]), nonsustained tachycardia (OR 3.40 [95% CI 1.03–11.20]), and complex ventricular ectopy (OR 1.75 [95% CI 1.11–2.74]),[175] with a fourfold increase in the prevalence of atrial fibrillation in patients with severe OSA.[175] It has

been shown that ventricular premature beats decreased by 58% after 1 month of CPAP treatment in OSA patients with CHF.[176] The mechanisms by which OSA induces ventricular arrhythmias are uncertain, but hypoxemia, bradyarrhythmias, and sympathetic activation induced by apneic events may play a critical important role. Initially, increased vagal tone is observed during apnea as a result of hypoxic stimulation of the carotid bodies during absent ventilation. Once respiration resumes, inflation of the lungs decreases vagal tone, while the hypoxic influences on sympathetic tone are unmasked with resulting tachycardia. These episodes of tachycardia and postapneic elevated blood pressure increase myocardial oxygen demand while hypoxemia exists, predisposing to ischemia and possibly tachyarrhythmias. In healthy subjects, sleep usually is a time of reduced tachyarrhythmias and ischemia, while patients with OSA may not enjoy this effect. In atrial fibrillation, hypoxemia, blood pressure changes, sympathetic activation, transmural pressor surges, and systemic inflammation are predisposing mechanisms to its development. The relationship between OSA and atrial fibrillation may also contribute indirectly to the increased risk of stroke in patients with OSA.

Coronary Artery Disease

Some studies suggest an independent association between OSA and CAD in middle-aged adults.[177] One study described not only the association between coronary artery calcification (CAC) and OSA, but also highlighted the association between CAC and increasing OSA severity. The OR for CAC increased with rising OSA severity: mild (OR 2.1 [50% CI 0.8–5.4]), moderate (OR 2.4 [75% CI 1.0–6.4]), and severe OSA (OR 3.3 [95% CI 1.2–9.4]).[178] The frequency of nocturnal oxygen desaturation correlated with the extent of coronary lesions and explained 13.4% of their variance, suggesting a pathophysiologic role of OSA in coronary atherosclerosis.[179] The chronic effects of OSA, such as systemic inflammation, oxidative stress, lymphocyte activation, vascular smooth cell activation, decrease in macrophages, increased lipid levels, lipid peroxidation, high-density lipoprotein dysfunction, and finally endothelial dysfunction, potentially trigger the formation of atherosclerotic plaques. Plaque rupture can be provoked by the acute effects of OSA, such as intermittent hypoxemia, acidosis, blood pressure surges, and systemic vasoconstriction, in conjunction with simultaneous changes in intrathoracic and transmural pressure.[166] Hence, the increased oxygen demand and reduced oxygen supply at night in OSA patients may trigger an attack of myocardial ischemia and resulting nocturnal angina. Nocturnal angina and ST depression have been described in OSA patients, but may be diminished after CPAP treatment.[180,181] However, another study did not find evidence of nocturnal myocardial injury based on measurements of cardiac troponin T in patients with established CAD and moderate to severe OSA.[182] In addition, observations of the occurrence of myocardial infarction (MI) in OSA patients found an altered time interval of nocturnal sudden death compared to the general population. In general, the likelihood of onset of MI is between 6 and 11 AM. In contrast, almost half of OSA patients have their onset of MI during the sleep hours, between 10 PM and 6 AM. This may implicate that OSA patients are prone to nocturnal MI.[183,184] Recently, a new provocative scenario has emerged to suggest that in some specific populations, OSA could be associated with a cardioprotective role. Epidemiological studies are also suggesting that protective mechanisms may be activated in a particular subset of patients with OSA.[185] In patients with acute MI and mild to moderate OSA, activated adaptive mechanisms were shown to improve endothelial function, hence providing cardioprotection in context of acute MI. Shah et al demonstrated that patients with OSA have less severe cardiac injury during an acute nonfatal MI when compared with similar patients without OSA. The protective role could become activated via ischemic preconditioning and supersedes the detrimental inflammatory and oxidative stress which is typically present in patients with relevant OSA.[186]

Subclinical Cardiocirculatory Impairment

One of the most important clinical findings in the recent years is the occurrence of atherosclerosis in overall healthy subjects with OSA, free of any cardiovascular morbidity and other cardiovascular risk factors.[167,187] This is part of subclinical cardiocirculatory impairment described in OSA, together with masked systemic hypertension,[188] increase in arterial stiffness,[189] diastolic dysfunction,[190,191] and left and right ventricle hypertrophy.[192] These early cardiovascular changes have been correlated with systemic inflammation,[193] related to intermittent hypoxemia.[194] About half of the cases presenting with clinically relevant heart failure have a normal left ventricular ejection fraction (so-called HFpEF), and left ventricular diastolic dysfunction is considered to be a common underlying pathology.[195] Studies have shown that impairment of the left ventricular diastolic function is very common in OSA patients, suggesting not only subclinical myocardial disease (that may account for the risk of heart failure),[196,197,198] but also a role of OSA in pulmonary hypertension. OSA appears to be associated with cardiac remodelling and altered diastolic function, and to exert an additive effect to that of elevated blood pressure in patients with both hypertension and OSA.[190] Cross-sectional data from the SHHS have shown a strong association of SDB in moderate and severe OSA with chronic heart failure (OR 2.38 [95% CI 1.22–4.62]) and a weaker association for mild OSA (OR 1.95 [75% CI 0.99–3.83]).[199]

Cardiovascular Mortality

Observational cohort studies indicate that untreated patients with OSA have an increased risk of nonfatal and fatal cardiovascular events, an increased risk of sudden cardiac death during the night, and a higher risk of stroke or death from any cause.[144,145] In an older study, the probability of cumulative 8-year survival was 0.96 for patients with an apnea index below 20 and 0.63 for those with an apnea index above 20. Difference in mortality related to apnea index was particularly accurate in patients younger than 50 years and in whom mortality from other causes is uncommon.[200] In the study of Marin et al, multivariate analysis, adjusted for potential confounders, showed that untreated severe OSA significantly increased the risk of fatal (OR 2.87 [95% CI 1.17–7.51]) cardiovascular events compared with healthy subjects.[25] Treatment with CPAP attenuated this risk.[144,200]

Since the group that received CPAP got more intensive follow-up during the first year after diagnosis (two additional visits), outcome could be improved in this group independent of the CPAP treatment itself. Moreover, these results were only valid in men. The occurrence of OSA was a significant predictor of premature death in patients with CAD and who are at increased risk of stroke.[201,202] These studies have the intrinsic limitation of lacking a randomized controlled design, which clearly limits the evidence level. In one prospective study, it was found that the apnea index was a predictor of excess mortality in the fourth and fifth decade, but not in aged population.[203] In some population-based cohorts, a decrease in survival was reported with increasing OSA severity, with an OR of 3.0 (95% CI 1.4–6.3) (Wisconsin) and 1.46 (1.14–1.86) (SHHS) in subjects with severe OSA compared with those in the normal range.[204,205] However, after stratification by age and gender in the SHHS, the OR remained only significant in males aged less than 70 years. Lavie and Lavie proposed a survival advantage in moderate OSA, suggesting, as a potential mechanism, that chronic intermittent hypoxemia during sleep may activate adaptive pathways in the elderly.[206] For example, older people have a reduced acute cardiovascular response to arousal from sleep, compared with younger subjects.[207] Hence, the poorer cardiovascular reactivity of aged adults may, paradoxically, reduce the impact of arousals from sleep and protect against cardiovascular morbidities and mortality. However, it has to be reminded that the cardiovascular consequences of sleep apnea in the aged population may also be influenced by survival bias, as middle-aged, hypertensive OSA patients may not survive into old age. Discrepancies between studies could probably be explained by the heterogeneity of the patients included in the elderly populations.

Metabolic Consequences

A number of metabolic consequences have been identified in OSA. Some studies found increased insulin resistance and impaired glucose tolerance, independent of body weight,[208,209,210] and a worsening of insulin resistance with increasing AHI.[211] However, other investigations failed to demonstrate an independent effect of AHI due to the major impact of obesity.[212] In cohorts of the general population, both the Wisconsin Cohort Study and the SHHS have identified OSA as an independent risk factor for insulin resistance, after adjustment for probable confounding variables, such as age, sex, and BMI.[213,214] However, individuals with an AHI above or equal to 15 did not differ significantly from those with an AHI below 5 when it came to the risk of developing diabetes over a 4-year period (OR 1.62 [95% CI 0.7–3.6]), after adjustment for age, sex, and BMI.[133] Recent data from the ESADA study demonstrated that sleep apnea severity independently predicts glycemic health in nondiabetic subjects. Following adjustment for confounding factors, AHI, along with nocturnal hypoxaemia, predicted HbA1c.[215] From the same group, it has been shown that increasing OSA severity is associated with increased likelihood of concomitant type 2 diabetes mellitus (T2DM) and worse diabetes control in patients with T2DM.[216] Intermittent hypoxia and sleep fragmentation seem to play a key role in the development of metabolic disturbances, through the activation of the sympathetic nervous system and proinflammatory pathways. It has been shown that even lower grade oxygen desaturations are convincingly linked with glycemic status abnormalities.[217] Furthermore, OSA has an increased risk for developing diabetes over time, independent of the decrease in arterial oxygen saturation.[218] Sleep fragmentation due to cortical and autonomic arousals accounts for alterations in sympathetic/parasympathetic balance, and the simultaneous presence of metabolic syndrome and OSA further increases sympathetic activity and worsens glycemic control, even after adjustment for BMI.[219] Alteration in glucose metabolism and sympathovagal activity has been observed previously in healthy subjects following two nights of experimental sleep fragmentation.[220] The impact of treatment of OSA on long-term diabetes and the diabetic complications remains to be unravelled.

Cognitive Deficits

It is not surprising that OSA with the consecutive sleep alterations has dramatic effects on cerebral function. Memory, concentration, and learning ability have been reported to be abnormal in selective OSA patients.[221,222,223,224] Both "lower-level" processes (alertness and arousal) and "higher-level" cognitive processes (e.g., executive attention) have been disturbed, including the ability to inhibit inappropriate behaviors and ideas, regulate attention, and plan and organize for the future.[225,226,227] Particular cognitive impairments (such as thinking, perception, memory, communication, or the ability to learn new information) are present in a high proportion of OSA patients.[228] Studies using positron emission tomography (PET) or functional MRI indicate sleep loss as the primary cause of neurocognitive deficits, mainly a basal slowing in information processing, more than hypoxemia.[226] Earlier studies have shown profound evidence for a role of hypoxemia.[229] Since the profound effects of decreased alertness on higher cognitive functioning mimic cerebral damage due to hypoxemia, it is more complex to evaluate whether there are only functional or anatomical sequels also of OSA. OSA can promote axonal dysfunction or loss and myelin metabolism impairment in the frontal periventricular white matter, related to cognitive executive dysfunction.[230] A therapeutic challenge with CPAP could be very attractive to learn that not all cognitive function alterations are reversible, and hence, may represent neuronal damage. Moreover, when cognitive function is preserved in OSA patients, functional brain imaging has revealed that brain activation is increased, compared with the activation that occurs in healthy subjects performing the same task. The association between preserved cognitive function and greater activation in OSA patients suggests that enhanced cerebral recruitment (overrecruitment) is required to maintain cognitive performance.[231,232] Currently, it is also well established that cognitive and attentional deficits appear in OSA in the absence of perceived subjective sleepiness.[233] It questions the sensitivity of the tools used to assess sleepiness. Moreover, attentional deficits may occur without objective sleepiness.[233] Reaction time, sustained and divided attention tasks may be influenced in the absence of sleepiness. It should further be studied whether these attentional deficits may impair driving ability and other social and professional skills. If confirmed, it raises the question of who should be considered for treatment, since the absence of perceived sleepiness would then not be required for treating OSA. Finally, a number of factors other than OSA contribute to daytime sleepiness, including behavioral sleep deprivation and medication side effects. There is also considerable variability in the susceptibility to develop sleepiness as a result of sleep fragmentation. Therefore, it should not be surprising that there is only a weak correlation between the AHI and subjective or objective measures. Moreover, it should also be stressed that effective treatment of sleepy OSA does not always abolish daytime sleepiness.

Malignancies

From population-based studies and large clinical cohorts from Spain and the United States, it has been shown that OSA is an independent risk for both incident cancer and for overall cancer mortality.[234,235] Increased overnight hypoxia (time SaO_2 < 90% [TSat90]) as a surrogate of OSA severity was associated with increased incidence of cancer, and this association was stronger in patients younger than 65 years. Patients who spent more than 12% of nighttime with SO_2 below 90% had a more than twofold greater adjusted risk of incident cancer, and even those who spent more than 1.2% of nighttime in this situation were at increased risk of cancer, compared to individuals who spent less than 1.2% of the time with SaO_2 < 90%. Increasing continuous TSat90 was associated with increasing cancer incidence with an adjusted hazard ratio (HR) of 1.07 (95% CI 1.02–1.13, per 10-unit increase in TSat90).

The AHI itself was not associated with cancer incidence in the adjusted analyses, except for patients younger than 65 years (adjusted HR for AHI > 43 vs <18.7 was 1.66; 95% CI 1.04–2.64). From an Australian study, estimates for cancer mortality in the moderate-to-severe range (adjusted HR 3.4) were consistent with those estimated from the Wisconsin Cohort, which reported the HR for moderate OSA of 2.0 and severe OSA of 4.8.[234,236] In a multicentre observational study in 82 consecutive patients diagnosed with cutaneous malignant melanoma (CMM), AHI (OR 1.08, 95% CI 1.02–1.14), ODI3% (OR 1.08, 95% CI 1.02–1.11), and ODI4% (OR 1.1, 95% CI 1.02–1.2) were independently associated with an increased melanoma growth rate. Furthermore, AHI, ODI4%, and ODI3% were significantly correlated with other aggressive factors of CMM, such as Breslow index, presence of ulceration, and mitotic index.[237] The effect of sleep apnea on cancer risk might also provide an additional mechanism by which obesity reduction is associated with reduced cancer risk.[238] Concerning the mechanisms likely to be involved in the development of cancer in patients with OSA, it can be hypothesized that various pathways triggered by hypoxia may play a key role. Research has found that elevation of reactive oxygen species during the reoxygenation periods of intermittent hypoxia can modify gene expression through the regulation of the activity of some transcription factors and signaling pathways involved in tumorigenesis.[239,240] Increased oxidative stress has been reported as a risk factor for developing some solid and hematologic cancers.[241,242,243] OSA has been recognized as an oxidative stress disorder,[194,244,245,246] and various parameters of OSA severity including several oximetric parameters have been shown to be correlated with oxidative stress.[244,247] In addition, both chronic and intermittent hypoxia and reactive oxygen species can activate transcription factors, such as hypoxia-inducible factor-1, which are known to promote angiogenesis and enhance tumor progression. Further data are needed to confirm the cancer association.

Economic Consequences

There is enough evidence pointing at a significant increase in medical consumption in OSA, and also in accidents on the road and at work due to excessive daytime sleepiness. Therefore, it is no surprise that economic models have clearly demonstrated the cost-effectiveness of interventions for OSA,[248,249,250] which gives support to screening for OSA.

Medical Consumption

Given the links between OSA and cardiometabolic pathologies, it is inevitable that OSA patients consume a significant amount of health care resources. OSA patients have increased number of hospitalizations, more emergency department visits, more ambulatory contacts, and a higher consumption of drugs.[251] Case-control studies have shown that OSA patients use more physician services and are admitted to hospital at greater rates in the years preceding the diagnosis when compared with healthy subjects.[252,253,254,255,256,257,258] Kryger et al estimated that health care utilization among patients with OSA was twice that of age- and sex-matched controls, and was especially high in pateints with severe OSA.[255] Data from another source demonstrated a dose-response relationship between OSA severity and health care use.[259] It was also shown that excessive daytime sleepiness is a risk factor for increased healthcare utilisation among patients referred for assessment of OSA. In a clinic-based cohort of 2,149 adults, sleepiness was associated with an increased rate of outpatient physician visits, after adjustment for demographic variables, comorbidities, OSA severity, sleep medication use compared to nonsleepy subjects.[260] Moreover, health care use was even higher among patients with severe OSA and sleepiness. This finding was confirmed by the SHHS that found an 11% increase in health care use among sleepy subjects versus those with no sleepiness.[261] Furthermore, Ronksley et al identified that measures of nocturnal hypoxemia derived from PSG or PG to be independent predictors of increased health care use in a large clinic-based cohort. Spending more than 12% of total sleep time at an SaO_2 less than 90% resulted in a 33% increase in the outpatient physician vists, irrespective of OSA severity.[260] Other contributory factors could be recognized as well, such as age and socioeconomic status. Tarasiuk et al figured out that health care use and costs are greater in elderly populations compared with middle-aged populations with OSA because of increased cardiovascular morbidities and need for prescription drugs.[262] Also, socioeconomic status has been shown to be an independent risk factor for cardiovascular disease and adherence to CPAP among OSA patients.[263,264] The reported subsequent cost associated with health care use in OSA patients is in line with this increased consumption, even over a period of 10-years before diagnosis.[257] Health care costs are approximately double than those in patients without OSA.[258,265] A relevant method to document the additional cost of OSA is the comparison of the costs before and after treatment. In a retrospective study, the overall hospitalization duration was evaluated 2 years before and 2 years after the start of CPAP therapy.[266] In a study of 88 patients, it was found that the number of in-hospital days was reduced from 413 in the 2 years before CPAP therapy to 54 in the 2 years following the start of therapy, which is a substantial effect. Reuveni et al reported similar findings in a cohort of young and middle-aged adults in a 5-year period before OSA diagnosis.[256] Moreover, it has also become clear that this cost-effectivity is not only related to the effects in males.[252] In females, a decrease in medical consumption could be achieved after the start of CPAP therapy. A gradual increase in medical consumption in the 2 years before diagnosis and a significant decrease in the 2 years following took place in females.[253] It was also revealed that the differences were only significant in the group of patients who reported being compliant with CPAP therapy.[252] Overall, the medical consumption seems to decrease after the start of an efficient therapy[265] however, it increases gradually in patients with untreated OSA. After appropriate diagnostic assessment and start of therapy, there was a decrease of 1.95 visits per year versus an increase of 0.48 visits in the control group. On the other hand, treatment with CPAP consumes resources, mostly in the first year of treatment, and direct medical costs may increase temporarily due to the cost of the device; however, these costs decline over subsequent years.[252,265,267,268,269,270] Moreover, presence of established comorbidities means that costs do not return to the levels seen in those without OSA, but costs are much lower in treated compared with untreated OSA.

However, a number of factors can be identified that limit evidence. The majority of case-control studies were unable to control for differences in BMI between OSA cases and controls, and so, increased health care use may have been driven by obesity-related differences between groups. Also factors associated with health care use could be a bias: subjects who seek health care more frequently may be more likely to be diagnosed with OSA compared with subjects who have less illness. More compelling evidence was obtained from population-based studies: the SHHS demonstrated in a sample of 6,440 adults an 18% increase in health care use in OSA subjects compared to those with no OSA, after adjusting for multiple clinical factors.[261] However, questions remain, since health care utilization was based on indirect measures, and may not reflect the true magnitude of the relationship between OSA and health care use.

Occupational Performance

The efficient and correct performance of tasks in an occupational setting has a great economic impact, although it is hard to measure this directly. In an earlier study, excessive daytime sleepiness at workplace was evaluated in workers without and with complaints of snoring. Snorers had four times more sleepiness than those who do not snore. Moreover, the ability to concentrate on new tasks and to learn and execute them was significantly worse.[271] Not only absence from work and lost productivity, but also presenteeism is now being considered in the estimation of cost.[272,273,274] When taking these indirect costs into account the societal costs of OSA are equivalent to those of stroke or CHF. In 2010, it was estimated that the annual cost of OSA in the United States was between $67 billion and $165 billion.[275]

Traffic Accidents

OSA also gives rise to motor vehicle accidents (MVAs) secondary to hypersomnolence, which varies between 2 and 7 times the general population risk in different

reports,[276,277] and the driving impairment in OSA patients has been reported as equivalent to driving while drunk.[278] A recent meta-analysis of published reports indicated that the overall increased risk of MVAs is 2.4 times that of the general population,[279] which exceeds the risk of MVA in many other clinical disorders already identified as at-risk.[280,281] Some studies also took into account possible confounding factors, such as the frequency of driving (distance driven per year), obesity, alcohol consumption, or the presence of visual defects. Accident recording also varies between reports with some studies focusing on recorded actual accidents presenting to emergency departments, whereas others used a prospective assessment of an epidemiologic sample. While reports differ in some way, the majority of evidence supports the principle that driving risk in OSA is more closely related to the degree of daytime sleepiness than the objective severity of OSA as measured by AHI.[282,283] The importance of sleepiness as the major contributing factor to MVA risk in OSA is supported by Karimi et al,[284] who demonstrated that excessive sleepiness based on an ESS greater than 15 significantly related to MVA rate, whereas AHI did not. On the other hand, the earlier report of Terán-Santos et al found that AHI was more closely related to accident risk than subjective sleepiness based on ESS in a group of 102 patients presenting to hospital following MVA when compared to a matched control group.[285] Furthermore, the recent report from the ESADA group also found that OSA severity based on AHI was superior to subjective sleepiness in predicting accident risk,[286] a finding also reported in an earlier Canadian study.[287] Other factors that can further increase sleepiness in an individual OSA patient include poor sleep hygiene habits, lack of sleep, time of day (early morning and afternoon), shift work, sedative medications, and alcohol use,[288] and these additional factors may be particularly important in commercial drivers.[289]

Patients with OSA not only have more accidents, but very often have repeated accidents.[290] Therefore, it may present a health hazard for pedestrians. Some years ago, the costs related to car accidents due to OSA in the United States were estimated to exceed $15 billion.[291] Many studies have demonstrated an effect of CPAP therapy on the costs related to accidents due to OSA. A study of 547 patients has shown that the number of effective accidents decreased from 1.6 to 1.1 per patient and the number of near-miss accidents from 4.5 to 1.8 per patient, taking into account the incidence of MVAs before and after the start of CPAP therapy.[292] The number of in-hospital days related to accidents, including occupational and domestic accidents, decreased from 885 to 84 days. In terms of resources, this could reduce the cost of $15 billion to almost $3 billion.[291] Economic models have shown a favorable cost per quality-adjusted life-years (QALY) for CPAP therapy: the cost per QALY related to MVAs amounts for only $3,354.[293,294] These values compare very favorably with other publicly funded therapies and are lower than the cost per QALY for the use of cholesterol-lowering therapy ($54,000–$1,4 million), the use of antihypertensives ($10,000–$57,000), the use of oral hypoglycaemics for diabetes ($34,000), the use of inhalation corticoids in COPD ($19,000), or for coronary reperfusion in ischemic heart disease ($18,000).[259,265,295,296]

Driving License Issues

The growing recognition of increased MVA risk in untreated patients with OSA together with the evidence that effective therapy substantially alleviates that risk has prompted many European countries to implement regulations that limit certain categories of OSA patients from holding a driving license.[297] These regulations vary in the degree of restriction imposed, but usually permit OSA patients complying with effective therapy to continue driving. Recently, a new EU Directive 2014/85/EU was accepted, indicating that patients with moderate to severe OSA (AHI > 15/h) associated with sleepiness should not drive until effectively treated.[298] The directive did not specifically indicate the severity of sleepiness required, but sleepiness while driving represents the most relevant criterion. Similar restrictions are applied to private and professional drivers, although the requirements for follow-up of treatment efficacy are more stringent in professional drivers. This Directive became mandatory for all EU member states on January 1, 2016. However, considerable variability has been identified among clinicians in the interpretation of this Directive, which compromises uniform implementation among patients with OSA.[299] A major concern is that such regulations may deter patients with a high likelihood of OSA from seeking medical attention leading to effective therapy, which could have a negative effect on road safety. Thus, a broad education campaign targeting patients, health care professionals, and the transport industry is required to facilitate sensible implementation of the new Directive and to minimize the possibility of driving OSA patients underground.[300] This possibility is a particular concern in commercial drivers who depend on retention of a driving licence for their income, and also represent the group where failure to diagnose and treat OSA carries the greatest risk to public safety on the highways.

High-Risk Populations

Epidemiological studies and large clinical cohorts provide strong evidence that OSA is highly prevalent in patients with systemic hypertension,[3,4] obesity,[1,301,302] diabetes mellitus,[9,11,303] metabolic syndrome,[12] cardiovascular disease,[5,304,305,306] and endocrinopathies.[9,13] Often, these patients suffer from the typical symptoms of OSA, while others remain asymptomatic. In the presence of other disorders, symptoms in OSA may not conform to the usual history and physical findings. Moreoover, sleepiness is a common symptom in the absence of OSA, and is thereby not a useful clinical symptom to suspect OSA in these patients. On the other hand, patients with medical disorders often express lack of energy, tiredness, or fatigue rather than sleepiness itself, which can be related to the medical disturbance, but can also be pathognomonic for an underlying OSA[14,15,16,17] or any other relevant sleep disorder. Their negative effects are more prevalent, rapid, and intensive if patients suffering from medical disorders suffer from OSA as well. Due to this coexistence of OSA and disorders of other systems, their consequences are mutually enforced, which accelerate disease progression, quality of life, and health care costs.[18]

Obesity

Obesity is strongly linked with OSA. According to various data, the simultaneous occurrence of obesity and OSA is approximately 25 to 50% and their mutual relationship is reciprocal. Deposition of fat, especially in the tongue and the neck area, contributes to upper airway obstruction and to easier development of obstructive apneas. Inconsistency remains as to whether specific anthropometric indices of body habitus, such as neck or waist circumference, are better predictors of OSA as compared to BMI alone.[4,303] However, despite the strong relationship with obesity, it is important to remember that not all subjects who are obese or have a fat neck suffer from relevant sleep apnea and that some one-third of OSA patients are not obese.[303]

Systemic Hypertension

Several large population-based cross-sectional studies have reported an independent link between systemic hypertension and OSA, when controlling for multiple potential confounding variables. OSA and systemic hypertension often coexist: OSA is present in at least 30% of hypertensive patients, while approximately half of OSA patients suffer from systemic hypertension.[166] In patients with drug-resistant hypertension, up to 85% have OSA, and the prevalence of systemic hypertension increases with OSA severity.[156,307,308,309,310,311,312,313] Currently, OSA is also considered a risk factor in the international hypertension guidelines.[4,314,315]

Chronic Heart Failure

Studies have suggested an increased prevalence of OSA as well as CSA in patients with CHF, even in patients with asymptomatic left ventricular dysfunction, between 20 and 50%, and half of these patients have moderate to severe OSA.[5,316] CHF with reduced left ventricular ejection fraction (HFrEF; systolic heart failure) and CHF with preserved ejection fraction (HFpEF; diastolic heart failure) is more vulnerable to stressors such as increased blood pressure (afterload) or sympathetic activation as compared with a healthy heart.[317,318] The severity of ventricular dysfunction increases the risk for central disturbances in both groups. Untreated OSA and central events are indendent risk factors for worse prognosis and deaths in CHF patients.[319,320,321,322] These data imply that strategies to recognize sleep apnea are highly warranted in CHF patients. Predictive factors for the presence of central apneas are male gender, daytime hypocapnia, the presence of atrial fibrillation, or age above 60 years. Predictors for OSA include an increased BMI (BMI > 35 kg/m²) in men and age above 60 years in women.[323] The majority of patients with CHF and comorbid OSA do not complain of excessive daytime sleepiness, possibly owing to chronically elevated sympathetic activity.[324] The 2010 Heart Failure Society of America Comprehensive Heart Failure guidelines[325] and the 2013 American College of Cardiology Foundation (ACCF)/American Heart Association (AHA) guidelines[326] recommend that CHF patients with OSA should receive appropriate treatment for OSA.

Atrial Fibrillation

OSA is highly prevalent in patients with tachyarrhythmias, particularly atrial fibrillation.

Gami et al compared patients with atrial fibrillation (n = 151) with patients having no history of atrial fibrillation in a general cardiology practice (n = 312) and concluded that the proportion of patients with OSA was 49% in the patients with atrial fibrillation versus 32% in the patients without atrial fibrillation (P = 0.0004), with adjusted OR for atrial fibrillation of 2.19 (P = 0006).[305] In a multivariate analysis, BMI, neck circumference, systemic hypertension, diabetes mellitus, and atrial fibrillation remained significantly associated with OSA, and the OR was largest for atrial fibrillation. The prevalence of OSA in patients with atrial fibrillation presenting for electrical cardioversion is approximately 75,[317] and a higher relapse rate of atrial fibrillation after cardioversion has also been reported in those with untreated OSA compared with those without OSA.[324,327] The effectiveness of antiarrhythmic drugs for the treatment of atrial fibrillation is also reduced in patients with severe OSA.[327] In a study of more than 10,000 patients referred to for PSG assessment of OSA, severe OSA was an independent and significant risk factor for sudden cardiac death at night. Moreover, it increased the risk of ventricular premature beats and nonsustained ventricular tachycardia.[175] Coexisting CHF and OSA also increases the risk of developing malignant ventricular arrhythmias.[328] Currenlty, proper treatment of OSA is recommended by the electrophysiological societies of Europe and North America.[329] Therefore, patients referred for evaluation of significant tachyarrhythmia or bradyarrhythmia should be immediately examined for symptoms of OSA.

Coronary Artery Disease

There is a high prevalence of OSA among patients with angiographically proven CAD and an increased incidence of CAD in patients free of coronary symptoms at the time of OSA diagnosis.[8,330,331,332,333,334,335] In a population of patients referred for coronary artery bypass graft surgery, up to 87% demonstrated OSA.[331] The prevalence of OSA in CAD is higher than that of the established risk factors, such as obesity, systemic hypertension, or diabetes mellitus,[336] even after adjustment for other risk factors such as smoking, dyslipidemia, and BMI.

CAD patients with OSA have a worse prognosis than those without OSA. Cardiovascular event rates over 5-years' follow-up were 37.5% in CAD patients with OSA versus 9.3% in those without (P = 0.018), and untreated OSA was a significant independent predictor of (cardiovascular) mortality.[202] In a study conducted by Yumino et al, OSA was identified as a strong independent predictor of major cardiac events (HR 11.62, P = 0.004) in patients with acute coronary syndromes, with a follow-up period of about 7 months.[337]

Therefore, patients with CAD should be particulary examined for symptoms and signs of sleep apnea. Patients should undergo a PSG if there is a suspicion of sleep apnea.[323]

Stroke

It has been shown that the prevalence of OSA in patients with stroke is about 70%, based on data from case-control studies.[159,338] It is also evident that OSA plays a significant role in the overall risk management of stroke patients, with OSA as an independent risk factor for stroke recurrence.[339] This warrants incorporation of PSG or PG as part of stroke assessment.

Endocrine and Metabolic Disorders

OSA is prevalent in many endocrine and metabolic conditions such as insuline resistance, T2DM, and the metabolic syndrome.[9,13,340] Specialists treating metabolic disorders should investigate their pateints for OSA, considering the high prevalence of OSA among these patients.

Hypothyroidism

OSA has been reported to occur often in patients with untreated hypothyroidism (50–100%), especially when myxoedema (dry hair and skin, loss of physical and mental vigor) is present.[341] However, so far, there are no conclusive studies since an association could largely be explained by coexisting obesity and male sex. No large prospective studies looking at the prevalence of OSA in patients with hypothyroidism are available. On the other hand, patients with hypothyroidism, especially when clinical signs are present, should be screened for the presence of OSA. Symptoms of sleep apnea in patients with hypothyroidism do not substantially differ from those with normal thyroid function.[9,340] Pathogenesis appears to involve both upper airway edema and myopathy.[342] Both median and maximal apnea duration, as well as maximum SaO$_2$, are significantly correlated with thyroxin levels and improve with substitution therapy. Hormone therapy also significantly improves AHI and arousal index. Some studies report persisting respiratory events despite adequate replacement therapy, which supports the view of a chance rather than causal association. In these circumstances, such patients continue to require regular nasal CPAP for an unlimited time.

Acromegaly

OSA is common in acromegaly, a condition resulting from excessive growth hormone, with variable prevalence rates, ranging from 12 to 75% in unselected patients.[343] Sleep apnea is more likely to occur with increased severity of acromegaly, greater neck circumference, higher age, greater initial tongue volume, presence of changes in craniofacial dimensions (predominantly of the mandible), and upper airway narrowing due to alterations in pharyngeal soft tissues.[344] Other factors involved are facial bone deformity, mucosal edema, hypertrophy of the pharyngeal and laryngeal cartilages, and rarely, the presence of nasal polyps. Increases in BMI in acromegaly may be due to increased muscle mass rather than increased body fat usually seen in obesity, while BMI is often normal.[345] There appears to be no relationship between OSA and biomarkers of disease activity such as growth hormone and insulin-like growth factor (IGF)-1 levels. OSA may persist despite normalization of growth hormone levels during therapy. Central events are also common and are associated with higher random growth hormone and IGF-1 levels than in OSA. Possible mechanisms for the development of central apneas in these patients include reflex inhibition of the respiratory center as a result of narrowing of the upper airways or due to an increase in the ventilatory response of the respiratory center to hypercapnia. It is yet to be studied that how many patients with both sleep apnea and acromegaly would have complete cure of their sleep apnea after resolution of acromegaly. Nevertheless, it is clear that sleep apnea does occur in cured acromegaly, due to slow resolution of the effects of acromegaly, due to coincidence, or there may be permanent effects on upper airway function or sleep-related regulation.[13,340]

Cushing's Syndrome

Patients with Cushing's syndrome (CS) produce an excess of adrenocorticosteroid hormones. Sleep complaints are frequent, including an increased incidence of OSA of approximately 18 to 32% in patients with CS (in those with pituitary disease).[346] In one study, all CS patients had an AHI above 5. Fat accumulation in the parapharyngeal area could play a role in the pathogenesis of OSA.[347] Patients with CS can also present with steroid-induced changes in sleep architecture including more fragmented sleep, poorer sleep maintenance, shortened REM sleep latency, a decrease in delta sleep, and an increased REM propensity, which may explain the insomnia and fatigue and possibly some of the psychiatric symptoms. These features can be aggravated by coexistent OSA.[13,17,47,348]

Diabetes Mellitus

The prevalence of both T2DM and OSA is about 3 to 5% of the general population and is increasing rapidly worldwide.[349] Therefore, it is not surprising that a significant number of patients suffer from both conditions. Recent reports have indicated that many patients with type 2 diabetes have OSA, but the relationship between OSA and metabolic disturbance is probably bidirectional, and at least partially independent of adiposity.[350,351,352] In type 2 diabetes with OSA, several studies have assessed the impact of CPAP treatment on glycemic control.[353] Recent observational studies using continuous glucose monitoring techniques have reported positive effects of CPAP on glycemic control, immediately present during the first night of treatment, as variability of glycemic values decreased compared with baseline conditions.[354] The reduction in HbA1c level was significantly correlated with CPAP compliance. In diabetic patients with autonomic neuropathy, OSA is also more prevalent (26%) than in those without, and diabetic neuropathy appears to be directly linked to OSA.[355] Altogether, screening for OSA in diabetes may help improve glycemic control, especially in insufficiently controlled type 2 diabetic patients, and is slowly being incorporated by endocrinologists in care paths for diabetes.[356,357]

Metabolic Syndrome

According to clinical and epidemiological studies, the cluster of risk factors known as the metabolic syndrome is associated with increased risk of diabetes, cardiovascular events, and even mortality in the general population.[358] Insuline resistance is considered the major metabolic abnormality and is usually associated with an increased amount of abdominal fat.[359,360] In some studies, a high prevalence of severe OSA (82%) has been reported in metabolic syndrome patients.[12] Prevalence of the metabolic syndrome is also higher in patients with OSA than in obese subjects without OSA or in the European general population (15–20%).[361] This indicates a bidirectional association between metabolic syndrome and OSA. Indeed, abdominal obesity and the cluster of the metabolic risk factors may lead to OSA, which in turn may accelerate these metabolic abnormalities, possibly through the induction of inflammatory pathways and oxidative stress.[12] Coexistence of these two conditions remarkably increases the risk of cardiovascular events and mortality, with higher blood pressure and sympathetic activity, compared to patients with metabolic syndrome without OSA. The need for screening of metabolic syndrome patients for OSA is furthermore emphasized by several studies demonstrating improvements in insulin sensitivity in patients with metabolic syndrome after successful treatment of comorbid OSA by CPAP.[362]

Chronic Obstructive Pulmonary Disease

Overall, patients with COPD sleep poorly compared with healthy subjects.[363] By coexistence they have a high prevalence of OSA. The incidence of disturbed sleep is related to the rates of respiratory symptoms in COPD patients.[363,364] However, compared to patients who only have COPD, those suffering from OSA have higher ESS scores, lower sleep efficiency, lower total sleep time, and higher arousal index.[365] The coexistence of COPD and OSA promotes the presence of daytime hypoxemia and can lead to earlier development of hypercapnia relative to the COPD severity class. Arousals may or may not be related to hypoxemia or hypercapnia.[340,366]

Chronic Kidney Disease

In end-stage renal disease, OSA is 10 times more prevalent than in the normal population and is improved by hemodialysis.[367] The pathophysiology of OSA in this particular population is mainly related to fluid overload, metabolic disturbances including uremia, dialysis treatments (with accompanying changes in serum electrolytes, osmolarity, and acid–base balance), and the production of somnogenic substances such as interleukin (IL)-1 and tumor necrosis factor (TNF)-α during dialysis. Patients with end-stage renal disease are generally not obese and do not often conform to the stereotypical presentation of OSA.[368,369] Patients with end-stage renal disease often have multiple sleep disturbances, which may complicate the clinical picture of OSA, and may result in underestimation of OSA in this population.[9,368]

Polycythemia

Hypoxemic states are often associated with increased hematocrit levels.[370] In OSA, it is thought that this hypoxemic stress might contribute to secondary polycythemia. The evidence is largely based on case reports, and there have been few studies that systematically examined this phenomenon.[371,372] However, after controlling for possible confounding variables, hematocrit is only weakly increased (just 2–3%; within the normal range) in patients with severe OSA, compared with controls. Hence, OSA doesn't seem to lead to clinically significant polycythemia. On the other hand, the search for the source of unexplained polycythemia anecdotally reveals the presence of OSA.

Moreover, the observation that successful treatment of OSA with nasal CPAP decreases hematocrit after 1 night, indicating an intimate relationship between polycythaemia and OSA.[373] An association with OSA will more often be found in the presence of respiratory morbidities, with hypoventilation and chronic nocturnal hypoxemia, for example, as present in obesity hypoventilation.[43]

2.1.10 Conclusions

OSA is a very widespread disorder and is characterized by substantial cardiovascular, metabolic, and neurocognitive morbidity. Untreated patients with OSA are at an increased risk of fatal cardiovascular events and death from any cause. Heavy snoring is the most prominent symptom. Often OSA is associated in chronic medical disorders.

Patients with OSA have increased utilization of health care resources, related to the severity of the disease and the associated comorbidities. These costs increase over time until diagnosis and decrease after administration of an appropriate treatment. Moreover, OSA represents a serious safety issue on the road. Altogether, current insights provide an excellent rationale for diagnosing and treating OSA and for the inclusion of OSA screening and treatment in disease management pathways for the chronic diseases with which OSA is often associated.

Therefore, early recognition is warranted and may reduce end-organ damage and economic burden.

2.2 Causes of Obstructive Sleep Apnea

Dirk Pevernagie and Nico de Vries

2.2.1 Introduction

OSA belongs to a range of respiratory disorders that occur during sleep, and these disorders are commonly referred to as SDB.[374] Other syndromes that fall under this category are CSA and sleep-related alveolar hypoventilation. Sleep is the common factor in the pathophysiology of all these, indicating that the respiratory disturbances are absent or less pronounced during wakefulness.

While several factors may contribute to its pathogenesis, SDB is mainly the result of altered control of breathing during sleep.[375] The sleep state is associated with decreased nervous output and relative hypotonia of the respiratory muscles, involving both the upper airway dilators and the respiratory pump musculature. Sleep is also characterized by a reduced responsiveness of the respiratory center to afferent stimuli from mechanoreceptors and chemoreceptors. Together, these changes induce a decrease in minute ventilation and an increase in upper airway resistance. A drop in respiratory drive is key to the cessation of breathing seen in CSA, whereas alveolar hypoventilation is associated with extended episodes of reduced breathing effort. Snoring, obstructive hypopneas, and apneas are the result of reduced activation of upper airway dilator muscles, for example, genioglossus, geniohyoideus, and tensor veli palatini. As a result, the pharyngeal lumen is narrowed and the resistance to airflow is increased.[376] In OSAs the airflow is completely blocked, whereas in obstructive hypopneas and snoring the airflow is significantly reduced. Arousal from sleep terminates obstructive respiratory events by reactivation of the dilator muscles, by which the patency of the upper airway is restored.[377,378] The remainder of this section deals with causes of obstructive respiratory events during sleep. While CSA and sleep-induced alveolar hypoventilation share features with OSA from a pathophysiological point of view, the discussion of these breathing disturbances is outside the scope of this chapter.

Until recently, OSA was mainly attributed to anatomic issues of the upper airway. It has been hypothesized that anomalies of craniofacial structure in combination with obesity and increased volume of pharyngeal tissue were the principal causes of sleep-related pharyngeal collapse. In this light, it was believed that the patency of the compromised upper airway was maintained during wakefulness by compensatory (hyper)activity of dilator muscles. During sleep, this compensatory mechanism would fall off and passive upper airway occlusion would ensue.[379] Many, but not all, OSA patients have some underlying anatomic predisposition to pharyngeal obstruction. This anatomic factor may be assessed by quantifying the collapsibility of the airway. The collapsibility is measured by lowering the intraluminal pressure until the airway is closed. The pressure at which collapse occurs, called the critical pressure (Pcrit), is a general measure for the anatomic characteristic of the pharynx.[380] In an anatomically compromised upper airway, Pcrit is typically situated above atmospheric pressure. In normal subjects, negative "suction" pressure must be applied in order to occlude the pharynx during sleep. However, nonanatomic factors such as instability of the respiratory control system and increased arousability may play an important role in the pathogenesis of OSA, at least in some individuals. Both anatomic and nonanatomic features seem to be involved in the phenotypic presentation of OSA.[381] These concepts are further discussed in the subsequent sections.

2.2.2 Anatomic Causes of Obstructive Sleep Apnea

Obstructive SDB may be caused or aggravated by any structure or mechanism that affects the patency of the oronasal airway. Examples are manifold such as polyposis nasi, tumors, mucosal congestion, secretions, hypertrophy of adenoids and tonsils, and bony malformations. Craniofacial abnormalities and increased upper airway tissue volume are commonly implicated in the pathophysiology of OSA.

Craniofacial Abnormalities

Bony structures of the cranium and jaws encase inner soft tissues surrounding the upper airway. The spatial relationship between the skeletal elements and the walls of the upper airway should be such that airflow is preserved during the entire breathing cycle in both wake and sleep states. In some patients, the morphological aspects of the skeletal frame and the enclosed tissues are disproportional.[382] The bony compartment may be relatively too small and/or the tissue compartment may be relatively too large. As a result, the size of the airway is reduced and airflow is obstructed when the force of the dilator muscles drops during sleep. Frequent findings with respect to skeletal anomalies are described in this section.

Lateral cephalometry is a standard diagnostic procedure to assess the skeleton of the head and neck. This technique has been used on a large scale for morphometric analysis of the upper airway and its bony enclosure in OSA patients. In a recent systematic review, it was pointed out that reduced lower facial height, caudal position of the hyoid bone, and reduced pharyngeal airway space are features commonly associated with OSA. Moreover, subjects with a small and retruded mandible are at higher risk of OSA, especially in the presence of other skeletal anomalies such as maxillary deficiency. Often, these anatomic peculiarities result in a reduced posterior airway space.[383]

Increased Upper Airway Tissue Volume

Various abnormalities of the soft tissues in the naso- and oropharynx are associated with increased collapsibility of the upper airway. These abnormalities include crowding, accumulation of fat, infiltration, congestion or edema of the walls, as well as hypertrophy of structures protruding into the lumen of the airway (e.g., tonsils and adenoids). MRI technology has been useful to study the characteristics of pharyngeal soft tissues in OSA patients. Three features have been found to be consistently present in these individuals: (1) increased tongue volume, (2) increased thickness of lateral pharyngeal walls, (3) and increased total soft tissue volume.[384]

All these conditions predispose to elevated intrinsic tissue pressure and to increased Pcrit.

The presence of enlarged tonsils is associated with an increased risk of OSA. This association persists after correction for body weight and neck circumference.[385] Tonsillar hypertrophy is of special interest in children and nonobese adults. Following tonsillectomy, short-term resolution of OSA has been observed.[386]

Macroglossia is also known to be implicated in the pathogenesis of OSA. When macroglossia is found on clinical examination, the patient should be scrutinized for underlying diseases such as amyloidosis, acromegaly, hypothyroidism, Down's syndrome, etc.[387,388,389] If treatment with CPAP should be contraindicated or should fail, surgical lingual plasty may be considered.[390]

In routine physical examinations, the Mallampati and Friedman scores are used to assess the size of the tongue in reference with the lower edge of the soft palate. Independent associations between these scores and presence and severity of OSA has been reported.[391,392] For the purpose of clinical tonsil size grading, different standards can be used, for example the Friedman and Brodsky scales.[393] Clinical inspection of the mouth and throat is an essential part of the physical examination in each subject suspected of OSA, considering the relevance of anatomic abnormalities.

Obesity is a major cause of OSA. Epidemiological studies have pointed out that OSA may be attributable to obesity in approximately 60% of subjects.[394] Even moderate changes in BMI seem to affect the severity of OSA: weight gain is associated with an increase in the AHI, whereas weight loss predicts a decrease in the AHI.[301] Central adiposity affects the respiratory function of the upper airway in several ways. Increased amounts of adipose tissue have been demonstrated in the collapsible segment of the upper airway, that is, lateral pharyngeal walls[384] and tongue base.[395] Increased volumes of pharyngeal fat may add to narrowing of the lumen. More importantly, however, central adiposity may increase the collapsibility of the upper airway via an indirect mechanism, which is decreased traction on the upper airway by the trachea. Release of tracheal tug reduces the stiffness of the upper airway. This mechanism was first shown in an animal model,[396,397] and subsequently confirmed in human studies.[398] It was found that Pcrit varies inversely with absolute end-expiratory lung volume.[399] In OSA patients, an increase in lung volume induced by applying negative extrathoracic pressure caused a substantial decrease in SDB during non-REM sleep.[400] Excessive abdominal adipose tissue reduces lung volume, especially when obese subjects sleep in the recumbent body position. This condition is associated with less caudal traction on the upper airway, which increases its collapsibility and elevates Pcrit.

Recently, the role of overnight fluid shift from the lower part of the body into the head and neck region has been emphasized.[401] Accumulation of interstitial fluid might enlarge the pharyngeal tissue volume and thus reduce the airway lumen. The prevalence of SDB is increased in patients with fluid retaining states, for example hypertension, heart failure, and renal failure. In these conditions, gravity induces fluid accumulation in the intravascular and interstitial spaces of the lower part of the body during the day. In the recumbent position at night, fluid is redistributed rostrally, again owing to gravity. This pathophysiological concept might open new perspectives for the treatment of OSA, such as prescription of diuretics, postural therapy, and application of compression stockings.[402]

2.2.3 Nonanatomic Causes of Obstructive Sleep Apnea

While collapsibility of the upper airway and Pcrit (its physiological measure) largely determine the anatomic features of OSA, ventilatory control mechanisms also play an important role in the pathogenesis of upper airway obstruction during sleep. The existence of nonanatomic factors can be inferred from the fact that AHI and Pcrit poorly correlate with each other,[403] and from the large overlap observed in OSA patients and normal controls regarding Pcrit values.[404] The nonanatomic factors consist of at least three phenomena: loop gain, arousal threshold, and responsiveness of upper airway dilator muscles. Together, these factors constitute the pathophysiological concept of ventilatory instability. Similarly as with Pcrit, nonanatomic causative factors can be derived from manipulating nasal pressure in OSA patients treated with CPAP.[381]

Loop Gain

Loop gain is an engineering term used to define the gain of the negative feedback loop that controls how ventilation responds to transient breathing disturbances. The loop gain is defined as the ratio of a ventilatory response to a ventilatory disturbance, induced by a sudden drop in nasal pressure. High loop gain is linked to an oversensitive ventilator control system and a large loop gain ratio indicates an unstable system prone to oscillations. High loop gain in combination with a modestly collapsible upper airway (i.e., Pcrit < −2 cm H_2O) is sufficient to cause clinically relevant OSA.

Arousal Threshold

In response to upper airway obstruction, respiratory drive increases and with each consecutive breath the intrathoracic pressure becomes progressively more negative. At a certain pressure level, a respiratory-induced arousal occurs and breathing resumes.[378,405] The arousal threshold can be quantified using an esophageal pressure probe and can be unveiled by applying a sudden drop in nasal pressure.[381] A low arousal threshold may be important in OSA pathogenesis for at least two reasons. Frequent arousals may prevent the occurrence of slow-wave sleep (which is characterized by more stable breathing) and may be associated with temporary hyperpnea, which tends to lower the $PaCO_2$ and to perpetuate the ventilatory instability.

Responsiveness of the Upper Airway Dilator Muscles

During upper airway obstruction in sleep, the genioglossus muscle and other dilator muscles are progressively activated with each consecutive breath. In some OSA patients, activation of these muscles is insufficient to maintain or restore the patency of the upper airway. This may be either due to poor neural drive or inadequate neuromechanical coupling. Adequate activation and movement of upper airway dilators is characterized by sufficient (re)opening of the pharynx in a way that arousal from sleep is averted.

Interaction Between Anatomic and Nonanatomic Traits

It is hypothesized that both anatomic and nonanatomic factors causal to OSA may interact independently. The result of these interactions, or emergent property, constitutes the pathophysiological phenotype of OSA.[381,406] Eckert et al used an innovative approach to assess these different factors and to render the phenotype into a composite PALM score (P, Pcrit; A, arousal; L, loop gain; M, muscle responsiveness).[381] The starting point in this study was the Pcrit. Based on this anatomic measure, the upper airway of OSA patients and controls was classified as: (1) highly collapsible (Pcrit > 2 cm H_2O), (2) moderately collapsible (Pcrit ≥ −2 and ≤ 2 cm H_2O), and (3) slightly collapsible or "vulnerable" (Pcrit < −2 cm H_2O). In the first subgroup, the anatomic factor is predominant and other factors have no or only a subordinate role. The second subgroup is divided into patients who have and who don't have associated nonanatomic traits. In the third subgroup, all of the subjects have at least one nonanatomic trait. Targeted therapies such as dampening of loop gain, inhibition of arousal, etc., may be devised for the patients in whom ventilatory instability is paramount.

A predominant anatomic trait should be treated with a mechanical intervention, that is, classical CPAP therapy, treatment with oral appliances, or surgical procedures. However, in subjects with predominant loop gain abnormality, anatomic interventions are likely to fail. Recently, Joosten et al showed that upper airway surgery most effectively resolves OSA in patients with lower loop gain.[407] Predicting the failure of surgical treatment, consequent to unstable ventilatory control, can be achieved with pathophysiological evaluation of the upper airway and may prove to become important in future preoperative assessment of OSA patients.

It must be noted that a big overlap exists between the subgroups described earlier. Therefore, treatment of OSA will remain empirical in nature, implying that trial-and-error will always be part of the medical management. Assessment of physiological phenotypes, however, may be efficient in selecting up-front the (set of) therapeutic intervention(s) that most likely will sort beneficial effects.

Joosten et al have conducted couple of studies exploring the physiological factor(s) that contribute to OSA in the context of therapeutic decision making.[408,409]

Position-Dependent OSA

The PALM model ignores the importance of body position in the etiology of SDB. This aspect has been neglected and overlooked for too long. Positional obstructive sleep apnea (POSA) is common and can be treated effectively with new forms of positional therapy.[410,411,412,413,414,415]

Over the years it has become clear that the role of gravity and body position are important factors to consider, especially in early stage of disease. Authors who have considered this factor have found that more than 50% of patients with mild OSA are sufferers of POSA; their AHI is at least twice as high in supine position as compared with the other sleep positions.[416,417,418] More often than not, POSA and mild OSA are synonymous. This percentage of positional patients is lower in moderate OSA and very low in severe OSA. In other words, the transition from mild to severe OSA is usually from mild POSA into severe nonpositional OSA. It has been observed that, in early stage of OSA, the AHI is high only in supine position; however, in the later stage the AHI is high in all positions. This phenomenon has been found to be reversible: after partial effective upper airway surgery,[419] after treatment with mandibular advancement device (MAD),[420] after bariatric surgery and weight loss,[421] and even after bimaxillary osteotomies in advanced disease. In all these populations, patients have been shown to reverse from serious nonpositional OSA to less severe POSA.

For sleep surgeons this is very important. Sleep surgeons should have thorough knowledge about positionality. Unexplained remarkable outcomes after sleep surgery, for example, better or worse outcome than expected, can often be explained by reconsidering differences in the percentage sleeping in supine position. It has also been found that after palatal surgery the effect on the AHI in lateral sleeping position is often more than in the supine position, therefore the positional effect after surgery is bigger. This opens channels for adjunctive positional therapy after partial effective upper airway surgery.

Published and ongoing studies show that new generation positional therapy is effective, patient-friendly, has no side effects, does not change sleep quality or may even improve it, is reversible, with good compliance, and with acceptable costs. Positional therapy can be a stand alone therapy or can be combined with other treatments such as oral device therapy or surgery. It can be used for patients with habitual snoring as well as in patients with OSA.

▶ Fig. 2.5 depicts a very archetypal patient with mild OSA, who sleeps 50% of the total sleeping time on his back. In this sleeping position, the AHI is 30, while the average AHI in non supine position is less than 10. This 50% of the total sleeping time in supine position is not unusual. Positional therapy is nothing more than elimination of the supine position. If this patient's OSA remains untreated then, since OSA is a progressive disease, it would develop from moderate to severe. The patient would then no longer be positional and the AHI would remain high in all sleeping positions.

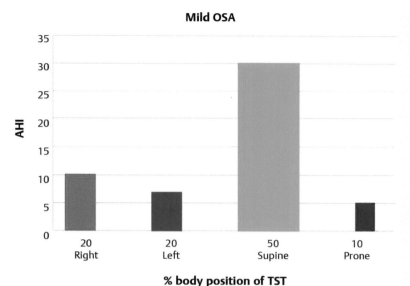

Fig. 2.5 Graph depicting a typical patient with mild obstructive sleep apnea (OSA).

References

[1] Young T, Peppard PE, Taheri S. Excess weight and sleep-disordered breathing. J Appl Physiol (1985). 2005; 99(4):1592–1599

[2] Ling IT, James AL, Hillman DR. Interrelationships between body mass, oxygen desaturation, and apnea-hypopnea indices in a sleep clinic population. Sleep. 2012; 35(1):89–96

[3] Cano-Pumarega I, Barbé F, Esteban A, Martínez-Alonso M, Egea C, Durán-Cantolla J; Spanish Sleep Network(*). Sleep apnea and hypertension: are there sex differences? The Vitoria Sleep Cohort. Chest. 2017; 152(4):742–750

[4] Chobanian AV, Bakris GL, Black HR, et al. Joint National Committee on Prevention, Detection, Evaluation, and Treatment of High Blood Pressure. National Heart, Lung, and Blood Institute. National High Blood Pressure Education Program Coordinating Committee. Seventh report of the Joint National Committee on Prevention, Detection, Evaluation, and Treatment of High Blood Pressure. Hypertension. 2003; 42(6):1206–1252

[5] Sin DD, Fitzgerald F, Parker JD, Newton G, Floras JS, Bradley TD. Risk factors for central and obstructive sleep apnea in 450 men and women with congestive heart failure. Am J Respir Crit Care Med. 1999; 160(4):1101–1106

[6] Shpilsky D, Erqou S, Patel SR, et al. Association of obstructive sleep apnea with microvascular endothelial dysfunction and subclinical coronary artery disease in a community-based population. Vasc Med. 2018:X18755003

[7] Kohno T, Kimura T, Fukunaga K, et al. Prevalence and clinical characteristics of obstructive- and central-dominant sleep apnea in candidates of catheter ablation for atrial fibrillation in Japan. Int J Cardiol. 2018; 260:99–102

[8] Alonderis A, Varoneckas G, Raskauskiene N, Brozaitiene J. Prevalence and predictors of sleep apnea in patients with stable coronary artery disease: a cross-sectional study. Ther Clin Risk Manag. 2017; 13:1031–1042

[9] Tkacova R, Dorkova Z. Clinical presentations of OSA in adults. Eur Respir Mon. 2010; 50:86–103

[10] Lindberg E. Epidemiology of OSA. Eur Respir Mon. 2010; 50:51–68

[11] Lévy P, Bonsignore MR, Eckel J. Sleep, sleep-disordered breathing and metabolic consequences. Eur Respir J. 2009; 34(1):243–260

[12] Angelico F, del Ben M, Augelletti T, et al. Obstructive sleep apnoea syndrome and the metabolic syndrome in an internal medicine setting. Eur J Intern Med. 2010; 21(3):191–195

[13] Grunstein R. Endocrine disorders. In: Kryger MH, Roth T, Dement W, eds. Principles and Practice of Sleep Medicine. Philadelphia, PA: Elsevier Saunders; 2005;105:1237–1245

[14] Fritschi C, Quinn L. Fatigue in patients with diabetes: a review. J Psychosom Res. 2010; 69(1):33–41

[15] Chotinaiwattarakul W, O'Brien LM, Fan L, Chervin RD. Fatigue, tiredness, and lack of energy improve with treatment for OSA. J Clin Sleep Med. 2009; 5(3):222–227

[16] Lewis G, Wessely S. The epidemiology of fatigue: more questions than answers. J Epidemiol Community Health. 1992; 46(2):92–97

[17] ASDA. Report of a Task Force of the American Academy of Sleep Medicine. Sleep-related breathing disorders in adults: recommendations for syndrome definition and measurement techniques in clinical research. Sleep. 1999; 22:667–689

[18] Trombetta IC, Somers VK, Maki-Nunes C, et al. Consequences of comorbid sleep apnea in the metabolic syndrome–implications for cardiovascular risk. Sleep. 2010; 33(9):1193–1199

[19] Young T, Palta M, Dempsey J, Skatrud J, Weber S, Badr S. The occurrence of sleep-disordered breathing among middle-aged adults. N Engl J Med. 1993; 328(17):1230–1235

[20] Bixler EO, Vgontzas AN, Lin HM, et al. Prevalence of sleep-disordered breathing in women: effects of gender. Am J Respir Crit Care Med. 2001; 163(3 Pt 1):608–613

[21] Durán J, Esnaola S, Rubio R, Iztueta A. Obstructive sleep apnea-hypopnea and related clinical features in a population-based sample of subjects aged 30 to 70 yr. Am J Respir Crit Care Med. 2001; 163(3 Pt 1):685–689

[22] Young T, Shahar E, Nieto FJ, et al. Sleep Heart Health Study Research Group. Predictors of sleep-disordered breathing in community-dwelling adults: the Sleep Heart Health Study. Arch Intern Med. 2002; 162(8):893–900

[23] Hrubos-Strøm H, Randby A, Namtvedt SK, et al. A Norwegian population-based study on the risk and prevalence of obstructive sleep apnea. The Akershus Sleep Apnea Project (ASAP). J Sleep Res. 2011; 20(1 Pt 2):162–170

[24] Franklin KA, Sahlin C, Stenlund H, Lindberg E. Sleep apnoea is a common occurrence in females. Eur Respir J. 2013; 41(3):610–615

[25] Ip MS, Lam B, Lauder IJ, et al. A community study of sleep-disordered breathing in middle-aged Chinese men in Hong Kong. Chest. 2001; 119(1):62–69

[26] Ip MS, Lam B, Tang LC, Lauder IJ, Ip TY, Lam WK. A community study of sleep-disordered breathing in middle-aged Chinese

women in Hong Kong: prevalence and gender differences. Chest. 2004; 125(1):127–134

[27] Kim J, In K, Kim J, et al. Prevalence of sleep-disordered breathing in middle-aged Korean men and women. Am J Respir Crit Care Med. 2004; 170(10):1108–1113

[28] Reddy EV, Kadhiravan T, Mishra HK, et al. Prevalence and risk factors of obstructive sleep apnea among middle-aged urban Indians: a community-based study. Sleep Med. 2009; 10(8):913–918

[29] Heinzer R, Vat S, Marques-Vidal P, et al. Prevalence of sleep-disordered breathing in the general population: the HypnoLaus study. Lancet Respir Med. 2015; 3(4):310–318

[30] The International Classification of Sleep Disorders. Diagnostic and Coding Manual. 3rd ed. Chicago, IL: American Academy of Sleep Medicine; 2005

[31] Verbraecken JA, De Backer WA. Upper airway mechanics. Respiration. 2009; 78(2):121–133

[32] Berry RB, Budhiraja R, Gottlieb DJ, et al. American Academy of Sleep Medicine. Deliberations of the Sleep Apnea Definitions Task Force of the American Academy of Sleep Medicine. Rules for scoring respiratory events in sleep: update of the 2007 AASM Manual for the Scoring of Sleep and Associated Events. J Clin Sleep Med. 2012; 8(5):597–619

[33] Epstein LJ, Kristo D, Strollo PJ Jr, et al. Adult Obstructive Sleep Apnea Task Force of the American Academy of Sleep Medicine. Clinical guideline for the evaluation, management and long-term care of obstructive sleep apnea in adults. J Clin Sleep Med. 2009; 5(3):263–276

[34] Iranzo A. Excessive daytime sleepiness in OSA. Eur Respir Mon. 2010; 50:17–30

[35] Silber MH, Krahn LE, Morgenthaler TI. Approach to the sleepy patient. In: Silber MH, Krahn LE, Morgenthaler TI, eds. Sleep Medicine in Clinical Practice. London/New York: Taylore & Francis; 2000;65–77

[36] Silber MH. The investigation of sleepiness. Sleep Med Clin. 2006; 1:1–8

[37] Ramar K, Guilleminault C. Excessive daytime sleepiness and obstructive sleep apnea syndrome. Sleep Med Clin. 2006; 1:63–78

[38] Ayappa I, Norman RG, Krieger AC, Rosen A, O'malley RL, Rapoport DM. Non-Invasive detection of respiratory effort-related arousals (RERas) by a nasal cannula/pressure transducer system. Sleep. 2000; 23(6):763–771

[39] Iber C, Ancoli-Israel S, Chesson AL, Jr. Quan SF. The AASM Manual for the Scoring of Sleep and Associated Events: Rules, Terminology and Technical Specifications. Westchester, IL: American Academy of Sleep Medicine; 2007

[40] Gold AR, Dipalo F, Gold MS, O'Hearn D. The symptoms and signs of upper airway resistance syndrome: a link to the functional somatic syndromes. Chest. 2003; 123(1):87–95

[41] Bao G, Guilleminault C. Upper airway resistance syndrome–one decade later. Curr Opin Pulm Med. 2004; 10(6):461–467

[42] Verbraecken J, McNicholas WT. Respiratory mechanics and ventilatory control in overlap syndrome and obesity hypoventilation. Respir Res. 2013; 14:132

[43] Piper AJ. Nocturnal hypoventilation - identifying and treating syndromes. Indian J Med Res. 2010; 131:350–365

[44] Mokhlesi B. Obesity hypoventilation syndrome: a state-of-the-art review. Respir Care. 2010; 55(10):1347–1362, discussion 1363–1365

[45] Berger KI, Goldring RM, Rapoport DM. Obesity hypoventilation syndrome. Semin Respir Crit Care Med. 2009; 30(3):253–261

[46] Berger KI, Ayappa I, Chatr-Amontri B, et al. Obesity hypoventilation syndrome as a spectrum of respiratory disturbances during sleep. Chest. 2001; 120(4):1231–1238

[47] Shepertycky MR, Banno K, Kryger MH. Differences between men and women in the clinical presentation of patients diagnosed with obstructive sleep apnea syndrome. Sleep. 2005; 28(3):309–314

[48] Peter JH, Koehler U, Grote L, Podszus T. Manifestations and consequences of obstructive sleep apnoea. Eur Respir J. 1995; 8(9):1572–1583

[49] Hoffstein V. Snoring. Chest. 1996; 109:201–222

[50] Hong SN, Yoo J, Song IS, et al. Does snoring time always reflect the severity of obstructive sleep apnea? Ann Otol Rhinol Laryngol. 2017; 126(10):693–696

[51] Guilleminault C, Stoohs R, Clerk A, Cetel M, Maistros P. A cause of excessive daytime sleepiness. The upper airway resistance syndrome. Chest. 1993; 104(3):781–787

[52] Lugaresi E, Cirignotta F, Coccagna G, Piana C. Some epidemiological data on snoring and cardiocirculatory disturbances. Sleep. 1980; 3(3–4):221–224

[53] Lindberg E, Taube A, Janson C, Gislason T, Svärdsudd K, Boman G. A 10-year follow-up of snoring in men. Chest. 1998; 114(4):1048–1055

[54] Ohayon MM, Guilleminault C, Priest RG, Caulet M. Snoring and breathing pauses during sleep: telephone interview survey of a United Kingdom population sample. BMJ. 1997; 314(7084):860–863

[55] Larsson LG, Lindberg A, Franklin KA, Lundbäck B. Gender differences in symptoms related to sleep apnea in a general population and in relation to referral to sleep clinic. Chest. 2003; 124(1):204–211

[56] Olson LG, King MT, Hensley MJ, Saunders NA. A community study of snoring and sleep-disordered breathing. Symptoms. Am J Respir Crit Care Med. 1995; 152(2):707–710

[57] Boudewyns A, Willemen M, De Cock W, et al. Does socially disturbing snoring and/or excessive daytime sleepiness warrant polysomnography? Clin Otolaryngol Allied Sci. 1997; 22(5):403–407

[58] Hoffstein V, Mateika S, Anderson D. Snoring: is it in the ear of the beholder? Sleep. 1994; 17(6):522–526

[59] McArdle N, Kingshott R, Engleman HM, Mackay TW, Douglas NJ. Partners of patients with sleep apnea/hypopnoea syndrome: effect of CPAP treatment on sleep quality and quality of life. Thorax. 2001; 56(7):513–518

[60] Roland MM, Baran AS, Richert AC. Sleep-related laryngospasm caused by gastroesophageal reflux. Sleep Med. 2008; 9(4):451–453

[61] Ohayon MM. Epidemiology of excessive daytime sleepiness. Sleep Med Clin. 2006; 1:9–16

[62] Hirshkowitz M, Gast H. Sleep-related breathing disorders and sleepiness. Sleep Med Clin. 2006; 1:491–498

[63] Littner MR, Kushida C, Wise M, et al. Standards of Practice Committee of the American Academy of Sleep Medicine. Practice parameters for clinical use of the multiple sleep latency test and the maintenance of wakefulness test. Sleep. 2005; 28(1):113–121

[64] Akerstedt T, Bassetti C, Cirignotta F. Sleepiness at the wheel [white paper] = La somnolence au volant [livre blanc]. Institut National du Sommeil et de la Vigilance (INSV); 2013 Available at: http://library.brrc.be/opac_css/index.php?lvl=notice_display&id=45078. Accessed September 11, 2013.

[65] Krieger J, McNicholas WT, Levy P, et al. ERS Task Force. European Respiratory Society. Public health and medicolegal implications of sleep apnoea. Eur Respir J. 2002; 20(6):1594–1609

[66] Engleman HM, Hirst WS, Douglas NJ. Under reporting of sleepiness and driving impairment in patients with sleep apnoea/hypopnoea syndrome. J Sleep Res. 1997; 6(4):272–275

[67] Monk TH. A Visual Analogue Scale technique to measure global vigor and affect. Psychiatry Res. 1989; 27(1):89–99

[68] Akerstedt T, Gillberg M. Subjective and objective sleepiness in the active individual. Int J Neurosci. 1990; 52(1–2):29–37

[69] Hoddes E, Zarcone V, Smythe H, Phillips R, Dement WC. Quantification of sleepiness: a new approach. Psychophysiology. 1973; 10(4):431–436

[70] Johns MW. A new method for measuring daytime sleepiness: the Epworth Sleepiness Scale. Sleep. 1991; 14(6):540–545

[71] Murray BJ. Subjective and objective assessment of hypersomnolence. Sleep Med Clin. 2017; 12(3):313–322

[72] Sullivan SS, Kushida CA. Multiple sleep latency test and maintenance of wakefulness test. Chest. 2008; 134(4):854–861

[73] Arand D, Bonnet M, Hurwitz T, Mitler M, Rosa R, Sangal RB. The clinical use of the MSLT and MWT. Sleep. 2005; 28(1):123–144

[74] Hein H. Objectifying sleepiness. In: Randerath W, Sanner BM, Somers VK, eds. Sleep Apnea: Current Diagnosis and Treatment. Basel: Karger; Prog Respir Res, 2006;35:43–46

[75] Martin SE, Engleman HM, Kingshott RN, Douglas NJ. Microarousals in patients with sleep apnoea/hypopnoea syndrome. J Sleep Res. 1997; 6(4):276–280

[76] Hosselet J, Ayappa I, Norman RG, Krieger AC, Rapoport DM. Classification of sleep-disordered breathing. Am J Respir Crit Care Med. 2001; 163(2):398–405

[77] Gottlieb DJ, Whitney CW, Bonekat WH, et al. Relation of sleepiness to respiratory disturbance index: the Sleep Heart Health Study. Am J Respir Crit Care Med. 1999; 159(2):502–507

[78] Koutsourelakis I, Perraki E, Economou NT, et al. Predictors of residual sleepiness in adequately treated obstructive sleep apnoea patients. Eur Respir J. 2009; 34(3):687–693

[79] Dongol EM, Williams AJ. Residual excessive sleepiness in patients with obstructive sleep apnea on treatment with continuous positive airway pressure. Curr Opin Pulm Med. 2016; 22(6):589–594

[80] Chapman JL, Serinel Y, Marshall NS, Grunstein RR. Residual daytime sleepiness in obstructive sleep apnea after continuous positive airway pressure optimization: causes and management. Sleep Med Clin. 2016; 11(3):353–363

[81] Bixler EO, Vgontzas AN, Lin HM, Calhoun SL, Vela-Bueno A, Kales A. Excessive daytime sleepiness in a general population sample: the role of sleep apnea, age, obesity, diabetes, and depression. J Clin Endocrinol Metab. 2005; 90(8):4510–4515

[82] Resnick HE, Carter EA, Aloia M, Phillips B. Cross-sectional relationship of reported fatigue to obesity, diet, and physical activity: results from the third national health and nutrition examination survey. J Clin Sleep Med. 2006; 2(2):163–169

[83] Basta M, Lin HM, Pejovic S, Sarrigiannidis A, Bixler E, Vgontzas AN. Lack of regular exercise, depression, and degree of apnea are predictors of excessive daytime sleepiness in patients with sleep apnea: sex differences. J Clin Sleep Med. 2008; 4(1):19–25

[84] Koutsourelakis I, Perraki E, Bonakis A, Vagiakis E, Roussos C, Zakynthinos S. Determinants of subjective sleepiness in suspected obstructive sleep apnoea. J Sleep Res. 2008; 17(4):437–443

[85] Stradling JR, Smith D, Crosby J. Post-CPAP sleepiness–a specific syndrome? J Sleep Res. 2007; 16(4):436–438

[86] Pépin JL, Viot-Blanc V, Escourrou P, et al. Prevalence of residual excessive sleepiness in CPAP-treated sleep apnoea patients: the French multicentre study. Eur Respir J. 2009; 33(5):1062–1067

[87] Verbruggen AE, Dieltjens M, Wouters K, et al. Prevalence of residual excessive sleepiness during effective oral appliance therapy for sleep-disordered breathing. Sleep Med. 2014; 15(2):269–272

[88] Shen J, Barbera J, Shapiro CM. Distinguishing sleepiness and fatigue: focus on definition and measurement. Sleep Med Rev. 2006; 10(1):63–76

[89] Mills PJ, Kim JH, Bardwell W, Hong S, Dimsdale JE. Predictors of fatigue in obstructive sleep apnea. Sleep Breath. 2008; 12(4):397–399

[90] Chervin RD. Sleepiness, fatigue, tiredness, and lack of energy in obstructive sleep apnea. Chest. 2000; 118(2):372–379

[91] Jackson ML, Stough C, Howard ME, Spong J, Downey LA, Thompson B. The contribution of fatigue and sleepiness to depression in patients attending the sleep laboratory for evaluation of obstructive sleep apnea. Sleep Breath. 2011; 15(3):439–445

[92] Bardwell WA, Ancoli-Israel S, Dimsdale JE. Comparison of the effects of depressive symptoms and apnea severity on fatigue

in patients with obstructive sleep apnea: a replication study. J Affect Disord. 2007; 97(1–3):181–186

[93] Stepnowsky CJ, Palau JJ, Zamora T, Ancoli-Israel S, Loredo JS. Fatigue in sleep apnea: the role of depressive symptoms and self-reported sleep quality. Sleep Med. 2011; 12(9):832–837

[94] Hossain JL, Ahmad P, Reinish LW, Kayumov L, Hossain NK, Shapiro CM. Subjective fatigue and subjective sleepiness: two independent consequences of sleep disorders? J Sleep Res. 2005; 14(3):245–253

[95] Sauter C, Asenbaum S, Popovic R, et al. Excessive daytime sleepiness in patients suffering from different levels of obstructive sleep apnoea syndrome. J Sleep Res. 2000; 9(3):293–301

[96] Bardwell WA, Moore P, Ancoli-Israel S, Dimsdale JE. Fatigue in obstructive sleep apnea: driven by depressive symptoms instead of apnea severity? Am J Psychiatry. 2003; 160(2):350–355

[97] McHorney CA, Ware JE Jr, Raczek AE. The MOS 36-Item Short-Form Health Survey (SF-36): II. Psychometric and clinical tests of validity in measuring physical and mental health constructs. Med Care. 1993; 31(3):247–263

[98] De Vries J, Pedersen S. The impact of sleep apnoea on fatigue: assessment issues for clinical practice. Int J Sleep Wakefulness. 2007; 1(2):66–69

[99] Jankowski JT, Seftel AD, Strohl KP. Erectile dysfunction and sleep related disorders. J Urol. 2008; 179(3):837–841

[100] Luyster FS, Buysse DJ, Strollo PJ Jr. Comorbid insomnia and obstructive sleep apnea: challenges for clinical practice and research. J Clin Sleep Med. 2010; 6(2):196–204

[101] Walters AS. Clinical identification of the simple sleep-related movement disorders. Chest. 2007; 131(4):1260–1266

[102] van Kerrebroeck P, Abrams P, Chaikin D, et al. Standardisation Sub-committee of the International Continence Society. The standardisation of terminology in nocturia: report from the Standardisation Sub-committee of the International Continence Society. Neurourol Urodyn. 2002; 21(2):179–183

[103] Rohrmann S, Nelson WG, Rifai N, et al. Serum sex steroid hormones and lower urinary tract symptoms in Third National Health and Nutrition Examination Survey (NHANES III). Urology. 2007; 69(4):708–713

[104] Krieger J, Petiau C, Sforza E, Delanoë C, Hecht MT, Chamouard V. Nocturnal pollakiuria is a symptom of obstructive sleep apnea. Urol Int. 1993; 50(2):93–97

[105] Guilleminault C, Lin CM, Gonçalves MA, Ramos E. A prospective study of nocturia and the quality of life of elderly patients with obstructive sleep apnea or sleep onset insomnia. J Psychosom Res. 2004; 56(5):511–515

[106] Umlauf MG, Chasens ER, Greevy RA, Arnold J, Burgio KL, Pillion DJ. Obstructive sleep apnea, nocturia and polyuria in older adults. Sleep. 2004; 27(1):139–144

[107] Fitzgerald MP, Mulligan M, Parthasarathy S. Nocturic frequency is related to severity of obstructive sleep apnea, improves with continuous positive airways treatment. Am J Obstet Gynecol. 2006; 194(5):1399–1403

[108] Oztura I, Kaynak D, Kaynak HC. Nocturia in sleep-disordered breathing. Sleep Med. 2006; 7(4):362–367

[109] Arai H, Furuta H, Kosaka K, et al. Polysomnographic and urodynamic changes in a case of obstructive sleep apnea syndrome with enuresis. Psychiatry Clin Neurosci. 1999; 53(2):319–320

[110] Bonsignore MR, McNicholas WT. Sleep-disordered breathing in the elderly. Eur Respir Mon. 2009; 43:179–204

[111] Quintana-Gallego E, Carmona-Bernal C, Capote F, et al. Gender differences in obstructive sleep apnea syndrome: a clinical study of 1166 patients. Respir Med. 2004; 98(10):984–989

[112] Browne HA, Adams L, Simonds AK, Morrell MJ. Sleep apnoea and daytime function in the elderly–what is the impact of arousal frequency? Respir Med. 2003; 97(10):1102–1108

[113] Mathur R, Douglas NJ. Frequency of EEG arousals from nocturnal sleep in normal subjects. Sleep. 1995; 18(5):330–333

[114] Boselli M, Parrino L, Smerieri A, Terzano MG. Effect of age on EEG arousals in normal sleep. Sleep. 1998; 21(4):351–357

[115] Bixler EO, Kales A, Jacoby JA, Soldatos CR, Vela-Bueno A. Nocturnal sleep and wakefulness: effects of age and sex in normal sleepers. Int J Neurosci. 1984; 23(1):33–42

[116] Redline S, Kirchner HL, Quan SF, Gottlieb DJ, Kapur V, Newman A. The effects of age, sex, ethnicity, and sleep-disordered breathing on sleep architecture. Arch Intern Med. 2004; 164(4):406–418

[117] Unruh ML, Redline S, An MW, et al. Subjective and objective sleep quality and aging in the Sleep Heart Health Study. J Am Geriatr Soc. 2008; 56(7):1218–1227

[118] Endeshaw Y. Clinical characteristics of obstructive sleep apnea in community-dwelling older adults. J Am Geriatr Soc. 2006; 54(11):1740–1744

[119] Browne HA, Adams L, Simonds AK, Morrell MJ. Ageing does not influence the sleep-related decrease in the hypercapnic ventilatory response. Eur Respir J. 2003; 21(3):523–529

[120] Chung S, Yoon IY, Lee CH, Kim JW. Effects of age on the clinical features of men with obstructive sleep apnea syndrome. Respiration. 2009; 78(1):23–29

[121] Ancoli-Israel S, Kripke DF, Klauber MR, Mason WJ, Fell R, Kaplan O. Sleep-disordered breathing in community-dwelling elderly. Sleep. 1991; 14(6):486–495

[122] McNicholas WT. COPD-OSA overlap syndrome: evolving evidence regarding epidemiology, clinical consequences, and management. Chest. 2017; 152(6):1318–1326

[123] Spruit MA, Vercoulen JH, Sprangers MAG, Wouters EFM; FAntasTIGUE consortium. Fatigue in COPD: an important yet ignored symptom. Lancet Respir Med. 2017; 5(7):542–544

[124] Flemons WW, Douglas NJ, Kuna ST, Rodenstein DO, Wheatley J. Access to diagnosis and treatment of patients with suspected sleep apnea. Am J Respir Crit Care Med. 2004; 169(6):668–672

[125] Bliwise DL, Nekich JC, Dement WC. Relative validity of self-reported snoring as a symptom of sleep apnea in a sleep clinic population. Chest. 1991; 99(3):600–608

[126] Martinez D, Breitenbach TC, Lumertz MS, et al. Repeating administration of Epworth Sleepiness Scale is clinically useful. Sleep Breath. 2011; 15(4):763–773

[127] Deegan PC, McNicholas WT. Predictive value of clinical features for the obstructive sleep apnoea syndrome. Eur Respir J. 1996; 9(1):117–124

[128] Verbraecken J, Hedner J, Penzel T. Pre-operative screening for obstructive sleep apnoea. Eur Respir Rev. 2017; 26(143):160012

[129] Horvath CM, Jossen J, Kröll D, et al. Prevalence and prediction of obstructive sleep apnea prior to bariatric surgery-gender-specific performance of four sleep questionnaires. Obes Surg. 2018

[130] Chung F, Ward B, Ho J, Yuan H, Kayumov L, Shapiro C. Preoperative identification of sleep apnea risk in elective surgical patients, using the Berlin questionnaire. J Clin Anesth. 2007; 19(2):130–134

[131] Gross JB, Bachenberg KL, Benumof JL, et al. American Society of Anesthesiologists Task Force on Perioperative Management. Practice guidelines for the perioperative management of patients with obstructive sleep apnea: a report by the American Society of Anesthesiologists Task Force on Perioperative Management of patients with obstructive sleep apnea. Anesthesiology. 2006; 104(5):1081–1093, quiz 1117–1118

[132] Chung F, Yegneswaran B, Liao P, et al. STOP questionnaire: a tool to screen patients for obstructive sleep apnea. Anesthesiology. 2008; 108(5):812–821

[133] Flemons WW, Whitelaw WA, Brant R, Remmers JE. Likelihood ratios for a sleep apnea clinical prediction rule. Am J Respir Crit Care Med. 1994; 150(5 Pt 1):1279–1285

[134] Rowley JA, Aboussouan LS, Badr MS. The use of clinical prediction formulas in the evaluation of obstructive sleep apnea. Sleep. 2000; 23(7):929–938

[135] Gali B, Whalen FX, Schroeder DR, Gay PC, Plevak DJ. Identification of patients at risk for postoperative respiratory complications using a preoperative obstructive sleep apnea screening tool and postanesthesia care assessment. Anesthesiology. 2009; 110(4):869–877

[136] Takegami M, Hayashino Y, Chin K, et al. Simple four-variable screening tool for identification of patients with sleep-disordered breathing. Sleep. 2009; 32(7):939–948

[137] Netzer NC, Stoohs RA, Netzer CM, Clark K, Strohl KP. Using the Berlin Questionnaire to identify patients at risk for the sleep apnea syndrome. Ann Intern Med. 1999; 131(7):485–491

[138] Finkel KJ, Searleman AC, Tymkew H, et al. Prevalence of undiagnosed obstructive sleep apnea among adult surgical patients in an academic medical center. Sleep Med. 2009; 10(7):753–758

[139] Enciso R, Clark GT. Comparing the Berlin and the ARES questionnaire to identify patients with obstructive sleep apnea in a dental setting. Sleep Breath. 2011; 15(1):83–89

[140] Chung F, Yegneswaran B, Liao P, et al. Validation of the Berlin questionnaire and American Society of Anesthesiologists checklist as screening tools for obstructive sleep apnea in surgical patients. Anesthesiology. 2008; 108(5):822–830

[141] Ong TH, Raudha S, Fook-Chong S, Lew N, Hsu AAL. Simplifying STOP-BANG: use of a simple questionnaire to screen for OSA in an Asian population. Sleep Breath. 2010; 14(4):371–376

[142] Chai-Coetzer CL, Antic NA, Rowland LS, et al. A simplified model of screening questionnaire and home monitoring for obstructive sleep apnoea in primary care. Thorax. 2011; 66(3):213–219

[143] Ramachandran SK, Kheterpal S, Consens F, et al. Derivation and validation of a simple perioperative sleep apnea prediction score. Anesth Analg. 2010; 110(4):1007–1015

[144] Marin JM, Carrizo SJ, Vicente E, Agusti AG. Long-term cardiovascular outcomes in men with obstructive sleep apnoea-hypopnoea with or without treatment with continuous positive airway pressure: an observational study. Lancet. 2005; 365(9464):1046–1053

[145] Gami AS, Howard DE, Olson EJ, Somers VK. Day-night pattern of sudden death in obstructive sleep apnea. N Engl J Med. 2005; 352(12):1206–1214

[146] Schipper MH, Jellema K, Thomassen BJW, Alvarez-Estevez D, Verbraecken J, Rijsman RM. Stroke and other cardiovascular events in patients with obstructive sleep apnea and the effect of continuous positive airway pressure. J Neurol. 2017; 264(6):1247–1253

[147] Durán-Cantolla J, Aizpuru F, Martínez-Null C, Barbé-Illa F. Obstructive sleep apnea/hypopnea and systemic hypertension. Sleep Med Rev. 2009; 13(5):323–331

[148] Veale D, Pépin JL, Lévy PA. Autonomic stress tests in obstructive sleep apnea syndrome and snoring. Sleep. 1992; 15(6):505–513

[149] Peker Y, Hedner J, Norum J, Kraiczi H, Carlson J. Increased incidence of cardiovascular disease in middle-aged men with obstructive sleep apnea: a 7-year follow-up. Am J Respir Crit Care Med. 2002; 166(2):159–165

[150] Silverberg DS, Oksenberg A. Are sleep-related breathing disorders important contributing factors to the production of essential hypertension? Curr Hypertens Rep. 2001; 3(3):209–215

[151] Hedner J, Bengtsson-Boström K, Peker Y, Grote L, Råstam L, Lindblad U. Hypertension prevalence in obstructive sleep apnoea and sex: a population-based case-control study. Eur Respir J. 2006; 27(3):564–570

[152] Suzuki M, Guilleminault C, Otsuka K, Shiomi T. Blood pressure "dipping" and "non-dipping" in obstructive sleep apnea syndrome patients. Sleep. 1996; 19(5):382–387

[153] Davies CW, Crosby JH, Mullins RL, Barbour C, Davies RJ, Stradling JR. Case-control study of 24 hour ambulatory blood pressure in patients with obstructive sleep apnoea and normal matched control subjects. Thorax. 2000; 55(9):736–740

[154] Young T, Peppard P, Palta M, et al. Population-based study of sleep-disordered breathing as a risk factor for hypertension. Arch Intern Med. 1997; 157(15):1746–1752

[155] Nieto FJ, Young TB, Lind BK, et al. Association of sleep-disordered breathing, sleep apnea, and hypertension in a large

community-based study. Sleep Heart Health Study. JAMA. 2000; 283(14):1829–1836

[156] Peppard PE, Young T, Palta M, Skatrud J. Prospective study of the association between sleep-disordered breathing and hypertension. N Engl J Med. 2000; 342(19):1378–1384

[157] Tkacova R, McNicholas WT, Javorsky M, et al. European Sleep Apnoea Database study collaborators. Nocturnal intermittent hypoxia predicts prevalent hypertension in the European Sleep Apnoea Database cohort study. Eur Respir J. 2014; 44(4): 931–941

[158] Yaggi HK, Concato J, Kernan WN, Lichtman JH, Brass LM, Mohsenin V. Obstructive sleep apnea as a risk factor for stroke and death. N Engl J Med. 2005; 353(19):2034–2041

[159] Arzt M, Young T, Finn L, Skatrud JB, Bradley TD. Association of sleep-disordered breathing and the occurrence of stroke. Am J Respir Crit Care Med. 2005; 172(11):1447–1451

[160] Redline S, Yenokyan G, Gottlieb DJ, et al. Obstructive sleep apnea-hypopnea and incident stroke: the Sleep Heart Health Study. Am J Respir Crit Care Med. 2010; 182(2):269–277

[161] Kiely JL, McNicholas WT. Cardiovascular risk factors in patients with obstructive sleep apnoea syndrome. Eur Respir J. 2000; 16(1):128–133

[162] Good DC, Henkle JQ, Gelber D, Welsh J, Verhulst S. Sleep-disordered breathing and poor functional outcome after stroke. Stroke. 1996; 27(2):252–259

[163] Bassetti CL, Milanova M, Gugger M. Sleep-disordered breathing and acute ischemic stroke: diagnosis, risk factors, treatment, evolution, and long-term clinical outcome. Stroke. 2006; 37(4):967–972

[164] Schipper MH, Jellema K, Rijsman RM. Occurrence of obstructive sleep apnea syndrome in patients with transient ischemic attack. J Stroke Cerebrovasc Dis. 2016; 25(5):1249–1253

[165] Wessendorf TE, Teschler H, Wang YM, Konietzko N, Thilmann AF. Sleep-disordered breathing among patients with first-ever stroke. J Neurol. 2000; 247(1):41–47

[166] Somers VK, White DP, Amin R, et al. American Heart Association Council for High Blood Pressure Research Professional Education Committee, Council on Clinical Cardiology. American Heart Association Stroke Council. American Heart Association Council on Cardiovascular Nursing. American College of Cardiology Foundation. Sleep apnea and cardiovascular disease: an American Heart Association/american College Of Cardiology Foundation Scientific Statement from the American Heart Association Council for High Blood Pressure Research Professional Education Committee, Council on Clinical Cardiology, Stroke Council, and Council on Cardiovascular Nursing. In collaboration with the National Heart, Lung, and Blood Institute National Center on Sleep Disorders Research (National Institutes of Health). Circulation. 2008; 118(10):1080–1111

[167] Baguet JP, Hammer L, Lévy P, et al. The severity of oxygen desaturation is predictive of carotid wall thickening and plaque occurrence. Chest. 2005; 128(5):3407–3412

[168] Suzuki T, Nakano H, Maekawa J, et al. Obstructive sleep apnea and carotid-artery intima-media thickness. Sleep. 2004; 27(1):129–133

[169] Parra O, Arboix A, Montserrat JM, Quintó L, Bechich S, García-Eroles L. Sleep-related breathing disorders: impact on mortality of cerebrovascular disease. Eur Respir J. 2004; 24(2):267–272

[170] Good DC, Henkle JQ, Gelber D, Welsh J, Verhulst S. Sleep-disordered breathing and poor functional outcome after stroke. Stroke. 1996; 27(2):252–259

[171] Johnson KG, Johnson DC. Frequency of sleep apnea in stroke and TIA patients: a meta-analysis. J Clin Sleep Med. 2010; 6(2):131–137

[172] Liston R, Deegan PC, McCreery C, McNicholas WT. Role of respiratory sleep disorders in the pathogenesis of nocturnal angina and arrhythmias. Postgrad Med J. 1994; 70(822):275–280

[173] Koehler U, Schäfer H. Is obstructive sleep apnea (OSA) a risk factor for myocardial infarction and cardiac arrhythmias in patients with coronary heart disease (CHD)? Sleep. 1996; 19(4):283–286

[174] Shepard JW Jr. Hypertension, cardiac arrhythmias, myocardial infarction, and stroke in relation to obstructive sleep apnea. Clin Chest Med. 1992; 13(3):437–458

[175] Mehra R, Benjamin EJ, Shahar E, et al. Sleep Heart Health Study. Association of nocturnal arrhythmias with sleep-disordered breathing: the Sleep Heart Health Study. Am J Respir Crit Care Med. 2006; 173(8):910–916

[176] Ryan CM, Usui K, Floras JS, Bradley TD. Effect of continuous positive airway pressure on ventricular ectopy in heart failure patients with obstructive sleep apnoea. Thorax. 2005; 60(9):781–785

[177] Peker Y, Kraiczi H, Hedner J, Löth S, Johansson A, Bende M. An independent association between obstructive sleep apnoea and coronary artery disease. Eur Respir J. 1999; 14(1):179–184

[178] Sorajja D, Gami AS, Somers VK, Behrenbeck TR, Garcia-Touchard A, Lopez-Jimenez F. Independent association between obstructive sleep apnea and subclinical coronary artery disease. Chest. 2008; 133(4):927–933

[179] Hayashi M, Fujimoto K, Urushibata K, Uchikawa S, Imamura H, Kubo K. Nocturnal oxygen desaturation correlates with the severity of coronary atherosclerosis in coronary artery disease. Chest. 2003; 124(3):936–941

[180] Franklin KA, Nilsson JB, Sahlin C, Näslund U. Sleep apnoea and nocturnal angina. Lancet. 1995; 345(8957):1085–1087

[181] Peled N, Abinader EG, Pillar G, Sharif D, Lavie P. Nocturnal ischemic events in patients with obstructive sleep apnea syndrome and ischemic heart disease: effects of continuous positive air pressure treatment. J Am Coll Cardiol. 1999; 34(6):1744–1749

[182] Gami AS, Svatikova A, Wolk R, et al. Cardiac troponin T in obstructive sleep apnea. Chest. 2004; 125(6):2097–2100

[183] Narkiewicz K, Montano N, Cogliati C, van de Borne PJ, Dyken ME, Somers VK. Altered cardiovascular variability in obstructive sleep apnea. Circulation. 1998; 98(11):1071–1077

[184] Kuniyoshi FH, Garcia-Touchard A, Gami AS, et al. Day-night variation of acute myocardial infarction in obstructive sleep apnea. J Am Coll Cardiol. 2008; 52(5):343–346

[185] Berger S, Aronson D, Lavie P, Lavie L. Endothelial progenitor cells in acute myocardial infarction and sleep-disordered breathing. Am J Respir Crit Care Med. 2013; 187(1):90–98

[186] Shah N, Redline S, Yaggi HK, et al. Obstructive sleep apnea and acute myocardial infarction severity: ischemic preconditioning? Sleep Breath. 2013; 17(2):819–826

[187] Drager LF, Bortolotto LA, Lorenzi MC, Figueiredo AC, Krieger EM, Lorenzi-Filho G. Early signs of atherosclerosis in obstructive sleep apnea. Am J Respir Crit Care Med. 2005; 172(5):613–618

[188] Baguet JP, Hammer L, Lévy P, et al. Night-time and diastolic hypertension are common and underestimated conditions in newly diagnosed apnoeic patients. J Hypertens. 2005; 23(3):521–527

[189] Tsioufis C, Thomopoulos K, Dimitriadis K, et al. The incremental effect of obstructive sleep apnoea syndrome on arterial stiffness in newly diagnosed essential hypertensive subjects. J Hypertens. 2007; 25(1):141–146

[190] Drager LF, Bortolotto LA, Figueiredo AC, Silva BC, Krieger EM, Lorenzi-Filho G. Obstructive sleep apnea, hypertension, and their interaction on arterial stiffness and heart remodeling. Chest. 2007; 131(5):1379–1386

[191] Alchanatis M, Tourkohoriti G, Kosmas EN, et al. Evidence for left ventricular dysfunction in patients with obstructive sleep apnoea syndrome. Eur Respir J. 2002; 20(5):1239–1245

[192] Shivalkar B, Van de Heyning C, Kerremans M, et al. Obstructive sleep apnea syndrome: more insights on structural and functional cardiac alterations, and the effects of treatment with continuous positive airway pressure. J Am Coll Cardiol. 2006; 47(7):1433–1439

[193] Minoguchi K, Yokoe T, Tazaki T, et al. Increased carotid intima-media thickness and serum inflammatory markers in obstructive sleep apnea. Am J Respir Crit Care Med. 2005; 172(5):625–630

[194] Lavie L. Obstructive sleep apnoea syndrome–an oxidative stress disorder. Sleep Med Rev. 2003; 7(1):35–51

[195] Aurigemma GP, Gaasch WH. Clinical practice. Diastolic heart failure. N Engl J Med. 2004; 351(11):1097–1105

[196] Chan J, Sanderson J, Chan W, et al. Prevalence of sleep-disordered breathing in diastolic heart failure. Chest. 1997; 111(6):1488–1493

[197] Fung JW, Li TS, Choy DK, et al. Severe obstructive sleep apnea is associated with left ventricular diastolic dysfunction. Chest. 2002; 121(2):422–429

[198] Arias MA, García-Río F, Alonso-Fernández A, Mediano O, Martínez I, Villamor J. Obstructive sleep apnea syndrome affects left ventricular diastolic function: effects of nasal continuous positive airway pressure in men. Circulation. 2005; 112(3):375–383

[199] Shahar E, Whitney CW, Redline S, et al. Sleep-disordered breathing and cardiovascular disease: cross-sectional results of the Sleep Heart Health Study. Am J Respir Crit Care Med. 2001; 163(1):19–25

[200] He J, Kryger MH, Zorick FJ, Conway W, Roth T. Mortality and apnea index in obstructive sleep apnea. Experience in 385 male patients. Chest. 1988; 94(1):9–14

[201] Sahlin C, Sandberg O, Gustafson Y, et al. Obstructive sleep apnea is a risk factor for death in patients with stroke: a 10-year follow-up. Arch Intern Med. 2008; 168(3):297–301

[202] Peker Y, Hedner J, Kraiczi H, Löth S. Respiratory disturbance index: an independent predictor of mortality in coronary artery disease. Am J Respir Crit Care Med. 2000; 162(1):81–86

[203] Lavie P, Herer P, Peled R, et al. Mortality in sleep apnea patients: a multivariate analysis of risk factors. Sleep. 1995; 18(3):149–157

[204] Young T, Finn L, Peppard PE, et al. Sleep disordered breathing and mortality: eighteen-year follow-up of the Wisconsin Sleep Cohort Study. Sleep. 2008; 31(8):1071–1078

[205] Punjabi NM, Caffo BS, Goodwin JL, et al. Sleep-disordered breathing and mortality: a prospective cohort study. PLoS Med. 2009; 6(8):e1000132

[206] Lavie P, Lavie L. Unexpected survival advantage in elderly people with moderate sleep apnoea. J Sleep Res. 2009; 18(4):397–403

[207] Goff EA, O'Driscoll DM, Simonds AK, Trinder J, Morrell MJ. The cardiovascular response to arousal from sleep decreases with age in healthy adults. Sleep. 2008; 31(7):1009–1017

[208] Strohl KP, Novak RD, Singer W, et al. Insulin levels, blood pressure and sleep apnea. Sleep. 1994; 17(7):614–618

[209] Ip MS, Lam B, Ng MM, Lam WK, Tsang KW, Lam KS. Obstructive sleep apnea is independently associated with insulin resistance. Am J Respir Crit Care Med. 2002; 165(5):670–676

[210] Vgontzas AN, Papanicolaou DA, Bixler EO, et al. Sleep apnea and daytime sleepiness and fatigue: relation to visceral obesity, insulin resistance, and hypercytokinemia. J Clin Endocrinol Metab. 2000; 85(3):1151–1158

[211] Punjabi NM, Sorkin JD, Katzel LI, Goldberg AP, Schwartz AR, Smith PL. Sleep-disordered breathing and insulin resistance in middle-aged and overweight men. Am J Respir Crit Care Med. 2002; 165(5):677–682

[212] Stoohs RA, Facchini F, Guilleminault C. Insulin resistance and sleep-disordered breathing in healthy humans. Am J Respir Crit Care Med. 1996; 154(1):170–174

[213] Punjabi NM, Shahar E, Redline S, Gottlieb DJ, Givelber R, Resnick HE; Sleep Heart Health Study Investigators. Sleep-disordered breathing, glucose intolerance, and hypertension: the Sleep Heart Health Study. Am J Epidemiol. 2004; 160(6):521–530

[214] Reichmuth KJ, Austin D, Skatrud JB, Young T. Association of sleep apnea and type II diabetes: a population-based study. Am J Respir Crit Care Med. 2005; 172(12):1590–1595

[215] Kent BD, Grote L, Bonsignore MR, et al. European Sleep Apnoea Database collaborators. Sleep apnoea severity independently predicts glycaemic health in nondiabetic subjects: the ESADA study. Eur Respir J. 2014; 44(1):130–139

[216] Kent BD, Grote L, Ryan S, et al. Diabetes mellitus prevalence and control in sleep-disordered breathing: the European Sleep Apnea Cohort (ESADA) study. Chest. 2014; 146(4):982–990

[217] Stamatakis K, Sanders MH, Caffo B, et al. Fasting glycemia in sleep disordered breathing: lowering the threshold on oxyhemoglobin desaturation. Sleep. 2008; 31(7):1018–1024

[218] Botros N, Concato J, Mohsenin V, Selim B, Doctor K, Yaggi HK. Obstructive sleep apnea as a risk factor for type 2 diabetes. Am J Med. 2009; 122(12):1122–1127

[219] Grassi G, Seravalle G, Quarti-Trevano F, et al. Reinforcement of the adrenergic overdrive in the metabolic syndrome complicated by obstructive sleep apnea. J Hypertens. 2010; 28(6):1313–1320

[220] Stamatakis KA, Punjabi NM. Effects of sleep fragmentation on glucose metabolism in normal subjects. Chest. 2010; 137(1):95–101

[221] Naëgelé B, Thouvard V, Pépin JL, et al. Deficits of cognitive executive functions in patients with sleep apnea syndrome. Sleep. 1995; 18(1):43–52

[222] Twigg GL, Papaioannou I, Jackson M, et al. Obstructive sleep apnea syndrome is associated with deficits in verbal but not visual memory. Am J Respir Crit Care Med. 2010; 182(1):98–103

[223] Naëgelé B, Launois SH, Mazza S, Feuerstein C, Pépin JL, Lévy P. Which memory processes are affected in patients with obstructive sleep apnea? An evaluation of 3 types of memory. Sleep. 2006; 29(4):533–544

[224] Quan SF, Wright R, Baldwin CM, et al. Obstructive sleep apnea-hypopnea and neurocognitive functioning in the Sleep Heart Health Study. Sleep Med. 2006; 7(6):498–507

[225] Banno K, Kryger MH. Sleep apnea: clinical investigations in humans. Sleep Med. 2007; 8(4):400–426

[226] Arnsten AF, Li BM. Neurobiology of executive functions: catecholamine influences on prefrontal cortical functions. Biol Psychiatry. 2005; 57(11):1377–1384

[227] Verstraeten E, Cluydts R. Executive control of attention in sleep apnea patients: theoretical concepts and methodological considerations. Sleep Med Rev. 2004; 8(4):257–267

[228] Kales A, Caldwell AB, Cadieux RJ, Vela-Bueno A, Ruch LG, Mayes SD. Severe obstructive sleep apnea–II: Associated psychopathology and psychosocial consequences. J Chronic Dis. 1985; 38(5):427–434

[229] Findley LJ, Barth JT, Powers DC, Wilhoit SC, Boyd DG, Suratt PM. Cognitive impairment in patients with obstructive sleep apnea and associated hypoxemia. Chest. 1986; 90(5):686–690

[230] Alchanatis M, Deligiorgis N, Zias N, et al. Frontal brain lobe impairment in obstructive sleep apnoea: a proton MR spectroscopy study. Eur Respir J. 2004; 24(6):980–986

[231] Ayalon L, Ancoli-Israel S, Klemfuss Z, Shalauta MD, Drummond SP. Increased brain activation during verbal learning in obstructive sleep apnea. Neuroimage. 2006; 31(4):1817–1825

[232] Glasser M, Bailey N, McMillan A, Goff E, Morrell MJ. Sleep apnoea in older people. Breathe. 2011; 7(3):249–256

[233] Mazza S, Pépin JL, Naëgelé B, et al. Driving ability in sleep apnoea patients before and after CPAP treatment: evaluation on a road safety platform. Eur Respir J. 2006; 28(5):1020–1028

[234] Nieto FJ, Peppard PE, Young T, Finn L, Hla KM, Farré R. Sleep-disordered breathing and cancer mortality: results from the Wisconsin Sleep Cohort Study. Am J Respir Crit Care Med. 2012; 186(2):190–194

[235] Campos-Rodriguez F, Martinez-Garcia MA, Martinez M, et al. Spanish Sleep Network. Association between obstructive sleep apnea and cancer incidence in a large multicenter Spanish cohort. Am J Respir Crit Care Med. 2013; 187(1):99–105

[236] Marshall NS, Wong KK, Cullen SR, Knuiman MW, Grunstein RR. Sleep apnea and 20-year follow-up for all-cause mortality, stroke, and cancer incidence and mortality in the Busselton Health Study cohort. J Clin Sleep Med. 2014; 10(4):355–362

[237] Martínez-García MÁ, Martorell-Calatayud A, Nagore E, et al. Association between sleep disordered breathing and aggressiveness markers of malignant cutaneous melanoma. Eur Respir J. 2014; 43(6):1661–1668

[238] Sjöström L, Gummesson A, Sjöström CD, et al. Swedish Obese Subjects Study. Effects of bariatric surgery on cancer incidence in obese patients in Sweden (Swedish Obese Subjects Study): a prospective, controlled intervention trial. Lancet Oncol. 2009; 10(7):653–662

[239] Toffoli S, Michiels C. Intermittent hypoxia is a key regulator of cancer cell and endothelial cell interplay in tumours. FEBS J. 2008; 275(12):2991–3002

[240] Reuter S, Gupta SC, Chaturvedi MM, Aggarwal BB. Oxidative stress, inflammation, and cancer: how are they linked? Free Radic Biol Med. 2010; 49(11):1603–1616

[241] Hole PS, Darley RL, Tonks A. Do reactive oxygen species play a role in myeloid leukemias? Blood. 2011; 117(22):5816–5826

[242] Sato T, Takeda H, Otake S, et al. Increased plasma levels of 8-hydroxydeoxyguanosine are associated with development of colorectal tumors. J Clin Biochem Nutr. 2010; 47(1):59–63

[243] Xue X, Taylor M, Anderson E, et al. Hypoxia-inducible factor-2α activation promotes colorectal cancer progression by dysregulating iron homeostasis Cancer Res. 2012; 72(9):2285–2293

[244] Gozal D, Kheirandish-Gozal L. Cardiovascular morbidity in obstructive sleep apnea: oxidative stress, inflammation, and much more. Am J Respir Crit Care Med. 2008; 177(4):369–375

[245] Alonso-Fernández A, García-Río F, Arias MA, et al. Effects of CPAP on oxidative stress and nitrate efficiency in sleep apnoea: a randomised trial. Thorax. 2009; 64(7):581–586

[246] Barceló A, Barbé F, de la Peña M, et al. Antioxidant status in patients with sleep apnoea and impact of continuous positive airway pressure treatment. Eur Respir J. 2006; 27(4):756–760

[247] Yamauchi M, Nakano H, Maekawa J, et al. Oxidative stress in obstructive sleep apnea. Chest. 2005; 127(5):1674–1679

[248] Ayas NT, FitzGerald JM, Fleetham JA, et al. Cost-effectiveness of continuous positive airway pressure therapy for moderate to severe obstructive sleep apnea/hypopnea. Arch Intern Med. 2006; 166(9):977–984

[249] Ayas NT, Marra C. Continuous positive airway pressure therapy for obstructive sleep apnea syndrome: do the dollars make sense? Sleep. 2005; 28(10):1211–1213

[250] Kapur VK, Alfonso-Cristancho R. Just a good deal or truly a steal? Medical cost savings and the impact on the cost-effectiveness of treating sleep apnea. Sleep. 2009; 32(2):135–136

[251] Tarasiuk A, Greenberg-Dotan S, Brin YS, Simon T, Tal A, Reuveni H. Determinants affecting health-care utilization in obstructive sleep apnea syndrome patients. Chest. 2005; 128(3):1310–1314

[252] Bahammam A, Delaive K, Ronald J, Manfreda J, Roos L, Kryger MH. Health care utilization in males with obstructive sleep apnea syndrome two years after diagnosis and treatment. Sleep. 1999; 22(6):740–747

[253] Banno K, Manfreda J, Walld R, Delaive K, Kryger MH. Healthcare utilization in women with obstructive sleep apnea syndrome 2 years after diagnosis and treatment. Sleep. 2006; 29(10):1307–1311

[254] Greenberg-Dotan S, Reuveni H, Simon-Tuval T, Oksenberg A, Tarasiuk A. Gender differences in morbidity and health care utilization among adult obstructive sleep apnea patients. Sleep. 2007; 30(9):1173–1180

[255] Kryger MH, Roos L, Delaive K, Walld R, Horrocks J. Utilization of health care services in patients with severe obstructive sleep apnea. Sleep. 1996; 19(9, Suppl):S111–S116

[256] Reuveni H, Greenberg-Dotan S, Simon-Tuval T, Oksenberg A, Tarasiuk A. Elevated healthcare utilisation in young adult males with obstructive sleep apnoea. Eur Respir J. 2008; 31(2): 273–279

[257] Ronald J, Delaive K, Roos L, Manfreda J, Bahammam A, Kryger MH. Health care utilization in the 10 years prior to diagnosis in obstructive sleep apnea syndrome patients. Sleep. 1999; 22(2):225–229

[258] Smith R, Ronald J, Delaive K, Walld R, Manfreda J, Kryger MH. What are obstructive sleep apnea patients being treated for prior to this diagnosis? Chest. 2002; 121(1):164–172

[259] Kapur V, Blough DK, Sandblom RE, et al. The medical cost of undiagnosed sleep apnea. Sleep. 1999; 22(7):749–755

[260] Ronksley PE, Hemmelgarn BR, Heitman SJ, et al. Excessive daytime sleepiness is associated with increased health care utilization among patients referred for assessment of OSA. Sleep. 2011; 34(3):363–370

[261] Kapur VK, Redline S, Nieto FJ, Young TB, Newman AB, Henderson JA; Sleep Heart Health Research Group. The relationship between chronically disrupted sleep and healthcare use. Sleep. 2002; 25(3):289–296

[262] Tarasiuk A, Greenberg-Dotan S, Simon-Tuval T, Oksenberg A, Reuveni H. The effect of obstructive sleep apnea on morbidity and health care utilization of middle-aged and older adults. J Am Geriatr Soc. 2008; 56(2):247–254

[263] Tarasiuk A, Greenberg-Dotan S, Simon T, Tal A, Oksenberg A, Reuveni H. Low socioeconomic status is a risk factor for cardiovascular disease among adult obstructive sleep apnea syndrome patients requiring treatment. Chest. 2006; 130(3):766–773

[264] Simon-Tuval T, Reuveni H, Greenberg-Dotan S, Oksenberg A, Tal A, Tarasiuk A. Low socioeconomic status is a risk factor for CPAP acceptance among adult OSAS patients requiring treatment. Sleep. 2009; 32(4):545–552

[265] Albarrak M, Banno K, Sabbagh AA, et al. Utilization of healthcare resources in obstructive sleep apnea syndrome: a 5-year follow-up study in men using CPAP. Sleep. 2005; 28(10):1306–1311

[266] Peker Y, Hedner J, Johansson A, Bende M. Reduced hospitalization with cardiovascular and pulmonary disease in obstructive sleep apnea patients on nasal CPAP treatment. Sleep. 1997; 20(8):645–653

[267] Jennum P, Kjellberg J. Health, social and economical consequences of sleep-disordered breathing: a controlled national study. Thorax. 2011; 66(7):560–566

[268] Cai Q, Tan H, Singer J. Impact of positive airway pressure among obstructive sleep apnea patients. Am J Manag Care. 2012; 18(6):e225–e233

[269] Hoffman B, Wingenbach DD, Kagey AN, Schaneman JL, Kasper D. The long-term health plan and disability cost benefit of obstructive sleep apnea treatment in a commercial motor vehicle driver population. J Occup Environ Med. 2010; 52(5):473–477

[270] Potts KJ, Butterfield DT, Sims P, Henderson M, Shames CB. Cost savings associated with an education campaign on the diagnosis and management of sleep-disordered breathing: a retrospective, claims-based US study. Popul Health Manag. 2013; 16(1):7–13

[271] Ulfberg J, Carter N, Talbäck M, Edling C. Excessive daytime sleepiness at work and subjective work performance in the general population and among heavy snorers and patients with obstructive sleep apnea. Chest. 1996; 110(3):659–663

[272] Omachi TA, Claman DM, Blanc PD, Eisner MD. Obstructive sleep apnea: a risk factor for work disability. Sleep. 2009; 32(6):791–798

[273] Sivertsen B, Overland S, Glozier N, Bjorvatn B, Maeland JG, Mykletun A. The effect of OSAS on sick leave and work disability. Eur Respir J. 2008; 32(6):1497–1503

[274] Sjösten N, Vahtera J, Salo P, et al. Increased risk of lost workdays prior to the diagnosis of sleep apnea. Chest. 2009; 136(1):130–136

[275] Harvard Medical School Division of Sleep Medicine. The price of fatigue: the surprising economic costs of unmanaged sleep apnea. Boston, MA: Harvard Medical School; 2010 Available at: http://sleep.med.harvard.edu/what-we-do/public-policy-research. Accessed on 10/04/2018

[276] Rodenstein D; Cost-B26 Action on Sleep Apnoea Syndrome. Driving in Europe: the need of a common policy for drivers with obstructive sleep apnoea syndrome. J Sleep Res. 2008; 17(3):281–284

[277] Strohl KP, Brown DB, Collop N, et al. ATS Ad Hoc Committee on Sleep Apnea, Sleepiness, and Driving Risk in Noncommercial Drivers. An official American Thoracic Society Clinical Practice Guideline: sleep apnea, sleepiness, and driving risk in noncommercial drivers. An update of a 1994 Statement. Am J Respir Crit Care Med. 2013; 187(11):1259–1266

[278] Tippin J. Driving impairment in patients with obstructive sleep apnea syndrome. Am J Electroneurodiagn Technol. 2007; 47(2):114–126

[279] Tregear S, Reston J, Schoelles K, Phillips B. Obstructive sleep apnea and risk of motor vehicle crash: systematic review and meta-analysis. J Clin Sleep Med. 2009; 5(6):573–581

[280] Marshall SC, Man-Son-Hing M. Multiple chronic medical conditions and associated driving risk: a systematic review. Traffic Inj Prev. 2011; 12(2):142–148

[281] Vaa T. Impairments, diseases, age and their relative risks of accident involvement: results from a meta-analysis. Oslo, Norway: Institute of Transport Economics; 2003

[282] Arita A, Sasanabe R, Hasegawa R, et al. Risk factors for automobile accidents caused by falling asleep while driving in obstructive sleep apnea syndrome. Sleep Breath. 2015; 19(4):1229–1234

[283] Ward KL, Hillman DR, James A, et al. Excessive daytime sleepiness increases the risk of motor vehicle crash in obstructive sleep apnea. J Clin Sleep Med. 2013; 9(10):1013–1021

[284] Karimi M, Hedner J, Häbel H, Nerman O, Grote L. Sleep apnea-related risk of motor vehicle accidents is reduced by continuous positive airway pressure: Swedish Traffic Accident Registry data. Sleep. 2015; 38(3):341–349

[285] Terán-Santos J, Jiménez-Gómez A, Cordero-Guevara J; Cooperative Group Burgos-Santander. The association between sleep apnea and the risk of traffic accidents. N Engl J Med. 1999; 340(11):847–851

[286] Karimi M, Hedner J, Lombardi C, et al. Esada Study Group. Driving habits and risk factors for traffic accidents among sleep apnea patients–a European multi-centre cohort study. J Sleep Res. 2014; 23(6):689–699

[287] Mulgrew AT, Nasvadi G, Butt A, et al. Risk and severity of motor vehicle crashes in patients with obstructive sleep apnoea/hypopnoea. Thorax. 2008; 63(6):536–541

[288] Di Milia L, Smolensky MH, Costa G, Howarth HD, Ohayon MM, Philip P. Demographic factors, fatigue, and driving accidents: An examination of the published literature. Accid Anal Prev. 2011; 43(2):516–532

[289] Stevenson MR, Elkington J, Sharwood L, et al. The role of sleepiness, sleep disorders, and the work environment on heavy-vehicle crashes in 2 Australian states. Am J Epidemiol. 2014; 179(5):594–601

[290] Young T, Blustein J, Finn L, Palta M. Sleep-disordered breathing and motor vehicle accidents in a population-based sample of employed adults. Sleep. 1997; 20(8):608–613

[291] Sassani A, Findley LJ, Kryger M, Goldlust E, George C, Davidson TM. Reducing motor-vehicle collisions, costs, and fatalities by treating obstructive sleep apnea syndrome. Sleep. 2004; 27(3):453–458

[292] Krieger J, Meslier N, Lebrun T, et al. Accidents in obstructive sleep apnea patients treated with nasal continuous positive airway pressure: a prospective study. The Working Group ANTADIR, Paris and CRESGE, Lille, France. Association Nationale de Traitement à Domicile des Insuffisants Respiratoires. Chest. 1997; 112(6):1561–1566

[293] Tousignant P, Cosio MG, Levy RD, Groome PA. Quality adjusted life years added by treatment of obstructive sleep apnea. Sleep. 1994; 17(1):52–60

[294] AlGhanim N, Comondore VR, Fleetham J, Marra CA, Ayas NT. The economic impact of obstructive sleep apnea. Lung. 2008; 186(1):7–12

[295] Prosser LA, Stinnett AA, Goldman PA, et al. Cost-effectiveness of cholesterol-lowering therapies according to selected patient characteristics. Ann Intern Med. 2000; 132(10):769–779

[296] Kapur VK. Obstructive sleep apnea: diagnosis, epidemiology, and economics. Respir Care. 2010; 55(9):1155–1167

[297] Alonderis A, Barbé F, Bonsignore M, et al. COST Action B-26. Medico-legal implications of sleep apnoea syndrome: driving license regulations in Europe. Sleep Med. 2008; 9(4):362–375

[298] Revision to Annex Iii of Eu Driving Licence Directive Regarding Obstructive Sleep Apnoea Syndrome. Available at: http://eur-lex.europa.eu/legal-content/EN/TXT/?uri=uriserv:OJ.L_.2014.194.01.0010.01.ENG (2014). Accessed 10/04/2018

[299] Dwarakanath A, Twiddy M, Ghosh D, Jamson SL, Baxter PD, Elliott MW; British Thoracic Society. Variability in clinicians' opinions regarding fitness to drive in patients with obstructive sleep apnoea syndrome (OSAS). Thorax. 2015; 70(5):495–497

[300] Bonsignore MR, Randerath W, Riha R, et al. New rules on driver licensing for patients with obstructive sleep apnoea: EU Directive 2014/85/EU. Eur Respir J. 2016; 47(1):39–41

[301] Peppard PE, Young T, Palta M, Dempsey J, Skatrud J. Longitudinal study of moderate weight change and sleep-disordered breathing. JAMA. 2000; 284(23):3015–3021

[302] Kositanurit W, Muntham D, Udomsawaengsup S, Chirakalwasan N. Prevalence and associated factors of obstructive sleep apnea in morbidly obese patients undergoing bariatric surgery. Sleep Breath. 2018; 22(1):251–256

[303] Amin A, Ali A, Altaf QA, et al. Prevalence and associations of obstructive sleep apnea in South Asians and White Europeans with type 2 diabetes: a cross-sectional study. J Clin Sleep Med. 2017; 13(4):583–589

[304] Vanderveken OM, Boudewyns A, Ni Q, et al. Cardiovascular implications in the treatment of obstructive sleep apnea. J Cardiovasc Transl Res. 2011; 4(1):53–60

[305] Gami AS, Pressman G, Caples SM, et al. Association of atrial fibrillation and obstructive sleep apnea. Circulation. 2004; 110(4):364–367

[306] Peker Y, Carlson J, Hedner J. Increased incidence of coronary artery disease in sleep apnoea: a long-term follow-up. Eur Respir J. 2006; 28(3):596–602

[307] Guillot M, Sforza E, Achour-Crawford E, et al. Association between severe obstructive sleep apnea and incident arterial hypertension in the older people population. Sleep Med. 2013; 14(9):838–842

[308] Hla KM, Young T, Finn L, Peppard PE, Szklo-Coxe M, Stubbs M. Longitudinal association of sleep-disordered breathing and nondipping of nocturnal blood pressure in the Wisconsin Sleep Cohort Study. Sleep. 2008; 31(6):795–800

[309] Hla KM, Young TB, Bidwell T, Palta M, Skatrud JB, Dempsey J. Sleep apnea and hypertension. A population-based study. Ann Intern Med. 1994; 120(5):382–388

[310] Lavie P, Herer P, Hoffstein V. Obstructive sleep apnoea syndrome as a risk factor for hypertension: population study. BMJ. 2000; 320(7233):479–482

[311] Marin JM, Agusti A, Villar I, et al. Association between treated and untreated obstructive sleep apnea and risk of hypertension. JAMA. 2012; 307(20):2169–2176

[312] Crinion SJ, Ryan S, McNicholas WT. Obstructive sleep apnoea as a cause of nocturnal nondipping blood pressure: recent evidence regarding clinical importance and underlying mechanisms. Eur Respir J. 2017; 49(1):1601818

[313] Muxfeldt ES, Margallo VS, Guimarães GM, Salles GF. Prevalence and associated factors of obstructive sleep apnea in patients with resistant hypertension. Am J Hypertens. 2014; 27(8):1069–1078

[314] Parati G, Lombardi C, Hedner J, et al. EU COST Action B26 members. Recommendations for the management of patients with obstructive sleep apnoea and hypertension. Eur Respir J. 2013; 41(3):523–538

[315] Mancia G, De Backer G, Dominiczak A, et al. Management of Arterial Hypertension of the European Society of Hypertension. European Society of Cardiology. 2007 Guidelines for the Management of Arterial Hypertension: The Task Force for the Management of Arterial Hypertension of the European Society of Hypertension (ESH) and of the European Society of Cardiology (ESC). J Hypertens. 2007; 25(6):1105–1187

[316] Randerath W, Verbraecken J, Andreas S, et al. Definition, discrimination, diagnosis and treatment of central breathing disturbances during sleep. Eur Respir J. 2017; 49(1):1600959

[317] Bitter T, Faber L, Hering D, Langer C, Horstkotte D, Oldenburg O. Sleep-disordered breathing in heart failure with normal left ventricular ejection fraction. Eur J Heart Fail. 2009; 11(6):602–608

[318] Oldenburg O, Lamp B, Faber L, Teschler H, Horstkotte D, Töpfer V. Sleep-disordered breathing in patients with symptomatic heart failure: a contemporary study of prevalence in and characteristics of 700 patients. Eur J Heart Fail. 2007; 9(3):251–257

[319] Javaheri S, Shukla R, Zeigler H, Wexler L. Central sleep apnea, right ventricular dysfunction, and low diastolic blood pressure are predictors of mortality in systolic heart failure. J Am Coll Cardiol. 2007; 49(20):2028–2034

[320] Jilek C, Krenn M, Sebah D, et al. Prognostic impact of sleep disordered breathing and its treatment in heart failure: an observational study. Eur J Heart Fail. 2011; 13(1):68–75

[321] Khayat R, Abraham W, Patt B, et al. Central sleep apnea is a predictor of cardiac readmission in hospitalized patients with systolic heart failure. J Card Fail. 2012; 18(7):534–540

[322] Wang H, Parker JD, Newton GE, et al. Influence of obstructive sleep apnea on mortality in patients with heart failure. J Am Coll Cardiol. 2007; 49(15):1625–1631

[323] Kushida CA, Littner MR, Morgenthaler T, et al. Practice parameters for the indications for polysomnography and related procedures: an update for 2005. Sleep. 2005; 28(4):499–521

[324] Kanagala R, Murali NS, Friedman PA, et al. Obstructive sleep apnea and the recurrence of atrial fibrillation. Circulation. 2003; 107(20):2589–2594

[325] Lindenfeld J, Albert NM, Boehmer JP, et al. Heart Failure Society of America. HFSA 2010 Comprehensive Heart Failure Practice Guideline. J Card Fail. 2010; 16(6):e1–e194

[326] Yancy CW, Jessup M, Bozkurt B, et al. WRITING COMMITTEE MEMBERS. American College of Cardiology Foundation/American Heart Association Task Force on Practice Guidelines. 2013 ACCF/AHA guideline for the management of heart failure: a report of the American College of Cardiology Foundation/American Heart Association Task Force on practice guidelines. Circulation. 2013; 128(16):e240–e327

[327] Monahan K, Brewster J, Wang L, et al. Relation of the severity of obstructive sleep apnea in response to anti-arrhythmic drugs in patients with atrial fibrillation or atrial flutter. Am J Cardiol. 2012; 110(3):369–372

[328] Bitter T, Westerheide N, Prinz C, et al. Cheyne-Stokes respiration and obstructive sleep apnoea are independent risk factors for malignant ventricular arrhythmias requiring appropriate cardioverter-defibrillator therapies in patients with congestive heart failure. Eur Heart J. 2011; 32(1):61–74

[329] Calkins H, Kuck KH, Cappato R, et al. Heart Rhythm Society Task Force on Catheter and Surgical Ablation of Atrial Fibrillation. 2012 HRS/EHRA/ECAS expert consensus statement on catheter and surgical ablation of atrial fibrillation: recommendations for patient selection, procedural techniques, patient management and follow-up, definitions, endpoints, and research trial design: a report of the Heart Rhythm Society (HRS) Task Force on Catheter and Surgical Ablation of Atrial Fibrillation. Developed in partnership with the European Heart Rhythm Association (EHRA), a registered branch of the European Society of Cardiology (ESC) and the European Cardiac Arrhythmia Society (ECAS); and in collaboration with the American College of Cardiology (ACC), American Heart Association (AHA), the Asia Pacific Heart Rhythm Society (APHRS), and the Society of Thoracic Surgeons (STS). Endorsed by the governing bodies of the American College of Cardiology Foundation, the American Heart Association, the European Cardiac Arrhythmia Society, the European Heart Rhythm Association, the Society of Thoracic Surgeons, the Asia Pacific Heart Rhythm Society, and the Heart Rhythm Society. Heart Rhythm. 2012; 9(4):632–696.e21

[330] Andreas S, Schulz R, Werner GS, Kreuzer H. Prevalence of obstructive sleep apnoea in patients with coronary artery disease. Coron Artery Dis. 1996; 7(7):541–545

[331] Danzi-Soares NJ, Genta PR, Nerbass FB, et al. Obstructive sleep apnea is common among patients referred for coronary artery bypass grafting and can be diagnosed by portable monitoring. Coron Artery Dis. 2012; 23(1):31–38

[332] Lee CH, Khoo SM, Tai BC, et al. Obstructive sleep apnea in patients admitted for acute myocardial infarction. Prevalence, predictors, and effect on microvascular perfusion. Chest. 2009; 135(6):1488–1495

[333] Mooe T, Rabben T, Wiklund U, Franklin KA, Eriksson P. Sleep-disordered breathing in men with coronary artery disease. Chest. 1996; 109(3):659–663

[334] Mooe T, Rabben T, Wiklund U, Franklin KA, Eriksson P. Sleep-disordered breathing in women: occurrence and association with coronary artery disease. Am J Med. 1996; 101(3):251–256

[335] Nakashima H, Katayama T, Takagi C, et al. Obstructive sleep apnoea inhibits the recovery of left ventricular function in patients with acute myocardial infarction. Eur Heart J. 2006; 27(19):2317–2322

[336] Glantz H, Thunström E, Herlitz J, et al. Occurrence and predictors of obstructive sleep apnea in a revascularized coronary artery disease cohort. Ann Am Thorac Soc. 2013; 10(4):350–356

[337] Yumino D, Tsurumi Y, Takagi A, Suzuki K, Kasanuki H. Impact of obstructive sleep apnea on clinical and angiographic outcomes following percutaneous coronary intervention in patients with acute coronary syndrome. Am J Cardiol. 2007; 99(1):26–30

[338] Im KB, Strader S, Dyken ME. Management of sleep disorders in stroke. Curr Treat Options Neurol. 2010; 12(5):379–395

[339] Dziewas R, Humpert M, Hopmann B, et al. Increased prevalence of sleep apnea in patients with recurring ischemic stroke compared with first stroke victims. J Neurol. 2005; 252(11):1394–1398

[340] Bansal A, Lee-chiong T. Sleep and medical disorders. In: Butkov N, Lee-Chiong T, eds. Fundamentals of Sleep Technology. Philadelphia, PA: Lippincott Williams & Wilkins; 2007;22:186–197

[341] Khawaja IT, Sayyed RT, Jaouni H. Obstructive sleep apnea: an unrecognized but prevalent condition. Compr Ther. 2000; 26(4):294–297

[342] Bottini P, Tantucci C. Sleep apnea syndrome in endocrine diseases. Respiration. 2003; 70(3):320–327

[343] Weiss V, Sonka K, Pretl M, et al. Prevalence of the sleep apnea syndrome in acromegaly population. J Endocrinol Invest. 2000; 23(8):515–519

[344] Bengtsson BA, Brummer RJ, Edén S, Bosaeus I. Body composition in acromegaly. Clin Endocrinol (Oxf). 1989; 30(2):121–130

[345] Isono S, Saeki N, Tanaka A, Nishino T. Collapsibility of passive pharynx in patients with acromegaly. Am J Respir Crit Care Med. 1999; 160(1):64–68

[346] Shipley JE, Schteingart DE, Tandon R, Starkman MN. Sleep architecture and sleep apnea in patients with Cushing's disease. Sleep. 1992; 15(6):514–518

[347] Yanovski JA, Cutler GB Jr. Glucocorticoid action and the clinical features of Cushing's syndrome. Endocrinol Metab Clin North Am. 1994; 23(3):487–509

[348] Rosenow F, McCarthy V, Caruso AC. Sleep apnoea in endocrine diseases. J Sleep Res. 1998; 7(1):3–11

[349] Harris MI, Flegal KM, Cowie CC, et al. Prevalence of diabetes, impaired fasting glucose, and impaired glucose tolerance in U.S. adults. The Third National Health and Nutrition Examination Survey, 1988–1994. Diabetes Care. 1998; 21(4):518–524

[350] West SD, Nicoll DJ, Stradling JR. Prevalence of obstructive sleep apnoea in men with type 2 diabetes. Thorax. 2006; 61(11):945–950

[351] Foster GD, Sanders MH, Millman R, et al. Sleep AHEAD Research Group. Obstructive sleep apnea among obese patients with type 2 diabetes. Diabetes Care. 2009; 32(6):1017–1019

[352] Resnick HE, Jones K, Ruotolo G, et al. Strong Heart Study. Insulin resistance, the metabolic syndrome, and risk of incident cardiovascular disease in nondiabetic american indians: the Strong Heart Study. Diabetes Care. 2003; 26(3):861–867

[353] Babu AR, Herdegen J, Fogelfeld L, Shott S, Mazzone T. Type 2 diabetes, glycemic control, and continuous positive airway pressure in obstructive sleep apnea. Arch Intern Med. 2005; 165(4):447–452

[354] Pallayova M, Donic V, Tomori Z. Beneficial effects of severe sleep apnea therapy on nocturnal glucose control in persons with type 2 diabetes mellitus. Diabetes Res Clin Pract. 2008; 81(1):e8–e11

[355] Ficker JH, Dertinger SH, Siegfried W, et al. Obstructive sleep apnoea and diabetes mellitus: the role of cardiovascular autonomic neuropathy. Eur Respir J. 1998; 11(1):14–19

[356] American Association of clinical endocrinologists medical guidelines for clinical practice for developing a diabetes mellitus comprehensive care plan. Available at: https://www.aace.com/file/dm-guidelines-ccp.pdf. Accessed 10/04/2018

[357] Shaw JE, Punjabi NM, Wilding JP, Alberti KG, Zimmet PZ; International Diabetes Federation Taskforce on Epidemiology and Prevention. Sleep-disordered breathing and type 2 diabetes:

a report from the International Diabetes Federation Taskforce on Epidemiology and Prevention. Diabetes Res Clin Pract. 2008; 81(1):2–12

[358] Park YW, Zhu S, Palaniappan L, Heshka S, Carnethon MR, Heymsfield SB. The metabolic syndrome: prevalence and associated risk factor findings in the US population from the Third National Health and Nutrition Examination Survey, 1988–1994. Arch Intern Med. 2003; 163(4):427–436

[359] Reaven G. Role of insulin resistance in human disease. Banting lecture. Diabetes. 1997; 37(12):1595–1607

[360] DeFronzo RA, Ferrannini E. Insulin resistance. A multifaceted syndrome responsible for NIDDM, obesity, hypertension, dyslipidemia, and atherosclerotic cardiovascular disease. Diabetes Care. 1991; 14(3):173–194

[361] Kahn R, Buse J, Ferrannini E, Stern M; American Diabetes Association. European Association for the Study of Diabetes. The metabolic syndrome: time for a critical appraisal: joint statement from the American Diabetes Association and the European Association for the Study of Diabetes. Diabetes Care. 2005; 28(9):2289–2304

[362] Dorkova Z, Petrasova D, Molcanyiova A, et al. Effects of CPAP on cardiovascular risk profile in patients with severe obstructive sleep apnea and metabolic syndrome. Chest. 2008; 134:686–692

[363] Klink ME, Dodge R, Quan SF. The relation of sleep complaints to respiratory symptoms in a general population. Chest. 1994; 105(1):151–154

[364] Agusti A, Hedner J, Marin JM, Barbé F, Cazzola M, Rennard S. Night-time symptoms: a forgotten dimension of COPD. Eur Respir Rev. 2011; 20(121):183–194

[365] Lee R, McNicholas WT. Obstructive sleep apnea in chronic obstructive pulmonary disease patients. Curr Opin Pulm Med. 2011; 17(2):79–83

[366] McNicholas WT, Verbraecken J, Marin JM. Sleep disorders in chronic obstructive pulmonary disease: the forgotten dimension. Eur Respir Rev. 2013; 22(129):365–375

[367] de Oliveira Rodrigues CJ, Marson O, Tufic S, et al. Relationship among end-stage renal disease, hypertension, and sleep apnea in nondiabetic dialysis patients. Am J Hypertens. 2005; 18(2 Pt 1):152–157

[368] Jean G, Piperno D, François B, Charra B. Sleep apnea incidence in maintenance hemodialysis patients: influence of dialysate buffer. Nephron. 1995; 71(2):138–142

[369] Beecroft JM, Pierratos A, Hanly PJ. Clinical presentation of obstructive sleep apnea in patients with end-stage renal disease. J Clin Sleep Med. 2009; 5(2):115–121

[370] Choi JB, Loredo JS, Norman D, et al. Does obstructive sleep apnea increase hematocrit? Sleep Breath. 2006; 10(3):155–160

[371] Moore-Gillon JC, Treacher DF, Gaminara EJ, Pearson TC, Cameron IR. Intermittent hypoxia in patients with unexplained polycythaemia. Br Med J (Clin Res Ed). 1986; 293(6547):588–590

[372] Carlson JT, Hedner J, Fagerberg B, Ejnell H, Magnusson B, Fyhrquist F. Secondary polycythaemia associated with nocturnal apnoea–a relationship not mediated by erythropoietin? J Intern Med. 1992; 231(4):381–387

[373] Krieger J, Sforza E, Delanoe C, Petiau C. Decrease in haematocrit with continuous positive airway pressure treatment in obstructive sleep apnoea patients. Eur Respir J. 1992; 5(2):228–233

[374] American Academy of Sleep Medicine. Obstructive sleep apnea, adult. In: Sateia M, editor. ICSD-3. Chicago, IL: AASM; 2014

[375] Dempsey JA, Xie A, Patz DS, Wang D. Physiology in medicine: obstructive sleep apnea pathogenesis and treatment–considerations beyond airway anatomy. J Appl Physiol (1985). 2014; 116(1):3–12

[376] Hudgel DW, Hendricks C. Palate and hypopharynx–sites of inspiratory narrowing of the upper airway during sleep. Am Rev Respir Dis. 1988; 138(6):1542–1547

[377] Remmers JE, deGroot WJ, Sauerland EK, Anch AM. Pathogenesis of upper airway occlusion during sleep. J Appl Physiol. 1978; 44(6):931–938

[378] Vincken W, Guilleminault C, Silvestri L, Cosio M, Grassino A. Inspiratory muscle activity as a trigger causing the airways to open in obstructive sleep apnea. Am Rev Respir Dis. 1987; 135(2):372–377

[379] Mezzanotte WS, Tangel DJ, White DP. Waking genioglossal electromyogram in sleep apnea patients versus normal controls (a neuromuscular compensatory mechanism). J Clin Invest. 1992; 89(5):1571–1579

[380] Smith PL, Wise RA, Gold AR, Schwartz AR, Permutt S. Upper airway pressure-flow relationships in obstructive sleep apnea. J Appl Physiol (1985). 1988; 64(2):789–795

[381] Eckert DJ, White DP, Jordan AS, Malhotra A, Wellman A. Defining phenotypic causes of obstructive sleep apnea. Identification of novel therapeutic targets. Am J Respir Crit Care Med. 2013; 188(8):996–1004

[382] Watanabe T, Isono S, Tanaka A, Tanzawa H, Nishino T. Contribution of body habitus and craniofacial characteristics to segmental closing pressures of the passive pharynx in patients with sleep-disordered breathing. Am J Respir Crit Care Med. 2002; 165(2):260–265

[383] Neelapu BC, Kharbanda OP, Sardana HK, et al. Craniofacial and upper airway morphology in adult obstructive sleep apnea patients: A systematic review and meta-analysis of cephalometric studies. Sleep Med Rev. 2017; 31:79–90

[384] Schwab RJ, Pasirstein M, Pierson R, et al. Identification of upper airway anatomic risk factors for obstructive sleep apnea with volumetric magnetic resonance imaging. Am J Respir Crit Care Med. 2003; 168(5):522–530

[385] Schellenberg JB, Maislin G, Schwab RJ. Physical findings and the risk for obstructive sleep apnea. The importance of oropharyngeal structures. Am J Respir Crit Care Med. 2000; 162(2 Pt 1):740–748

[386] Marcus CL. Tonsillectomy for short-term benefit in obstructive sleep-disordered breathing. J Pediatr. 2017; 186:209–212

[387] Xavier SD, Bussoloti IF, Müller H. Macroglossia secondary to systemic amyloidosis: case report and literature review. Ear Nose Throat J. 2005; 84(6):358–361

[388] Wittmann AL. Macroglossia in acromegaly and hypothyroidism. Virchows Arch A Pathol Anat Histol. 1977; 373(4):353–360

[389] Guimaraes CV, Donnelly LF, Shott SR, Amin RS, Kalra M. Relative rather than absolute macroglossia in patients with Down syndrome: implications for treatment of obstructive sleep apnea. Pediatr Radiol. 2008; 38(10):1062–1067

[390] Gunawardena I, Robinson S, MacKay S, et al. Submucosal lingualplasty for adult obstructive sleep apnea. Otolaryngol Head Neck Surg. 2013; 148(1):157–165

[391] Nuckton TJ, Glidden DV, Browner WS, Claman DM. Physical examination: Mallampati score as an independent predictor of obstructive sleep apnea. Sleep. 2006; 29(7):903–908

[392] Friedman M, Hamilton C, Samuelson CG, Lundgren ME, Pott T. Diagnostic value of the Friedman tongue position and Mallampati classification for obstructive sleep apnea: a meta-analysis. Otolaryngol Head Neck Surg. 2013; 148(4):540–547

[393] Kumar DS, Valenzuela D, Kozak FK, et al. The reliability of clinical tonsil size grading in children. JAMA Otolaryngol Head Neck Surg. 2014; 140(11):1034–1037

[394] Newman AB, Foster G, Givelber R, Nieto FJ, Redline S, Young T. Progression and regression of sleep-disordered breathing with changes in weight: the Sleep Heart Health Study. Arch Intern Med. 2005; 165(20):2408–2413

[395] Nashi N, Kang S, Barkdull GC, Lucas J, Davidson TM. Lingual fat at autopsy. Laryngoscope. 2007; 117(8):1467–1473

[396] Van de Graaff WB. Thoracic influence on upper airway patency. J Appl Physiol (1985). 1988; 65(5):2124–2131

[397] Van de Graaff WB. Thoracic traction on the trachea: mechanisms and magnitude. J Appl Physiol (1985). 1991; 70(3):1328–1336

[398] Schwartz AR, Smith PL, Schneider H, Patil SP, Kirkness JP. Invited editorial on "lung volume and upper airway collapsibility: what does it tell us about pathogenic mechanisms?". J Appl Physiol (1985). 2012; 113(5):689–690

[399] Squier SB, Patil SP, Schneider H, Kirkness JP, Smith PL, Schwartz AR. Effect of end-expiratory lung volume on upper airway collapsibility in sleeping men and women. J Appl Physiol (1985). 2010; 109(4):977–985

[400] Heinzer RC, Stanchina ML, Malhotra A, et al. Effect of increased lung volume on sleep disordered breathing in patients with sleep apnoea. Thorax. 2006; 61(5):435–439

[401] Redolfi S, Yumino D, Ruttanaumpawan P, et al. Relationship between overnight rostral fluid shift and obstructive sleep apnea in nonobese men. Am J Respir Crit Care Med. 2009; 179(3):241–246

[402] White LH, Bradley TD. Role of nocturnal rostral fluid shift in the pathogenesis of obstructive and central sleep apnoea. J Physiol. 2013; 591(5):1179–1193

[403] Younes M. Contributions of upper airway mechanics and control mechanisms to severity of obstructive apnea. Am J Respir Crit Care Med. 2003; 168(6):645–658

[404] Isono S, Remmers JE, Tanaka A, Sho Y, Sato J, Nishino T. Anatomy of pharynx in patients with obstructive sleep apnea and in normal subjects. J Appl Physiol (1985). 1997; 82(4):1319–1326

[405] Gleeson K, Zwillich CW, White DP. The influence of increasing ventilatory effort on arousal from sleep. Am Rev Respir Dis. 1990; 142(2):295–300

[406] Parthasarathy S. Emergence of obstructive sleep apnea phenotyping. From weak to strong! Am J Respir Crit Care Med. 2013; 188(8):898–900

[407] Joosten SA, Leong P, Landry SA, et al. Loop gain predicts the response to upper airway surgery in patients with obstructive sleep apnoea: Ventilatory control abnormalities predict surgical responsiveness. Sleep. 2017

[408] Joosten SA, O'Driscoll DM, Berger PJ, Hamilton GS. Supine position related obstructive sleep apnea in adults: pathogenesis and treatment. Sleep Med Rev. 2014; 18(1):7–17

[409] Joosten SA, Edwards BA, Wellman A, et al. The effect of body position on physiological factors that contribute to obstructive sleep apnea. Sleep. 2015; 38(9):1469–1478

[410] Bignold JJ, Mercer JD, Antic NA, McEvoy RD, Catcheside PG. Accurate position monitoring and improved supine-dependent obstructive sleep apnea with a new position recording and supine avoidance device. J Clin Sleep Med. 2011; 7(4):376–383

[411] Eijsvogel MM, Ubbink R, Dekker J, et al. Sleep position trainer versus tennis ball technique in positional obstructive sleep apnea syndrome. J Clin Sleep Med. 2015; 11(2):139–147

[412] van Maanen JP, Meester KA, Dun LN, et al. The sleep position trainer: a new treatment for positional obstructive sleep apnoea. Sleep Breath. 2013; 17(2):771–779

[413] van Maanen JP, de Vries N. Long-term effectiveness and compliance of positional therapy with the sleep position trainer in the treatment of positional obstructive sleep apnea syndrome. Sleep. 2014; 37(7):1209–1215

[414] Benoist L, de Ruiter M, de Lange J, de Vries N. A randomized, controlled trial of positional therapy versus oral appliance therapy for position-dependent sleep apnea. Sleep Med. 2017; 34:109–117

[415] Ravesloot MJ, van Maanen JP, Dun L, de Vries N. The undervalued potential of positional therapy in position-dependent snoring and obstructive sleep apnea-a review of the literature. Sleep Breath. 2013; 17(1):39–49

[416] Oksenberg A, Silverberg DS, Arons E, Radwan H. Positional vs nonpositional obstructive sleep apnea patients: anthropomorphic, nocturnal polysomnographic, and multiple sleep latency test data. Chest. 1997; 112(3):629–639

[417] Richard W, Kox D, den Herder C, Laman M, van Tinteren H, de Vries N. The role of sleep position in obstructive sleep apnea syndrome. Eur Arch Otorhinolaryngol. 2006; 263(10):946–950

[418] Mador MJ, Kufel TJ, Magalang UJ, Rajesh SK, Watwe V, Grant BJ. Prevalence of positional sleep apnea in patients undergoing polysomnography. Chest. 2005; 128(4):2130–2137

[419] Benoist LB, Verhagen M, Torensma B, van Maanen JP, de Vries N. Positional therapy in patients with residual positional obstructive sleep apnea after upper airway surgery. Sleep Breath. 2016

[420] Dieltjens M, Vroegop AV, Verbruggen AE, et al. A promising concept of combination therapy for positional obstructive sleep apnea. Sleep Breath. 2015; 19(2):637–644

[421] Morong S, Benoist LB, Ravesloot MJ, Laman DM, de Vries N. The effect of weight loss on OSA severity and position dependence in the bariatric population. Sleep Breath. 2014; 18(4):851–856

3 Diagnosis of Sleep-Disordered Breathing

Abstract

This chapter focuses on the workup of a patient with sleep-disordered breathing. As in all domains of medicine, the workup starts with the medical history (anamnesis). Clinical evaluation includes a general as well as an OSA-specific evaluation, evaluation of the mouth and upper airway. Next, a sleep study is needed. There are several forms of sleep studies, all with their own pros and cons. They can be performed in the sleep lab as well as at home. After the sleep study, a differential diagnosis can be established. In case treatment other than CPAP is considered, a sleep study is often not sufficient for definitive treatment planning. Clinical investigations also include questionnaires. For sleep surgeons specifically, an insight of awake endoscopy, Müller's maneuver, and drug-induced sleep endoscopy (DISE) is pivotal. To score DISE findings, several systems have been proposed. The VOTE system is the mostly wide used system and is discussed in detail, with regards to organization, logistics and staff, indication, patient selection, sedation protocol, and how to translate the various findings into treatment planning.

Keywords: OSA, history, evaluation, sleep study, questionnaires, DISE, VOTE, SDB clinical evaluation, upper airway evaluation, awake nasopharyngoscopy, Müller's maneuver

3.1 History Taking

Nico de Vries and Thomas Verse

The medical history, as in all domains of medicine, is always pivotal and determines the level of suspicion in obstructive sleep apnea (OSA) to a large extent. Although the most striking features of the history as socially unacceptable snoring and witnessed apneic events are already often known from the referral letter from the general physician, it remains important to have a preferably standardized comprehensive own assessment.

It is beneficial if the bed partner accompanies the patient to double check the complaints. It is not unusual if the complaints noticed by the bed partner and the complaints reported by the patient vary considerably, where the bed partner often scores a twice as high severity. For example, the irritability, length and loudness of snoring, and the presence and length of apneas are best noticed by the bed partner. The position also influences the sleep: are the snoring and apneic events present in all sleep positions, or are they only present or more pronounced in supine position? In particular men are inclined to downgrade their snoring level in particular and severity of complaints in general. For surgical purposes it has been strongly recommended to let the bed partner score his/her grade of being disturbed by his/her bed partner's snoring. For this grading a 10-point visual analogue (VAS) scale is used. VAS grading provides the possibility of comparing pre- and postoperative results, providing the fact, that the patient still has the same bed partner. We all know that the annoyance of snoring depends on the particular individual. Another fact that needs to be kept in mind is that most patients are compelled by their bed partners to undergo painful surgical treatment for snoring, else they would get expelled from the joint bedroom. After a painful palatal surgery we ask the bed partner in presence of the patient about the success. This often affects the answers, resulting in a lower postoperative VAS score. Maybe this is why many scientific papers present highly significant VAS scores about snoring intensity. However, VAS provides a quick and easy-to-perform instrument to measure surgical success.

Many sleep clinics routinely use specific questionnaires regarding sleepiness and different levels of quality of life (QoL) such as the Epworth Sleepiness Scale (ESS)[1] and Functional Outcomes of Sleep Questionnaire (FOSQ).[2] ▶Table 3.1 summarizes the recently used QoL test instruments in sleep surgery. It should be considered that patients filled in these questionnaires electronically in soft copy before the first clinic visit so that

▶Table 3.1 Quality-of-life instruments recently used in sleep surgery

Instrument	Level	Target	Number of items
SF-36[3]	Health-related	General health	36
FOSQ[2]	Disease-specific	Sleep quality	10–30
PQSI[4]	Disease-specific	Sleep quality and disturbances over the past several months	17
SOS[5]	Disease-specific	Snoring	8
ESS[1]	Symptom-related	Daytime sleepiness	8
NOSE[7]	Symptom-related	Nasal obstruction	7
SCL-90[8]	Symptom-related	Psychological disturbances for the past 7 days	9

Abbreviations: ESS, Epworth Sleepiness Scale; FOSQ, Functional Outcome of Sleep Questionnaire; NOSE, Nasal Obstruction Symptom Evaluation; PQSI, Pittsburgh Sleep Quality Index; SF-36, Short-Form 36; SOS, Snore Outcome Survey; SSI, Snore Symptom Inventory; SCL-90, Symptom Checklist-90.

their responses can be recorded in electronic files. This system of electronic data collection before the actual visit works only if patients have access to Internet and have no language barriers. As an alternative, patients and bed partners may fill in these questionnaires in the waiting room before meeting the physician. Based on the level of suspicion, a first triage for further diagnostics can be considered, for example, in case of high pretest likelihood of OSA only polygraphy might be ordered first, while in case of lower levels of suspicion, full polysomnography should be considered. It has been noted from the earlier studies that more than 50% of patients visiting sleep centers because of severe snoring and possible OSA, had confirmation of OSA in the sleep registration. Sometimes the history makes OSA less likely (such as in case of tiredness in young lean individuals, no history of snoring, etc.) and no sleep study is performed, or, in case of suspicion of narcolepsy, another form of sleep study is ordered.

It is important to realize that the medical history obtained either from the patient or as noted by the bed partner is far from a 100% reliable positive or negative predictor of the presence of OSA. The possibility of OSA cannot be ruled out if the bed partner does not notice apneic events. In particular, hypopneas (and respiratory-related arousals) can easily be missed. The bed partner is not awake during the night and has no information about the various sleep stages and sleep positions or combinations of sleep stage and sleep position. Bed partners may provide a proof of OSA through video recordings; however, subsequent confirmation by a sleep study is mandatory. Oftentimes the reverse also happens where the medical history told by patient and bed partner makes the presence of witnessed apneas possible, but the subsequent sleep study does not confirm sufficient hypopneic and apneic events to establish the diagnosis.

Nowadays there are various applications that promise to analyze sleep; however, all of them are not validated and require verification by sleep studies.

Many patients do not have the full-blown syndrome of socially unacceptable snoring, witnessed apneas, extreme tiredness, and hypersomnolence. This is in particular true for early stage disease, mild and moderate OSA; but even in case of severe OSA, and in case of apnea–hypopnea index (AHI) above 60, patients might experience remarkably little complaints. Others such as professional drivers, who are concerned about their permission to drive, might deliberately minimize their complaints of sleepiness. Therefore sleep studies remain the gold standard to confirm the clinical suspicion of OSA.

Signs and symptoms that should be included in (electronic) checklists can be divided into complaints during wakefulness (▶ Table 3.2) and during sleep (▶ Table 3.3).

Socially unacceptable loud snoring is the most suspicious alarming symptom, but apneas and hypopneas are also very ominous signs but not always noticed. In particular, nycturia is typical for OSA. It is due to a lack of sufficient deep sleep.

Sleepiness and never feeling rested after sleep are suspicious symptoms. Many other signs and symptoms during the day are atypical and might be due to other causes as well. This is one of the reasons that the diagnosis of OSA is often missed, or patients are misdiagnosed as having a depression or burnout. OSA is a gradual progressive disease and many complaints might gradually become worse if OSA is left untreated. A subtle change in character may be noticed by partners, family members, or colleagues; for example, irritability, loss of focus, and less intellectual and sexual performance. These symptoms are often attributed to increasing age and social issues, while they in fact are due to the development of OSA. In retrospect many patients have had complaints for several years before the diagnosis is established. It is the combination of nocturnal symptoms with signs occurring during the day that should lead to the suspicion of OSA.

Daytime sleepiness is mostly scored by means of ESS (▶ Table 3.4).

The ESS consists of eight questions with four answer categories. Scores vary from 0 (never, or not applicable), 1 (sometimes), 2 (usually), to 3 (always). The maximum score is 24, and a score of 10 or more is regarded as abnormal. The average score in healthy people is around 6. It is clear that the positive and negative predictive values of the ESS are moderate, but it does give a first indication of the level of sleepiness. One should be aware of its limitations; for example, patients who do not drive a motor vehicle or have never visited a theatre or meeting cannot

▶ Table 3.2 Signs and symptoms during wakefulness

Sleepiness
Falls asleep easily
Tiredness
Painful muscles and joints
Loss of concentration/focus
Difficulty with staying awake when driving
Lack of energy
Painful feeling in the chest
Easily irritated
Decreased memory and cognitive functioning

▶ Table 3.3 Signs and symptoms during sleep

Severe snoring
Witnessed apneic events by patient or bed partner
Awakenings with feeling of choking
Decreased sexual performance and/or impotence
Transpiration during sleep
Nycturia
Dry mouth after awakening
Morning headache

▶ Table 3.4 Epworth Sleepiness Scale

Situation	0	1	2	3
Sit and read				
Watching television				
In a theatre or meeting				
As passenger in a car during a hour without pause				
Resting during the afternoon				
Sitting and having a conversation				
After dinner without alcohol				
In a car, before a traffic light waiting				
Total score				

reach maximal high scores. With all its limitations, the ESS is still often used in the clinical setting as well as in research projects.

Other questions that should be included concern sleep hygiene and rhythm, lifestyle, alcohol consumption and smoking, medication, and weight loss and weight gain. In case of work shifts, irregular working hours, other sleeping disorders, and too little sleeping hours might be present. Some patients have more than one reason for being sleepy. Alcohol consumption before bedtime induces muscle relaxation and thereby OSA. Smoking is thought to induce edema of the upper airway and is regarded as a cofactor. Its role is not as important as alcohol consumption. Medication, such as sleeping pills and muscle relaxants, should be asked for while taking medical history.

In the authors' opinion, it is very important to collect the biometric data of each patient such as patient's weight (and height for calculation of body mass index [BMI]) and history of recent weight gain. Weight gain might lead to the development or worsening of OSA, but the reverse should also be considered: OSA might lead to weight gain.

In authors' opinion, patients should be asked about their sleep habits before treatment. Do the patient and his/her bed partner still sleep together or does the bed partner go to bed earlier to avoid not being able to fall asleep because of the loud snoring? Does the bed partner use ear plugs, or is sleeping together no longer possible at all? Do other family members complain? How is the sleep in hotels, on camping grounds, and in airplanes? Does the snoring wake up the patient? How do the complaints exist? Are the complaints always present or present in specific situations and circumstances? Are the complaints due to specific sleeping positions (mostly supine) or present in all sleeping positions? Is the patient forced to sleep on the back because of specific medical conditions such as hip, back, or shoulder complaints?

Another crucial issue is to record patient's comorbidities. The patient's health condition is relevant to decide, whether the patient may undergo a surgical treatment, and how to organize the perioperative care (please refer to Chapter 10 for more details). Please check for high blood pressure.

Patients should be asked about other sleep disturbances. OSA is only 1 out of about 80 diseases that may cause restless sleep. One should refer to the International Classification of Sleep Disorders (ICSD, Quelle), that is updated by the American Academy of Sleep Disorders every few years. Is the patient less focused, does he/she experience loss of concentration, less intellectual performance, mood changes, transpiration during sleep with several awakenings for urinating during the night, does the patient have a dry mouth when waking up, doe he/she has a morning headache, does he/she feel refreshed/rested after sleep at all? Is the patient less alert, irritable, and depressive? Has the sexual performance deteriorated or is there overt sexual impotence?

It is important to know if there is a history of teeth grinding (bruxism?) or other oral diseases to consider treatment options. This fact might interfere with an oral appliance treatment.

Another crucial thing to know is what has already been done to treat the patient's OSA or snoring. Has the patient had other previous attempts to treat the snoring and OSA complaints, such as attempts to improve nasal breathing either by means of medication or surgery? Are the complaints worse in case of blocked nose as because of hay fever, seasonal rhinitis, other allergies, during common colds, or because of nasal polyps, or anatomical reasons such as septal deviation or hypertrophic inferior turbinates. In case of nasal pathology, specific questionnaire for nasal pathologies, such as the Nose Obstruction Symptom Evaluation (NOSE) might be helpful.[4] Have there been any attempts to solve the snoring problem either with over-the-counter antisnoring measures, of boil and bite or custom-made oral devices; have there been previous sleep studies, sleep surgery, CPAP use?

The variety of questions addressed in previous sections makes us think that every sleep surgery center should use a comprehensive and surgery-specific OSA questionnaire. Unfortunately there is no standard questionnaire, which means that every center should create its own. In authors' opinion, the questionnaire should at least include biometric data, questions about sleep habits, comorbidities, dental health, and past sleep-related treatments.

The authors expect that smartphone applications will gain relevance within the next couple of years. Earlier they did not enter daily routine.

3.1.1 Conclusion

The medical history determines the level of suspicion in OSA to a large extent. The most striking features of the history are socially unacceptable snoring and witnessed apneic events, but there are many nocturnal and wakeful signs and symptoms that can be attributed to OSA as well. The use of standardized comprehensive OSA-specific questionnaires is strongly recommended.

3.2 Clinical Evaluation of Patients with (Suspected) Sleep-Disordered Breathing

Marina Carrasco-Llatas and Nico de Vries

3.2.1 Introduction

Physical and clinical evaluations are essential for the assessment of the patient with SDB. The findings contribute to the treatment advice to the patient. The doctor and patient can only take a shared decision about a treatment plan after all information has been obtained about the severity (mild, moderate, severe) and the type (obstructive, mixed, central) of the OSA. As obstruction is almost always in the upper airway, level(s), severity, and configuration (or direction) of the obstruction(s) are also analyzed. OSA, the most common type of SDB, is a complex syndrome due to many different factors, both anatomical and functional. It can originate from different and multiple segments of the upper airway; therefore, the entire upper airway from the entrance of the nose to the level of the vocal cords should be examined during the evaluation.

An ideal clinical evaluation would be predictive of the site(s) of obstruction and would be cost effective and reproducible. Unfortunately, clinical evaluation is subjective and it is usually performed while awake, which does not represent the situation when asleep. While it provides valuable information in a glance, some general anatomical facts can be easily obtained (e.g., an edentulous patient will not be treated with a mandibular advancement device [MAD], patients with a high body mass index [BMI] are not the best surgical candidates, the combination of large tonsils and small tongue is more attractive from a surgical point of view than vice versa). General ear, nose, and throat (ENT) examination in awake situation is not the preferred workup for a patient in whom surgery is considered. In this chapter OSA-specific ENT examination, as performed in the examination room, is discussed keeping its reservations and limitations in mind.

3.2.2 Anamnesis

A thorough medical history is essential. The use of standardized OSA-specific questionnaires, to be filled in by the patient and bed partner, can be extremely helpful in this regard. Questions should include snoring (frequency, loudness, sleep position), witnessed apneas, sleepiness, tiredness, morning headache, character changes, sexual dysfunction, etc. Often, these questions are better answered by the bed partner. Bed partners can provide information about witnessed apneas and sleep characteristics.

There is also a need to collect data on the surgical history, specially related to the upper airway (e.g., previous tonsillectomy, nasal surgery, etc.) including orthodontic treatment, tobacco and alcohol consumption, as well as comorbidities that can increase cardiovascular risk (hypertension, dyslipidemia, diabetes, arrhythmias, previous stroke) and the use of medication that could alter sleep or decrease upper airway muscle tone while sleeping (sedatives, muscle relaxants, sleeping medication). Family history of snoring and sleep apnea should be evaluated as well, as there might be familial aggregation.

Sleep habits, shift-work, driving performance, occupation of the patient, and questions related to sleep quality and fatigue/sleepiness are also mandatory. The ESS, a self-administered questionnaire consisting eight questions (▶Table 3.5), is the most common scale used to assess sleepiness. The patient scores from 0 to 3 depending on the chance of dozing. A score of more than 10 is considered excessive daytime sleepiness. OSA is not the only cause of sleepiness: sleep deprivation, shift-work, occupation, and lifestyle are also common factors. Although not every patient with OSA is sleepy, and sleepiness is not related to the severity of sleep apnea, if present, it is one of the symptoms that usually improve in case of successful treatment.

Questions about quality of life (QoL) should be included as well. Snoring, sleepiness, and QoL scales help monitor any improvement in the patient after treatment.

3.2.3 General Evaluation

As in all diseases, after taking the history, a clinical evaluation follows. OSA-specific examination differs from standard ENT examination. It is essential that the exploration is systematic and that one pays attention to all the details.

It starts with the general aspect of the patient. Males have a higher probability of suffering from OSA than females. The male:female ratio is approximately 2:1. Prevalence increases with BMI.[9] Height, weight, and BMI (measured as weight in kilogram divided by height squared in meters) are essential. Neck circumference is related to the probability of having OSA. There are increased chances of having OSA if neck circumference is more than 42 cm in men and more than 37 cm in women.

Some studies suggest that neck–height ratio correlates better with AHI than BMI.[10,11] Fat deposition both around the pharynx and within upper airway dilator muscles, such as the genioglossus, decreases airway lumen size and causes detrimental changes to upper airway muscle function. Abdominal obesity compresses the abdomen and thoracic cavities, reducing lung volume and possibly causing rostral shifting of the diaphragm, which reduces tracheal tension and thus impairs pharyngeal mechanism. Therefore, fat deposition around the pharynx and trunk both increase airway collapsibility.[12]

Face profile may indicate box problems. A person has retrognathia if the menton is more than 2 mm behind the vertical line that starts at the anterior nasal spine. A patient with a long face, also called dolichofacial, will also have a smaller upper airway. In such patients activation of the genioglossus muscle during sleep after apneic or hypopneic events will not widen the lumen of the upper airway as compared with patients having a wide face. (▶Fig. 3.1) A lower position of the hyoid bone will lead to a longer upper airway that is more collapsible than a shorter one.

3.2.4 Upper Airway Evaluation

A systematic upper airway evaluation starts with examination of the nose. Most of the resistance in the upper airway is generated in this area. One looks for nasal valve collapse, septal deviation, possible septal perforation, synechiae, hypertrophy of the inferior turbinates, a concha media bullosa, mucosal swelling due to allergy or aspecific hypersensitivity, nasal polyps, and hypertrophy of the adenoid. Although correction of decreased nasal breathing, either medically or surgically, might

▶Table 3.5 Epworth Sleepiness Scale[a]

Situations	0 Never doze	1 Slight chance of dozing	2 Moderate chance of dozing	3 High chance of dozing
Sitting and reading				
Watching television				
Sitting inactive in a public place (theater, meeting)				
As a passenger in a car for 1 h without break				
Lying down to rest in the afternoon				
Sitting and talking to someone				
Sitting quickly after lunch (without alcohol)				
In a car while stopped in a traffic				

[a]Patients are asked to grade from 0 to 3 their likelihood of falling sleep in contrast to just feeling tired in certain situations. The total score will be between 0 and 24.

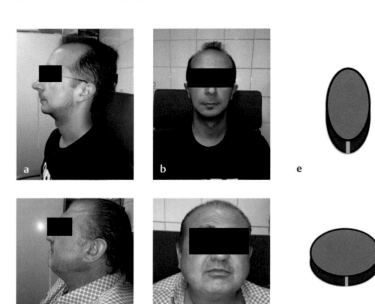

Fig. 3.1 The pictures show two different OSAS patients. (a, b) Patient with a long face and retrognathia (vertical line is drawn for better visualization).
(c, d) Obese patient, without significant craniofacial problems. (e, f) Circles represent the UA of a patient with a long face and a wide face, when there is an obstruction and genioglossus muscle is activated, the patient with a wide face will have a bigger UA due to the inherent morphology of the UA. The line represents the same movement of the genioglossus muscle.

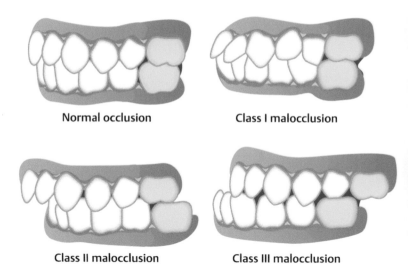

Normal occlusion   Class I malocclusion

Class II malocclusion   Class III malocclusion

Fig. 3.2 Angle's occlusion classification.

improve quality of sleep, it will usually not lead to a significant improvement of the AHI or other sleep-study parameters. A patent nose might also improve CPAP and MAD adherence. Surgery of the nose is very rarely the first-line treatment in OSA. The role of the nose in OSA is less important than previously thought. That said, an obstructed nose should be fixed; although one should not expect a resolution of the snoring or apneas, it is true that SDB will be cured in some rare cases. Please refer to Chapter 7.2 for more information.

Subsequently, the surgeon should examine the patient's mouth to assess the dental status. Gums and teeth should be checked. Occlusion is classified with Angle's classification (▶Fig. 3.2). Type 2 occlusion is often linked to retrognathia and denotes a smaller upper airway at the level of the tongue base. Type 3 patients are not good candidates for treatment with a MAD (see Chapter 4). In order to use an MAD, the gums and teeth must be in good condition. Surgeons should also check the maximum mouth opening. If it is limited then problems may arise during intubation and surgery. For example, if a patient cannot open his/her mouth, then it is best to use the laser for lingual tonsillectomy instead of the coblator. Sometimes it is better to intubate nasally.

The hard palate can be narrow. This is frequently seen in people with a history of oral breathing during childhood and will lead to a narrow upper airway and a long palate. This might have consequences for performing surgery. One can suspect a narrow palate if the patient has a long face.

Presence of crowded teeth can make the surgeons think about a small box problem. If the tongue has edge crenations (▶Fig. 3.3) caused by teeth pressure, this can be related to a small box, a (relative) macroglossia (big tongue), or both. The presence of these tongue crenations has been related to presence of obstructive sleep apnea syndrome (OSAS).[13]

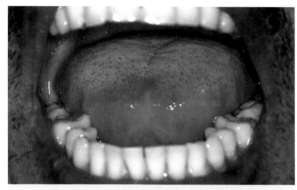

Fig. 3.3 Edge crenations in the lateral sides of the tongue: the tongue is too wide.

The relative position of the palate and the tongue can be assessed using two scales: the Mallampati classification (▶Fig. 3.4) and Friedman palate classification, previously called modified Mallampati index (MMI) (▶Fig. 3.5). The patient is asked to breathe through the nose to avoid elevation of the palate that would decrease the degree. In the Mallampati classification, the patient is asked to protrude the tongue, whereas in the Friedman classification, the tongue has to stay inside the mouth without elevating it and without depressing it with a tongue spatula. Therefore, both classifications are not equal and might have a different degree.

The Friedman staging system is a combination of two classifications and BMI (▶Table 3.6). One classification is the MMI; the other is the tonsil hypertrophy classification from 0 (if a previous tonsillectomy was performed) to 4 (kissing tonsils touching in the midline) (▶Fig. 3.4, ▶Fig. 3.5, ▶Fig. 3.6, ▶Fig. 3.7).

Stage 1 is any patient with big tonsils (grade 3 and 4) and a small tongue (grade 1 or 2). In this type of patients,

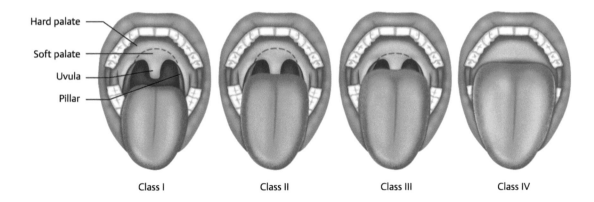

Hard palate
Soft palate
Uvula
Pillar

Class I   Class II   Class III   Class IV

Fig. 3.4 Mallampati classification.

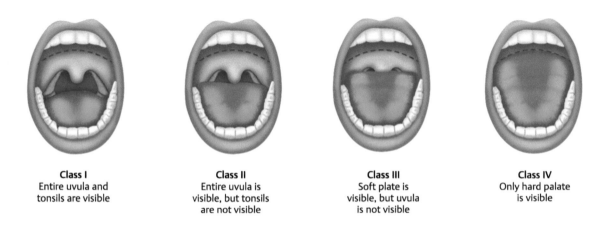

Class I
Entire uvula and
tonsils are visible

Class II
Entire uvula is
visible, but tonsils
are not visible

Class III
Soft plate is
visible, but uvula
is not visible

Class IV
Only hard palate
is visible

Fig. 3.5 Modified Mallampati index.

▶ **Table 3.6** Friedman Staging System

Stage	MMI	Tonsil size	BMI
Stage I	1	3–4	<40
	2	3–4	
Stage 2	1–2	1–2	<40
	3–4	3–4	
Stage 3	3–4	0,1,2	<40
Stage 4	1,2,3,4	0,1,2,3,4	>40
All patients with significant craniofacial or other anatomic deformities			

Abbreviations: BMI, body mass index; MMI, modified Mallampati index.

which occurs in less than 15% of patients with OSA,[14] surgical success of uvulopalatopharyngoplasty (UPPP) assessed by Sher's criteria (AHI <20, and more reduction of the AHI >50%) is more than 80%.[7] Patients categorized in stage 2 share two characteristics: big tonsils with big tongues or small tonsils with small tongues. In this group, 40% of the patients achieve success after UPPP. Stage 3 patients have a big tongue and small tonsils or tonsillectomies and UPPP success is 8%.[15] Stage 4 is for patients with a BMI greater than 40 or with craniofacial deformities

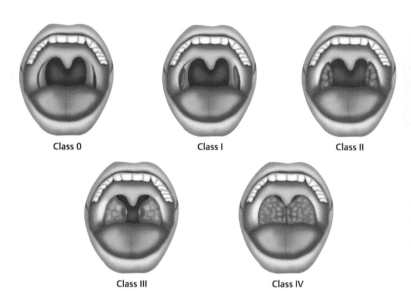

Fig. 3.6 Tonsil size classification.

Class 0 Class I Class II

Class III Class IV

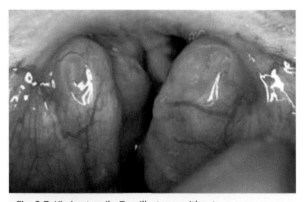

Fig. 3.7 Kissing tonsils: Tonsillectomy without uvulopalatopharyngoplasty (UPPP) might be sufficient.

such as severe retrognathia. Surgery is not recommended for stage 4 patients. In a later study, Friedman reported higher surgical success rates, performing tongue base surgery, especially in stage 2 patients but not in stage 3.[16]

Although earlier studies have given first information about which patients are suitable for sleep surgery, there are some serious concerns about the use of these forms of clinical examination in an awake situation. The authors are concerned whether the clinical assessment alone in an awake situation is sufficient for a careful surgical planning or not. Some of the concerns and limitations are discussed further.

3.2.5 Limitations

First, stage 1 patients can be cured with a simple tonsillectomy without performing UPPP. To the best of our knowledge, there are no studies comparing tonsillectomy with tonsillectomy and UPPP, but there is a meta-analysis showing that tonsillectomy alone can be useful.[17]

Second, in these studies, classical UPPP or Friedman's Z-palatoplasty was performed. There are studies suggesting that more recent pharyngeal techniques addressing the lateral pharyngeal walls in a different way have better surgical results.[18,19] These new techniques are discussed in Chapter 8.

Third, the tongue base surgery performed was interstitial radiofrequency treatment (RFT). RFT turned out to be less effective in reducing the AHI. Nowadays, with the use of new technologies, such as coblation, midline glossectomy, or submucosal minimally invasive lingual excision (SMILE), results are better in patients with grade 3 or 4 Mallampati.[20,21,22]

Besides, although Friedman argues that by using his classification, there is less subjectivity and a good agreement in classifying patients; however, in authors' experience, patients often unintentionally elevate the tongue when they are asked to open their mouth. The size of the tongue can thus be overestimated, while the contrary also happens. The patient might depress the tongue leading to underestimation of its size. This experience has been recently corroborated by Sundman et al.[23] They recruited 4 ENT specialists and 11 ENT residents who scored themselves and there were 210 observations. The median kappa was 0.36 (first and third quartile, 0.23 and 0.42), corresponding to only a slight agreement. This study concluded that the Friedman tongue position demonstrated only a slight inter-examiner agreement among 15 medical doctors, indicating that the method is difficult to perform and could be an uncertain method to select patients for UPPP.

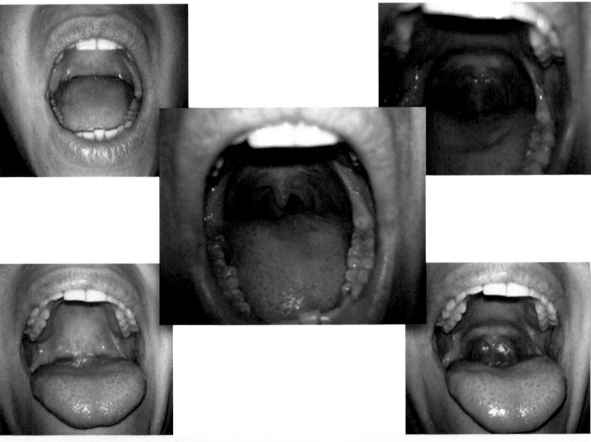

Fig. 3.8 Same individual presenting different "tongue sizes."

For demonstration purposes, an example of the same individual is shown (▶ Fig. 3.8), in which all four stages are demonstrated depending on the tongue and palate position.

Moreover, a higher MMI does not always imply more collapse at the tongue base during sedation or natural sleep.[16,17,18,19,24,25,26,27] A big tongue can push the palate against the posterior wall causing a retropalatal obstruction. Small tongues can have retroglossal collapse due to lingual tonsil hypertrophy or loss of muscle tone. This has been discussed in other sections of this chapter (see Chapter 3.4.2).

In both the Friedman and Mallampati classifications the shape, position, and length of palate and uvula are not further specified. In authors' view this is another important limitation of both systems.

▶ Fig. 3.9 shows a "normal" palate. Although a clear consensus is lacking on the definition of the normal palate. If the length of the uvula is less than 15 mm and the width is less than 10 mm, the palate is considered normal.

In contrast, ▶ Fig. 3.10 shows a long palate and uvula.

▶ Fig. 3.11 shows examples of isolated long uvulae (uvula elongata), whereas ▶ Fig. 3.12 shows a uvula which is both wide and long.

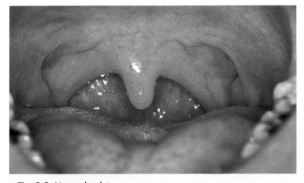

Fig. 3.9 Normal palate.

The mildest form of cleft palate, uvula bifida (▶ Fig. 3.13), has been occasionally seen as well. Palatal surgery has the risk of velopharyngeal insufficiency and rhinolalia aperta.

In the Middle East and North Africa, there is a traditional practice to remove uvula soon after the birth of a child (ritual uvulectomy, ▶ Fig. 3.14). This intervention is thought to protect against throat disease.[27] This

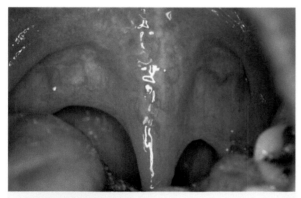

Fig. 3.10 Long palate and uvula.

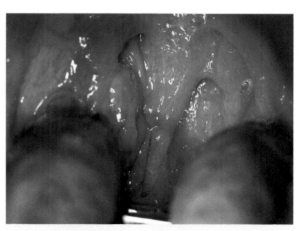

Fig. 3.11 Uvula elongate.

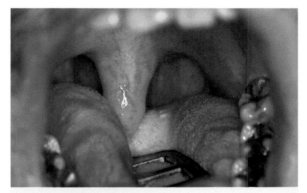

Fig. 3.12 Uvula is both wide and long.

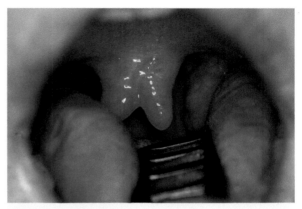

Fig. 3.13 Uvula bifida.

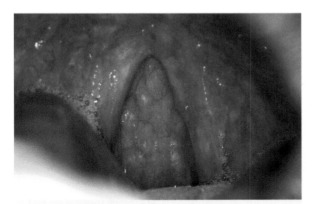

Fig. 3.14 Stenotic palate after ritual uvulectomy.

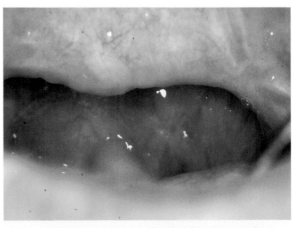

Fig. 3.15 Postoperative status of uvulopalatopharyngoplasty (UPPP).

procedure, in addition to many other complications, might accidentally lead to palatal stenosis.

▸Fig. 3.15 shows a status after UPPP, with a visual good result, with a wide opening and sufficient distance between the palate and the posterior pharyngeal wall.

▸Fig. 3.16 shows the situation after Zetaplasty. The fibrotic tissue in the anterolateral direction ("the scar tissue works for you") can be clearly seen.

▸Fig. 3.17, ▸Fig. 3.18, and ▸Fig. 3.19 show several degrees of palatal stenosis after incorrectly performed palatal techniques. Such unfortunate situations might

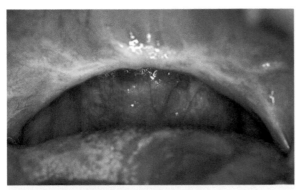

Fig. 3.16 Postoperative status of Zetaplasty.

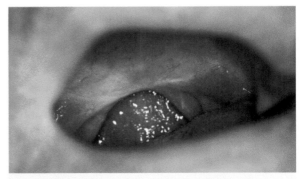

Fig. 3.17 Stenotic palate after uvulopalatopharyngoplasty (UPPP), without tonsillectomy.

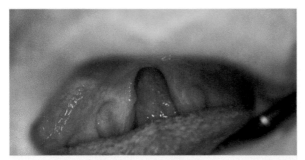

Fig. 3.18 Stenotic palate, after uvulopalatopharyngoplasty (UPPP).

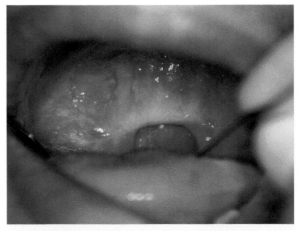

Fig. 3.19 Stenotic palate after uvulopalatopharyngoplasty (UPPP).

occur if the surgeon places his/her suture under too much tension or leaves the tonsils in situ, hoping to reduce pain for the patient. These iatrogenic complications should be avoided at all costs.

Palatal stenosis is scored in 3 grades (▶ Fig. 3.20). Often grades I and II can be improved by a modified Zetaplasty to some extent, while grade II needs to be treated by (LASER) excision and the long-term use of an obturator. This situation is extremely rare.

A possible collapse of the epiglottis can be missed with awake examination. Isolated epiglottis collapse is only assessed by DISE and will be discussed in the next section.

3.2.6 Conclusion

The workup of a patient with suspected OSA begins with taking a medical history and performing a physical examination. General examination of the head and neck area and trunk, (height, length, BMI, neck circumference), external examination of the head and neck area, (shape of the face, position of the mandible), and an internal examination of the upper airway, including dental status,

are performed. The Friedman and Mallampati classifications are used to assess the upper airway, providing a first general impression of tonsil and tongue size. However, both are insufficient for a careful assessment, in particular when surgery is considered. They both provide common information, with a rough first impression of the anatomical situation of the upper airway. In particular, they do not provide information on dental status, or of the length, shape, and position of the palate and uvula, neither of possible epiglottis collapse. There may be practical reasons to rely on clinical examination only, such as when insurance companies do not reimburse drug-induced sleep endoscopy (DISE). But in our philosophy, in the ideal situation, in case other treatment than CPAP (surgery, MAD, combined treatment) is considered, additional DISE is indicated (discussed in Chapter 3.4.2). A patient who considers upper airway surgery for OSA has a right to a careful and comprehensive workup.

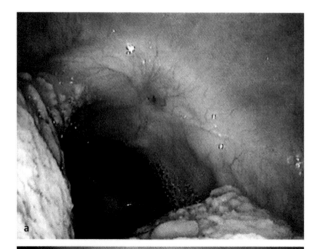

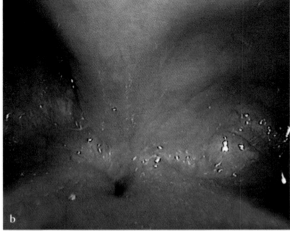

Fig. 3.20 Nasopharyngeal stenosis. **(a)** Transoral preoperative view. **(b)** Transnasal view. Reproduced from Bernal-Sprekelsen M, Carrau R, Dazert S, et al. Complications in Otolaryngology—Head and Neck Surgery. Thieme 2013.

3.3 Sleep Studies

Simon Herkenrath, Alessandra Castrogiovanni, Carla Miltz, and Winfried J. Randerath

Sleep studies summarize various parameters on sleep, ventilation, oxygen saturation, and limb movement. They help evaluate the sleep profile and identify sleep-associated diseases. Sleep studies are typically divided into four categories based on the number of channels and presence or absence of attendance during the procedure. The attended PSG (Level 1) is the gold standard for diagnosis of sleep-related breathing disturbances (SRBDs), and allows a reliable diagnosis taking into account all aspects obtained in the differential diagnosis. Attended PSG is recommended in patients with comorbidities such as chronic obstructive pulmonary disease, heart failure,

or renal failure, in patients with low pretest probability, and in patients suspected of sleep-related diseases other than OSA. A third-level device (polygraphy) is sufficient to confirm the diagnosis in patients with a high pretest probability for OSA. Third and fourth level devices are screening tools to evaluate the pretest probability of the presence or absence of SRBD, but they are not suitable for final diagnosis.

SRBDs are present in three major entities, differing substantially in pathophysiological and therapeutical aspects. They comprise obstructive and central sleep apnea (CSA) as well as alveolar hypoventilation syndromes. The detection, differentiation, and clinical evaluation of SRBD requires profound anamnesis and physical examination along with extensive medical tests, including specific questionnaires, as well as electrophysiological and instrument-based tests.

3.3.1 Differential Diagnosis in Sleep-Related Breathing Disturbances

With an incidence of 90%, OSA is the most common phenotype of SRBD. The prevalence of OSA increases with age and BMI and is associated with a restriction of the upper airways.[28] There is a higher prevalence in men (13%) as compared to women (6%).[29] Skeletal dysmorphias of the facial skull, enlarged tonsils and tongue, fat deposits at the soft tissues of the neck as well as cranial movement of the pulmonic-bronchial-tracheal system predispose to upper airway obstruction. Dilating muscles compensate upper airway obstruction during daytime, but muscle relaxation during sleep supports a reduction or complete interruption of respiratory flow.[30,31] One major aspect in the distinction toward CSA is the continuation of respiratory effort in case of OSA.

CSA represents about 10% of SRBD. Within the group of patients suffering from neurological diseases (e.g., stroke), renal failure, and especially systolic heart failure, prevalence of CSA is estimated at 21 to 37%.[32,33] CSA is characterized by the cessation of airflow and accompanying absence of respiratory effort. The pathogenesis of CSA is still object of research, so by now the classification of CSA is based on the etiology (e.g., CSA due to medication, high altitude, systolic heart failure, etc.).[34] However, the "loop gain" idea in patients with periodic breathing due to systolic heart failure represents a key concept in understanding the phenomenon of CSA.[35] The loop gain is based on a model known from engineering, defining the response of the respiratory system to changes of $PaCO_2$. Patients with systolic heart failure show an increased left atrial pressure and an accompanying tendency to chronic hyperventilation. In addition, overreacting chemoreceptors support an overshoot of ventilation in case of slight fluctuations of $PaCO_2$, which are quite common during the transition from wakefulness to sleep. An additional reduction of $PaCO_2$ is followed by a decrease of respiratory drive, which leads to apneas or hypopneas and an increase of $PaCO_2$ again. Thus, overreacting chemoreceptors result in alternating conditions of hyper- and hypoventilation (waxing and waning).[35]

Alveolar hypoventilation syndromes are characterized by a reduction of minute ventilation leading to chronic hypercapnia. Various diseases induce alveolar hypoventilation including diseases of respiratory drive, for example, obesity hypoventilation syndrome (OHS), failure of the neuromuscular or skeletal system (e.g., muscular dystrophy, diaphragm paralysis, or scoliosis), and pulmonary disorders such as the chronic obstructive lung disease. As minute ventilation during sleep is reduced in healthy persons by 10 to 15%, chronic ventilatory failure unmasks at first during sleep. Typical characteristics include an increase of $PaCO_2$ with a subsidiary sustained decrease of oxygen saturation. Alveolar hypoventilation syndromes often remain undetected in sleep medicine, as a continuous reduction of flow and effort may be overseen in PSG and necessary PCO_2 measurements (e.g., transcutaneous capnometry) are not performed routinely.

Especially, OHS often coexists with OSA (9–14%) and is defined by a BMI greater than or equal to 30 kg/m² and $PaCO_2$ greater than or equal to 45 mm Hg when awake.[36,37,38] Other diseases causing hypoventilation need to be excluded. OHS is estimated in about 10% of patients with a BMI between 30 and 35 kg/m². The prevalence rises to 50% in patients with a BMI greater than 50 kg/m².[36,37,39] Obesity requires increased respiratory work due to the larger body mass. Obese patients present with reduced diaphragm mobility, increased oxygen demand, restriction of the upper airways, and increased ventilation/perfusion-mismatch. OHS patients are not able to maintain the increased respiratory work and present with dampened ventilatory response to hypoxia and changes of $PaCO_2$ levels. [40,41,42]

Multiple studies have shown that all entities of SRBD are associated with an increased mortality and morbidity.[39,43,44,45,46] OSA has proven to be an independent risk factor of arterial hypertension, atrial fibrillation, systolic and diastolic heart failure as well as cerebrovascular events.[47,48] Patients suffering from OHS have poorer quality of life and have a higher risk of developing pulmonary hypertension (PH)[49] compared with OSA patients. The consequences of CSA on the cardiovascular system are less clear, but besides an increased mortality there is evidence that patients with CSA show a higher risk for heart transplantation than patients without SRBD.[39]

An early and profound distinction between the entities of SRBD is of crucial importance due to the differences in pathophysiology and therapeutic approach.

3.3.2 Clinical Investigations

Patients' Approach

The ICSD includes 60 specific diagnoses and 6 major categories including SRBD, insomnia, parasomnia, and sleep-related movement disorders. The latest edition, ICSD-3, was released in 2014.[34]

SRBD are associated with cyclic oxygen desaturations and catecholamine release, inducing arousals, systemic inflammation, and oxidative stress.[50] Arousals result in fragmented sleep and therefore prevent slow wave and rapid eye movement (REM) sleep. As a consequence the recovery effect is reduced and sleepiness during the day is increased. Typical symptoms of OSA and OHS include snoring, witnessed apneas, daytime sleepiness, reduced concentration, momentary nodding off, morning headaches, depression, and nocturnal dyspnea (▶Table 3.7). CSA is not associated with any specific symptoms, but can be accompanied by unspecific symptoms such as fatigue and daytime sleepiness.[39]

The ICSD-3 defines insomnia as "a repeated difficulty with sleep initiation, duration, consolidation, or quality that occurs despite adequate opportunity and circumstances for sleep, and results in some form of daytime impairment."[34] Anxiety, frustration, irritability, and mood changes during daytime are accompanying phenomena.

Parasomnia includes episodes of dream-enacting behavior during REM sleep as well as episodes of inconsolable screaming and amnesia during the first third of the night. Information from the bed partner on parasomnia can be of crucial importance for the evaluation of abnormal events during sleep.

Sleep-related movement disorders comprise restless legs syndrome (RLS) and periodic limb movements (PLM). Typical symptoms include discomfort or pain shortly before sleep onset (RLS) in addition to daytime sleepiness and fatigue (PLM).[34]

Physical Examination

Physical examination includes evaluation of the oral cavity, skeletal status, and soft tissue factors. The Mallampati

▶Table 3.7 Symptoms of sleep-related breathing disorders

During sleep	Awake
Nonrestorative sleep	Daytime sleepiness
Apneas witnessed by bed partner	Lack of concentration
	Cognitive deficits
Awaking with choking	Changes in mood
Nocturnal restlessness	Morning headaches
Vivid dreams	Dry mouth
Gastroesophageal reflux	Impotence or decreased libido
Nocturia	
Diaphoresis	
Hypersalivation	
Insomnia with frequent awakenings	

score identifies patients with restrictions of the oropharyngeal cavity.[51] Liistro et al found that the visualization of the soft palate (Grade I–IV) is an associated risk factor for OSA (▶Fig. 3.4).[52]

Maxillary and/or mandibular hypoplasia as well as the retroposition and inferior displacement of the hyoid reduce the diameter of the posterior airway space. Cephalometry (▶Fig. 3.21) visualizes and evaluates the anatomy of the upper airways.

Abnormalities of the soft tissue include adenotonsillar hypertrophy, macroglossia, fat deposition, pharyngeal inflammation, and edema. CT of head and throat[31] as well as acoustic pharyngometry quantify the geometry of oral cavity.

Thus, Young et al showed that body weight, neck circumference, and BMI correlate with the presence and severity of OSA.[53] Moreover, any signs of heart failure (e.g., edema of the lower leg) or neurological diseases (e.g., sensorimotor deficits) can be a first indicator for CSA.

Questionnaires

Questionnaires help detect and quantify SRBD as well as other entities of sleep-associated diseases. Although not predictive, they can be used as a first indicator for SRBD. The most important questionnaires used today are the ESS, the Berlin questionnaire, and the STOP-BANG questionnaire.

The ESS is the most common instrument to evaluate sleepiness. It assesses the patient's probability of falling asleep in eight different everyday situations. Numerical values ranging from 0 ("I never fall asleep") to 3 ("I have a high probability of falling asleep") are used to quantify sleepiness. A score above or equal to 10 is indicative for daytime sleepiness and requires further investigation.[1]

The Berlin questionnaire identifies OSA patients in primary care and general population. It is characterized by 10 questions divided into 3 categories investigating the severity of snoring, daytime sleepiness, and history of high blood pressure or obesity. Predefined questions are assigned to a certain score. SRBD becomes very likely if two categories are classified positive.[54] The specificity and sensitivity of the Berlin questionnaire to detect OSA is 80% and 40%, respectively.[55]

The STOP-BANG questionnaire was originally developed for preoperative situations.[56] It consists of two domains: A self-assessment questionnaire evaluating snoring, tiredness, witnessed apneas, and treatment of arterial hypertension. The second part collects anthropometric data including BMI, age, neck circumference, and sex. The score is calculated by assigning one point to each positive answer (BMI >35 kg/m², male gender, neck circumference >40 cm, and age >50 years). A score above or equal to 3 indicates a high probability for OSA. Compared to the Berlin questionnaire, STOP-BANG is more sensitive (87%) in identifying subjects with moderate to severe SRBD and is gaining clinical acceptance.[57]

Electrophysiological Tests

The most common electrophysiological tests to objectify central nervous activation and daytime sleepiness are the multiple sleep latency test (MSLT), the multiple wakefulness test (MWT), and the Oxford Sleep Resistance (OSLER) test.[58]

The MSLT evaluates daytime sleep latency at five standardized times during the day, based on electroencephalogram (EEG), electro-oculogram (EOG), and electromyogram (EMG), assuming that sleep latency decreases with sleepiness. The American Sleep Disorders Association (ASDA) evaluated degrees of severity based on experience and defined age-dependent norms.[58] While mean sleep latency at the age of 20 is 10.4 minutes, it is 12.1 minutes at the age of 50, and 15.2 minutes at the age of 80. REM sleep less than 10 minutes after sleep onset in combination with a reduced sleep latency (<8 minutes) indicates narcolepsy (see ICSD3).[34]

The MWT evaluates sleepiness that overpowers a patients' ability to stay awake in a sleep-promoting

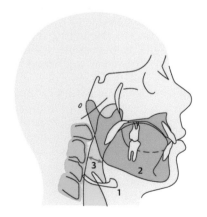
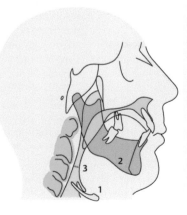

Fig. 3.21 Cephalometry evaluates soft tissue and skeletal relationships including posterior airway space, hyoid position, and length of the soft palate. Caudal hyoid bone (1) and retropositioned mandible (2) predispose to a reduction of posterior airway space (3) and obstructive sleep apnea (OSA).

environment. Its results correlate with the severity of OSA and reflect improvement during treatment.[59,60] The Atlas Task Force of American Academy of Sleep Medicine (AASM) defined guidelines for the protocol of the procedure. In four 40-minute sessions separated by 2-hour intervals, patients are observed by EEG, EOG, and EMG. Sleep latency, total sleep time (TST), and sleep stages are evaluated.[61] The AASM refers to data of healthy people in a clinical trial performed by Doghramji et al from 1997 to define standard values.[62] Sleep onset below 13 minutes is defined pathological.

The OSLER test is a modification of the MWT. In addition to the setup of the MWT, patients are instructed to respond to a dim light flash at 3-second intervals during a 40-minute period by hitting a button on a portable device.[63] Missing responses for 21 seconds (e.g., 7 consecutive flashes) suggest that the person has fallen asleep and the test is finished.[64]

These three tests are of crucial relevance in the evaluation of daytime sleepiness and central nervous activation. Although there is a limited validity of each test alone, they represent a beneficial tool in the diagnostical algorithm in addition to a comprehensive patient history and PSG.

3.3.3 Computer-Based Tests of Vigilance and Attention

Computer-based tests such as Carda, driving simulation tests, or the Pupillographic Sleepiness Test evaluate qualities of attention and vigilance.

Carda is a computer-assisted response test to evaluate sustained attention. The image of a road is projected on a black background and patients are required to respond to obstacles. They are visible for 20 milliseconds and randomly appear on the road about 100 times in 10 minutes.[65]

Driving-simulation tests focus on different components of attention, especially divided attention or sustained attention. Reaction time and directional stability represent target parameters.[66] Risser et al found higher error rates in OSA patients as compared with healthy controls. Sufficient therapy reduced failures significantly.[67]

The Pupillographic Sleepiness Test is based on the correlation of fluctuations of the pupil width and daytime sleepiness.[58] The pupil behavior is recorded by an infrared-sensitive camera. Target variables are the pupillary unrest index (PUI) in millimeters per minute and the amplitude spectrum. Based on the data of 349 healthy people, unusual values were defined starting from a PUI more than or equal to 1.89 mm/min, pathological values from a PUI more than or equal to 2.28 mm/min.[68]

In the setting of the Quatember Maly test, patients observe a moving point inside a circle and respond to double jumps. Seven missed or false reactions are considered pathological. Rühle et al found that the Quatember

Maly test shows the best sensitivity (61.9%) and specificity (72.2%) as compared to the PUI (47.6%/57.9%) or the Carda test (23.8%/21.1%).[69]

Although instrument-based tests have no specific validity, they help evaluate the ability to concentrate, reaction time, attention during monotonous activities, and objectify therapy responsiveness during the course of the disease.

3.3.4 Evaluation of Sleep and Breathing Disturbances During Sleep

Various parameters on sleep, ventilation, oxygen saturation, and limb movement help evaluate the sleep profile and identify sleep-associated diseases. Sleep studies summarize these parameters and are typically divided into four categories based on the number of channels and presence or absence of attendance during the procedure.

The attended PSG (Level 1) is the gold standard for diagnosis of SRBD, which includes a minimum of seven and a maximum of nine channels supervised by a technician in a sleep laboratory. The unattended PSG is considered a second level study. Both, attended and unattended PSG include neurologic, cardiac, and respiratory parameters, in particular, EEG, EOG, EMG, thoracoabdominal effort, air flow (via nasal cannula, thermistor, or thermocouple), oxygen saturation, heart rate, electrocardiogram (ECG), snoring (via microphone), and body position.[70]

A third-level study comprises at least four parameters, and a fourth-level study measures at least one. Both do not record EEG, EOG, and EMG and thus do not allow for evaluating sleep or limb movement. A third level study focuses on breathing, ECG, and oxygen saturation, while a fourth level study measures airflow and/or oxygen saturation only.[70]

The attended PSG represents the reference method for the differential diagnosis of sleep disorders. Especially in low pretest probability for OSA, PSG is indispensable and enables the differentiation between entities of SRBD and other diseases such as insomnia, parasomnia, movement disorders during sleep, and rare types of epilepsy. In the presence of comorbidities such as pulmonary, psychiatric, or other neurologic, and neuromuscular diseases, simple devices do not sufficiently allow to diagnose or exclude SRBD.[70]

Third- and fourth-level devices can be useful for screening SRBD in asymptomatic patients. As known from various studies, particularly patients with cardiovascular comorbidities cannot sufficiently be identified based on symptoms and history.[39] Third- and fourth-level devices can be used as a screening tool to evaluate the pretest probability of the presence or absence of SRBD; however, they are not suitable for final diagnosis.

The German guidelines suggest a third-level device (polygraphy) to confirm the diagnosis in patients with a high pretest probability for OSA. A high pretest probability is defined by the coexistence of snoring, daytime sleepiness, and witnessed apneas.[39]

Thus, a PSG is recommended in patients with comorbidities such as chronic obstructive pulmonary disease, heart failure, or renal failure, in patients with low pretest probability, and in patients suspected of having sleep-related diseases other than OSA.[39] The AASM Task Force issued recommendations on the use of limited studies (portable monitoring) in 2007[71] (▸Table 3.8).

Special sleep studies, based on the overnight pulse oximetry were developed to describe the effect of SRBD on the cardiovascular system. The two methods that are widely used in clinical trials are plethysmographic arterial tonometry (PAT) and pulse wave attenuation index (PWAI).

The PAT allows for the measurement of the pulsatile blood volume by generating signals from a pulse oximeter and a digital pneumatic system at constant volume and variable pressure. A battery-powered, wrist-mounted device, which records PAT signal, pulse rate derived from PAT signal, oxyhemoglobin saturation, and wrist activity (derived from actigraphy), has been proven to accurately describe vasoconstriction caused by hypopneas and apneas and detects OSA sufficiently.[72]

In addition, the plethysmographic technique allows to analyze specific components of the pulse wave.[73]

▸ **Table 3.8** Recommendations of the AASM Task Force 2007

- The diagnosis of OSA using portable monitoring should be carried out only after an overall assessment of sleep.

- The clinical evaluation of respiratory disorders using portable monitoring should always be supervised by a certified expert in sleep medicine or by an individual who meets the criteria for certification.

- Portable devices are an alternative to PSG in patients with high pretest probability of moderate to severe OSA.

- Portable monitoring for the diagnosis of OSA may be indicated when PSG in the laboratory is impossible due to immobility or critical medical condition.

- Portable monitoring may be indicated for follow-up of patients not using CPAP after weight loss or UA surgery or using MADs.

- "Limited" studies are not appropriate for the diagnosis of OSA in subjects suspected for sleep disorders other than OSA (central apnea, periodic leg movements, insomnia, parasomnias, narcolepsy).

- The portable devices are not indicated for the diagnosis in patients with comorbidities that would reduce the accuracy of the examination, including heart failure, neuromuscular disease, and moderate to severe pulmonary disease.

- Portable monitors are inappropriate for general screening in the asymptomatic population.

Abbreviations: AASM, American Academy of Sleep Medicine; CPAP, continuous positive airway pressure; MADs, mandibular advancement devices; OSA, obstructive sleep apnea; PSG, polysomnography; UA, upper airway.

A composite biosignal score for the individual cardiovascular risk is derived from the information of the single parameters. The output is a number between 0 (low risk) and 1 (high risk), which was validated against the cardiovascular risk matrix of the European Society of Hypertension/European Society of Cardiology (ESH/ESC).[74]

The diagnosis of sleep-associated alveolar hypoventilation requires the examination of arterial blood gases during sleep.[34] The measurement of transcutaneous PCO_2 or the assessment of exhaled CO_2 represent viable alternatives. The diagnostic criteria for a relevant alveolar hypoventilation in adults include: (1) increase of arterial PCO_2 more than or equal to 55 mm Hg for more than or equal to 10 minutes; (2) increase of arterial PCO_2 more than or equal to 10 mm Hg during sleep (compared to a recorded value when awake) more than or equal to 50 mm Hg for more than or equal to 10 minutes.[75]

3.3.5 Parameters of Sleep Studies

The most important parameters of sleep studies are categorized by sleep, breathing, oxygen saturation, and limb movement (▸Table 3.9). The evaluation of sleep is based on EEG, EOG, and EMG. Sleep can be distinguished into nonrapid eye movement (NREM) sleep, including sleep stages 1, 2, 3, and REM sleep. Sleep stage NREM1 is associated with the transition from wakefulness to sleep. The EEG shows a change from beta (12–30 Hz) and gamma (25–100 Hz) waves to alpha (8–13 Hz) and theta (4–7 Hz) waves (▸Fig. 3.22). NREM2 comprises 50% of the TST and is accompanied by a decrease of muscle tone. It follows NREM1 and is dominated by theta waves. Two specific phenomena characterize NREM2: sleep spindles (▸Fig. 3.23) and K-complexes (▸Fig. 3.24). Sleep spindles are short bursts with a frequency of 12 to 14 Hz and duration of 0.5 second. K-complexes last about 1 to 2 seconds and are characterized by a short negative high voltage peak, followed by a slower positive complex and a negative peak in the end.[76]

NREM3 (▸Fig. 3.25) is considered "deep sleep" or "slow-wave sleep" and comprises about 15 to 20% of TST. The EEG shows delta waves with a frequency of 0.5 to 4 Hz. Sleep spindles can occur in NREM3, however, rarely as compared to NREM2.

REM sleep (▸Fig. 3.26) is characterized by a further reduction of muscle tone and rapid side to side movement of the closed eyes. The EEG is dominated by alpha, beta, and theta waves, where beta waves can present as "sawtooth" pattern. REM sleep returns cyclically every 90 to 120 minutes following NREM3 (▸Fig. 3.27).

Arousals are defined as a return of alpha or theta rhythm for more than or equal to 3 seconds (▸Fig. 3.28). EMG tone elevations are required during arousals in REM sleep, but are not mandatory in NREM. Arousals are associated with respiratory disturbances, limb movement, or vegetative activations. They fragment sleep, diminish sleep stages NREM3 and REM, and reduce the recreational effect of sleep.[34]

▶Table 3.9 Parameters of sleep studies according to AASM and Randerath[7,51]

Sleep	
TIB	Time from "lights out" to "lights on," independent from sleep or wakefulness.
TST	Amount of actual sleep between "lights out" and "lights on," including NREM and REM.
Sleep latency	Duration from "lights out," or "bedtime," to the onset of sleep.
REM latency	Duration from "lights out," or "bedtime" to REM sleep.
Sleep efficiency	Proportion of sleep in comparison to the time in bed (i.e., ratio of TST to TIB)
Arousal index	Amount of arousals in 1 h of TST. Normal values change with age.
Breathing	
Apnea	Reduction of air flow ≥90% compared to the pre-event amplitude plus duration ≥10 s.
Obstructive apnea	Characteristics of apnea plus persistence of thoracoabdominal effort (▶Fig. 3.29)
Central apnea	Characteristics of apnea plus absence of thoracoabdominal effort (▶Fig. 3.30).
Mixed apnea	Apnea plus central phenotype in the beginning and obstructive phenotype in the end of one apnea (▶Fig. 3.31).
Hypopnea	Reduction of air flow ≥30% compared to pre-event amplitude plus duration ≥10 s; additionally either oxygen desaturation ≥3% compared to pre-event basis SpO_2 or occurrence of an arousal.
Obstructive hypopnea	Hypopnea plus characteristics such as flattening of the flow curve, paradoxical movement of thorax and abdomen, or sharp increase of ventilation at end of event, often associated with an arousal (▶Fig. 3.32).
Central hypopnea	Hypopnea plus characteristics such as reduction of thoraco-abdominal movements without paradoxical breathing, waxing ventilation at end of respiratory event, often associated with an arousal during maximum ventilation peak (▶Fig. 3.33).
Periodic breathing	Three or more central apneas or hypopneas separated by waxing and waning flow pattern (crescendo–decrescendo) plus a cycle length of ≥40 s. Duration of cycle defined by central event duration plus duration of recovery respiratory phase, (▶Fig. 3.34). Additionally, a minimum of five central apneas or hypopneas per hour of sleep with crescendo–decrescendo ventilation within 2 h of monitoring are required.
Ataxic breathing (Biot's respiration)	Irregular breathing pattern with rhythmical pauses lasting 10–30 s and sometimes alternating periods of apnea and tachypnea (▶Fig. 3.35).
RERA	Series of breaths characterized by flow-limitation associated with increased respiratory effort lasting ≥10 s plus arousal at the end of event (▶Fig. 3.36).
RDI	Numerical value describing respiratory disturbances per hour of TST, including apneas, hypopneas, and RERA.
AHI	Number of apneas and hypopneas in relation to 1 h of TST.
SpO_2	
Average SpO_2	Average SpO_2 in healthy adults 96.5 ± 1.5%. Normal values lower with increasing age.
Cumulative percentage of time spent at oxygen saturations below 90% (CT90%)	Parameter to estimate global degree of hypoxemia.
Lowest SpO_2	Lowest oxygen saturation value during recording time. Artificial influences need to be excluded carefully.
ODI	Number of desaturations ≥ 3% in 1 h of TST.
Limb movement	
Periodic limb movement	Repetitive episodes of muscle contraction (0.5–5 s) separated by an interval of 20–40 s.

Abbreviations: AASM, American Academy of Sleep Medicine; AHI, apnea–hypopnea index; NREM, nonrapid eye movement; ODI, oxygen desaturation index; RDI, respiratory disturbance index; REM, rapid eye movement; RERA, respiratory effort related arousal; TIB, time in bed; TST, total sleep time.

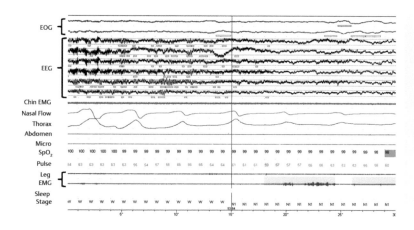

Fig. 3.22 Transition from wake to sleep stage N1. A 30-second screenshot of a polysomnography (PSG): Sleep stage nonrapid eye movement (NREM1) is associated with the transition from wakefulness to sleep. The electroencephalogram (EEG) shows a change from beta (12–30 Hz) and gamma (25–100 Hz) waves to alpha (8–13 Hz) and theta (4–7 Hz) waves.

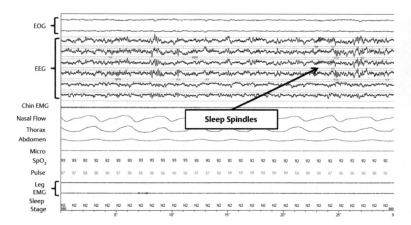

Fig. 3.23 Sleep stage N2: Sleep spindles. A 30-second screenshot of a polysomnography (PSG): N2 is characterized by theta waves (4–7 Hz) in addition to sleep spindles (short bursts with a frequency of 12–14 Hz and a duration of 0.5 second).

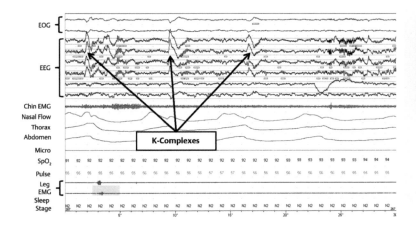

Fig. 3.24 Sleep stage N2: K-complexes. A 30-second screenshot of a polysomnography (PSG): N2 is dominated by theta waves (4–7 Hz) and K-complexes (short negative high voltage peak, followed by a slower positive complex and a negative peak at the end, duration 1–2 seconds).

Breathing is evaluated based on the respiratory flow as well as the thoracic and abdominal movement as parameters for respiratory effort. EMG, EEG (arousals), and SpO_2 (desaturations), allow to define and distinguish between apneas and hypopneas of central or obstructive origin. Respiratory events can be classified according to the AASM and noninvasive algorithm by Randerath et al.[77] (▶Table 3.9; ▶Fig. 3.27b, ▶Fig. 3.28, ▶Fig. 3.29, ▶Fig. 3.30, ▶Fig. 3.31, ▶Fig. 3.32, ▶Fig. 3.33, ▶Fig. 3.34, ▶Fig. 3.35, ▶Fig. 3.36). The severity of SRBD is quantified by the AHI that describes the number of apneas and hypopneas in relation to 1 hour of TST. It is widely used in clinical practice, clinical trials, and epidemiological studies. Three degrees of severity are distinguished: mild

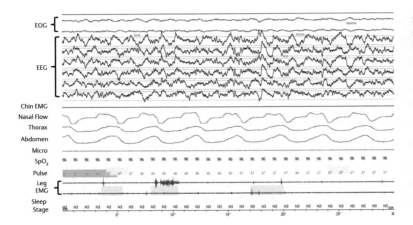

Fig. 3.25 Sleep stage N3. A 30-second screenshot of a polysomnography (PSG): N3 is characterized by delta waves (0.5–4 Hz). Sleep spindles can occur.

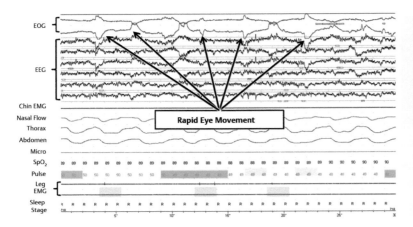

Fig. 3.26 Rapid eye movement (REM) sleep. A 30-second screenshot of a polysomnography (PSG): REM sleep is characterized by a complete paralysis of muscle tone and rapid side to side movement of the closed eyes. The electroencephalogram (EEG) is dominated by alpha (8–13 Hz), beta (12–30 Hz), and theta waves (4–7 Hz).

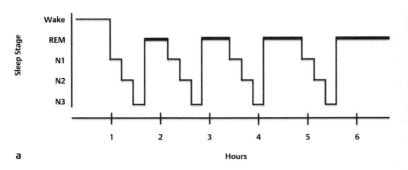

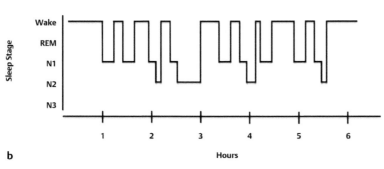

Fig. 3.27 Sleep stages and transitions are illustrated by the hypnogram using an analog plot of sleep–wake stages. **(a)** A normal hypnogram with 4 REM/NREM stages, a cycle duration of 90 minutes and prolonging REM phases during sleep. **(b)** A pathologic hypnogram with disrupted sleep, missing sleep stages N3 and REM as well as recurring awake states.

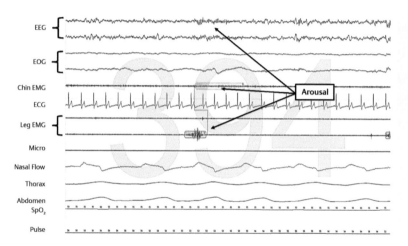

Fig. 3.28 A 30-second polysomnography (PSG) screenshot showing an arousal. Arousals are defined as a return of alpha or theta rhythm for more than or equal to 3 seconds. Electromyography tone elevations are required in rapid eye movement (REM) sleep, but not mandatory in nonrapid eye movement (NREM).

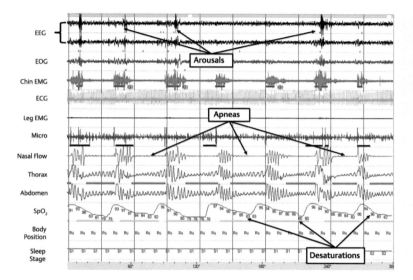

Fig. 3.29 A 5-minute screenshot of a polysomnography (PSG) showing recurring obstructive apneas. They are characterized by a reduction of air flow of more than or equal to 90% compared to the pre-event amplitude, a duration of more than or equal to 10 seconds and persistence of thoracoabdominal effort.

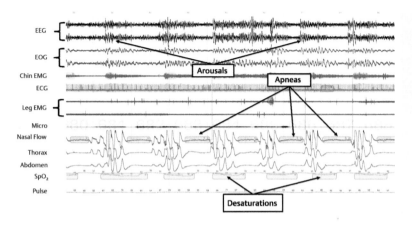

Fig. 3.30 A 5-minute screenshot of a polysomnography (PSG) showing recurrent central apneas. They are characterized by a reduction of airflow greater than or equal to 90% compared to the pre-event amplitude, a duration greater than or equal to 10 seconds and absence of thoracoabdominal effort.

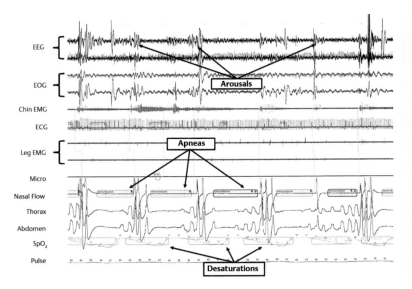

Fig. 3.31 A 5-minute screenshot of a polysomnography (PSG) showing recurring mixed apneas. They are characterized by a reduction of the air flow greater than or equal to 90% compared to the pre-event amplitude, a duration greater than or equal to 10 seconds and a central phenotype in the beginning and obstructive phenotype in the end of one apnea.

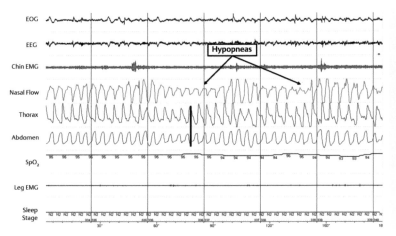

Fig. 3.32 A 3-minute screenshot of a polysomnography (PSG) showing recurring obstructive hypopneas. They are characterized by a reduction of the air flow greater than or equal to 30% compared to the pre-event amplitude, a duration greater than or equal to 10 seconds, an oxygen desaturation greater than or equal to 3%, and/or the occurrence of an arousal. Typical obstructive characteristics are flattening of the flow curve and paradoxical movement of thorax and abdomen (*black vertical line*).

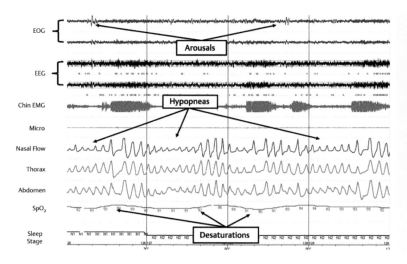

Fig. 3.33 A 2-minute screenshot of a polysomnography (PSG) showing central hypopnea. They are characterized by a reduction of the air flow greater than or equal to 30% compared to the pre-event amplitude, a duration greater than or equal to 10 seconds, an oxygen desaturation greater than or equal to 3%, and/or the occurrence of an arousal. Typical characteristics are a reduction of thoracoabdominal movements without paradoxical breathing, waxing ventilation at the end of a respiratory event, and an association with an arousal during the maximum ventilation.

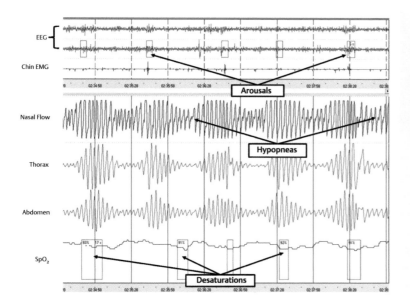

Fig. 3.34 A 4-minute screenshot of a polysomnography (PSG) showing periodic breathing with central hypopneas. They are characterized by three or more central apneas or hypopneas separated by waxing and waning flow pattern (crescendo–decrescendo), a cycle length of more than or equal to 40 seconds, and an arousal during the maximum ventilation peak.

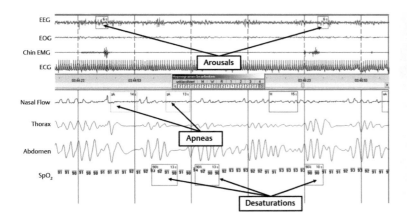

Fig. 3.35 A 3-minute screenshot of a polysomnography (PSG) showing ataxic breathing with irregular central respiratory events. The breathing pattern is irregular, rapid, and shows periods of apnea and tachypnea.

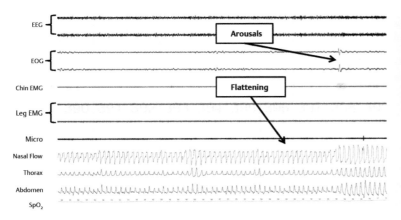

Fig. 3.36 A 5-minute screenshot of a polysomnography (PSG) showing respiratory effort-related arousals (RERAs). They are characterized by flow limitation associated with increased respiratory effort lasting for more than 10 seconds and an arousal at the end of the event.

SRBD, AHI 5 to 14/h; moderate SRBD, AHI 15 to 29/h; and severe SRBD, AHI greater than or equal to 30/h.[34]

The impact of respiratory instability on oxygen saturation is measured by pulse oximetry, evaluating the extent of desaturations and mean oxygen saturation. The average SpO_2 in healthy adults is 96.5 ± 1.5%, but normal values lower with increasing age.[78] In general, longer lasting SpO_2 below 90% cannot be explained by sleep apnea, therefore comorbidities such as ventilatory failure or diffusion impairment need to be investigated.

An EMG delivers information on muscle tone. It is generally derived from an electrode on chin and tibia and enables the evaluation of sleep stages, arousals, and limb movement disorders.[7]

3.3.6 Case Reports
Severe Obstructive Sleep Apnea

A 38-year-old male truck driver presents with witnessed apneas, snoring, daytime sleepiness, and reduced performance status. Comorbidities: arterial hypertension and severe obesity (BMI 46 kg/m²). See ▶Fig. 3.37, ▶Fig. 3.38, ▶Fig. 3.39, ▶Fig. 3.40.

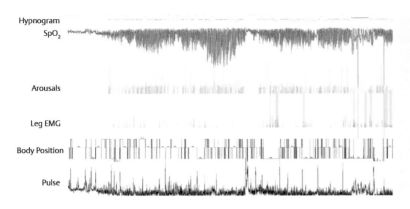

Fig. 3.37 A 7-hour screenshot of a polysomnography (PSG) showing destructed sleep architecture, recurring relevant desaturations, multiple arousals, and changes of body position.

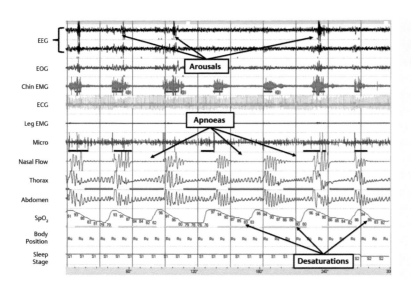

Fig. 3.38 A 5-minute screenshot of a polysomnography (PSG) showing recurring obstructive apneas associated with arousals and relevant desaturations.

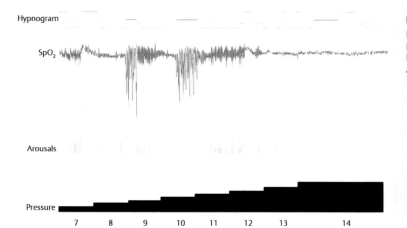

Hypnogram

SpO₂

Arousals

Pressure

7   8   9   10   11   12   13   14

Fig. 3.39 A 7-hour screenshot of a polysomnography (PSG) under continuous positive airway pressure (CPAP) therapy. Respiratory events are suppressed under a positive airway pressure of more than 13 mbar.

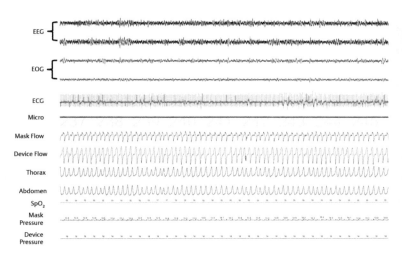

EEG

EOG

ECG

Micro

Mask Flow

Device Flow

Thorax

Abdomen

SpO₂

Mask Pressure

Device Pressure

Fig. 3.40 A 5-minute screenshot of a polysomnography (PSG) showing a sufficient suppression of obstructive respiratory events under a positive airway pressure of 14 mbar.

Central Sleep Apnea

A 64-year-old overweight male (BMI 28.5 kg/m²), who is a sales representative, presents with ankle edema, nycturia, daytime sleepiness, and fatigue. Comorbidities: arterial hypertension, hypertensive cardiomyopathy, and atrial fibrillation. See ▶ Fig. 3.41, ▶ Fig. 3.42, ▶ Fig. 3.43.

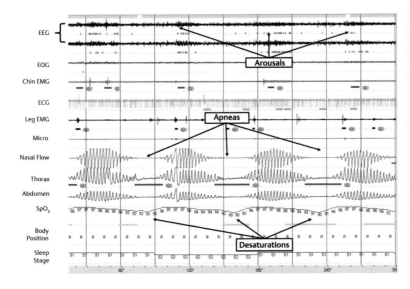

Fig. 3.41 A 5-minute screenshot of a polysomnography (PSG) showing a periodic breathing pattern with central apneas and arousals during maximum ventilatory peak.

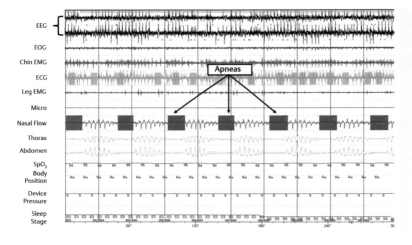

Fig. 3.42 A 5-minute screenshot of a polysomnography (PSG) showing a persistence of central sleep apnea during initial continuous positive airway pressure (CPAP) therapy.

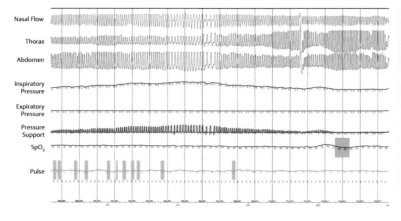

Fig. 3.43 A 5-minute screenshot of a polysomnography (PSG) showing successful adaptive servo ventilation (ASV) therapy with resolution of periodic breathing and stabilization of respiratory drive.

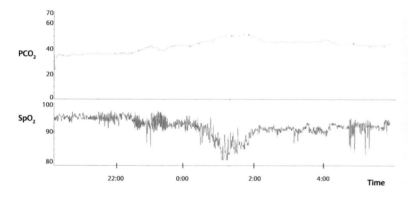

Fig. 3.44 A 7-hour screenshot of a transcutaneous PCO_2 measurement under CPAP therapy showing a relevant hypoventilation with deep and prolonged oxygen desaturations associated with an inverse increase of PCO_2. A continuous increase of PCO_2 throughout the recording can be seen. Clusters of short-term desaturations suggest the coexistence of sleep apnea.

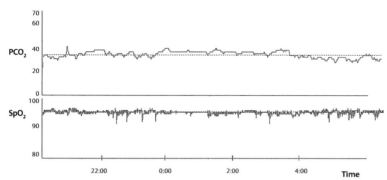

Fig. 3.45 A 7-hour screenshot of a transcutaneous PCO_2 measurement under noninvasive ventilation showing a stabilization of PCO_2 and oxygen saturation.

Obesity Hypoventilation Syndrome

A 55-year-old male insurance salesman, presents with snoring, fatigue, poor sleep quality, severe obesity (BMI 46.6 kg/m^2), and a moderate restrictive ventilation disorder in the body plethysmography. Comorbidities: Diabetes mellitus type II and arterial hypertension. Arterial blood gas analysis shows PCO_2 is 52 mm Hg in the early morning. See ▶ Fig. 3.44, ▶ Fig. 3.45.

3.4 Topo Diagnosis of Obstruction Site(s)

3.4.1 Awake Nasopharyngoscopy

Nico de Vries, Peter van Maanen, and Linda B. L. Benoist

Introduction

The workup of a patient with suspected OSA includes a careful history and physical examination. In addition to general examination and an internal examination of the upper airway, awake nasopharyngoscopy might be performed. Its routine performance is debatable. It does not provide information on the essential differences in the awake situation and during sleep, of the collapsible segment of the upper airway. If DISE will be performed later, awake nasopharyngoscopy might be considered superfluous. If DISE will not be performed, awake nasopharyngoscopy might be of

use to assess the whole upper airway in order to rule out any (rare) abnormalities in the upper airway that could be overlooked with routine ENT investigation. It is also useful in anxious patients and patients with high gag reflexes.

SDB is caused by a combination and variety of factors, such as neurological factors, insufficient respiratory drive, increased collapsibility of the collapsible segment of the upper airway, and wrong sleep position. Local anatomical variations in the upper airway and facial skeleton, associated with neuromuscular alterations in the pharynx are among these causes. To assess the anatomical causes and subsequent treatment options of SDB, an evaluation of the upper airway, from entrance of the nose to the level of the vocal cords is mandatory. In addition to OSA-specific clinical ENT investigation, awake nasopharyngoscopy is a diagnostic modality that is often performed. Its routine performance is, however, debatable. In this section, the technique, indication, and limitations of awake nasopharyngoscopy will be discussed.

Methods of Airway Evaluation

There is a whole spectrum of diagnostic modalities available to assess the upper airway in general ENT examination. Which modalities are of use and make sense, depends on the specific disease that is being evaluated. For example, biopsies and imaging are of major importance in oncology. In sinus disease, nasendoscopy and CT scans are pivotal. In SBD, most of these techniques are of little or no value.

In evaluation of the upper airway in the patient with SBD, in addition to clinical examination in the office, a wide range of specific diagnostic modalities—such as awake endoscopy (with or without the Müller's maneuver), lateral cephalometry, CT scanning and MR imaging (both awake and during natural sleep), video-endoscopy during spontaneous sleep, DISE, and critical closing pressure measurements—have been used and described to quantify obstruction and collapsibility of the different sites of the upper airway. Presently most of these techniques have been abandoned and no longer have a role in routine clinical practice. They are mostly of research interest and have little role in the routine assessment of the upper airway of the patient with SDB.

The most important limitation of CT and MR scanning is that they assess the anatomical and collapsible situation in the upper airway in an awake patient, while the real goal is to assess the situation during sleep. The limitation is that the evaluations are carried out with the patient awake, when his/her muscle tone is maintained, but during sleep there is a progressive hypotonia, reaching maximum muscle relaxation during REM sleep.

Interesting research has been, and is being performed with imaging, both with CT scans and MRI scans, during natural sleep. Apparently, some patients are able, when given sufficient time to adapt to the situation, to sleep in a loud MR machine, with or even without the use of earplugs. These techniques, although of research interest, will in our opinion never make it to routine use, as they are time consuming and therefore expensive.

This chapter aims to be a guide for upper airway evaluation, as could be used in the workup of patients with SBD. But the aim is not comprehensiveness or description of everything that has ever been tried, and presently abandoned by most. The goal is rather clinical usefulness. In this book we deliberately focus on these diagnostic modalities that are of use in routine practice. The cornerstones are OSA-specific ENT examination and DISE, in case treatment other than CPAP is considered, while imaging is hardly ever indicated.

Awake Endoscopy

Awake endoscopy is a test that is performed routinely by some while others consider this of little value, in particular if DISE is scheduled later. The important difference between awake endoscopy and DISE is the awake versus sleeping condition. Awake endoscopy does provide insight in the anatomy of the upper airway, from the level of the entrance of the nose up to vocal cord level. The endoscopy can be performed with or without local anesthesia and decongestion of the nose. The test can be performed in sitting, supine, and lateral positions. Passive and active maneuvers, such as chin lift and mouth closure, can be performed in the different positions during awake nasopharyngoscopy, hoping that these maneuvers might provide some predictive value for various therapeutic interventions. There is, however, little evidence for this. One of these techniques is the so-called Müller's maneuver.

Müller's Maneuver

The Müller's maneuver, introduced in 1983, is a simple test that has been used in evaluation of the upper airway in patients with SDB.

With Müller's maneuver, the patient undergoes a forced inhaling effort, after a forced expiration, with both the nose and mouth closed.[79] The negative pressure in the chest and lungs becomes subatmospheric; a reversed Valsalva maneuver. The flexible laryngoscope is placed in the retrolingual region to assess the lateral and anteroposterior (AP) narrowing of the pharyngeal walls. The maneuver is then repeated with the device placed in the retropalatal region. In the past, it was hoped that a positive Müller's maneuver result would indicate that the site of upper airway collapse was below the level of the soft palate, and the patient would probably not benefit from a UPPP, while patients with retropalatal collapse would be the best candidates for UPPP.[80,81,82,83,84] There is now evidence that the sites of obstruction with Müller's maneuver do not reliably represent the sites of obstruction during normal sleep.[80,81,82,83,84] Its value can therefore be questioned. There is serious doubt whether the sites of obstruction as seen with the Müller's maneuver do reflect the site(s) of obstruction during sleep. Results of UPPP with the Müller's maneuver as a tool for patient selection are not better than without using it. In summary, the use of the Müller's maneuver is not advised. In spite of being technically easy to perform and inexpensive, it is also unspecific and subjective (▶Table 3.10).

Indications and Limitations of Awake Nasopharyngoscopy

The technique can be applied to rule out anatomical structures that can sometimes be missed by routine ENT investigation, such as obstruction in the nasopharynx, or lower, at laryngeal level. Usually, these are not the levels that are of highest interest, as these levels are rarely the sites of obstruction during sleep. They are no part of the collapsible upper airway segment. These sites can usually be visualized by routine anterior and posterior

▶Table 3.10 Incidence of severe airway collapse

Technique	Incidence
Retropalatal DISE	94.7%
Retropalatal MM	65.57%
Retrolingual DISE	69.56%
Retrolingual MM	28.98%

Abbreviations: DISE, drug-induced sleep endoscopy; MM, Müller's maneuver. Data based on Zerpa Zerpa V et al.[25]

rhinoscopy and indirect laryngoscopy using mirrors. In anxious patients or patients with high gag reflexes, awake nasopharyngoscopy might be used.

Awake nasopharyngoscopy provides insight in the anatomy of the nose, nasopharynx, pharynx, and larynx. Some of the sites, such as the nose, nasopharynx, and vocal cords, are not collapsible and so the situation during wakefulness and sleep is not different; for example, a straight nasal septum is not suddenly deviated during sleep, whether there is an obstruction in the nasopharynx or not, vocal cords are mobile or not, and have irregularities such as cysts, polyps, tumors, or not. In addition, such abnormalities become apparent because they cause other (nasal or voice) complaints that are present during wakefulness as well.

In contrast, the other sites such as velum, oropharynx, base of tongue, and epiglottis are collapsible. But in whichever position awake nasopharyngoscopy is performed, with or without maneuvers such as chin lift and mouth closure, it does not provide any information on the change in collapse pattern of the collapsible segment of the upper airway during sleep. That is why DISE is more reliable.

Therefore, in case treatment other than CPAP is considered, DISE will be performed (see Chapter 3.4.2) as awake nasopharyngoscopy does not provide any information that DISE cannot reveal. Hence, one could argue that awake nasopharyngoscopy can be regarded superfluous, unless the upper airway cannot be investigated in a proper way without it.

In case CPAP treatment is planned and DISE will not be performed, awake nasopharyngoscopy might be of value to rule out any rare findings. However, routine ENT investigation will also almost always reveal these abnormalities. Patients who are very anxious to undergo awake nasopharyngoscopy or patients with high gag reflexes are exceptions.

Conclusion

The workup of a patient with suspected OSA starts with careful history taking and physical examination. This might include awake nasopharyngoscopy. Its routine performance is debatable in case DISE is planned later. The Müller's maneuver is obsolete and not advised. There may be a role for awake nasopharyngoscopy in patients who cannot have DISE, especially anxious patients or patients with high gag reflexes.

3.4.2 Drug-Induced Sleep Endoscopy

Nico de Vries, Peter van Maanen, and Linda B. L. Benoist

It is the philosophy of this book, that in patients with SDB in whom treatment other than CPAP is considered, DISE should be performed. Such other treatments include sleep surgery, combined treatments (e.g., surgery and positional therapy), and treatment with an oral device (somewhat controversial). In this section the use of DISE and, in particular, the VOTE classification system will be discussed.

Introduction

DISE is a rapidly growing diagnostic tool to evaluate airway collapse in patients who might have non-CPAP therapies for SDB. DISE is an evaluation technique using fiberoptic nasopharyngoscopy to examine the upper airway that involves assessment of individuals under pharmacological sedation designed to mimic the situation during natural sleep as closely as possible. Sedative drugs such as midazolam, propofol, or combinations are usually used.

In 1978, Borowiecki introduced sleep endoscopy during natural sleep.[85] The method was cumbersome. In 1991, Croft and Pringle reported on sleep endoscopy in SDB under sedation.[86] The sedation allows assessment of the upper airway without waking the patient.

During DISE, the whole upper airway from entrance of the nose up to vocal cord level is assessed. The nasal passage, nasopharynx and velum, base of tongue, epiglottis, and endolarynx are examined.

Clinical and scientific interest in DISE is growing. For example, in the past few years, the number of scientific publications on DISE is equal to the number of earlier publications from all the years.[87] The evidence is also growing that certain DISE findings do have predictive value for surgery and other forms of treatment. DISE therefor is pivotal in treatment planning, in case other treatment than CPAP is considered.

It is the philosophy of this book, that in patients with SDB in whom other treatment than CPAP is considered, DISE should be performed. Such other treatments include sleep surgery, combined treatments (e.g., surgery and positional therapy) and, somewhat more controversial, treatment with an oral device. The first exception of this concept is positional therapy. In patients with positional OSA who can be cured with positional therapy alone, there is no need to perform DISE first. In case treatment with an MAD is considered, it is not clear whether DISE should be performed first. The first approach is to prescribe an MAD and not perform DISE. Insufficient effect of the MAD treatment would cost money and effort. The alternative approach is to perform DISE first, and if there is insufficient reaction to chin lift, then MAD is not recommended. The performance of DISE would also cost money. This is the topic of ongoing cost-effectiveness research.

European Position Paper on DISE

Since consensus on how to perform and score DISE was lacking, in 2014 an European working group was established in the hope to construct a consensus document. This led to the development of the "European position paper on DISE."[87] In this paper by De Vito et al, a proposal of the DISE procedure standardization has been brought forward with a general agreement concerning the terminology, indications, contraindications, required preliminary examinations, setting, required technical equipment and staffing, local anesthesia and nasal decongestion, patient positioning, basic and special passive diagnostic maneuvers, sedation drugs, and observation windows and required number of breathing cycles. The working group obtained consensus on many aspects, but failed to reach consensus on other aspects. The large number of variables when performing DISE might have blocked the development so far of a universal accepted scoring and classification system. This is unfortunate, but presently a clinical reality. Standardization of DISE would enable researchers and clinicians worldwide to compare findings and results of treatment.

One of the issues where no consensus was reached was the actual scoring system, how many and which levels or structures to score, and how to describe and quantify them? The authors of this chapter were involved in the development of one of the classification and scoring systems, the VOTE system and have extensive experience with it.[88] VOTE is presently the most used scoring system worldwide and will be discussed in more detail. Although there are other systems highlighted in De Vito et al's European position paper, the authors have deliberately not discussed them in this chapter to avoid confusion.

VOTE

Some scoring systems are complex and may be over comprehensive, while others group sites and structures together in various combinations, making them difficult to use and elaborate, with limited reproducibility and limited inter and intra-rater agreement. To overcome these drawbacks of some of earlier systems, the VOTE classification was proposed.[88] The VOTE classification is a scoring

method for describing DISE findings that focusses on specific sites and structures that contribute to obstruction. VOTE is an acronym. These structures include the collapsible segment of the upper airway: the Velum (palate and uvula), the Oropharyngeal lateral walls, including tonsils, base of Tongue, and Epiglottis. The VOTE concept consists of these four levels, of which the degree of obstruction and the configuration or direction is assessed.

The degree of obstruction involves three categories:

1. No obstruction: 50% narrowing.
2. Partial obstruction: 50 to 75% narrowing.
3. Complete obstruction: More than 75% narrowing.

The configuration or direction also has three possibilities:

1. AP
2. Concentric
3. Lateral

All forms of obstruction are not possible on all levels: on Velum level AP, lateral, and concentric are possible, but in general the obstruction at this level is either AP or concentric. Obstruction on oropharyngeal level is usually lateral (tonsils) but never AP; tongue base is usually AP but never lateral, epiglottis is either AP or lateral, but never concentric. Therefore the VOTE table is often used with closed options (▶ Fig. 3.46).

The clinical value of DISE is that we now know that certain findings are less attractive for surgery than others:

For instance, AP collapse is more favorable than concentric; unilevel collapse is more favorable than multilevel; partial collapse is better than complete.[9] With DISE, not infrequently, abnormalities such as an epiglottis collapse or complete concentric collapse at palatal level are found, that would not have been found with other diagnostic methods ▶ Fig. 3.47, ▶ Fig. 3.48, ▶ Fig. 3.49). In the upper airway stimulation STAR trial complete concentric collapse (▶ Fig. 3.50)

Fig. 3.46 VOTE classification.

LEVEL	DIRECTION		
	a-p	lateral	concentric
Velum			
Oropharynx, tonsils			
Tongue Base			
Epiglottis + Larynx			

on palatal level was an exclusion criterion, actually the first time that the FDA approved of DISE as a tool for patient selection.[89] Some more examples of static DISE findings are shown in ▶ Fig. 3.51, ▶ Fig. 3.52, ▶ Fig. 3.53, ▶ Fig. 3.54, ▶ Fig. 3.55, ▶ Fig. 3.56, ▶ Fig. 3.57 and ▶ Fig. 3.58.

Organization

The growing number of DISEs has consequences for the organization of clinical practice. When DISE is performed occasionally it can be incorporated in a regular operation

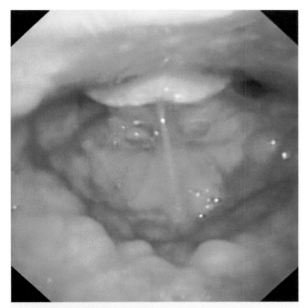

Fig. 3.47 Complete anteroposterior (AP) epiglottis collapse isolated (not secondary to tongue base collapse).

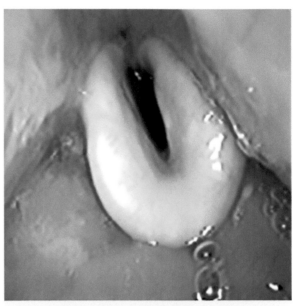

Fig. 3.48 Complete lateral collapse of the epiglottis.

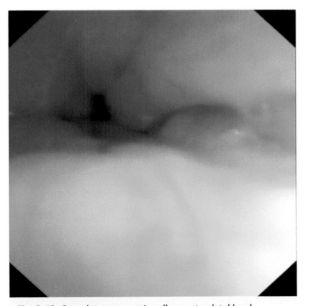

Fig. 3.49 Complete concentric collapse at palatal level.

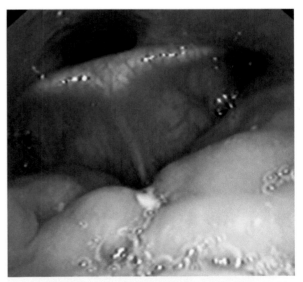

Fig. 3.50 Primary partial collapse of the epiglottis (not secondary to tongue base collapse).

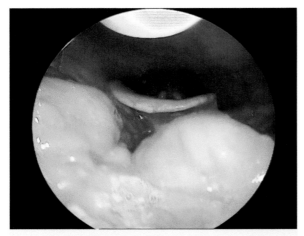

Fig. 3.51 No collapse of the epiglottis but the base of tongue is filled, vallecula is not visible.

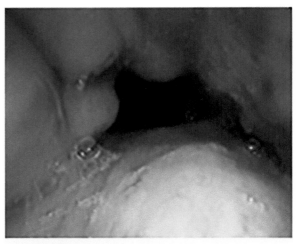

Fig. 3.52 Partial concentric collapse at palate.

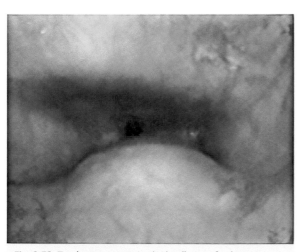

Fig. 3.53 Total anteroposterior (AP) collapse of palate.

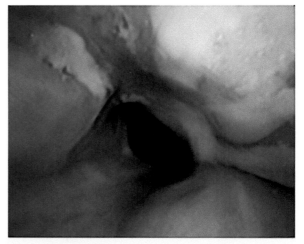

Fig. 3.54 Partial concentric collapse at palate.

room (OR) schedule. However, if DISEs are performed frequently on a weekly basis, other efficient forms of organizations might be preferable and would have to be organized.

Several organizational and logistical issues should be considered.[90] Based on authors' experience with hundreds of DISEs per year in recent years, they are of the opinion that DISE does not need to be performed by the same surgeon who would perform the sleep surgery later. DISE can also be performed by a medical resident/fellow without the presence of a senior staff member. It is not necessary to perform DISE in the OR, and it can be safely done in an outpatient setting. The presence of an anesthesiologist is also not necessary and sedation can be provided by a nurse anesthetist. It is not necessary that the endoscopist (or person who performs the DISE) performs the consultation with the patient after the DISE. Someone else from the care team can do the consultation and discuss the findings and

the recommended treatment or various treatment options. The post-DISE consultation can be done on the same day, but the patient and bed partner might come back later for a separate consultation as well.

Patient Indication for Drug-Induced Sleep Endoscopy

Selection criteria for DISE are mild to moderate OSA (i.e., AHI between 5 and 30/h sleep), or severe OSA and CPAP failure, BMI (arbitrarily) less than 32 kg/m², possible surgery, combined treatment or oral device candidates, and American Society of Anesthesiologists (ASA) class I or II. Patients with ASA 3 and severe cardiovascular comorbidity are a relative contraindication for the outpatient endoscopy setting. These patients have their DISE performed in the OR. As a rule, selecting lower BMI

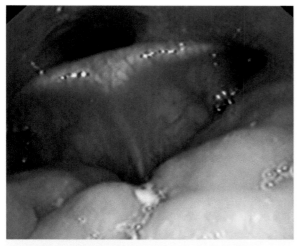

Fig. 3.55 Total anteroposterior (AP) collapse of the tongue base, epiglottis not visible.

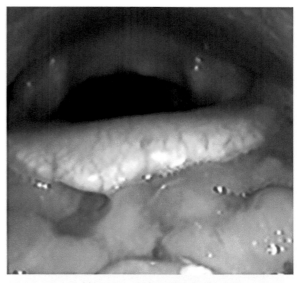

Fig. 3.56 Arguably no or partial epiglottis collapse, compare with ▶ Fig. 3.57.

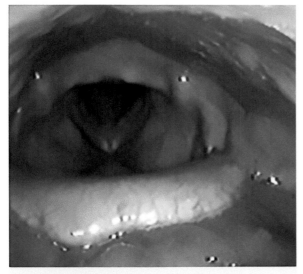

Fig. 3.57 Same patient as in ▶ Fig. 3.56. Effect of jaw thrust: complete opening of the airway.

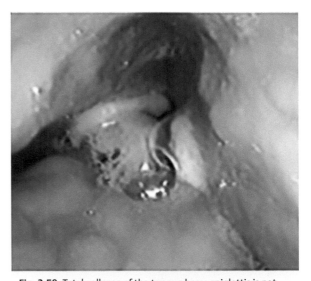

Fig. 3.58 Total collapse of the tongue base; epiglottis is not visible.

is important as it has been shown that surgery and oral devices have lower success rates above this BMI threshold.[91,92,93]

Staff

Since the beginning of January 2013, the authors switched from having an ENT staff performing DISE in the OR to performing the DISE in an outpatient endoscopy setting. The DISE is performed by an ENT resident or fellow, with a trained nurse anesthetist managing sedation. The other personnel present in the room is the ENT doctor's assistant, who arranges the flexible endoscope, operates the video recording system, and assists with minimizing patient movement during the examination. After DISE, patients go into a recovery area where a recovery nurse monitors blood pressure, saturation levels, and gives oxygen as needed.

Sedation Protocol

In the outpatient endoscopy setting, blood pressure, pulse oximetry, and ECG during DISE are monitored. To preoxygenate the patient, 100% oxygen is applied by a face mask. In the past Midazolam sedation was used, but authors have stopped doing this because of the amnesia caused by midazolam, which excludes the possibility to discuss the DISE outcome with the patient on the same day. Currently, we use intravenous (IV) propofol with the sedation rate controlled by a target controlled infusion (TCI) pump.

The sedation starts by setting the TCI pump according to height, age, and body weight of the patient. Before propofol, 2 cc Lidocaine intravenously is administered to prevent pain caused by the infusion of propofol. In some patients glycopyrrolate (antisecretory drug) through the IV might be indicated to avoid excessive secretions that may interfere with the quality of the imaging. The initial sedation starts with a small bolus of propofol (20–50 mg) and is subsequently maintained by the TCI pump. When the patient does not respond to the eyelash reflex and to verbal commands and/or starts snoring, the flexible nasopharyngoscopy is introduced through the nose. Adverse effects of the DISE procedure are rare; the authors have never encountered severe side effects or emergency situations.

Logistics

It is possible to perform DISE on 16 to 20 patients per day in an outpatient endoscopy setting.[89] Patients may undergo DISE in series; that is, one patient comes in for DISE as the last patient goes to the postanesthesia recovery room. In this way it is possible to perform 10 cases in half-day session. On average, the typical DISE lasts for 15 minutes.

DISE is historically performed in supine position. Since several years, in positional patients, the authors have performed DISE in lateral position as well. Research by Safiruddin et al has shown that the DISE findings in left and right lateral position are the same, while turning of the head alone and head and trunk combined, is almost the same.[94,95,96,97] This implicates that in positional patients, DISE does not have to be performed in five positions (head and trunk to the left, head only to the left, supine, head and trunk to the right, head only to the right), but only in two positions: supine and the head turned to one side.

In case MAD treatment is open as treatment option, chin lift will be performed as well. Chin lift is regarded as a predictor for the effect of an MAD to a certain extent. The precise positive and negative predictive values remain to be established, but it is reasonable to assume that when maximum chin lift does not open the airway sufficiently, the prescription of a MAD is not logical.

After DISE, patients spend on average 60 to 90 minutes in the recovery room, and are sufficiently awake to go for an office consultation to discuss the DISE findings and therapeutic options. Patients who come from outside the region are offered a same day consultation with the sleep surgeon to discuss the results and treatment options. Patients who live nearby might have a repeat consultation on another day.

DISE Report

After DISE, the ENT resident prepares a report that includes the following:

1. Results of the previous PSG containing a minimum the total AHI (obstructive, mixed, central), and the AHIs in each sleeping position; and amount of time spent in the various sleep positions.
2. BMI and ENT investigation findings, including nasal examination and dental status.
3. The VOTE score is used to classify the upper airway collapse pattern during DISE, which is also video recorded for later review if needed.[88,95] In case an MAD is considered as treatment option, a chin lift is performed and VOTE is scored. Similarly, if positional therapy may be considered, the DISE will also be performed with the patient's head turned to the side and the VOTE table is again filled out.[94,95] In case a combination of an oral device and positional therapy is considered, chin lift may be performed in lateral position. The VOTE table is again filled out.
4. The resident's or fellow's treatment proposal, which may include conservative measures, CPAP, oral device, positional therapy, various forms of surgery (including upper airway stimulation), participation in clinical trials, or combined therapies.[98,99,100,101] This report allows the supervisor to check the resident's progress at diagnosis and treating the patient.

Consequences of DISE Findings

In authors' view, the DISE findings, in combination with PSG outcome and patient's preference, dictate the treatment options to a large extent. Usually the PSG and DISE findings have a moderate to reasonable correlation. In case of a low AHI at PSG, limited obstruction is encountered during DISE (more often unilevel than multilevel, more often partial than complete, more often AP than concentric); with high AHIs, this is usually the other way around. Whenever one experiences an inconsistency between AHI and DISE that is not well understood, one should be alert whether one of the two studies is incorrect. In doubtful cases, either the PSG or DISE should be repeated. Which one of the two needs to be repeated depends on which test is not representative of the clinical situation; for example, in a patient with complaints of severe OSA and more severe, multilevel obstruction but low AHI during DISE, it would make sense to repeat the PSG. One should also always be aware of too low or too deep sedation level during DISE.

In case the PSG and DISE scores align well, any surgical approach should be based on the levels, severity, and configuration of obstruction. This implies that in case of multilevel obstruction, a multilevel surgery should be offered. Patients with multilevel obstruction sometimes request to perform only one surgery to start with, but authors strongly avoid doing so as multilevel obstruction cannot be corrected with a one-level surgery. Similarly, in case of only partial obstruction of base of the tongue level, a minimal invasive intervention (e.g., radiofrequent ablation) would be offered, while in complete obstruction this would not be sufficient and a more aggressive approach (e.g., radiofrequent ablation combined with hyoid suspension) would be indicated. In case of a complete concentric palatal collapse, patients would not be eligible for several modern treatments such as upper airway stimulation, while participation in some trials with tongue implants would also not be possible. In expert opinion, a case of complete concentric palatal collapse needs a special surgical technique such as expansion sphincter pharyngoplasty that addresses the lateral pharyngeal wall, rather than traditional UPPP. Sometimes patients present with severe OSA, but with obstruction at only one level, for example, limited to the palate. In such a case, the authors would still consequently follow the DISE findings and, in spite of the severe OSA, start with surgery on the level where the obstruction was found.

Conclusion

In the philosophy of this book, DISE is a standard diagnostic tool for patients with OSA where non-CPAP therapies are considered. Because of the large numbers of patients scheduled for DISE, organization of procedure logistics is critically important. DISE can be easily performed by an ENT resident or fellow, and nurse anesthetist in an outpatient endoscopy setting. The use of a standardized DISE scoring system such as the VOTE score allows a common framework for sharing findings between the endoscopist (who may be an ENT resident/fellow) and the ENT surgeon. In some cases, further discussion of the DISE findings between the resident/fellow and staff surgeon might be indicated, for example, in case of complete circular palatal collapse versus AP collapse, as this might have consequences for eligibility for certain forms of surgery, such as upper airway stimulation. In these circumstances, the

DISE video recordings can be reassessed by the resident/fellow, surgeon, or a larger group in order to reach consensus. From a teaching perspective, there's also an advantage of delegating DISE to the resident. This system allows the supervisor to monitor the resident's train of thought, logic, and learning curve while performing a large number of DISEs, as it's been well established that high-procedure volume is important for proper medical training.

Acknowledgment

The authors would like to thank the nurse anesthetists for their help and valuable support during the DISE procedures: P. Karlas, E. van Aalst and A. van Limburg-Brouwer.

3.4.3 Upper Airway Imaging in Sleep-Disordered Breathing

Jolien Beyers, Olivier M. Vanderveken, Johan Verbraecken, Robert Poirrier, and Anne-Lise Poirrier

Most cases of SDB, if not all, include a partial or a total obstruction of the upper airway, at the retropalatal or retroglossal regions.[102,103,104,105]

This phenomenon is causal in simple snoring, upper airway resistance syndrome, and OSAS, and has been demonstrated since two to four decades by radio cinematography associated with fluoroscopy.[106,107,108,109] Oscillations in the permeability of the upper airway may also contribute to the pathophysiology of periodic breathing and CSA syndromes.[110,111] The temporal pattern of patency reduction of the upper airway may vary from permanent flow limitation to intermittent collapses of at least 10 seconds in any stage of sleep.

OSA is the most common SDB in referred populations; pathophysiologic studies have shown that upper airway obstruction results from structural and functional factors (▶ Fig. 3.59). The structural (or anatomical)

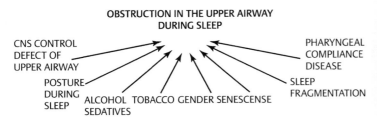

Fig. 3.59 Main structural and functional factors that may impinge on the upper airway during sleep in sleep-disordered breathing (SDB).

abnormalities provide a static component, while the functional abnormalities provide a dynamic component. A combination of a collapsible tube interfering with muscle and brain control activities explains the temporal distribution of events. Brain control acts by inducing a more or less pronounced pharyngeal dilator muscle tone during the different sleep stages as well as recurrent arousals.[112]

The genuine complexity of the pharynx—with very mobile anterior and compliant lateral parts, contrasting with relatively stiff posterior walls, the lack of anatomical normative data, and the intermingling of dynamic processes—explains why the diagnosis of SDB still depends essentially on PSG and less on imaging procedures. However, this situation could rapidly change, as new computer methods evolve, allowing three-dimensional image processing and digital analysis of fluid behavior through the collapsible pharynx.[113]

Nevertheless, in daily practice, some imaging techniques may provide interesting clues for understanding the main factors that contribute to obstruction of the upper airway in a given patient. These techniques could eventually help decide which treatments are most beneficial to the patient. Practically, three techniques offer the best quality price ratio: cephalometry, videoendoscopy, and acoustic reflectometry of the upper airway.

Cephalometry

Cephalometric analysis is used by orthodontics to measure the size and spatial relationship of the teeth, jaw, and facial subcranial volumes. The resulting information allows an appropriate correction of tooth arrangement. Classically, a set of landmarks are identified on lateral radiographs of an individual (▶Fig. 3.60, ▶Fig. 3.61). Between these landmarks distances, angles, or surfaces are measured and compared to normative data, taking into account potential radiological magnification factors. Such radiography is usually performed during wakefulness, patient sitting with the gaze fixed on a plane parallel to the ground, teeth in contact, while lips being relaxed.

Between 1983 and 1986, the Stanford University group, relying on a pathogenic theory that postulated that the bone enclosure of the upper airway must be abnormally reduced in SDB, compared the results of cephalometric analyses obtained in small series of OSA patients with anatomical anthropometric data. These first publications showed three abnormalities: a retroposition of the mandible relative to the upper maxilla, a long soft palate, and a too low position of the hyoid bone relative to the floor of the mandible.[114,115]

In 1986, Lowe et al showed a frequent steep mandibular plane angle and a maxilla that could also be in an abnormal posterior position.[116] In addition, Bacon et al in 1988 observed a shortening of the anterior skull base in some of their OSA patients, by measuring the distance between the center of the sella and the nasion (SN).[117]

Since these pioneer works, numerous other studies have demonstrated the relevance of these observations by multiplying the anthropometric marking methods on radiographs in lateral view and by increasing their statistical validities.[118,119,120,121,122,123,124,125,126,127,128,129,130] Others have pointed out ethnic characteristics in African-Americans,[131,132] East-Asians,[133] South-Asians,[134] and Polynesians[135] communities.

Frontal or AP cephalometry was developed in the early 2000s (▶Fig. 3.60).[135,136,137] This approach complements the data obtained by the lateral X-ray, showing that the maxilla could play a key role in the development of OSA. A growth deficiency of this bone is probably linked to long-standing oral breathing frequently observed in these patients.[138,139]

More recently, cone beam computed tomography (CBCT) was shown to integrate three-dimensional landmarks derived from cephalometry with a reasonable irradiation cost. CBCT is able to improve OSA diagnosis, mainly by quickly assessing the three dimensions of the upper airway.[140,141,142]

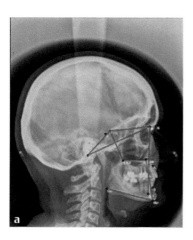
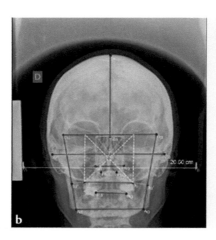

Fig. 3.60 Lateral **(a)** and frontal **(b)** radiographs with cranial and facial identifications of key cephalometric landmarks.

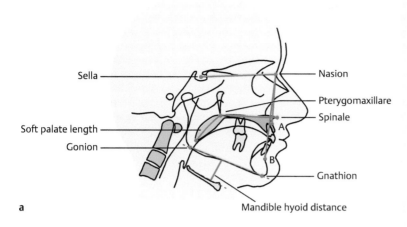

Fig. 3.61 Cone beam computed tomography (CBCT) with main cephalometric landmarks from a normal subject **(a)** and a patient with obstructive sleep apnea (OSA) **(b)**.

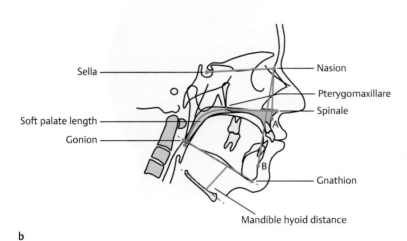

One of the most interesting aspects of cephalometric studies is their contribution to the understanding of OSA pathogenesis. Besides the mechanisms of obesity, it provides information on the nature of any deficits of the bone enclosure growth factors. A reduction of the anterior sagittal distance of the skull (SN) reflects a growth deficit of ethmoid or sphenoid bones. These bones belong to the chondrocranium and their final dimension is mainly genetically determined, while the maxillary and mandibular bones contain a large proportion of desmocranium. The growth of the latter is largely dependent on postnatal factors. In this way, cephalometric analysis can show different phenotypes, susceptible to develop upper airway SDB.

Soft tissues are also accessible to cephalometrics. The caliber of the upper airway, the length and shape of the soft palate,[143] the distance between the floor and mandibular hyoid bone are among the most commonly reported parameters, while soft tissues remain most difficult to characterize because they depend more on patient cooperation and intensity of radiation exposure.

Recently, Denolf et al reviewed the contribution of cephalometry in the prediction of outcome from OSA treatments, depending on the upper airway morphology in their mechanisms of action. Until now, isolated cephalometric parameters cannot be used for such predictions for treatment outcome of mandibular advancement therapy and various surgical methods for OSA. However, extreme or outlying values of cephalometric parameters might rather be used as contraindicators instead.[144]

In summary, studies using conventional and CBCT cephalometries have demonstrated the role of craniofacial bone development in sleep apnea. In particular, maxilla volume reduction plays a key role in sleep apnea development and severity. Other factors are reductions in mandibular body length (with or without retrognathia), restriction in the upper airway caliber, inferiorly positioned hyoid bone, and shortening of the anterior skull base.[145] All these features are schematically presented in ▸ Fig. 3.61.

Upper Airway Videoendoscopy

A need for credible alternative treatments to CPAP in OSA has increased, as its recognition has grown in populations. This is due, in part, to the progressive apprehension of its pathogenic role in cardiovascular disorders, diabetes mellitus, depression, etc., and in part to the better accessibility to diagnosis with the expanded use of simpler and easier portable monitoring systems. OSA is not only common but also presents as a broad spectrum of severity. In this context, a concern for more targeted treatments has emerged, at least for the less severe or earliest forms of the disease, as well as for the clinical conditions where CPAP is unsuccessful.

In these situations, it can be, a priori, estimated that surgical treatments of the soft palate or tonsils are more specifically justified when upper airway collapse is limited to the retropalatal pharynx. On the contrary, treatments with orthodontic devices, ensuring a mandibular advancement and a closing of the mouth, could be better indicated when the collapse takes place in the retrolingual region. The same has to be considered for a predictable efficiency of placing a stimulator on the motor nerve of the tongue. Consequently, surgical and prosthetic procedures are more dependent than CPAP to a clear knowledge of the abnormal behavior that has to be amended in the upper airway.

Upper airway videoendoscopy, before or during sleep, is a classical diagnostic approach in OSA, even if it is not systematically used. It can visualize permanent or intermittent obstacles in the lumen. Its main limitation is that it can neither assess the surrounding anatomical structures nor determine, consequently, their role. In this last context, drug-induced sleep videoendoscopy may represent a promising avenue.

Upper airway videoendoscopy during wakefulness is used to rule out any permanent and threatening narrowing, in the nose and pharynx, due to anatomical or anatomopathological abnormalities. However, in the most common OSA cases, the obstruction site is only discernible during sleep. The Müller's maneuver has been proposed in an attempt to predict the level at which collapse could occur in the upper airway.[83] It consists of a forced voluntary inspiratory effort against a closed mouth and nose. The endoscope is inserted through one of the nostrils, while the patient is supine and awake. The retropalatal, retrolingual, and epiglottic behavior of the pharynx can be investigated during this maneuver. However, it remains highly questionable to be sure that such behavior is identical to what happens during sleep. As the maneuver is voluntary, the muscular tone and respiratory drive

are different from what can be observed during sleep. Confrontation of results for the sites of obstruction by this method, with a multilevel pressure-transducer catheter method during sleep has shown that identical places of collapse by both methods were obtained in only one patient in four.[146] This could explain the generally poor results of UPPP when the Müller's maneuver is considered a predictor of outcome.[83,84,147]

Natural sleep videoendoscopy (NSVE) aims to determine the location, extent, and structural aspects (concentric or one-sided collapse) of an obstruction under the most realistic circumstances. It is technically limited by the need to insert or maintain an endoscope into the upper airway and wait for the occurrence of natural sleep stages, in a favorable environment. This is very difficult to obtain because the endoscope has to be handled and can therefore disturb sleep. A variant has been proposed, in which such intervention is realized while the patient is under treatment with CPAP. The administered pressure is reduced for a single breath. Digitized images of the lumen are recorded and the cross-sectional areas of the upper airway can be measured at different levels. This method has been found to be accurate within 10%.[148,149] The modalities of upper airway NSVE keep two limitations for a development as routine examination: (1) it is not possible to study different levels simultaneously, and (2) the method remains time- and instrument-consuming.

Drug-induced sleep videoendoscopy (DISVE) has the same objectives. It is assumed that neither the endoscope nor the drug may significantly disturb or influence breathing patterns or airway obstruction during the test. Indeed, such procedure is able to initiate snoring and upper airway obstruction.

The most frequently used anesthetic agents are the IV drugs midazolam, diazepam, and propofol. These are substances that enhance GABA neuron activity in the brain. This pharmacological action is closest to the recognized mechanisms of slow-wave sleep. DISVE by using IV midazolam was first reported in children,[150] then in adults.[86] It was performed on 71 patients. The authors successfully demonstrated the site of snoring and/or collapse in 56 patients (79%). Sadaoka et al[151] could demonstrate that during a 3-hour videoendoscopy under sedation with diazepam, only the longest apnea and the portion of REM sleep showed statistically significant differences compared to natural sleep. The severity of the underlying disorder appears comparable to natural sleep, although snoring sounds seem different.

Recent studies propose methods for scoring sites, degrees, and patterns of upper airway closure[88,95,152] and yields good results in predicting success or failure of various therapeutic interventions.[95,153,154] These observational or cross-sectional studies do still carry on relatively small series. More recently, a large observational study was conducted by Vroegop et al, providing an overview of upper airway collapse patterns.[101] The authors concluded that the associations found in the study might indicate that the collapse patterns observed during DISVE cannot be fully explained by selected baseline PSG and anthropometric characteristics.

In conclusion, DISVE has given new insight in the control of upper airway during sleep.

Upper Airway Reflectometry

Since the pioneering work of Fredberg et al[155] and Bradley et al[156] on acoustic reflectometry of the upper airway, this technique has known an eclipse. Probably, because of the fact that compared with videoendoscopy, it allows only a two-dimensional vision. More than the videoendoscopy, upper airway reflectometry gives access to pharynx-compliance measurements at different levels; however, the results have not always been encouraging.[157]

However, in recent years, sensitive technological improvements have allowed to measure the cross-sectional surfaces of the pharynx at all distances from the mouth. Patients are examined awake, sitting, or lying down in a comfortable position. Preliminary studies have shown that simple snorers can be easily differentiated from snorers with obstructive apneas. The method, also called acoustic pharyngometry, seems accurate and reproducible.[158,159] Therefore, it could be very useful to assess difficult diagnosis, such as the upper airway resistance syndrome. A recent cohort study confirms the use of acoustic pharyngometry as a quick and easily performed screening tool in awake subjects.[160] However, the authors of this study conclude that it is probably of no clinical utility in its current setting.

An interesting variation of acoustic reflectometry is the forced oscillation technique (FOT). It was first developed by DuBois et al in 1956.[161] It involves measuring the reflection of a pressure wave (usually 5 Hz) superimposed on the administration of air and to deduce the values of resistance in the different regions of the airways. FOT has been proposed for automatic titration of CPAP in OSAS,[162,163,164] but also to simply assess pharyngeal patency continuously and noninvasively during sleep.[165,166]

Conclusions

The popularity of upper airway imaging methods is largely determined by their contribution to the success of predictive models for alternative therapeutic treatment to CPAP, in OSA. Even though there is still not enough evidence that they can improve the outcome of snoring and sleep apnea surgery, it is clear that considerable progress can be expected in the coming years with technological and digital advancements. The cephalometric analysis will certainly benefit from the three-dimensional analytical capacity of tissue densities provided by CBCT.[167] Videoendoscopy could be largely improved by endoscopic long-range optical coherence tomography.[168] At last, novel imaging techniques using computer methods

for the prediction of the upper airway will also be of considerable help in decision making in patients with SDB.[113]

3.4.4 Analysis of Snoring Sounds

Michael Herzog

Background

Since the beginning of acoustic snoring noise analysis in the 80s and 90s, the focus was to distinguish between different types of snoring.[169,170,171,172,173] Snoring can occur as a symptom of OSA or as simple snoring without accompanying apneas. From the diagnostic point of view a differentiation between apneic and nonapneic snoring was relatively easy to perform by using the PSG parameters (e.g., AHI) as definition criteria.[174,175,176,177,178] In fact different types of snoring sounds could be differentiated by their spectral parameters. In the majority of publications an increase of the AHI is correlated with an increase of the fundamental frequency or frequency of maximum intensity. In general, there is consensus that apneic snoring predominantly has maxima frequency spectrum above 400 Hz, whereas nonapneic snoring is defined by maxima below 200 Hz. The discrimination is mostly based on frequency analyses (fast Fourier transformation [FFT]) creating frequency spectra of high or low intensity over a certain period of time.

Acoustic Information about the Obstruction Site

The differentiation of snoring sounds on the basis of the site of origin is an interesting aspect in the clinical use. DISE provides an alternative method to obtain combined acoustical and visual information because of the enormous difficulties of direct visualization of the upper airway during natural sleep. DISE became popular in the early 90s parallel to the snoring sound analysis and several authors applied both techniques.[179,180] It needs to be kept in mind that medically induced sleep does not match natural sleep and snoring sounds vary between natural and induced sleep even when produced at the same site.[181,182] Despite this restriction DISE is nowadays generally accepted as the method of choice to detect the site(s), severity, and patterns of obstruction. These patterns and sites obtained by DISE can be adapted for snoring sound analyses.

Sound Analysis during Drug-Induced Sleep Endoscopy

Applying the widely used VOTE classification of obstruction sites and patterns during DISE the different anatomic structures create individual snoring sounds which can be differentiated by sound analysis.[183] From the clinical aspect, the velum vibration is predominantly in AP direction. This fluttering type of snoring creates a low frequency-dominated sound (80–200 Hz) with accompanying harmonic spectra (►Fig. 3.62). Oropharyngeal obstructions can occur lateral or concentric with or without hyperplastic tonsils. Mostly, an oropharyngeal collapse has a higher obstructive component resulting in a raised frequency spectrum (100–500 Hz) (►Fig. 3.63). Tongue base obstruction is caused by a dorsal movement of the whole body of the tongue or by hyperplastic tongue base tonsils. The obstructive component is higher at velar or oropharyngeal level. The more obstructive a tongue base relapse is the higher the frequency spectrum (300–700 Hz). Additionally, harmonic spectra are reduced and disharmonic frequencies dominate the spectral analyses (►Fig. 3.64). A collapse caused by an epiglottal collapse often creates a subtotal or complete obstruction of the airway, resulting in a disharmonic

noise similar to a tongue base obstruction but with less intensity (►Fig. 3.65).

For ►Fig. 3.62, ►Fig. 3.63, ►Fig. 3.64, and ►Fig. 3.65, snoring samples have been obtained during DISE. The site and pattern of vibration/obstruction is visually classified (velum, ►Fig. 3.62; tonsil, ►Fig. 3.63; tongue, ►Fig. 3.64; epiglottis, ►Fig. 3.65). At the top of each of these figures, the endoscopic images are displayed. Three images at the left demonstrate exemplarily the movement of the anatomic structure. The image on the right side provides the pattern of obstruction by included arrows. The large image displays the spectral view of the specific snoring episode over the time (x-axis). The frequency is given in the y-axis. The intensity of a specific frequency is displayed by the brightness of the colors (black = weak intensity; white = high intensity).

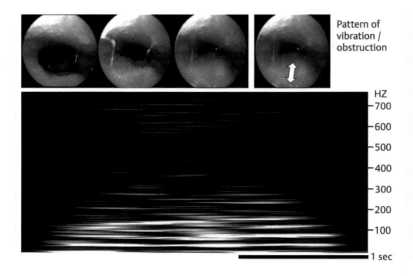

Pattern of vibration / obstruction

Fig. 3.62 Velar snoring. Snoring is induced by anterioposterior (AP) movement of the uvula. The frequency spectrum is dominated by intensities of low frequencies (below 200 Hz) and parallel harmonics.

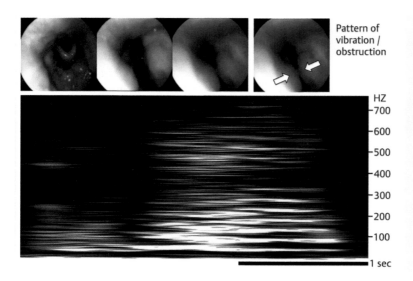

Pattern of vibration / obstruction

Fig. 3.63 Tonsillar snoring. Snoring is induced by lateral convergence of the tonsils indicated by arrows. The frequency spectrum is dominated by intensities of low frequencies (below 300 Hz) and parallel harmonics. Additionally higher frequencies (400–700 Hz) are present representing the obstructive character of the snoring noise.

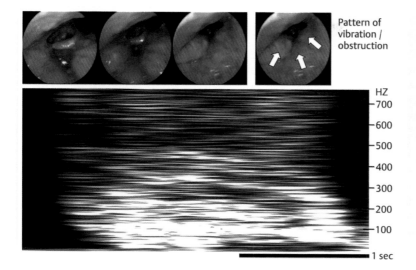

Pattern of vibration / obstruction

HZ
-700
-600
-500
-400
-300
-200
-100

1 sec

Fig. 3.64 Tongue base snoring. Snoring is induced by dorsal movement of the enlarged tongue base tonsils indicated by arrows. The frequency spectrum is dominated by intensities over a wide range of frequencies (50–700 Hz). No parallel harmonics are detectable as an indication for the obstructive character of the snoring noise induced by a big mass (tongue base).

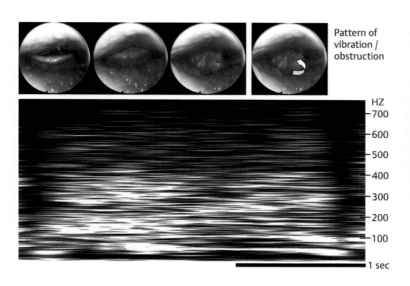

Pattern of vibration / obstruction

HZ
-700
-600
-500
-400
-300
-200
-100

1 sec

Fig. 3.65 Epiglottic snoring. Snoring is induced by relapse of the epiglottis indicated by arrows. The frequency spectrum is dominated by intensities over a wide range of frequencies (50–400 Hz). No parallel harmonics are detectable as an indication for the obstructive character of the snoring noise. Compared to tongue base snoring frequencies spectra above 400 Hz are low which indicates an induction by relatively small mass of the epiglottis (compared to ▶ Fig. 3.64, tongue as a big mass).

Acoustic Characteristics of Snoring Sounds

Despite a large variety of sound characters, some common assumptions can be stated:

1. Vibrations cause parallel harmonics (e.g., uvula or tonsils).
2. Obstructions reveal broad spectra of noise without harmonics (e.g., epiglottis or tongue base).
3. The lower the volume or the mass of the vibrating structure the lower the fundamental frequency spectrum (e.g., uvula lowers fundamental frequency than tonsils).
4. The higher the mass of the obstructing anatomic structure the wider the frequency spectra (e.g., epiglottis smaller spectrum than tongue base).

Future Perspectives

Nowadays psychoacoustic parameters have been investigated to provide a more clinical focus of sound analysis.[184,185,186,187] The background of this novel approach is the desire of otolaryngological surgeons to have an objective tool for measurement of annoyance of a specific snoring noise as annoyance is a major influence on surgery to be performed. Apparently, high-frequency dominated snoring noises are more annoying than lower ones. It can be assumed that the information about the degree and hazardousness of an airway obstruction is encoded in its frequency spectrum which is instinctively interpreted by the bed partner.

Despite all approaches to define anatomic structures causing vibrations and obstructions by their acoustic information a routine application is still not available.

This variety of snoring sounds is too heterogenic and often several sites and patterns of obstruction contribute to an individual snoring noise. Recent publications are based on a visual classification of the obstruction sites and the snoring sound was investigated accordingly. Only limited numbers of individuals can be investigated by this method. In order to classify different acoustic subpatterns a larger amount of samples need to be classified. Recent publications report this promising approach by self-learning neuronal networks.[188,189,190,191] As soon as reliable algorithms are defined, snoring sounds analyses can easily be conducted via small devices, smart phones, or even the Internet.[192,193] Novel technological options will extract even more information from snoring noises and might influence our diagnostic and therapeutic procedure for snoring and sleep apnea in the future.

References

[1] Johns MW. A new method for measuring daytime sleepiness: the Epworth sleepiness scale. Sleep. 1991; 14(6):540–545

[2] Weaver TE, Laizner AM, Evans LK, et al. An instrument to measure functional status outcomes for disorders of excessive sleepiness. Sleep. 1997; 20(10):835–843

[3] McHorney CA, Ware JE, Jr, Raczek AE. The MOS 36-Item Short-Form Health Survey (SF-36): II. Psychometric and clinical tests of validity in measuring physical and mental health constructs. Med Care. 1993; 31(3):247–263

[4] Buysse DJ, Reynolds CF, III, Monk TH, Berman SR, Kupfer DJ. The Pittsburgh Sleep Quality Index: a new instrument for psychiatric practice and research. Psychiatry Res. 1989; 28(2):193–213

[5] Gliklich RE, Wang PC. Validation of the snore outcomes survey for patients with sleep-disordered breathing. Arch Otolaryngol Head Neck Surg. 2002; 128(7):819–824

[6] Douglas SA, Webster S, El Badawey MR, et al. The development of a snoring symptoms inventory. Otolaryngol Head Neck Surg. 2006; 134(1):56–62

[7] Stewart MG, Witsell DL, Smith TL, Weaver EM, Yueh B, Hannley MT. Development and validation of the Nasal Obstruction Symptom Evaluation (NOSE) scale. Otolaryngol Head Neck Surg. 2004; 130(2):157–163

[8] Roskin M, Dasberg H. On the validity of the Symptom Check List-90 (SCL90): a comparison of diagnostic self-ratings in general practice patients and 'normals', based on the Hebrew version. Int J Soc Psychiatry. 1983; 29(3):225–230

[9] Koutsourelakis I, Safiruddin F, Ravesloot M, Zakynthinos S, de Vries N. Surgery for obstructive sleep apnea: sleep endoscopy determinants of outcome. Laryngoscope. 2012; 122(11):2587–2591

[10] Dancey DR, Hanly PJ, Soong C, Lee B, Shepard J, Jr, Hoffstein V. Gender differences in sleep apnea: the role of neck circumference. Chest. 2003; 123(5):1544–1550

[11] Davies RJ, Ali NJ, Stradling JR. Neck circumference and other clinical features in the diagnosis of the obstructive sleep apnoea syndrome. Thorax. 1992; 47(2):101–105

[12] Deacon NL, Jen R, Li Y, Malhotra A. Treatment of obstructive sleep apnea: prospects for personalized combined modality therapy. Ann Am Thorac Soc. 2016; 13:101–108

[13] Zonato AI, Bittencourt LR, Martinho FL, Júnior JFS, Gregório LC, Tufik S. Association of systematic head and neck physical examination with severity of obstructive sleep apnea-hypopnea syndrome. Laryngoscope. 2003; 113(6):973–980

[14] Rotenberg BW, Theriault J, Gottesman S. Redefining the timing of surgery for obstructive sleep apnea in anatomically favorable patients. Laryngoscope. 2014; 124(Suppl 4):S1–S9

[15] Friedman M, Ibrahim H, Bass L. Clinical staging for sleep-disordered breathing. Otolaryngol Head Neck Surg. 2002; 127(1):13–21

[16] Friedman M, Ibrahim H, Joseph NJ. Staging of obstructive sleep apnea/hypopnea syndrome: a guide to appropriate treatment. Laryngoscope. 2004; 114(3):454–459

[17] Camacho M, Li D, Kawai M, et al. Tonsillectomy for adult obstructive sleep apnea: A systematic review and meta-analysis. Laryngoscope. 2016; 126(9):2176–2186

[18] Vicini C, Montevecchi F, Pang K, et al. Combined transoral robotic tongue base surgery and palate surgery in obstructive sleep apnea-hypopnea syndrome: expansion sphincter pharyngoplasty versus uvulopalatopharyngoplasty. Head Neck. 2014; 36(1):77–83

[19] Pang KP, Pang EB, Win MTM, Pang KA, Woodson BT. Expansion sphincter pharyngoplasty for the treatment of OSA: a systemic review and meta-analysis. Eur Arch Otorhinolaryngol. 2016; 273(9):2329–2333

[20] Suh GD. Evaluation of open midline glossectomy in the multilevel surgical management of obstructive sleep apnea syndrome. Otolaryngol Head Neck Surg. 2013; 148(1):166–171

[21] Murphey AW, Kandl JA, Nguyen SA, Weber AC, Gillespie MB. The effect of glossectomy for obstructive sleep apnea: a systematic review and meta-analysis. Otolaryngol Head Neck Surg. 2015; 153(3):334–342

[22] Hou J, Yan J, Wang B, et al. Treatment of obstructive sleep apnea-hypopnea syndrome with combined uvulopalatopharyngoplasty and midline glossectomy: outcomes from a 5-year study. Respir Care. 2012; 57(12):2104–2110

[23] Sundman J, Bring J, Friberg D. Poor interexaminer agreement on Friedman tongue position. Acta Otolaryngol. 2016:1–3

[24] den Herder C, van Tinteren H, de Vries N. Sleep endoscopy versus modified Mallampati score in sleep apnea and snoring. Laryngoscope. 2005; 115(4):735–739

[25] Zerpa Zerpa V, Carrasco Llatas M, Agostini Porras G, Dalmau Galofre J. Drug-induced sedation endoscopy versus clinical exploration for the diagnosis of severe upper airway obstruction in OSAHS patients. Sleep Breath. 2015; 19(4):1367–1372

[26] Chen X, Sun J, Yuan W, Li J. OSAHS obstructive plane localization: comparative study between ag200 and Friedman classification. Int J Clin Exp Med. 2015; 8(2):2240–2246

[27] Lee CH, Won TB, Cha W, Yoon IY, Chung S, Kim JW. Obstructive site localization using multisensor manometry versus the Friedman staging system in obstructive sleep apnea. Eur Arch Otorhinolaryngol. 2008; 265(2):171–177

[28] Abrishami A, Khajehdehi A, Chung F. A systematic review of screening questionnaires for obstructive sleep apnea. Can J Anaesth. 2010; 57(5):423–438

[29] Peppard PE, Young T, Barnet JH, Palta M, Hagen EW, Hla KM. Increased prevalence of sleep-disordered breathing in adults. Am J Epidemiol. 2013; 177(9):1006–1014

[30] Remmers JE, deGroot WJ, Sauerland EK, Anch AM. Pathogenesis of upper airway occlusion during sleep. J Appl Physiol. 1978; 44(6):931–938

[31] Fogel RB, Malhotra A, Shea SA, Edwards JK, White DP. Reduced genioglossal activity with upper airway anesthesia in awake patients with OSA. J Appl Physiol (1985). 2000; 88(4):1346–1354

[32] Sin DD, Fitzgerald F, Parker JD, Newton G, Floras JS, Bradley TD. Risk factors for central and obstructive sleep apnea in 450 men and women with congestive heart failure. Am J Respir Crit Care Med. 1999; 160(4):1101–1106

[33] Javaheri S. Sleep disorders in systolic heart failure: a prospective study of 100 male patients. The final report. Int J Cardiol. 2006; 106(1):21–28

[34] American Academy of Sleep Medicine. International Classification of Sleep Disorders—Third Edition (ICSD-3). Westchester, IL: American Academy of Sleep Medicine; 2014

[35] Sands SA, Edwards BA, Kee K, et al. Loop gain as a means to predict a positive airway pressure suppression of Cheyne-Stokes respiration in patients with heart failure. Am J Respir Crit Care Med. 2011; 184(9):1067–1075

[36] Manuel AR, Hart N, Stradling JR. Correlates of obesity-related chronic ventilatory failure. BMJ Open Respir Res. 2016; 3(1):e000110

[37] Piper A. Obesity hypoventilation syndrome: weighing in on therapy options. Chest. 2016; 149(3):856–868

[38] German Society for Sleep Research and Sleep Medicine (DGSM). [S3-Guideline: Non- Restorative Sleep. Chapter: Sleep Related Breathing Disturbances] Somnologie (Berl) 2017; 20(Suppl s2):S97–S180

[39] Randerath WJ. Obesity hypoventilation syndrome. Somnologie (Berl). 2012; 16(3):154–159

[40] Steier J, Jolley CJ, Seymour J, Roughton M, Polkey MI, Moxham J. Neural respiratory drive in obesity. Thorax. 2009; 64(8):719–725

[41] Macavei VM, Spurling KJ, Loft J, Makker HK. Diagnostic predictors of obesity-hypoventilation syndrome in patients suspected of having sleep disordered breathing. J Clin Sleep Med. 2013; 9(9):879–884

[42] Zwillich CW, Sutton FD, Pierson DJ, Greagh EM, Weil JV. Decreased hypoxic ventilatory drive in the obesity-hypoventilation syndrome. Am J Med. 1975; 59(3):343–348

[43] Dong JY, Zhang YH, Qin LQ. Obstructive sleep apnea and cardiovascular risk: meta-analysis of prospective cohort studies. Atherosclerosis. 2013; 229(2):489–495

[44] Gami AS, Hodge DO, Herges RM, et al. Obstructive sleep apnea, obesity, and the risk of incident atrial fibrillation. J Am Coll Cardiol. 2007; 49(5):565–571

[45] Corrà U, Pistono M, Mezzani A, et al. Sleep and exertional periodic breathing in chronic heart failure: prognostic importance and interdependence. Circulation. 2006; 113(1):44–50

[46] Damy T, Margarit L, Noroc A, et al. Prognostic impact of sleep-disordered breathing and its treatment with nocturnal ventilation for chronic heart failure. Eur J Heart Fail. 2012; 14(9):1009–1019

[47] Young T, Finn L, Peppard PE, et al. Sleep disordered breathing and mortality: eighteen-year follow-up of the Wisconsin sleep cohort. Sleep. 2008; 31(8):1071–1078

[48] Marin JM, Carrizo SJ, Vicente E, Agusti AG. Long-term cardiovascular outcomes in men with obstructive sleep apnoea-hypopnoea with or without treatment with continuous positive airway pressure: an observational study. Lancet. 2005; 365(9464):1046–1053

[49] Kauppert CA, Dvorak I, Kollert F, et al. Pulmonary hypertension in obesity-hypoventilation syndrome. Respir Med. 2013; 107(12):2061–2070

[50] Javaheri S, Barbe F, Campos-Rodriguez F, et al. Sleep Apnea: Types, Mechanisms, and Clinical Cardiovascular Consequences. J Am Coll Cardiol. 2017; 69(7):841–858

[51] Samsoon GL, Young JR. Difficult tracheal intubation: a retrospective study. Anaesthesia. 1987; 42(5):487–490

[52] Liistro G, Rombaux P, Belge C, Dury M, Aubert G, Rodenstein DO. High Mallampati score and nasal obstruction are associated risk factors for obstructive sleep apnoea. Eur Respir J. 2003; 21(2):248–252

[53] Young T, Palta M, Dempsey J, Skatrud J, Weber S, Badr S. The occurrence of sleep-disordered breathing among middle-aged adults. N Engl J Med. 1993; 328(17):1230–1235

[54] Netzer NC, Stoohs RA, Netzer CM, Clark K, Strohl KP. Using the Berlin questionnaire to identify patients at risk for the sleep apnea syndrome. Ann Intern Med. 1999; 131(7):485–491

[55] Ahmadi N, Chung SA, Gibbs A, Shapiro CM. The Berlin questionnaire for sleep apnea in a sleep clinic population: relationship to polysomnographic measurement of respiratory disturbance. Sleep Breath. 2008; 12(1):39–45

[56] Chung F, Elsaid H. Screening for obstructive sleep apnea before surgery: why is it important? Curr Opin Anaesthesiol. 2009; 22(3):405–411

[57] Chung F, Subramanyam R, Liao P, Sasaki E, Shapiro C, Sun Y. High STOP-Bang score indicates a high probability of obstructive sleep apnoea. Br J Anaesth. 2012; 108(5):768–775

[58] Thorpy MJ. The clinical use of the Multiple Sleep Latency Test. The Standards of Practice Committee of the American Sleep Disorders Association. Sleep. 1992; 15(3):268–276

[59] Sangal RB, Thomas L, Mitler MM. Maintenance of wakefulness test and multiple sleep latency test. Measurement of different abilities in patients with sleep disorders. Chest. 1992; 101(4):898–902

[60] Poceta JS, Timms RM, Jeong DU, Ho SL, Erman MK, Mitler MM. Maintenance of wakefulness test in obstructive sleep apnea syndrome. Chest. 1992; 101(4):893–897

[61] Littner MR, Kushida C, Wise M, et al; Standards of Practice Committee of the American Academy of Sleep Medicine. Practice parameters for clinical use of the multiple sleep latency test and the maintenance of wakefulness test. Sleep. 2005; 28(1):113–121

[62] Doghramji K, Mitler MM, Sangal RB, et al. A normative study of the maintenance of wakefulness test (MWT). Electroencephalogr Clin Neurophysiol. 1997; 103(5):554–562

[63] Mazza S, Pepin JL, Deschaux C, Naegele B, Levy P. Analysis of error profiles occurring during the OSLER test: a sensitive mean of detecting fluctuations in vigilance in patients with obstructive sleep apnea syndrome. Am J Respir Crit Care Med. 2002; 166(4):474–478

[64] Alakuijala A, Maasilta P, Bachour A. The oxford sleep resistance test (OSLER) is sensitive in showing modifications in vigilance with CPAP therapy in sleep apnea patients. Sleep Med. 2013; 14(Supplement 1):e57

[65] Büttner A, Randerath W, Rühle KH. [Two simulation programs to measure continuous attention in obstructive sleep apnea syndrome] Pneumologie. 2003; 57(12):722–728

[66] Haraldsson PO, Carenfelt C, Laurell H, Törnros J. Driving vigilance simulator test. Acta Otolaryngol. 1990; 110(1–2):136–140

[67] Risser MR, Ware JC, Freeman FG. Driving simulation with EEG monitoring in normal and obstructive sleep apnea patients. Sleep. 2000; 23(3):393–398

[68] Wilhelm B, Wilhelm H, Lüdtke H, Streicher P, Adler M. Pupillographic assessment of sleepiness in sleep-deprived healthy subjects. Sleep. 1998; 21(3):258–265

[69] Rühle KH, Erle A, Nilius G. Vergleichende Untersuchungen von subjektiven und objektiven Schläfrigkeitstests beim obstruktiven Schlafapnoesyndrom. Pneumologie. 2007; 61(08):A16

[70] Kapur VK, Auckley DH, Chowdhuri S, et al. Clinical Practice Guideline for Diagnostic Testing for Adult Obstructive Sleep Apnea: an American Academy of Sleep Medicine Clinical Practice Guideline. J Clin Sleep Med. 2017; 13(3):479–504

[71] Collop NA, Anderson WM, Boehlecke B, et al. Portable Monitoring Task Force of the American Academy of Sleep Medicine. Clinical guidelines for the use of unattended portable monitors in the diagnosis of obstructive sleep apnea in adult patients. J Clin Sleep Med. 2007; 3(7):737–747

[72] Penzel T, Kesper K, Pinnow I, Becker HF, Vogelmeier C. Peripheral arterial tonometry, oximetry and actigraphy for ambulatory recording of sleep apnea. Physiol Meas. 2004; 25(4):1025–1036

[73] Grote L. [Invasive and noninvasive techniques for analysis of cardiovascular effects of sleep apnea] Biomed Tech (Berl). 2003; 48(7–8):190–196

[74] Sommermeyer D, Zou D, Grote L, Hedner J. Detection of sleep disordered breathing and its central/obstructive character using nasal cannula and finger pulse oximeter. J Clin Sleep Med. 2012; 8(5):527–533

[75] Berry RB, Budhiraja R, Gottlieb DJ, et al. American Academy of Sleep Medicine. Deliberations of the Sleep Apnea Definitions Task Force of the American Academy of Sleep Medicine. Rules for scoring respiratory events in sleep: update of the 2007 AASM Manual for the Scoring of Sleep and Associated Events. J Clin Sleep Med. 2012; 8(5):597–619

[76] Moser D, Anderer P, Gruber G, et al. Sleep classification according to AASM and Rechtschaffen & Kales: effects on sleep scoring parameters. Sleep. 2009; 32(2):139–149

[77] Randerath WJ, Treml M, Priegnitz C, Stieglitz S, Hagmeyer L, Morgenstern C. Evaluation of a noninvasive algorithm for differentiation of obstructive and central hypopneas. Sleep. 2013; 36(3):363–368

[78] Gries RE, Brooks LJ. Normal oxyhemoglobin saturation during sleep. How low does it go? Chest. 1996; 110(6):1489–1492

[79] Borowiecki BD, Sassin JF. Surgical treatment of sleep apnea. Arch Otolaryngol. 1983; 109(8):508–512

[80] Sher AE, Schechtman KB, Piccirillo JF. The efficacy of surgical modifications of the upper airway in adults with obstructive sleep apnea syndrome. Sleep. 1996; 19(2):156–177

[81] American Sleep Disorders Association Report. Practice parameters for the treatment of obstructive sleep apnea in adults: the efficacy of surgical modifications of upper airway. Sleep. 1996; 19(2):152–155

[82] Sher AE, Thorpy MJ, Shprintzen RJ, Spielman AJ, Burack B, McGregor PA. Predictive value of Müller maneuver in selection of patients for uvulopalatopharyngoplasty. Laryngoscope. 1985; 95(12):1483–1487

[83] Katsantonis GP, Maas CS, Walsh JK. The predictive efficacy of the Müller maneuver in uvulopalatopharyngoplasty. Laryngoscope. 1989; 99(7 Pt 1):677–680

[84] Petri N, Suadicani P, Wildschiødtz G, Bjørn-Jørgensen J. Predictive value of Müller maneuver, cephalometry and clinical features for the outcome of uvulopalatopharyngoplasty. Evaluation of predictive factors using discriminant analysis in 30 sleep apnea patients. Acta Otolaryngol. 1994; 114(5):565–571

[85] Borowiecki B, Pollak CP, Weitzman ED, Rakoff S, Imperato J. Fibro-optic study of pharyngeal airway during sleep in patients with hypersomnia obstructive sleep-apnea syndrome. Laryngoscope. 1978; 88(8 Pt 1):1310–1313

[86] Croft CB, Pringle M. Sleep nasendoscopy: a technique of assessment in snoring and obstructive sleep apnoea. Clin Otolaryngol Allied Sci. 1991; 16(5):504–509

[87] De Vito A, Carrasco Llatas M, Vanni A, et al. European position paper on drug-induced sedation endoscopy (DISE). Sleep Breath. 2014; 18(3):453–465

[88] Kezirian EJ, Hohenhorst W, de Vries N. Drug-induced sleep endoscopy: the VOTE classification. Eur Arch Otorhinolaryngol. 2011; 268(8):1233–1236

[89] Vanderveken OM, Maurer JT, Hohenhorst W, et al. Evaluation of drug-induced sleep endoscopy as a patient selection tool for implanted upper airway stimulation for obstructive sleep apnea. J Clin Sleep Med. 2013; 9(5):433–438

[90] Benoist LB, de Vries N. Organization and logistics of drug-induced sleep endoscopy in a training hospital. Eur Arch Otorhinolaryngol. 2015; 272(9):2557–2559

[91] Gislason T, Lindholm CE, Almqvist M, et al. Uvulopalatopharyngoplasty in the sleep apnea syndrome. Predictors of results. Arch Otolaryngol Head Neck Surg. 1988; 114(1):45–51

[92] Kezirian EJ, Goldberg AN. Hypopharyngeal surgery in obstructive sleep apnea: an evidence-based medicine review. Arch Otolaryngol Head Neck Surg. 2006; 132(2):206–213

[93] Kezirian EJ, Malhotra A, Goldberg AN, White DP. Changes in obstructive sleep apnea severity, biomarkers, and quality of life after multilevel surgery. Laryngoscope. 2010; 120(7):1481–1488

[94] Ravesloot MJL, van Maanen JP, Dun L, de Vries N. The undervalued potential of positional therapy in position-dependent snoring and obstructive sleep apnea-a review of the literature. Sleep Breath. 2013; 17(1):39–49

[95] Ravesloot MJL, de Vries N. One hundred consecutive patients undergoing drug-induced sleep endoscopy: results and evaluation. Laryngoscope. 2011; 121(12):2710–2716

[96] Safiruddin F, Koutsourelakis I, de Vries N. Analysis of the influence of head rotation during drug-induced sleep endoscopy in obstructive sleep apnea. Laryngoscope. 2014; 124(9):2195–2199

[97] Safiruddin F, Koutsourelakis I, de Vries N. Upper airway collapse during drug induced sleep endoscopy: head rotation in supine position compared with lateral head and trunk position. Eur Arch Otorhinolaryngol. 2014

[98] Strollo PJ Jr, Soose RJ, Maurer JT, et al. STAR Trial Group. Upper-airway stimulation for obstructive sleep apnea. N Engl J Med. 2014; 370(2):139–149

[99] van Maanen JP, Meester KA, Dun LN, et al. The sleep position trainer: a new treatment for positional obstructive sleep apnoea. Sleep Breath. 2013; 17(2):771–779

[100] van Maanen JP, Richard W, Van Kesteren ER, et al. Evaluation of a new simple treatment for positional sleep apnoea patients. J Sleep Res. 2012; 21(3):322–329

[101] Vroegop AV, Vanderveken OM, Boudewyns AN, et al. Drug-induced sleep endoscopy in sleep-disordered breathing: report on 1,249 cases. Laryngoscope. 2014; 124(3):797–802

[102] Isono S, Remmers JE, Tanaka A, Sho Y, Sato J, Nishino T. Anatomy of pharynx in patients with obstructive sleep apnea and in normal subjects. J Appl Physiol (1985). 1997; 82(4):1319–1326

[103] Schwab RJ. Upper airway imaging. Clin Chest Med. 1998; 19(1):33–54

[104] Isono S. Obesity and obstructive sleep apnoea: mechanisms for increased collapsibility of the passive pharyngeal airway. Respirology. 2012; 17(1):32–42

[105] Chen NH, Li KK, Li SY, et al. Airway assessment by volumetric computed tomography in snorers and subjects with obstructive sleep apnea in a Far-East Asian population (Chinese). Laryngoscope. 2002; 112(4):721–726

[106] Schwartz BA, Escande JP. [Cineradiographic study of hypnic Pickwickian respiration] Rev Neurol (Paris). 1967; 116(6):677–678

[107] Smith TH, Baska RE, Francisco CB, McCray GM, Kunz S. Sleep apnea syndrome: diagnosis of upper airway obstruction by fluoroscopy. J Pediatr. 1978; 93(5):891–892

[108] Suratt PM, Dee P, Atkinson RL, Armstrong P, Wilhoit SC. Fluoroscopic and computed tomographic features of the pharyngeal airway in obstructive sleep apnea. Am Rev Respir Dis. 1983; 127(4):487–492

[109] Pepin JL, Ferretti G, Veale D, et al. Somnofluoroscopy, computed tomography, and cephalometry in the assessment of the airway in obstructive sleep apnoea. Thorax. 1992; 47(3):150–156

[110] Kurtz D, Krieger J. Les arrêts respiratoires au cours du sommeil. Faits et hypothèses. Rev Neurol (Paris). 1978; 134(1):11–22

[111] Verbraecken JA, De Backer WA. Upper airway mechanics. Respiration. 2009; 78(2):121–133

[112] Susarla SM, Thomas RJ, Abramson ZR, Kaban LB. Biomechanics of the upper airway: changing concepts in the pathogenesis of obstructive sleep apnea. Int J Oral Maxillofac Surg. 2010; 39(12):1149–1159

[113] De Backer JW, Vos WG, Verhulst SL, De Backer W. Novel imaging techniques using computer methods for the evaluation of the upper airway in patients with sleep-disordered breathing: a comprehensive review. Sleep Med Rev. 2008; 114(6):437–447

[114] Riley R, Guilleminault C, Herran J, Powell N. Cephalometric analyses and flow-volume loops in obstructive sleep apnea patients. Sleep. 1983; 6(4):303–311

[115] Jamieson A, Guilleminault C, Partinen M, Quera-Salva MA. Obstructive sleep apneic patients have craniomandibular abnormalities. Sleep. 1986; 9(4):469–477

[116] Lowe AA, Santamaria JD, Fleetham JA, Price C. Facial morphology and obstructive sleep apnea. Am J Orthod Dentofacial Orthop. 1986; 90(6):484–491

[117] Bacon WH, Krieger J, Turlot JC, Stierle JL. Craniofacial characteristics in patients with obstructive sleep apneas syndrome. Cleft Palate J. 1988; 25(4):374–378

[118] deBerry-Borowiecki B, Kukwa A, Blanks RH. Cephalometric analysis for diagnosis and treatment of obstructive sleep apnea. Laryngoscope. 1988; 98(2):226–234

[119] Andersson L, Brattström V. Cephalometric analysis of permanently snoring patients with and without obstructive sleep

apnea syndrome. Int J Oral Maxillofac Surg. 1991; 20(3): 159–162

[120] Raskin S, Limme M. [Obstructive sleep apnea syndrome: the orthodontist's viewpoint] Rev Belge Med Dent. 1991; 46(4):33–37

[121] Lowe AA, Fleetham JA, Adachi S, Ryan CF. Cephalometric and computed tomographic predictors of obstructive sleep apnea severity. Am J Orthod Dentofacial Orthop. 1995; 107(6):589–595

[122] Johnson LM, Arnett GW, Tamborello JA, Binder A. Airway changes in relationship to mandibular posturing. Otolaryngol Head Neck Surg. 1992; 106(2):143–148

[123] Miles PG, Vig PS, Weyant RJ, Forrest TD, Rockette HE, Jr. Craniofacial structure and obstructive sleep apnea syndrome: a qualitative analysis and meta-analysis of the literature. Am J Orthod Dentofacial Orthop. 1996; 109(2):163–172

[124] Lowe AA, Ono T, Ferguson KA, Pae EK, Ryan CF, Fleetham JA. Cephalometric comparisons of craniofacial and upper airway structure by skeletal subtype and gender in patients with obstructive sleep apnea. Am J Orthod Dentofacial Orthop. 1996; 110(6):653–664

[125] Battagel JM, L'Estrange PR. The cephalometric morphology of patients with obstructive sleep apnoea (OSA). Eur J Orthod. 1996; 18(6):557–569

[126] Nelson S, Hans M. Contribution of craniofacial risk factors in increasing apneic activity among obese and nonobese habitual snorers. Chest. 1997; 111(1):154–162

[127] Zucconi M, Ferini-Strambi L, Palazzi S, Curci C, Cucchi E, Smirne S. Craniofacial cephalometric evaluation in habitual snorers with and without obstructive sleep apnea. Otolaryngol Head Neck Surg. 1993; 109(6):1007–1013

[128] Dostálová S, Smahel Z, Sonka K. Craniofacial abnormalities in sleep apnoea syndrome. Acta Chir Plast. 1998; 40(2):49–53

[129] Tangugsorn V, Krogstad O, Espeland L, Lyberg T. Obstructive sleep apnoea: multiple comparisons of cephalometric variables of obese and non-obese patients. J Craniomaxillofac Surg. 2000; 28(4):204–212

[130] Verin E, Tardif C, Buffet X, et al. Comparison between anatomy and resistance of upper airway in normal subjects, snorers and OSAS patients. Respir Physiol. 2002; 129(3):335–343

[131] Will MJ, Ester MS, Ramirez SG, Tiner BD, McAnear JT, Epstein L. Comparison of cephalometric analysis with ethnicity in obstructive sleep apnea syndrome. Sleep. 1995; 18(10):873–875

[132] Redline S, Tishler PV, Hans MG, Tosteson TD, Strohl KP, Spry K. Racial differences in sleep-disordered breathing in African-Americans and Caucasians. Am J Respir Crit Care Med. 1997; 155(1):186–192

[133] Li KK, Kushida C, Powell NB, Riley RW, Guilleminault C. Obstructive sleep apnea syndrome: a comparison between Far-East Asian and white men. Laryngoscope. 2000; 110(10 Pt 1): 1689–1693

[134] Wong ML, Sandham A, Ang PK, Wong DC, Tan WC, Huggare J. Craniofacial morphology, head posture, and nasal respiratory resistance in obstructive sleep apnoea: an inter-ethnic comparison. Eur J Orthod. 2005; 27(1):91–97

[135] Coltman R, Taylor DR, Whyte K, Harkness M. Craniofacial form and obstructive sleep apnea in Polynesian and Caucasian men. Sleep. 2000; 23(7):943–950

[136] Finkelstein Y, Wexler D, Horowitz E, et al. Frontal and lateral cephalometry in patients with sleep-disordered breathing. Laryngoscope. 2001; 111(4 Pt 1):634–641

[137] Poirrier AL, Pire S, Raskin S, Limme M, Poirrier R. Contribution of postero-anterior cephalometry in obstructive sleep apnea. Laryngoscope. 2012; 122(10):2350–2354

[138] Linder-Aronson S. Nasorespiratory function and craniofacial growth. In: McNamara JA, ed. Monograph 9, Craniofacial Growth Series. 8th ed. Center for Human Growth and Development. University of Michigan: Ann Arbor, MI; 1979:121–147

[139] Guilleminault C, Stoohs R. From apnea of infancy to obstructive sleep apnea syndrome in the young child. Chest. 1992; 102(4):1065–1071

[140] Alsufyani NA, Al-Saleh MA, Major PW. CBCT assessment of upper airway changes and treatment outcomes of obstructive sleep apnoea: a systematic review. Sleep Breath. 2013; 17(3):911–923

[141] Bruwier A, Poirrier R, Albert A, et al. Three-dimensional analysis of craniofacial bones and soft tissues in obstructive sleep apnea using cone beam computed tomography. Int Orthod. 2016; 14(4):449–461

[142] Momany SM, AlJamal G, Shugaa-Addin B, Khader YS. Cone beam computed tomography analysis of upper airway measurements in patients with obstructive sleep apnea. Am J Med Sci. 2016; 352(4):376–384

[143] Pépin JL, Veale D, Ferretti GR, Mayer P, Lévy PA. Obstructive sleep apnea syndrome: hooked appearance of the soft palate in awake patients–cephalometric and CT findings. Radiology. 1999; 210(1):163–170

[144] Denolf PL, Vanderveken OM, Marklund ME, Braem MJ. The status of cephalometry in the prediction of non-CPAP treatment outcome in obstructive sleep apnea patients. Sleep Med Rev. 2016; 27:56–73

[145] Poirrier AL, Fanielle J, Bruwier A, Chakar B, Poirrier R. Upper airway imaging in sleep-disordered breathing. Acta Neurol Belg. 2014; 114(2):87–93

[146] Skatvedt O. Localization of site of obstruction in snorers and patients with obstructive sleep apnea syndrome: a comparison of fiberoptic nasopharyngoscopy and pressure measurements. Acta Otolaryngol. 1993; 113(2):206–209

[147] Doghramji K, Jabourian ZH, Pilla M, Farole A, Lindholm RN. Predictors of outcome for uvulopalatopharyngoplasty. Laryngoscope. 1995; 105(3 Pt 1):311–314

[148] Remmers JE, Launois S, Feroah T, Whitelaw WA. Mechanics of the pharynx in patients with obstructive sleep apnea. Prog Clin Biol Res. 1990; 345:261–268, discussion 269–271

[149] Launois SH, Feroah TR, Campbell WN, et al. Site of pharyngeal narrowing predicts outcome of surgery for obstructive sleep apnea. Am Rev Respir Dis. 1993; 147(1):182–189

[150] Croft CB, Thomson HG, Samuels MP, Southall DP. Endoscopic evaluation and treatment of sleep-associated upper airway obstruction in infants and young children. Clin Otolaryngol Allied Sci. 1990; 15(3):209–216

[151] Sadaoka T, Kakitsuba N, Fujiwara Y, Kanai R, Takahashi H. The value of sleep nasendoscopy in the evaluation of patients with suspected sleep-related breathing disorders. Clin Otolaryngol Allied Sci. 1996; 21(6):485–489

[152] Bachar G, Nageris B, Feinmesser R, et al. Novel grading system for quantifying upper-airway obstruction on sleep endoscopy. Lung. 2012; 190(3):313–318

[153] Kezirian EJ. Nonresponders to pharyngeal surgery for obstructive sleep apnea: insights from drug-induced sleep endoscopy. Laryngoscope. 2011; 121(6):1320–1326

[154] van Maanen JP, Ravesloot MJ, Witte BI, Grijseels M, de Vries N. Exploration of the relationship between sleep position and isolated tongue base or multilevel surgery in obstructive sleep apnea. Eur Arch Otorhinolaryngol. 2012; 269(9):2129–2136

[155] Fredberg JJ, Wohl ME, Glass GM, Dorkin HL. Airway area by acoustic reflections measured at the mouth. J Appl Physiol. 1980; 48(5):749–758

[156] Bradley TD, Brown IG, Grossman RF, et al. Pharyngeal size in snorers, nonsnorers, and patients with obstructive sleep apnea. N Engl J Med. 1986; 315(21):1327–1331

[157] Hoffstein V, Wright S, Zamel N, Bradley TD. Pharyngeal function and snoring characteristics in apneic and nonapneic snorers. Am Rev Respir Dis. 1991; 143(6):1294–1299

[158] Kamal I. Acoustic pharyngometry patterns of snoring and obstructive sleep apnea patients. Otolaryngol Head Neck Surg. 2004; 130(1):58–66

[159] Kamal I. Test-retest validity of acoustic pharyngometry measurements. Otolaryngol Head Neck Surg. 2004; 130(2):223–228

[160] Kendzerska T, Grewal M, Ryan CM. Utility of acoustic pharyngometry for the diagnosis of obstructive sleep apnea. Ann Am Thorac Soc. 2016; 13(11):2019–2026

[161] Dubois AB, Brody AW, Lewis DH, Burgess BF, Jr. Oscillation mechanics of lungs and chest in man. J Appl Physiol. 1956; 8(6):587–594

[162] Randerath WJ, Parys K, Feldmeyer F, Sanner B, Rühle KH. Self-adjusting nasal continuous positive airway pressure therapy based on measurement of impedance: A comparison of two different maximum pressure levels. Chest. 1999; 116(4):991–999

[163] Farré R, Rigau J, Montserrat JM, Ballester E, Navajas D. Evaluation of a simplified oscillation technique for assessing airway obstruction in sleep apnoea. Eur Respir J. 2001; 17(3):456–461

[164] Farré R, Mancini M, Rotger M, Ferrer M, Roca J, Navajas D. Oscillatory resistance measured during noninvasive proportional assist ventilation. Am J Respir Crit Care Med. 2001; 164(5):790–794

[165] Badia JR, Farré R, Montserrat JM, et al. Forced oscillation technique for the evaluation of severe sleep apnoea/hypopnoea syndrome: a pilot study. Eur Respir J. 1998; 11(5):1128–1134

[166] Vanderveken OM, Oostveen E, Boudewyns AN, Verbraecken JA, Van de Heyning PH, De Backer WA. Quantification of pharyngeal patency in patients with sleep-disordered breathing. ORL J Otorhinolaryngol Relat Spec. 2005; 67(3):168–179

[167] Guijarro-Martínez R, Swennen GR. Cone-beam computerized tomography imaging and analysis of the upper airway: a systematic review of the literature. Int J Oral Maxillofac Surg. 2011; 40(11):1227–1237

[168] Armstrong J, Leigh M, Walton I, et al. In vivo size and shape measurement of the human upper airway using endoscopic longrange optical coherence tomography. Opt Express. 2003; 11(15):1817–1826

[169] Schäfer J. Ein einfaches Verfahren zur quantitativen und zeitcodierten Erfassung von Schnarchgeräuschen bei Apnoikern und Schnarchern. Laryngol Rhinol Otol (Stuttg). 1988; 67(9):449–452

[170] Schäfer J. Wie erkennt man einen Velum-Schnarcher? Laryngorhinootologie. 1989; 68(5):290–294

[171] Schäfer J, Pirsig W. Digital signal analysis of snoring sounds in children. Int J Pediatr Otorhinolaryngol. 1990; 20(3):193–202

[172] Dalmasso F, Benedetto G, Pogolotti R, Righini G, Spagnolo R. Digital processing of snoring sounds. Eur Respir J Suppl. 1990; 11:528s–532s

[173] Perez-Padilla JR, Slawinski E, Difrancesco LM, Feige RR, Remmers JE, Whitelaw WA. Characteristics of the snoring noise in patients with and without occlusive sleep apnea. Am Rev Respir Dis. 1993; 147(3):635–644

[174] Fiz JA, Abad J, Jané R, et al. Acoustic analysis of snoring sound in patients with simple snoring and obstructive sleep apnoea. Eur Respir J. 1996; 9(11):2365–2370

[175] Hara H, Murakami N, Miyauchi Y, Yamashita H. Acoustic analysis of snoring sounds by a multidimensional voice program. Laryngoscope. 2006; 116(3):379–381

[176] Herzog M, Schmidt A, Bremert T, Herzog B, Hosemann W, Kaftan H. Analysed snoring sounds correlate to obstructive sleep disordered breathing. Eur Arch Otorhinolaryngol. 2008; 265(1):105–113

[177] Sola-Soler J, Jane R, Fiz JA, Morera J. Automatic classification of subjects with and without sleep apnea through snoring analysis. IEEE Eng Med Biol Soc. 2007:6094–6097

[178] Miyazaki S, Itasaka Y, Ishikawa K, Togawa K. Acoustic analysis of snoring and the site of airway obstruction in sleep related respiratory disorders. Acta Otolaryngol Suppl. 1998; 537:47–51

[179] Quinn SJ, Huang L, Ellis PD, Williams JE. The differentiation of snoring mechanisms using sound analysis. Clin Otolaryngol Allied Sci. 1996; 21(2):119–123

[180] Hill PD, Lee BW, Osborne JE, Osman EZ. Palatal snoring identified by acoustic crest factor analysis. Physiol Meas. 1999; 20(2):167–174

[181] Hill PD, Osman EZ, Osborne JE, Lee BW. Changes in snoring during natural sleep identified by acoustic crest factor analysis at different times of night. Clin Otolaryngol Allied Sci. 2000; 25(6):507–510

[182] Agrawal S, Stone P, McGuinness K, Morris J, Camilleri AE. Sound frequency analysis and the site of snoring in natural and induced sleep. Clin Otolaryngol Allied Sci. 2002; 27(3):162–166

[183] Kezirian EJ, Hohenhorst W, de Vries N. Drug-induced sleep endoscopy: the VOTE classification. Eur Arch Otorhinolaryngol. 2011; 268(8):1233–1236

[184] Herzog M, Plößl S, Glien A, et al. Evaluation of acoustic characteristics of snoring sounds obtained during drug-induced sleep endoscopy. Sleep Breath. 2015; 19(3):1011–1019

[185] Fischer R, Kuehnel TS, Merz AK, Ettl T, Herzog M, Rohrmeier C. Calculating annoyance: an option to proof efficacy in ENT treatment of snoring? Eur Arch Otorhinolaryngol. 2016; 273(12):4607–4613

[186] Rohrmeier C, Fischer R, Merz AK, Ettl T, Herzog M, Kuehnel TS. Are subjective assessments of snoring sounds reliable? Eur Arch Otorhinolaryngol. 2015; 272(1):233–240

[187] Rohrmeier C, Herzog M, Haubner F, Kuehnel TS. The annoyance of snoring and psychoacoustic parameters: a step towards an objective measurement. Eur Arch Otorhinolaryngol. 2012; 269(5):1537–1543

[188] Qian K, Janott C, Pandit V, et al. Classification of the excitation location of snore sounds in the upper airway by acoustic multifeature analysis. IEEE Trans Biomed Eng. 2017; 64(8):1731–1741

[189] Nguyen TL, Won Y. Sleep snoring detection using multilayer neural networks. Biomed Mater Eng. 2015; 26 (Suppl 1):S1749–S1755

[190] Emoto T, Abeyratne UR, Akutagawa M, Nagashino H, Kinouchi Y. Feature extraction for snore sound via neural network processing. IEEE Eng Med Biol Soc 2007:5477–5480

[191] Emoto T, Abeyratne UR, Chen Y, Kawata I, Akutagawa M, Kinouchi Y. Artificial neural networks for breathing and snoring episode detection in sleep sounds. Physiol Meas. 2012; 33(10):1675–1689

[192] Qian K, Guo J, Xu H, Zhu Z, Zhang G. Snore related signals processing in a private cloud computing system. Interdiscip Sci. 2014; 6(3):216–221

[193] Seren E, Ilhanlı I, Bayar Muluk N, Cingi C, Hanci D. Telephonic analysis of the snoring sound spectrum. Ann Otol Rhinol Laryngol. 2014; 123(11):758–764

4 Nonsurgical Treatment: Lifestyle, Weight Loss, Positional Therapy, Mandibular Advancement Devices, Continuous Positive Airway Pressure, Multimodality Treatment

Nico de Vries, Peter van Maanen, Linda B. L. Benoist, and Aarnoud Hoekema

Abstract

This chapter is devoted to nonsurgical treatment: in particular, lifestyle interventions when applicable (physical activity and exercise in order to increase genioglossal muscle tone; avoidance of alcohol, smoking, and sedatives) are discussed first. Weight management is important but it is a clinical reality that this is very difficult for the vast majority of patients. The majority of cases with early stage/beginning obstructive sleep apnea (OSA), the mild-to-moderate OSA disease severity category, are positional; the number of events is much higher when sleeping on the back as compared to other sleeping positions. Positional therapy with new generation positional devices is highlighted. Positional therapy is an important adjunctive to sleep surgery. Oral appliances are discussed subsequently. Results are often good in mild-to-moderate OSA. Approximately one-third of patients have a contraindication to it. CPAP is gold standard therapy, in particular in moderate-to-severe OSA. CPAP is unfortunately often hampered by poor compliance. Multimodality treatment has not yet gained the attention it deserves. Combined treatments are often better than one treatment modality alone.

Keywords: lifestyle, physical activity, weight loss, positional therapy, oral appliances, CPAP, multimodality therapy

4.1 Introduction

In the general population, it is estimated that 3.3 to 7.5% of men and 1.2 to 3.2% of women meet the diagnostic criteria for obstructive sleep apnea (OSA) syndrome as described previously (see Chapter 2). Yet, the number of patients who are asymptomatic but have an apnea–hypopnea index (AHI) greater than or equal to 5 is significantly higher: 17 to 27% in men and 5 to 28% in women. The estimated prevalence of an AHI greater than or equal to 15, ranges from 7 to 14% in men and 1.2 to 7% in women. It should be noted that comparison of the results of these epidemiology studies is limited by methodological differences, including variation in used criteria, sleep registration techniques, and study methods (e.g., sampling schedules).

On the basis of these prevalence estimates, roughly 1 of every 5 adults has at least an AHI greater than or equal to 5 and 1 of every 15 adults at least an AHI greater than or equal to 15. It is estimated that nearly 80% of men and 93% of women with moderate to severe OSA remain undiagnosed.[1,2,3,4,5,6,7,8,9,10,11]

At present, the therapeutic armamentarium for obstructive sleep apnea (OSA) comprises several treatment options. To provide effective treatment for OSA, careful consideration of the individual patient, available medical and surgical therapies, and inherent risks and complications of those interventions must be taken into account. While this book focuses on surgical treatment of OSA, an overview of conservative treatment measures is crucial. Many of these treatment modalities can be applied as single therapy or as combination therapy, which is gaining momentum.

Physicians and surgeons treating patients with OSA should be up-to-date with the modern therapeutic armamentarium for OSA. The approach to treating OSA is steadily moving from a continuous positive airway pressure (CPAP) centered one-size-fits-all approach to individualized treatment of upper airway obstruction during sleep.

Treatment of OSA is approached in a stepwise manner and begins with lifestyle alterations, indicated for all patients with a modifiable risk factor, such as weight reduction and avoidance of alcohol and sedatives. In case of supine-position dependency, avoidance of the supine sleeping position is recommended. Conservative treatment options include CPAP, oral appliances, and active positional therapy. All treatment modalities have their own specific indications, contraindications, and side effects. So far, no drugs have been identified to help against obstructive sleep apnea syndrome (OSAS), but pharmaceutical companies are working hard to develop them.[12]

4.2 Lifestyle Intervention

Lifestyle interventions include weight reduction; physical activity and exercise to increase genioglossal muscle tone; and avoidance of alcohol, smoking, and sedatives.

Body weight is pivotal in OSA. Not everyone with OSA is obese, but most patients with morbid obesity have OSA. Even modest weight loss can be effective in reducing OSA severity, but there is a poor correlation between the amount of weight loss and the clinical response.

The exact pathophysiology of OSA in obese patients remains poorly understood; but it is thought that, in these patients, local fatty tissue deposition in the neck results in reduction of the lumen of the upper airway thereby reducing airflow and inducing airway collapse.[13,14] Most OSA patients are overweight and weight loss, even modest, can be effective in reducing OSA severity, with a clear relation between BMI and AHI.[15,16,17] Unfortunately, losing weight is particularly taxing in patients with OSA. Daytime hypersomnolence, an important symptom of

OSA, reduces the motivation for physical activity and dieting. Secondly, OSA is thought to induce weight gain. Sleep deprivation and intermittent hypoxia cause impaired glucose metabolism, hyperphagia, and imbalances of leptin, ghrelin, and orexin levels.[18,19] Therefore, on the whole, conservative treatment fails more often in obese patients with OSA; in obese patients bariatric surgery (BS) can be considered. BS is not only the most effective treatment modality in obese patients to lose weight, producing durable weight loss, it is also known to have a positive effect on comorbidities. BS is therefore becoming increasingly popular.[20]

The likelihood of OSA increases with increasing body weight. It cannot be stressed enough that this works in both directions: OSA leads to weight gain as well. The reason for this is probably twofold: (1) patients with OSA tend to be relatively less active and might gradually lose their motivation for physical exercise, which will contribute to weight gain; (2) OSA can influence the production of leptin and ghrelin—hormones responsible for hunger and satiety. Lack of oxygen affects the insulin balance as well. Sugars are not burned effectively, but might be converted to fat.

Body shape and fat distribution might differ considerably from person to person. In terms of OSA risk, the neck circumference might be a better metric than body mass index (BMI). It is not completely clear as to how far it matters if the neck circumference is big because of fat or because of muscle mass.

It is important, however, to realize that while we all should advise our patients with OSA and increased body weight to try to lose weight, but for the vast majority of patients this is easier said than done. In the majority of patients it takes many years before the actual diagnosis is established. Patients often have complaints for an average of 5 to 8 years and in the meantime have been misdiagnosed as having a burnout or depression. When the diagnosis is finally established and the caregiver recommends patients to lose weight then their first reaction is often: "Do you really think I have not tried that?" In contrast, patients would appreciate if the doctor understands their frustrating situation and explains to them that weight loss in general is difficult, and with OSA it is even more difficult, but not impossible. This mutual understanding is essential for a good patient-doctor relation. Only a few percent of patients with OSA who are advised to lose weight actually manage to do so and subsequently are able to maintain this more healthy body weight.

4.2.1 Didgeridoo and Physical Therapy

A disproportionally high amount of attention has been paid to practicing didgeridoo as treatment of sleep-disordered breathing. Playing didgeridoo indeed has an effect on the AHI, most likely because of improvement in the muscle tone of the genioglossus muscle, but the effect is very limited. For bed partners the question remains what is worse: the sound of the didgeridoo or the snoring sound? The effects of physical therapy and speech therapy have also been shown in recent research. Some exercises have shown positive effect in improving the muscle tone of the tongue and muscles of the oral cavity and floor of mouth, but these exercises are not alternative for other established treatments.

4.2.2 Alcohol, Tobacco, and Sedative Abstinence, Sleep Hygiene

Doctors should advise their patients to quit smoking. Studies have shown that there is a positive association between tobacco smoking and the presence of OSA. Tobacco smoking is a risk factor for the presence of OSA, but there is no evidence that cessation is effective in reducing apneic events.[2,21,22,23,24] The situation gets complex where the patients with OSA often gain weight after quitting smoking and subsequently their OSA deteriorates.

The use of sedatives and medication with muscle relaxing properties needs to be avoided. Both sedatives and alcohol are considered important risk factors for OSA because they cause a reduction in muscle tone and depression of the central nervous system, adversely affecting ventilatory response to hypoxia.

Alcohol has muscle relaxing properties and its use should be restricted as far as possible, especially before bedtime. Studies have shown that alcohol consumption aggravates OSA: an increase in frequency and duration of hypopneic or apneic events.[21,22,23,24,25,26,27,28,29,30,31,32,33,34,35,36,37,38] Therefore abstinence is recommended.

Good sleep hygiene is important and should be encouraged. Sleep hygiene advice includes attention to regularity in the circadian sleep rhythm, adequate sleep hours, and optimization of the sleep environment. Late-night dinners, consumption of caffeine at night, and strenuous activities before bedtime should be avoided.

Several drugs are used in the treatment of OSAS. Intranasal steroids might be used as additional therapy in case of decreased nasal breathing due to allergies, hypertrophic turbinates, chronic rhinosinusitis, or nasal polyps. Drug treatment of gastroesophageal reflux can be of value in case of hypertrophic lingual tonsils.

4.3 Positional Therapy

The majority of patients with mild to moderate OSA have more apneic events in the supine position, as compared with nonsupine positions.[39,40,41,42,43,44] Positional OSA (POSA) was originally defined as an AHI that is at least twice as high in supine position as compared with nonsupine positions.[41] In approximately 56 to 75% of patients with OSA, the frequency and duration of apneas are influenced by body position. This is particularly true for patients with mild or moderate OSA.

Patients can be treated by simply avoiding the worst sleeping position, most often the supine position.[39,40,41,42,43,44,45,46,47,48,49,50,51]

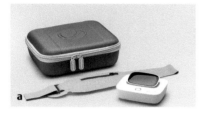
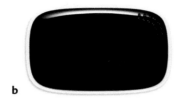

Fig. 4.1 (a, b) Small, light-weight sleep position therapy solution, NightBalance Lunoa. Courtesy of Philips.

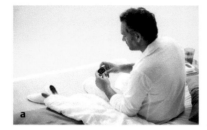
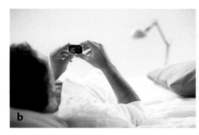

Fig. 4.2 (a, b) NightBalance Lunoa sleep position therapy solution. Courtesy of Philips.

Until recently, positional therapy (PT) consisted of suturing tennis balls, squash balls, (inflatable) bulky masses, or other such devices in the back side of a pajama or t-shirt in order to prevent patients from adopting the supine sleeping position.[39]

Promising results have recently been reported for active PT with a small device attached to either the neck or chest, which prevents the patient from adopting the supine position through a subtle vibrating stimulus[45,46,47,48,49,50,51] (▶Fig. 4.1a, b; ▶Fig. 4.2).

There is strong evidence that active PT is effective in reducing the AHI.[45,46,47,48,49,50,51] Furthermore, it is simple, relatively inexpensive, well tolerated, and reversible. Not only is PT successful, but it is also effective because of its high compliance.[47,49]

Further long-term high-quality studies are needed to confirm the promising role of PT as a single or as a combination treatment modality for many OSA patients.

4.4 Oral Appliances

The use of oral appliances for the treatment of sleep-related breathing disorders is not a new phenomenon. In 1902, the French physician Pierre Robin introduced oral appliance therapy for the treatment of tongue base obstruction in children with Pierre Robin sequence. The role of oral appliances to treat adult patients with OSA was first explored in the late 1970s.

Nowadays, mandibular advancement devices (MADs), a form of oral appliance therapy, are the leading alternative to the treatment with CPAP. Confusingly several synonyms for MAD are used including mandibular repositioning appliances (MRAs) and mandibular advancement splints (MASs) to describe the same type of appliance.[52,53,54,55,56,57,58,59] MADs are worn intraorally by attaching to the upper and lower dental arches to hold the mandible in a forward position (▶Fig. 4.3, ▶Fig. 4.4).

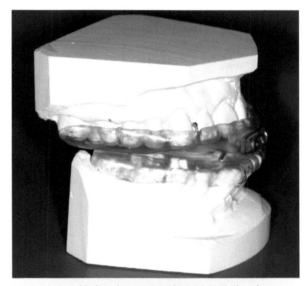

Fig. 4.3 Mandibular advancement device (MAD) placed on plaster casts following the construction in a dental laboratory.

The degree of forward movement is usually between 50 and 80% of the patient's maximum protrusion of the lower jaw. Other types of oral appliances are not recommended in the treatment of OSA because MADs are comparatively more effective.

4.4.1 Mechanism of Action

MADs have an anatomic effect on the pharyngeal airway and reduce upper airway collapsibility, thus increasing space in the velopharyngeal region, predominantly in the lateral dimension.[60] The anterior movement of the mandible and tongue facilitated by the MAD presumably stretches soft tissue connections between the pharyngeal walls and the mandible, preventing collapse of the tongue into the upper airway and increasing the caliber of the pharynx (▶Fig. 4.5).

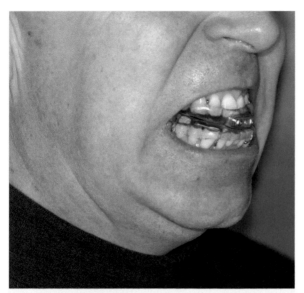

Fig. 4.4 Patient wearing the mandibular advancement device (MAD). The appliance secures the mandible in an anterior position. (Used with permission from Hoekema A, Wijkstra PJ, Buiter CT, van der Hoeven JH, Meinesz AF, de Bont LGM. Treatment of the obstructive sleep-apnoea syndrome in adults. Ned Tijdschr Geneeskd 2003;147:2407–2412.)

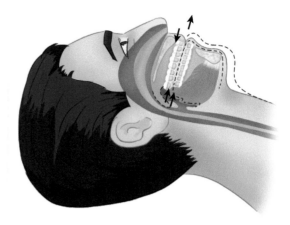

Fig. 4.5 Effects of a mandibular advancement device (MAD) on upper airway patency and dentition. The illustration shows the increase in upper airway dimensions following repositioning of the mandible with MAD therapy. The arrows on the teeth indicate the reciprocal forces that are generated by holding the mandible in a forward and vertically opened position. These forces transmit in a labial direction against the lower incisors and in a palatal direction against the upper incisors. In the long term, this may change the inclination and position of teeth, affect the position of the mandible, and increase the loading of the craniomandibular complex.

4.4.2 Outcomes

MADs have demonstrated efficacy in reducing OSA with associated improvements in health outcomes. The reported mean reduction in AHI ranges between 24 and 72%, and mean proportion of OSA patients who resolve completely (AHI < 5 events/h) with MAD treatment ranges between 29 and 71%.[60] Definition of OSA treatment success is, however, a major factor that influences the reported efficacy. MADs reduce snoring and improve polysomnographic indices including AHI, oxygen saturation, and sleep fragmentation compared with placebo devices (oral appliances that provide no mandibular advancement).[60,61,62] Excessive daytime sleepiness (EDS), measured both subjectively and objectively, is also reduced following MAS treatment.[60] MADs improve general and disease-specific measures of quality of life (QoL) assessed by questionnaire. MAS improves diastolic and systolic 24-hour mean arterial blood pressure (especially in hypertensive patients).[60] Long-term follow-up of MAD's efficacy on OSA patients have indicated that reduction in AHI is sustained after 6 months up to 4 years of treatment.[60]

Randomized studies have consistently shown CPAP to be more efficient in reducing respiratory events and completely resolving OSA. However, the superior efficacy of CPAP in improving polysomnographic indices compared to MADs does not seem to lead to better health outcomes. Additionally, MADs and CPAP are found to equally improve morning diastolic and 24-hour mean arterial blood pressure. Many patients with mild and moderate OSA prefer an MAD over CPAP.[63,64,65,66,67,68,69] Adherence to

MAD is, therefore, usually better than to CPAP. This may explain why therapeutic effectiveness of MAD and CPAP in patients with mild and moderate OSA is comparable.[61,62] In the treatment of severe OSA, MAD treatment remains a secondary line of treatment due to the superior effects of CPAP.

4.4.3 Side Effects

The side effects of MAD treatment in the beginning are usually mild and temporary. They often remain limited to sialorrhea, xerostomia, toothaches, gingival irritation, headaches, and temporomandibular joint (TMJ) pain.[60] Most adverse effects improve over time, and completely resolve 3 to 6 months after treatment, including TMJ pain. The adverse effects of long-term MAD use on the TMJs seem limited. In contrast, orthodontic effects have been described in many cases as a result of prolonged use of an MAD. Common dental changes include decrease in overbite and overjet, retroclination of the upper incisor and proclination of the lower incisors, reduction in the number of occlusal contacts, and increase in mandibular plane angle (▶ Fig. 4.5).[60] These findings highlight the importance of regular (dental) checkup visits during treatment with MADs.

4.4.4 Patient Selection

Treatment with MADs requires an extended period (2–3 months) of acclimatization to achieve the maximum therapeutic benefit. Therefore, MAD treatment is not suitable for patients with comorbidities and severe daytime sleepiness, and especially for sleepy drivers who require immediate intervention. MADs are not suitable for patients requiring major dental work because MAD fitting may be disturbed by the changes in dental shape. MADs are also not recommended to patients with major teeth loss because a solid base is needed to anchor them. Overall, one-third of OSA patients are not eligible for MAD treatment because of dental contraindications. In patients with a complete dental prosthesis, an MAD may be applied after placing dental implants in the lower and, possibly, the upper jaw.

Another barrier for implementing MAD treatment clinically is the interindividual variability of OSA patients' response to treatment. Therefore, much attention has been devoted to understand the reasons for treatment variability and to find predictors of successful treatment outcome. Several prediction tools have been proposed in the literature to enhance patient selection for MAD treatment. However, most of these are inadequate for routine clinical use due to inaccuracy, lack of prospective validation, high cost, and/or complexity. Suitable candidates, however, may be selected by means of procedures such as drug-induced sleep endoscopy. The use of an MAD appears to be indicated as primary intervention for the treatment of snoring up to mild and moderate OSA (AHI < 30). After fitting an MRA, repeat sleep studies are recommended in patients with AHI greater than 15.

4.5 Continuous Positive Airway Pressure

First introduced by Sullivan in 1981, CPAP is regarded as the gold standard in treatment of moderate and severe cases, and is the most efficacious treatment modality of OSA[70] (▶ Fig. 4.6, ▶ Fig. 4.7, ▶ Fig. 4.8). CPAP has the firmest evidence base in the treatment of OSA.

CPAP functions as a pneumatic splint to maintain upper airway patency. CPAP use is considered successful when the AHI reduces to below 5. In a meta-analysis of the Cochrane Collaboration, compared with control, CPAP was shown to be significantly effective in reducing the AHI as well as in improving measurements of QoL, cognitive function, and objective and subjective measures of sleepiness.

However, despite the efficacy of CPAP, it is a clinical reality that the use of CPAP is not suited for every patient. Patients seem to either tolerate the device well or not at all—a bimodal distribution. Studies have shown that 29 to 83% of patients are nonadherent, when adherence is defined as at least 4 hours of CPAP use per night.[71] More support and care is needed to improve compliance, especially on a long-term basis, such as addressing CPAP side effects. Possible side effects can be related to the interface (skin abrasion from contact with the mask, claustrophobia, mask leak, irritated eyes), pressure (nasal congestion and rhinorrhea with dryness or irritation of the nasal and pharyngeal membranes, sneezing, gastric and bowel distension, recurrent ear and sinus infections), and negative social factors.

In spite of continuing efforts by the CPAP industry to increase compliance, the percentage of nonacceptance is presently not better than that in the 1980s.

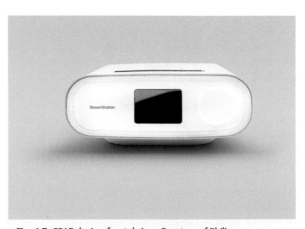

Fig. 4.7 CPAP device, frontal view. Courtesy of Philips.

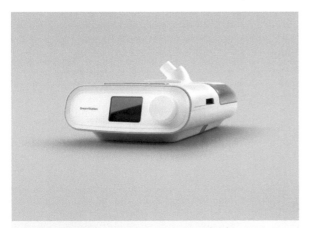

Fig. 4.6 CPAP device, lateral view. Courtesy of Philips.

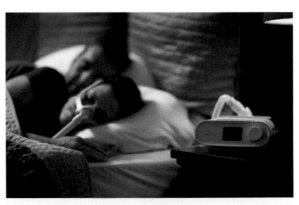

Fig. 4.8 CPAP in use. Courtesy of Philips.

The effectiveness of conservative treatment regarding the reduction of AHI depends both on its impact on airway obstruction and compliance. The approach to treating OSA is steadily moving from a CPAP-centered one-size-fits-all approach to individualized treatment of upper airway obstruction during sleep.

Millions of people all over the world use CPAP and it is a multibillion business. While some CPAP protagonists are still of the opinion that CPAP is the only treatment of OSA, others are more realistic and accept that CPAP is only effective when used sufficiently. CPAP is mostly used in moderate to severe OSA. It is less indicated in mild disease. In this particular group of patients, low motivation to use CPAP is an important limitation.

In conclusion, CPAP has a disadvantage because it works only when used. Many young patients in particular find the perspective unattractive to sleep with CPAP for the rest of their lives and want to be well informed about treatment alternatives.

4.6 Multimodality Treatment

In diseases such as hypertension and acquired immunodeficiency syndrome (AIDS), the use of drug combinations results in more robust outcomes as compared with single-drug therapy. Especially in AIDS, the transition from single-drug treatment to multiple-drug regimen is the quantum leap from deadly disease to chronic nonlethal disease. Still, multimodality treatment in OSA is uncommon. For many patients, a combination of different treatment modalities for OSA is indicated. For example, MAD and CPAP, surgery of the nose, and CPAP and PT in combination with either surgery or MAD treatment.[50,72] Patients with severe nonpositional OSA might improve to moderate or mild POSA (because sometimes the effect of surgery on the AHI is more robust in lateral position as compared to supine sleeping position). In such cases PT before surgery would make no sense, but additional PT after partial successful surgery would be helpful. Others have considered CPAP a failure because of intolerance to high pressures. The combination of CPAP with MAD might lead to lower pressures needed, resulting in better compliance.

The purpose of this text is not to advocate the use of surgery as the only treatment, but rather to also incorporate surgery into a multimodality treatment algorithm, if indicated.

References

[1] American Academy of Sleep Medicine. International classification of sleep disorders: diagnostic and coding manual. 2nd ed. Westchester, IL: American Academy of Sleep Medicine; 2005

[2] Young T, Peppard PE, Gottlieb DJ. Epidemiology of obstructive sleep apnea: a population health perspective. Am J Respir Crit Care Med. 2002; 165(9):1217–1239

[3] Punjabi NM. The epidemiology of adult obstructive sleep apnea. Proc Am Thorac Soc. 2008; 5(2):136–143

[4] Somers VK, White DP, Amin R, et al; American Heart Association Council for High Blood Pressure Research Professional Education Committee, Council on Clinical Cardiology. American Heart Association Stroke Council. American Heart Association Council on Cardiovascular Nursing. American College of Cardiology Foundation. Sleep apnea and cardiovascular disease: an American Heart Association/American College of Cardiology Foundation Scientific Statement from the American Heart Association Council for High Blood Pressure Research Professional Education Committee, Council on Clinical Cardiology, Stroke Council, and Council on Cardiovascular Nursing. In collaboration with the National Heart, Lung, and Blood Institute National Center on Sleep Disorders Research (National Institutes of Health). Circulation. 2008; 118(10):1080–1111

[5] Young T, Palta M, Dempsey J, Skatrud J, Weber S, Badr S. The occurrence of sleep-disordered breathing among middle-aged adults. N Engl J Med. 1993; 328(17):1230–1235

[6] Peppard PE, Young T, Barnet JH, Palta M, Hagen EW, Hla KM. Increased prevalence of sleep-disordered breathing in adults. Am J Epidemiol. 2013; 177(9):1006–1014

[7] Marin JM, Carrizo SJ, Vicente E, Agusti AG. Long-term cardiovascular outcomes in men with obstructive sleep apnoea-hypopnoea with or without treatment with continuous positive airway pressure: an observational study. Lancet. 2005; 365(9464): 1046–1053

[8] Redline S, Yenokyan G, Gottlieb DJ, et al. Obstructive sleep apnea-hypopnea and incident stroke: the sleep heart health study. Am J Respir Crit Care Med. 2010; 182(2):269–277

[9] Kendzerska T, Mollayeva T, Gershon AS, Leung RS, Hawker G, Tomlinson G. Untreated obstructive sleep apnea and the risk for serious long-term adverse outcomes: a systematic review. Sleep Med Rev. 2014; 18(1):49–59

[10] McNicholas WT, Bonsignore MR, eds. European Respiratory Society Monograph 50: Sleep Apnoea European Respiratory Society Journals; 2010

[11] Young T, Evans L, Finn L, Palta M. Estimation of the clinically diagnosed proportion of sleep apnea syndrome in middle-aged men and women. Sleep. 1997; 20(9):705–706

[12] Mason M, Welsh EJ, Smith I. Drug therapy for obstructive sleep apnoea in adults. Cochrane Database Syst Rev 2013;5:CD003002

[13] Maciel Santos ME, Rocha NS, Laureano Filho JR, Ferraz EM, Campos JM. Obstructive sleep apnea-hypopnea syndrome-the role of bariatric and maxillofacial surgeries. Obes Surg. 2009; 19(6): 796–801

[14] Hallowell PT, Stellato TA, Schuster M, et al. Potentially life-threatening sleep apnea is unrecognized without aggressive evaluation. Am J Surg. 2007; 193(3):364–367, discussion 367

[15] Suratt PM, McTier RF, Findley LJ, Pohl SL, Wilhoit SC. Effect of very-low-calorie diets with weight loss on obstructive sleep apnea. Am J Clin Nutr. 1992; 56(1, Suppl):182S–184S

[16] Browman CP, Sampson MG, Yolles SF, et al. Obstructive sleep apnea and body weight. Chest. 1984; 85(3):435–438

[17] Loube DI, Loube AA, Mitler MM. Weight loss for obstructive sleep apnea: the optimal therapy for obese patients. J Am Diet Assoc. 1994; 94(11):1291–1295

[18] Everson CA. Functional consequences of sustained sleep deprivation in the rat. Behav Brain Res. 1995; 69(1–2):43–54

[19] Pillar G, Shehadeh N. Abdominal fat and sleep apnea: the chicken or the egg? Diabetes Care. 2008; 31(Suppl 2):S303–S309

[20] SAGES Guidelines Committee. SAGES guideline for clinical application of laparoscopic bariatric surgery. Surg Endosc 2008; 22:2281–2300

[21] Jennum P, Hein HO, Suadicani P, Gyntelberg F. Cardiovascular risk factors in snorers. A cross-sectional study of 3,323 men aged 54 to 74 years: the Copenhagen Male Study. Chest. 1992; 102(5):1371–1376

[22] Jennum P, Sjøl A. Snoring, sleep apnoea and cardiovascular risk factors: the MONICA II Study. Int J Epidemiol. 1993; 22(3):439–444

[23] Stradling JR, Crosby JH. Predictors and prevalence of obstructive sleep apnoea and snoring in 1001 middle aged men. Thorax. 1991; 46(2):85–90

[24] Schmidt-Nowara WW, Coultas DB, Wiggins C, Skipper BE, Samet JM. Snoring in a Hispanic-American population. Risk factors and association with hypertension and other morbidity. Arch Intern Med. 1990; 150(3):597–601

[25] Scanlan MF, Roebuck T, Little PJ, Redman JR, Naughton MT. Effect of moderate alcohol upon obstructive sleep apnoea. Eur Respir J. 2000; 16(5):909–913

[26] Mitler MM, Dawson A, Henriksen SJ, Sobers M, Bloom FE. Bedtime ethanol increases resistance of upper airways and produces sleep apneas in asymptomatic snorers. Alcohol Clin Exp Res. 1988; 12(6):801–805

[27] Dawson A, Lehr P, Bigby BG, Mitler MM. Effect of bedtime ethanol on total inspiratory resistance and respiratory drive in normal nonsnoring men. Alcohol Clin Exp Res. 1993; 17(2):256–262

[28] Tanigawa T, Tachibana N, Yamagishi K, et al. Usual alcohol consumption and arterial oxygen desaturation during sleep. JAMA. 2004; 292(8):923–925

[29] Peppard PE, Austin D, Brown RL. Association of alcohol consumption and sleep disordered breathing in men and women. J Clin Sleep Med. 2007; 3(3):265–270

[30] Taasan VC, Block AJ, Boysen PG, Wynne JW. Alcohol increases sleep apnea and oxygen desaturation in asymptomatic men. Am J Med. 1981; 71(2):240–245

[31] Tsutsumi W, Miyazaki S, Itasaka Y, Togawa K. Influence of alcohol on respiratory disturbance during sleep. Psychiatry Clin Neurosci. 2000; 54(3):332–333

[32] Issa FG, Sullivan CE. Alcohol, snoring and sleep apnea. J Neurol Neurosurg Psychiatry. 1982; 45(4):353–359

[33] Berry RB, Desa MM, Light RW. Effect of ethanol on the efficacy of nasal continuous positive airway pressure as a treatment for obstructive sleep apnea. Chest. 1991; 99(2):339–343

[34] Scrima L, Hartman PG, Hiller FC. Effect of three alcohol doses on breathing during sleep in 30–49 year old nonobese snorers and nonsnorers. Alcohol Clin Exp Res. 1989; 13(3):420–427

[35] Enright PL, Newman AB, Wahl PW, Manolio TA, Haponik EF, Boyle PJ. Prevalence and correlates of snoring and observed apneas in 5,201 older adults. Sleep. 1996; 19(7):531–538

[36] Bearpark H, Elliott L, Grunstein R, et al. Snoring and sleep apnea. A population study in Australian men. Am J Respir Crit Care Med. 1995; 151(5):1459–1465

[37] Olson LG, King MT, Hensley MJ, Saunders NA. A community study of snoring and sleep-disordered breathing. Prevalence. Am J Respir Crit Care Med. 1995; 152(2):711–716

[38] Dawson A, Bigby BG, Poceta JS, Mitler MM. Effect of bedtime alcohol on inspiratory resistance and respiratory drive in snoring and nonsnoring men. Alcohol Clin Exp Res. 1997; 21(2):183–190

[39] Ravesloot MJ, van Maanen JP, Dun L, de Vries N. The undervalued potential of positional therapy in position-dependent snoring and obstructive sleep apnea-a review of the literature. Sleep Breath. 2013; 17(1):39–49

[40] Ravesloot MJ, Frank MH, van Maanen JP, Verhagen EA, de Lange J, de Vries N. Positional OSA part 2: retrospective cohort analysis with a new classification system (APOC). Sleep Breath. 2016; 20(2):881–888

[41] Cartwright RD. Effect of sleep position on sleep apnea severity. Sleep. 1984; 7(2):110–114

[42] Oksenberg A, Silverberg DS, Arons E, Radwan H. Positional vs nonpositional obstructive sleep apnea patients: anthropomorphic, nocturnal polysomnographic, and multiple sleep latency test data. Chest. 1997; 112(3):629–639

[43] Richard W, Kox D, den Herder C, Laman M, van Tinteren H, de Vries N. The role of sleep position in obstructive sleep apnea syndrome. European archives of oto-rhino-laryngology: official journal of the European Federation of Oto-Rhino-Laryngological Societies (EUFOS): affiliated with the German Society for Oto-Rhino-Laryngology—Head Neck Surg. 2006; 263(10):946–950

[44] Mador MJ, Kufel TJ, Magalang UJ, Rajesh SK, Watwe V, Grant BJ. Prevalence of positional sleep apnea in patients undergoing polysomnography. Chest. 2005; 128(4):2130–2137

[45] van Maanen JP, Richard W, Van Kesteren ER, et al. Evaluation of a new simple treatment for positional sleep apnoea patients. J Sleep Res. 2012; 21(3):322–329

[46] Bignold JJ, Mercer JD, Antic NA, McEvoy RD, Catcheside PG. Accurate position monitoring and improved supine-dependent obstructive sleep apnea with a new position recording and supine avoidance device. J Clin Sleep Med. 2011; 7(4):376–383

[47] Eijsvogel MM, Ubbink R, Dekker J, et al. Sleep position trainer versus tennis ball technique in positional obstructive sleep apnea syndrome. J Clin Sleep Med. 2015; 11(2):139–147

[48] van Maanen JP, Meester KA, Dun LN, et al. The sleep position trainer: a new treatment for positional obstructive sleep apnoea. Sleep Breath. 2013; 17(2):771–779

[49] van Maanen JP, de Vries N. Long-term effectiveness and compliance of positional therapy with the sleep position trainer in the treatment of positional obstructive sleep apnea syndrome. Sleep. 2014; 37(7):1209–1215

[50] Dieltjens M, Vroegop AV, Verbruggen AE, et al. A promising concept of combination therapy for positional obstructive sleep apnea. Sleep Breath. 2015; 19(2):637–644

[51] Levendowski DJ, Seagraves S, Popovic D, Westbrook PR. Assessment of a neck-based treatment and monitoring device for positional obstructive sleep apnea. J Clin Sleep Med. 2014; 10(8):863–871

[52] Hoekema A. Efficacy and comorbidity of oral appliances in the treatment of obstructive sleep apnea-hypopnea: a systematic review and preliminary results of a randomized trial. Sleep Breath. 2006; 10(2):102–103

[53] Lim J, Lasserson TJ, Fleetham J, Wright J. Oral appliances for obstructive sleep apnoea. Cochrane Database Syst Rev. 2006; (1):CD004435

[54] Phillips CL, Grunstein RR, Darendeliler MA, et al. Health outcomes of continuous positive airway pressure versus oral appliance treatment for obstructive sleep apnea: a randomized controlled trial. Am J Respir Crit Care Med. 2013; 187(8):879–887

[55] Petit FX, Pépin JL, Bettega G, Sadek H, Raphaël B, Lévy P. Mandibular advancement devices: rate of contraindications in 100 consecutive obstructive sleep apnea patients. Am J Respir Crit Care Med. 2002; 166(3):274–278

[56] Chung JW, Enciso R, Levendowski DJ, Morgan TD, Westbrook PR, Clark GT. Treatment outcomes of mandibular advancement devices in positional and nonpositional OSA patients. Oral Surg Oral Med Oral Pathol Oral Radiol Endod. 2010; 109(5):724–731

[57] Lindman R, Bondemark L. A review of oral devices in the treatment of habitual snoring and obstructive sleep apnoea. Swed Dent J. 2001; 25(1):39–51

[58] Rose E, Staats R, Schulte-Mönting J, Ridder GJ, Jonas IE. [Long term compliance with an oral protrusive appliance in patients with obstructive sleep apnoea] Dtsch Med Wochenschr. 2002; 127(23):1245–1249

[59] McGown AD, Makker HK, Battagel JM, L'Estrange PR, Grant HR, Spiro SG. Long-term use of mandibular advancement splints for snoring and obstructive sleep apnoea: a questionnaire survey. Eur Respir J. 2001; 17(3):462–466

[60] Bamagoos AA, Sutherland K, Cistulli PA. Mandibular advancement splints. Sleep Med Clin. 2016; 11(3):343–352

[61] Sutherland K, Phillips CL, Cistulli P. Efficacy versus effectiveness in the treatment of obstructive sleep apnea: CPAP and oral appliances. Journal Of Dental Sleep Medicine. 2015; 2(4):175–181

[62] Vanderveken OM, Dieltjens M, Wouters K, De Backer WA, Van de Heyning PH, Braem MJ. Objective measurement of compliance during oral appliance therapy for sleep-disordered breathing. Thorax. 2013; 68(1):91–96

[63] George PT. Selecting sleep-disordered-breathing appliances. Biomechanical considerations. J Am Dent Assoc. 2001;132 (3):339–347

[64] Schott TC, Göz G. Applicative characteristics of new microelectronic sensors Smart Retainer® and TheraMon® for measuring wear time. J Orofac Orthop. 2010; 71(5):339–347

[65] Sutherland K, Vanderveken OM, Tsuda H, et al. Oral appliance treatment for obstructive sleep apnea: an update. J Clin Sleep Med. 2014; 10(2):215–227

[66] Dieltjens M, Braem MJ, Vroegop AVMT, et al. Objectively measured vs. self-reported compliance during oral appliance therapy for sleep-disordered breathing. Chest. 2013; 144(5):1495–1502

[67] Pépin JL, Krieger J, Rodenstein D, et al. Effective compliance during the first 3 months of continuous positive airway pressure. A European prospective study of 121 patients. Am J Respir Crit Care Med. 1999; 160(4):1124–1129

[68] Engleman HM, Wild MR. Improving CPAP use by patients with the sleep apnoea/hypopnoea syndrome (SAHS). Sleep Med Rev. 2003; 7(1):81–99

[69] Weaver TE, Grunstein RR. Adherence to continuous positive airway pressure therapy: the challenge to effective treatment. Proc Am Thorac Soc. 2008; 5(2):173–178

[70] Sullivan CE, Issa FG, Berthon-Jones M, Eves L. Reversal of obstructive sleep apnoea by continuous positive airway pressure applied through the nares. Lancet. 1981; 1(8225):862–865

[71] Richard W, Venker J, den Herder C, et al. Acceptance and long-term compliance of nCPAP in obstructive sleep apnea. Eur Arch Otorhinolaryngol. 2007; 264(9):1081–1086

[72] Benoist LB, Verhagen M, Torensma B, van Maanen JP, de Vries N. Positional therapy in patients with residual positional obstructive sleep apnea after upper airway surgery. Sleep Breath. 2016:[Epub ahead of print]

5 Surgical Principles

Abstract

This chapter focuses on surgical principles in sleep-disordered breathing that might help select suitable patients for surgery. Factors that need to be addressed after extensive counseling include comorbidities, first- and second-line treatments, staged surgery versus multiple procedures at the same time, and the invasiveness of the procedure(s). In patients who are on CPAP, one should be aware of a possible washout phenomenon when preparing a sleep study. Finally, this chapter will address how to score and compare surgical and nonsurgical therapies. The real life effect of all nonsurgical treatments should take compliance into account as well. Mathematical formulas are provided for precise comparison.

Keywords: OSA, counseling, comorbidity, CPAP wash out, compliance, effectiveness

5.1 Patient Selection

Thomas Verse and Nico de Vries

5.1.1 Introduction

The most important issue in all kinds of surgery is to select suitable patients for the particular surgical procedure and vice versa. This chapter will focus on issues that might help select suitable patients for surgery for sleep-disordered breathing (SDB), as we are convinced that good patient selection improves surgical outcome.

Extensive Counseling

First of all, patients should be comprehensively informed about conservative alternatives to surgery. Devices such as positive airway pressure (PAP) machines, dental appliances, or positional devices (in positional obstructive sleep apnea [POSA]) can be recommended. If the patient feels fine with the device, he/she can decide to keep on using it. A conservative treatment can usually be stopped without long-lasting side effects. In contrast, surgery is not reversible in most cases. Once a tonsil is removed, it cannot be replaced. Furthermore, some complications of surgery are serious and may not be completely resolved. The individual effect of sleep surgery arises 2 to 3 months after surgery. In case it is not sufficient, further treatment might be necessary. This is why we advise our patients to try conservative treatment first (if there is any promising option) before undergoing surgery.

On the other hand, the best thing about successful surgery is that the disease gets completely resolved. In case of PAP users, obstructive sleep apnea (OSA) is only corrected as long as the patient uses his/her machine.

Therefore, in our opinion, it is crucial to inform the patient about advantages and disadvantages of any treatment beforehand.

The treatment of SDB is not necessarily a question of surgical versus nonsurgical measures. Often a combination of treatments finally helps the patients.

Comorbidities

As there are nonsurgical alternatives to surgery in OSA treatment, a surgeon should focus on the patient's specific comorbidities first. There is an increased perioperative risk for OSA patients undergoing any kind of surgery.[1,2,3,4] Various complications have been described in (▶ Table 5.1).

In sleep apnea surgery, an additional factor to be dealt with is any wound(s) within the upper airway that might cause bleeding, swelling, and airway compromise. This implicates that OSA surgery should be indicated with care in patients with severe comorbidities, and only in case of failure of conservative treatment.

If a patient with severe cardiorespiratory comorbidities is selected for upper airway surgery, surgery should only be performed as an inpatient procedure. If possible, the patient should be put on CPAP treatment prior to surgery with the treatment being continued during the perioperative phase. Overnight monitoring should be available in these cases. Please refer to Chapter 10 for further information.

Apart from these aspects, it is also mandatory to check for anticoagulative medication that might be stopped or bridged before surgery. Another important point is to look for signs of difficult intubation, such as micrognathia, male gender, age older than 50 years, body mass index (BMI) greater than 35 kg/m^2, and neck circumference greater than 40 cm.[6] In case a difficult intubation is expected, the anesthesiologist should be informed occasionally.

▶ Table 5.1 Postoperative complications in OSA patients[5]

Lung	Hypoxia, hypercapnia, atelectasis, bronchospasm, need for noninvasive ventilation or reintubation, pulmonary embolism, pneumonia, ARDS
Heart	Arrhythmia, ischemia, myocardial infarction, lung edema
Brain	Delirium, encephalopathia, stroke
Other complications	Gastrointestinal bleedings, wound infection, unscheduled increase in patient-centered care level, prolonged treatment

Abbreviations: ARDS, acute respiratory distress syndrome; OSA, obstructive sleep apnea.

First- or Second-Line Treatment

As stated previously, all kinds of sleep apnea treatments have certain failure rates. These failure rates vary substantially between different treatment modalities. In the case of surgery, we know that cure rates decrease with baseline BMI and apnea–hypopnea index (AHI) (▶Fig. 5.1).

As a consequence authors recommend surgery as a first-line procedure if the AHI is below 30 and the BMI is below 34 kg/m². These cut-off values are not supported by evidence-based medicine data from the literature but are based on authors' clinical experience of more than 20 years. However, exceptions to the rule are always possible. For example, the authors recently performed combined surgery of uvulopalatopharyngoplasty (UPPP) and tonsillectomy, and radiofrequency treatment (RFT) of the base of tongue in a patient with an AHI of 73 and cured the disease. In other words, if there is a pathoanatomical finding (e.g., massively enlarged tonsils) that is regarded as the origin of the airway obstruction and can be easily treated by surgery, first-line surgery may work well.

Multilevel or Staged Surgery

The authors use drug-induced sleep endoscopy (DISE) in addition to the ear, nose, and throat (ENT) examination (when the patient is awake) to determine the site(s) of obstruction. We prefer the VOTE-classification[8] that distinguishes four levels of obstruction, namely, velo-, oro-, hypopharynx, and epiglottis. If multilevel obstruction is detected, we need to decide whether surgeries can be combined at different levels within the same operation or if staged surgery should be recommended for treating every level separately.

In authors' opinion, multilevel surgery within a single operation is one step further than "staged surgery." The authors do not recommend performing surgery only one level at a time in case DISE shows obstruction at more levels. Multilevel surgery has proven to be safe, if the patients are selected carefully and monitored thoroughly

in the perioperative period. For perioperative monitoring please refer to Chapter 10. In mild OSA, however, the authors do not advocate the use of multilevel surgery in combination with unexpected and unexplained severe DISE findings.

In this context, the authors would like to stress that combinations of pharyngeal and nasal surgeries often lead to increased postoperative morbidity as the patients are forced to breath from their mouth. The loss of nasal climatization and humidification of the breathed air causes discomfort for a couple of days even without the use of nasal dressings. This is why authors do not recommend performing combined nasal and pharyngeal surgeries.

Invasiveness

Minimal invasiveness can be defined as surgery that can be performed under local anesthesia, as an outpatient procedure that causes little intra- and postoperative morbidity, and is affected with low complication rates. According to authors the following procedures can be regarded as minimally invasive: interstitially applied RFTs (turbinates, palate, tonsils, base of tongue, or any combination), and palatal implants. Other soft palate surgery such as uvulopalatoplasty, in its different modifications, causes substantial postoperative pain, but fulfills all the other criteria. Tongue implants (i.e., ReVent) require general anesthesia and is affected with low morbidity.

Minimal invasive techniques have limited effect on AHI. This fact limits the indication of these surgeries to either simple snoring or to mild OSA. The success rates of minimally invasive surgeries are low when the sleep apnea is severe. So the surgeons need to choose more invasive surgeries to be successful in case of severe disease.

Authors would like to exemplify this aspect. In a case with mainly oropharyngeal and limited hypopharyngeal obstruction during DISE authors would recommend a modified UPPP plus tonsillectomy in combination with an RFT of the base of tongue in mild OSA, while preferring a midline glossectomy instead of RFT in of severe OSA.

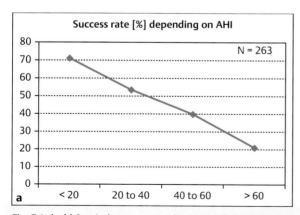
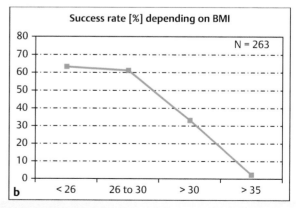

Fig. 5.1 **(a, b)** Surgical success rates decrease with increasing AHI and BMI. Success rate defined as reduction in AHI by 50% below an absolute value of less than 15. AHI, apnea–hypopnea index; BMI, body mass index. (Data taken from Verse.[7])

Another example could be palatal and oropharyngeal obstruction only. In snorers and mild apneics authors would recommend radiofrequency-assisted uvulopalatoplasty (RF-UPP) in combination with RFT of the tonsils, while recommending UPPP plus tonsillectomy in moderate to severe OSA.

The surgical principle that more severe OSA requires more invasive surgery has been postulated by Moore in 2000.[9] The authors are still convinced that this approach is partly correct, although technical developments and new surgical instruments have helped reduce postoperative morbidity substantially.

To sum it up, authors recommend to select surgeries with limited invasiveness (i.e., limited complication rates, limited morbidity, limited complexity for patient and surgeon) whenever possible while keeping the number of surgeries lesser. A single surgery is often better than repeated surgeries. As outcome in sleep apnea surgery is very difficult to predict, selection of the best surgical technique for the individual patient remains one of the biggest challenges in sleep surgery.

5.1.2 Continuous Positive Airway Pressure Washout

Anneclaire Vroegop, Jim Smithuis, Linda B. L. Benoist, Olivier M. Vanderveken, and Nico de Vries

Introduction

Patients who fail to use CPAP compliantly often visit surgeons for an alternative OSA treatment. Such patients might still use their CPAP machine until their visit to the outpatient clinic. Reevaluation of the severity of the disease is often necessary. This will include not only medical history taking and performing a thorough clinical ENT examination including DISE, but also polysomnographic (PSG) reevaluation in case no recent sleep study is available. The primary PSG often dates back to more than 1 year ago and one cannot assume the disease severity to remain stable over time.

The question then arises if patients should be advised to stop their CPAP use before the repeat PSG. Both ethical and medicolegal issues of CPAP cessation might arise. Recent literature suggests that CPAP might have a temporary residual effect on OSA after withdrawal from therapy. This is called the "washout period."[10] Therefore, it has been claimed that patients should stop their CPAP at least several days before the PSG is repeated. It has been suggested that without this washout period, the PSG result could be an underestimated level of the OSA severity. This washout phenomenon is an important issue from both theoretical and clinical perspective. This chapter aims to provide an overview of the available literature on this topic.

Material and Methods

A literature search was run electronically in the MEDLINE and EMBASE databases, based on the following main search terms: (CPAP OR nCPAP) and (OSA OR apnea) and (withdrawal OR residual), leaving 561 articles. In addition, articles were identified from the reference lists of these papers. For the comparison of pre-CPAP and post-CPAP outcome, relevant articles were included and analyzed when they enclosed information on OSA parameters before and after withdrawal from CPAP therapy. Studies in which long-term CPAP use (>1 month) was missing were excluded, resulting in a set of 13 studies that met the search criteria and were further evaluated. The studies within the present search criteria investigated different objective and subjective outcome parameters. In order to compare these studies, an analysis was performed focusing on the AHI as reported in the studies.

Results

Overview of the Evidence

The majority of the studies analyzed the severity of OSA during CPAP treatment and after CPAP withdrawal. Since not all studies provided the same data, the studies were split up into different sets. Studies in which there was no significant BMI change before and after CPAP therapy were separated from studies that found a statistically significant reduction of the BMI, or failed to report BMI changes entirely. Studies that calculated the significance for the mean AHI or respiratory disturbance index (RDI) or oxygen desaturation index (ODI) differences between pre- and post-CPAP were separated from those that did not report these calculations. An overview of these studies can be found in ▶ Table 5.2, with a bubble chart (▶ Fig. 5.2) visualizing the number of nights off CPAP (x-axis), delta AHI/RDI (change in AHI/RDI; y-axis), and number of patients included in each study (circle area).

CPAP Withdrawal Studies with No Significant BMI Change

Significant AHI/RDI Reduction after CPAP Withdrawal

Leech et al[22] included 17 patients on CPAP therapy for a median period of 6 months. PSG on the night off CPAP showed a significant improved average RDI (55/h sleep) compared with before the initiation of treatment (91/h sleep). Along with this finding, a significant improvement of the mean daytime oxygenation (PaO$_2$ in mm Hg) was found before treatment with CPAP (69 mm Hg) compared with after withdrawal (82 mm Hg).

Kribbs et al[21] performed a multiple sleep latency test (MSLT) in 15 patients with moderate to severe OSA after CPAP withdrawal. These patients received CPAP therapy for an average of 2 to 3 months, after which a PSG was conducted 1 night after CPAP cessation. The mean RDI post-CPAP (36.8/h sleep) was significantly lower than before initiation of therapy (56.6/h sleep).

Bonsignore et al[14] compared 29 untreated OSA patients, 10 OSA patients on CPAP, and 11 controls. Within the

▶ Table 5.2 Literature on AHI pre-CPAP versus post-CPAP

Study	Year	No. of patients studied (total)	BMI change ($P < 0.05$)	AHI/RDI pre-CPAP	Mean AHI/RDI on CPAP	Mean AHI/RDI post-CPAP	P value (mean AHI/RDI pre-CPAP vs. post-CPAP)	Duration of CPAP treatment (months)	Nights of withdrawal on which PSGs were performed	AHI definition according to AASM1[11]
Young et al[10]	2013	20 (42)	No	77.6	2.9	61.9	$P < 0.005$	4	2	No[a]
Kohler et al[12]	2011	21 (41)	Unknown	45.3	2.2	36.0	Unknown	>12	14	No[a]
Phillips et al[13]	2007	20	Unknown	46	0.7	26.7; 39.0	Unknown	>12	1, 7	Yes
Bonsignore et al[14]	2002	10 (29)	No	82	–	63	$P < 0.05$	5.5	1	Yes
Yang et al[15]	2006	20	No	47	2.7	50; 50	Unknown	>12	1, 7	Yes
Pankow et al[16]	2004	12	Unknown	43.0	3.7	32.3	Unknown	35	7–9	Yes
Marrone et al[17]	2003	13	Yes	80.1	–	64.6	$P < 0.05$	5	1	Yes
Fiz et al[18]	1998	10	No	47.0	5.4	40.5; 44.1; 42.2; 35.8	Unknown	24	1–4[b]	Yes
Boudewyns et al[19]	1996	25	No	93.6	–	94.1	NS	12	1	No[e]
Sforza and Lugaresi[20]	1995	30	Yes	74.4	1.2	61.1	$P < 0.005$	13	1	Yes
Kribbs et al[21]	1993	15	No	56.6	2.5	36.8	$P < 0.0001$	2.5	1	Yes
Leech et al[22]	1992	17	No	91	–	55	$P < 0.0001$	6[c]	1[d]	No[f]
Rauscher et al[23]	1991	21	No	53.9	–	28.7	NS	8	4 h	No[g]

Abbreviations: AASM, American Academy of Sleep Medicine; AHI, apnea–hypopnea index; BMI, body mass index; CPAP, continuous positive airway pressure; NS, nonsignificant; PSGs, polysomnographies; RDI, respiratory disturbance index.

[a]Hypopnea defined as airflow reduction > 30% for more than 10 s with a fall in oxygen saturation (SaO_2).
[b]Consecutive nights.
[c]Median.
[d]Presumably the PSG was conducted at the first night of withdrawal.
[e]Hypopneas were defined as a 50% drop in tidal volume from its value in quiet wakefulness prior to sleep onset.
[f]Definition of hypopnea not noted in study.
[g]Hypopneas were defined as a reduction in rib cage and abdominal movements to 50% or less compared to the preceding five breaths for longer than 10 s accompanied by a fall in SaO_2 to 92% or lower if baseline was equal or above 94% or a fall in SaO_2 of 3% or more if baseline was 93% or lower upon withdrawal (pre-CPAP: 77.6/h sleep, post-CPAP: 61.9/h sleep).

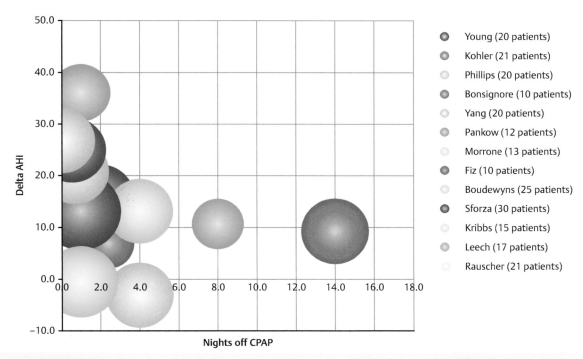

Fig. 5.2 Bubble chart displaying three data dimensions: the number of nights "off CPAP" (x axis) and the delta AHI or RDI (y axis), with the circle areas proportional to the amount of patients included. AHI, apnea–hypopnea index; CPAP, continuous positive airway pressure; RDI, respiratory disturbance index.

group of 10 OSA patients on CPAP (mean treatment duration 5.5 months), a significant better mean AHI after 1 night without CPAP (63/h sleep) was found compared to before treatment (82/h sleep).

Young et al[10] evaluated 42 OSA patients on CPAP for an average of 4 months, dividing them into subgroups of mild/moderate (n = 22) and severe OSA (n = 20). On the test night (second night of withdrawal), there was no significant difference in the mild/moderate group in the mean AHI (pre-CPAP: 15.7/h sleep, post-CPAP: 16.7/h sleep). However, within the severe OSA group, patients showed significantly better AHI values.

Insignificant AHI Reduction after CPAP Withdrawal

Contrary to these findings, Boudewyns et al[19] (n = 25) found no significant difference in AHI after stopping CPAP. On the first night of withdrawal, after 1 year of therapy, patients showed a comparable AHI (94.1 vs 93.6/h sleep) before and after CPAP.

Rauscher et al also found no statistical difference in 21 patients before and after CPAP therapy.[23] Patients using therapy for an average of 8 months were given CPAP for only the first part of the night. In the hours of sleep after using CPAP for the first part of the night a better improvement of the RDI (28.7/h sleep) compared to the hours of sleep before treatment with partial CPAP therapy (53.9/h sleep). The difference was not significant.

Fiz et al[18] studied 10 OSA patients, after 2 years of CPAP therapy, on first 4 nights after withdrawal from therapy. On the first night after stopping CPAP, the mean AHI level rose to severe OSA (40.5/h sleep) but the severity was less as compared to pretreatment (47.0/h sleep). On first 4 nights following CPAP withdrawal, AHI levels did not rise (i.e., night 1: 40.5/h sleep; night 2: 44.1/h sleep; night 3: 42.2/h sleep; night 4: 35.8/h sleep).

Yang et al reported even higher RDI levels in 20 patients after withdrawal (pre-CPAP: 47/h sleep, post-CPAP: 50/h sleep) compared to before treatment. There was no deterioration after further nights without CPAP; on the seventh night of withdrawal the AHI was 50/h sleep.

CPAP Withdrawal Studies with a Significant BMI Change or without Sufficient BMI Data

AHI Reduction after CPAP Withdrawal

Sforza and Lugaresi[20] studied 30 patients on CPAP for at least 1 year. The mean AHI before CPAP treatment (74.4/h sleep) was significantly higher compared with the first night of CPAP withdrawal (61.1/h sleep). However, the patients also had a significant lower BMI (pre-CPAP: 33.3 kg/m^2; post-CPAP: 31.3 kg/m^2; $P < 0.001$).

In a randomized controlled study Kohler et al[12] investigated 41 CPAP users, 21 of which were randomized to subtherapeutic CPAP use. The 2-week period on subtherapeutic

CPAP (AHI 33.8/h sleep) was associated with a significant increase in AHI, ODI, and number of arousals compared with the results of the therapeutic (continued CPAP) group (AHI 0.4/h sleep). During the first few nights a rapid increase in AHI in patients withdrawn from CPAP was noted. The mean pretreatment AHI in the therapeutic group was lower (36.0/h sleep) than the subtherapeutic group (45.3/h sleep), although not significant ($P = 0.155$).

Phillips et al[13] studied changes in inflammatory parameters in response to withdrawal from CPAP in 20 patients. The results showed a difference in the mean RDI on the first night of withdrawal (26.7/h sleep) as compared with before CPAP treatment (46/h sleep). The study was short, so changes in fat stores or BMI could be excluded. Sleeping without CPAP for another 6 nights showed a significant deterioration of the mean AHI compared with the first night without CPAP (seventh night: AHI 39.0/h sleep, $P < 0.005$).

Pankow et al[16] studied the effect of discontinuation of CPAP on blood pressure in 12 male patients with OSA and arterial hypertension. Baseline PSG showed a median AHI of 43.0/h sleep; the median AHI was 3.7/h sleep while on CPAP. After CPAP withdrawal for 7 to 9 days, there was a recurrence of the AHI to a median of 32.0/h sleep. No data on BMI differences were supplied.

Marrone et al[17] found a significant improvement of the mean AHI in 13 patients after 1 night of CPAP withdrawal (64.6/h sleep) as compared with the AHI before treatment (80.1/h sleep). However, the authors also reported a significant decrease of the mean BMI (pre-CPAP: 33.7/h sleep; post-CPAP: 32.6/h sleep; $P < 0.05$).

Discussion

A total of 13 studies on CPAP withdrawal were assessed, focusing on AHI and/or RDI, before and after withdrawal from long-term CPAP treatment (>1 month). Of these, three studies failed to report BMI changes during this period, while two studies found significant reductions in mean BMI after CPAP use. All these five studies showed an improvement in the AHI after withdrawal from CPAP compared with before treatment, of which two reported a significant drop in AHI. Importantly, these two studies were also the studies in which a significant decrease of the BMI was reported.

Of the remaining eight studies reporting no significant change in BMI, six showed improved AHI levels post-CPAP compared with AHI levels before treatment, of which four reported significant differences.[10,14,21,22] Young et al found statistical difference only in the severe, but not the mild/moderate OSA subgroup.[10] Two studies showed an increase in the AHI after CPAP withdrawal compared with before treatment.[15,19] The reported increase in AHI in these two studies was limited (0.5–3/h sleep).

A few studies have been performed with the goal of evaluating the difference in OSA severity (using AHI or RDI) before and after treatment with CPAP. A total of six studies[10,12,18,21,22,23] used AHI or RDI as primary outcome measure. Other studies reported the pre- and post-CPAP AHI level, but used MSLT,[20] respiratory effort,[19] neurobehavioral performance,[15] or cardiovascular parameters[13,14,16,17] as primary outcome parameters.

Studies that did not mention the AHI or RDI before and after CPAP treatment were excluded. Some of these studies described pre- and post-CPAP differences but focused on parameters such as hypoxemia,[24] stress hormones,[25] blood pressure,[26] snoring characteristics,[27] and driving performance.[28,29] Another study[30] was not included because patients did not receive long-term CPAP treatment before the investigation.

From the 13 studies matching the search criteria comparing AHI before and after CPAP use, long-term use of CPAP showed to have an acute residual effect after withdrawal from therapy. Of these 13 studies, decreased AHI after CPAP withdrawal was reported in 11 studies with significant decrease of AHI in 6 studies.

There are several important considerations to be made in order to interpret these results. Most studies were small (n = 10 to 30). Studies in which the BMI could have played a role in the AHI improvement were not excluded. Although we are aware that OSA severity is related to BMI,[31,32] for the sake of comprehensiveness these papers were also taken into account. All six studies that showed a significant difference in OSA severity between pre- and post-CPAP, conducted the PSG on the first or second night of withdrawal. This suggests that it is likely that the AHI is lower immediately after withdrawal and a washout effect is indeed to be expected.

There are three studies that report results of the AHI on multiple days after withdrawal from CPAP. Yang et al[15] conducted PSGs on the first and seventh night of withdrawal. Fiz et al[18] repeated PSGs on first 4 nights after withdrawal. Both studies did not show a deterioration of OSA after multiple days of withholding CPAP. In contrast to these results, Phillips et al[13] found a significant deterioration of OSA comparing the first and seventh night post-CPAP.

How long it takes before OSA reaches a reliable and stable level after quitting CPAP therapy remains unclear and might vary per individual. As one study showed a significant difference between first and seventh nights of CPAP withdrawal, it could be advised to withdraw treatment for at least 8 days before conducting a PSG.

There may be several explanations for this residual effect of CPAP after withdrawal. Various structures in the upper airway can contribute to upper airway obstruction in OSA. The upper airway anatomy and its response to differences in the pharyngeal pressure is one of the key factors in the pathogenesis of OSA.[33,34] During CPAP treatment, pharyngeal size increases,[35] thus facilitating airflow. Several articles suggest that a structural change in airway anatomy due to long-term CPAP use is the main reason for the presence of a residual effect after therapy.[10,23] Because of extended friction of the upper airway in OSA, pharyngeal edema might develop, thereby further decreasing the airway lumen. This edema would disappear with long-term use of CPAP. Ryan et al[35] performed an MRI study pre- and post-CPAP in five OSA patients and found a significant increase in oropharyngeal volume following CPAP therapy. Another study[36] screened 24 OSA patients using cephalometry before and after CPAP treatment. The mean posterior airway space was significantly increased in supine, but not in erect position. Unfortunately, this study did not use MRI. In contrast, Collop et al[37] who investigated pharyngeal volumes using MRI, found no pre- and post-CPAP difference in 12 patients with OSA. As these results show, there is limited data on the change of upper airway anatomy due to CPAP use. As a result, no definitive conclusion can be drawn about the possible existence of a difference between pharyngeal volume before and after CPAP treatment.

Another possible mechanism for the extended effect of CPAP on the AHI is an increased ventilation control mechanism in response to CPAP therapy. According to this theory, long-term exposure induces low oxygen levels in OSA. Patients would blunt their arousal responses to hypoxemic episodes. This lowered threshold in the central nervous system would result in altered responses to obstructive events.

Kimoff et al[38] showed that long-term OSA resulted in a reduction of breathing frequencies in response to hypoxia. Ventilation control mechanisms also seem to be impaired in individuals at high altitude with chronic hypoxemia.[39] A study by White et al[40] showed how sleep deprivation significantly decreased ventilation responses to hypoxia. These findings suggest that long-term use of CPAP could counter the altered neuronal threshold for arousal responses by reducing oxygen desaturation and facilitating sleep. This seems plausible regarding the dynamics of neuroplasticity and could play an essential role in the cause of a washout effect after acute withdrawal from long-term CPAP therapy.

It is interesting to evaluate this matter from the sleep surgeon's perspective in particular, as residual effects of non-CPAP therapies, for example, upper airway stimulation[41] or oral appliances (OAs), are not observed during DISE. The effect of these therapies seems to immediately disappear after the upper airway stimulation therapy is switched off or the OA is taken out. The same holds true for jaw thrust, chin lift, or similar maneuvers—these effects do not last. One hypothesis could be that, in the studies evaluated in the present paper, CPAP was used for more than 1 month and therefore a more prolonged effect on upper airway structures and behavior could be anticipated.

Atkins et al presented in a study that assessment of the quality of evidence and strength of recommendations by means of the Grading of Recommendations Assessment, Development and Evaluation (GRADE) system accentuates the lack of randomized controlled trials, limited study populations, imprecision because of different outcome measures, and the inconsistency of study results.[42] Moreover, the main research focus of the present study was mostly a secondary outcome in the majority of the

studies included. Furthermore, the balance between health benefits and harms of CPAP cessation and duration thereof was not explicitly considered in any of the included studies. This implies a relatively low quality of currently available evidence to substantiate a solid recommendation on this topic, resulting in a 2C grade of recommendation. Further research, preferable by means of randomized clinical trials, could contribute to more robust recommendations.

Generalization of study results is cumbersome because the studies included only small numbers of subjects, presented variable measurements of respiratory events, discussed different periods of time to assess CPAP washout, and only a few of the included studies took BMI into account. However, addressing the initial research question, even though within the limitations as previously mentioned, remains of clinical importance for any clinician treating OSA patients who failed or refused to use CPAP.

In conclusion, there is some evidence that CPAP washout exists in patients with a stable BMI throughout the follow-up period. However, the intensity and duration of this effect remain unclear.

The studies assessed in this section described rather small patient populations and to what extent other reasons for night-to-night variability were controlled for (e.g., sleep position in POSA, changes in the percentage of obstructive, mixed, and central events), is uncertain. Within these limitations, based on currently available literature, it might be reasonable to maintain a washout period, with approximately 1 week being a possible advisable period, in case alternative OSA treatment options are considered and especially when a baseline PSG (and a follow-up PSG after treatment) is needed in case of clinical trials.

5.2 How to Score and Compare Surgical Results with Those of Nonsurgical Treatment

Madeline Ravesloot and Nico de Vries

5.2.1 Introduction

The goals of treatment of OSA are:
- Elimination or improvement of symptoms.
- Normalization or improvement of sleep study parameters.
- Risk reduction in the longer term. This is especially true for severe OSA or for mild to moderate OSA starting at younger age.
- Reduction of perioperative risk in case of surgical patients.

PSG is the gold diagnostic standard in case of suspicion of OSA, for assessment of the severity and as control of the effect of treatment. Although according to the definition of OSA there must be an abnormal P(S)G in the presence of symptoms,[43] in clinical practice the severity of OSA is often expressed in the AHI (RDI or ODI) alone. Improvement in signs and symptoms and quality of life (QoL) are also important treatment outcomes, both in patients with mild, moderate, or severe OSA.

CPAP is an effective treatment for severe OSA as measured by improvement of the AHI, Epworth Sleepiness Scale (ESS), MSLT, reaction tests, and QoL questionnaires. For other forms of treatment and for milder forms of OSA treated with CPAP, the effect on these parameters is less pronounced. This can be partly explained by the fact, that unlike CPAP therapy, in mandibular reposition appliance (MRA) therapy and surgical therapy few randomized studies were performed.

The relationship between complaints (such as hypersomnolence) and outcomes of ESS, MSLT, QoL questionnaires, and PSG parameters (such as AHI and arousal index) is often moderate. Hypersomnolence is only moderately correlated with relevant P(S)G parameters. Perhaps this can be explained by assuming that a certain degree of sleep disturbance because of individual differences of basic fitness causes different degrees of sleepiness. However, instruments to assess basic fitness and alertness in clinical practice are lacking. It is a clinical reality that some patients with mild OSA have severe complaints, while others with severe abnormalities in sleep studies (high AHI, low oxygen levels) might have remarkably less complaints.

In scientific research different treatment outcome measures are used for CPAP, MRA, and surgical treatment. The objective effect of (surgical) therapy is expressed as change in P(S)G parameters, especially the AHI (and apnea index [AI]), and effect on average oxygen saturation, the lowest oxygen saturation, number of arousals (arousal index), and improvement in sleep architecture.

5.2.2 How to Compare the Different Treatment Options?

CPAP is regarded as the gold standard treatment of moderate to severe OSA, with oral device therapy or surgery reserved for CPAP failures or patients who desire a permanent solution.[44,45,46] In mild to moderate OSA, oral devices and surgery can be considered as first-line treatment in selected patients. Since more than 50% of patients with mild OSA have POSA, these patients can be treated with positional therapy as well.

Discussions about "the best treatment" might occur between CPAP protagonists, defenders of the merits of oral devices, and surgeons. Some CPAP advocates, (un)intentionally provocative, state that OSA can be treated without any surgery; lack of evidence from randomized controlled trials supporting surgical practices strengthens this perspective.[47] On the other hand it is believed that, in well-selected patients having obvious anatomical correctable features, surgery might be a viable alternative

to lifelong CPAP therapy. The issue is confused by the fact that different definitions of successful therapy are being used for different treatment options. Surgeons are being forced by the AHI classification to compete on an uneven playing field.

Traditionally, success in surgery was defined as a postoperative reduction of AHI to less than 20 and more than 50%.[48] Others have later proposed to tighten these criteria to a postoperative reduction of AHI to less than 15 (regarded as "clinically relevant" OSA), less than 10, and even less than 5 (as in CPAP therapy).[49] Some have added "response" as reduction of the AHI between 20 and 50%.[50] The same discussion regarding success criteria has surfaced in oral device therapy. Without external validation, any arbitrary definition of success will be incorrect. Furthermore, the cutoff point at which the AHI becomes harmful remains unclear. The cutoff point might also be dependent on the age of onset of the disease, duration of OSA, and for how long it was left untreated. He et al reported higher risk levels when the AHI is above 20 to 25.[51]

A patient is regarded "cured" when the AHI after treatment reaches below 5. Therefore CPAP therapy is considered successful if the AHI drops below 5 when CPAP is used. However, it is a clinical reality that the use of CPAP is cumbersome and it is often not used for 8 h/night for 7 consecutive nights. Patients seem to either tolerate the CPAP device well or not at all—a bimodal distribution, with an average of approximately 4 hours.[52] Hence the terms "compliance" or "adherence" were introduced. In the CPAP literature, existing trends define compliance or adherence observed as 4 h/night as an average on all nights. Another, even more lenient, definition is CPAP use for 4 h/night for 5 consecutive nights. Scientific proof for these arbitrary definitions is completely lacking.

The validity of such CPAP compliance criteria can be questioned, in the same manner as the validity of surgical success criteria has often been questioned.

For example, simple calculations show that given an average sleeping time of 8/24 h, the total sleeping time (TST) per week is 56 hours. With a minimal compliance of 4 h/wk, the mean AHI of a patient with an AHI of 60 before treatment would only drop to 32.5 (during 50% of the TST, the AHI would be 5; but during the remaining 50%, the AHI would still be 60). In a similar way, an AHI of 40 would only decrease to 22.5, an AHI of 30 to 17.5, and an AHI of 20 to 12.5, respectively.

Using the other definition, the change in AHI would even be less if the CPAP is used for 4 hours for 5 consecutive nights, (only 20 of the total 56 hours).

Such moderate decreases in AHI can often be reached with contemporary surgical techniques in well-selected patients, and are not in the range of the traditional liberal surgical success criteria of Sher (success would be reduction of the AHI of 60 to <20, AHI of 40 to <20, AHI of 30 to <15, and AHI of 20 to <10).

In order to avoid nonscientific and emotional discussions, there is need for objective criteria to compare the effects of successful surgery and nonsurgical therapy (be it oral device, CPAP, positional therapy, or combination treatments). Such equations were until recently lacking.

Ravesloot and de Vries were interested to see if mathematical formulas and graphs could be developed to compare the expected mean drop in AHI in case of surgery and CPAP therapy. In other words, how can nonoptimal use of optimal therapy (CPAP) be compared with the continuous effect (100%) of nonoptimal therapy (surgery).[53] The same principle is applicable to all other forms of nonsurgical treatment: MRA, positional therapy, and multimodality treatment.

In this chapter, mathematical formulas are provided that help compare suboptimal use of "highly effective CPAP treatment" with 100% TST effect of "subtherapeutic" surgical treatment effect.

5.2.3 Formulas

Using the mathematical formulas explained in this chapter, the effect on the AHI (or RDI, ODI, and so on) of various treatment modalities and their respective compliance and success criteria can be calculated.

Formula 5.1: Calculation of Mean AHI and Percentage AHI Reduction during Compliant CPAP Use

First of all, a patient must use CPAP for more than 4 hours per night to be deemed compliant or adherent. While using CPAP (HOURSonCPAP) ideally, the AHI is reduced to 0, 1, 2, 3, 4, or 5 (AHIonCPAP). While not using CPAP (HOURSoffCPAP = TST − HOURSonCPAP), the AHI can be assumed to remain stable (AHIoffCPAP). Ideally, we sleep 8 hours each night (TST); the average AHI per night can be calculated using the following formula:

$$MeanAHIforCPAP = \left[\frac{NIGHTSonCPAP}{week} \right.$$
$$\times \left(\frac{(HOURSonCPAP \times AHIonCPAP) + \left[(TST - HOURSonCPAP) \times AHIoffCPAP \right]}{TST} \right) \right]$$
$$+ \left[\frac{NIGHTSoffCPAP}{week} \times AHIoffCPAP \right]$$

For example, if we take a patient with an AHI of 19 (AHIoffCPAP), using the compliance criteria cutoff (4 h/wk) discussed, this patient sleeps using CPAP 7 nights per week (NIGHTSonCPAP). The AHI (AHIoffCPAP) is reduced to 5 (AHIonCPAP) during 4 hours, using the compliance cutoff criteria discussed (HOURSonCPAP). During the residual 4 hours (HOURSoffCPAP), the AHI remains 19. We can calculate the mean AHI during compliant use of CPAP by using the generalized formula given and the parameters for this patient:

$$MeanAHIforCPAP = \left[\frac{7}{7} \times \left(\frac{(4 \times 5) + (4 \times 19)}{8} \right) \right] = 12$$

The mean AHI is 12, so the AHI is reduced by 36.84%.

Formula 5.2: Percentage of TST during which CPAP Must Be Used to Reduce AHI to Less Than 5

To be *cured* of OSAS, the mean AHI must be less than 5. What would be the minimum percentage of TST during which CPAP must be used to reduce the AHI to < 5?

$$\left(\frac{(AHIonCPAP \times HOURSonCPAP) + \left[(TST - HOURSonCPAP) \times AHIoffCPAP \right]}{TST} \right)$$
$$= AHI_{<5}$$

$$HOURSonCPAP = \frac{TST \times (AHI_{<5} - AHIoffCPAP)}{AHIonCPAP - AHIoffCPAP}$$

Multiplied by 100 and divided by the TST, one can calculate the percentage of time (AHIonCPAP$_\%$).

For example, in a patient with an AHI of 19, the AHI is reduced to 4 while using CPAP. Using the following general and specific parameters for this patient—TST: 8 hours, AHIonCPAP: 4, AHIoffCPAP: 19, and AHI$_{<5}$—one can calculate that CPAP must be used more than or equal to 7 hours, 27 minutes (which is ≥ 93.33% of TST) to reach a mean AHI of less than 5.

$$HOURSonCPAP_\% = \left\{ \frac{8 \times (4.9 - 19)}{4 - 19} \right\} \times \frac{100}{8} = 93.33\%$$

One can use this formula to measure the minimum percentage of TST during which CPAP must be used to reduce the initial AHI number by simply replacing AHI$_{<5}$ by the other number, for example, AHI$_{<10}$ (9.9).

Formula 5.3: Percentage of TST during which CPAP Must Be Used to Reduce AHI by a Certain Percentage

The next question is: what is the minimum percentage of TST during which CPAP must be used to reduce the initial AHI by a certain percentage (%reduction)?

$$\left(\frac{AHIonCPAP \times HOURSonCPAP + \left[(TST - HOURSonCPAP) \times AHIoffCPAP \right]}{TST} \right)$$
$$= (100\% - \%reduction) \times AHIoffCPAP$$

$$HOURSonCPAP_\% = \left(\frac{-(\%reduction) \times AHIoffCPAP}{AHIonCPAP - AHIoffCPAP} \right) \times 100$$

For example, in a patient with an initial AHI of 77 *(AHIoff-CPAP)*, AHI is reduced to 5 while using CPAP *(AHIonCPAP)*: He/she must use CPAP more than or equal to 96.25% of TST to reduce the mean AHI by 90% *(%reduction)*.

When the AHI while using CPAP *(AHIonCPAP)* is reduced to 0, the formula reduces to:

$$HOURSonCPAP_\% = \%reduction \times 100$$

Therefore, for example, in this case to reach an 80% reduction in AHI, CPAP must be worn 80% of the time. But when the *AHIonCPAP* is more than 0, the *HOURSonCPAP$_\%$* will be higher than the *%reduction*.

Formula 5.4: Percentage of TST during which CPAP Must be Used to Meet Sher's Success Criteria

A 50% of the AHI is a straightforward division calculation, but from an AHI of 40 onward, a 50% reduction is insufficient to meet surgical success criteria; the AHI must be lower than 5.2.

What is the minimum percentage of TST during which CPAP must be used to reach Sher's surgical success criteria?

Using various formulas shown earlier:

In case of an initial AHI less than 40, one can use the following formula:

$$HOURSonCPAP_\% = \frac{\left(-50\%reduction \times AHIoffCPAP\right)}{\left(AHIonCPAP - AHIoffCPAP\right)} \times 100$$

and from an initial AHI of 40:

$$HOURSonCPAP_\% = \frac{\left(AHI_{<20} - AHIoffCPAP\right)}{AHIonCPAP - AHIoffCPAP} \times 100$$

Graphs

Percentage AHI Reduction during Compliant Use of CPAP

Again assuming that on average, people sleep 8 hours per night, and using the 4 hours per night compliance/adherence criteria, patients must use CPAP during more than or equal to 50% of TST (▶Fig. 5.3). As the initial AHI increases, so does the percentage of AHI reduction. Maximum AHI reduction stagnates at 50% when the AHI while using CPAP is 0 or initial AHI nears infinity. The lower the AHI while using CPAP (0–5), the more AHI reduction is attained (as shown in ▶Fig. 5.4). Patients with mild OSA (AHI 5–15) reduce their AHI by a minimum of 0 to 46.7% (AHI while using CPAP 1–5); those with moderate OSA (15–30) reduce their AHI by 33.3 to 48.3% (AHI while using CPAP 1–5); and those with severe OSA (AHI >30) reduce their AHI by 41.7% (AHI while using CPAP 1–5).

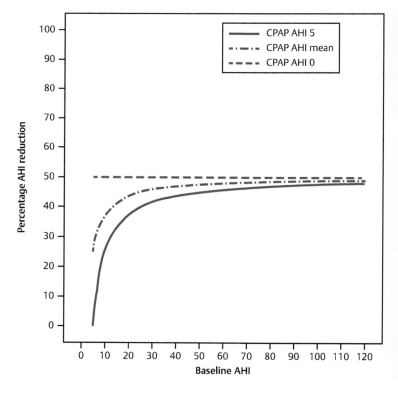

Fig. 5.3 Percentage AHI reduction when using CPAP 4 hours per night. This graph depicts the results when applying Formula 5.1, "Calculation of Mean AHI and Percentage AHI Reduction during Compliant CPAP Use." While using CPAP, ideally the AHI is reduced to 0–5. AHI, apnea–hypopnea index; CPAP, continuous positive airway pressure.

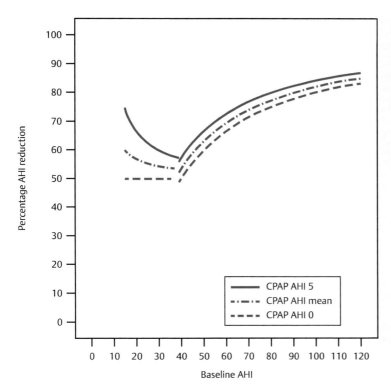

Fig. 5.4 The minimum percentage of TST during which CPAP must be used to reach Sher's surgical success criteria. The traditional criteria for a successful surgical outcome, was defined by Sher et al as a decrease ≥50% in postoperative AHI and a postoperative AHI <20 in patients whose preoperative AHI was >5.2. This graph depicts the results of Formula 5.4, "Percentage TST during which CPAP must be used to meet Sher's success criteria." AHI, apnea–hypopnea index; CPAP, continuous positive airway pressure; TST, total sleep time.

5.2.4 Percentage of TST during which CPAP Must Be Used to Meet Sher's Success Criteria

The traditional criteria for a successful surgical outcome, was originally defined by Sher et al as a decrease of more than or equal to 50% in postoperative AHI, and a postoperative AHI less than 20 in patients whose preoperative AHI was less than 5.2.[48]

Keeping these traditional "successful surgery" criteria into consideration, what is the minimal percentage of CPAP use needed per night to attain the same result? Up to an AHI of 40, CPAP must be used for at least 50% of the sleeping time; thereafter, the percentage quickly curves upward to reach a minimal percentage of 83.3% (initial AHI 120, AHI while using CPAP 0). These percentages surpass the 35.71% of the CPAP compliance criteria considerably and are therefore significantly harder to reach.

Elshaug et al debate whether the definition for surgical success should be redefined as a postoperative AHI less than 10 or even 5.[49,54]

5.2.5 Percentage of TST during which CPAP Must Be Used to Reduce AHI to Below 10

Concentrating on the first definition, to reach an average AHI less than 10, CPAP must be used for at least 33.3 to 66.7% per night, in patients with moderate OSA and an AHI of 0 while using CPAP. When the AHI is 5 while using CPAP, CPAP must be used minimally for 50% of the TST. In patients with severe OSA, a minimum of 67.4% of nightly use is necessary when the AHI is 0 while using CPAP, but 80% when the AHI is 5 while using CPAP.

5.2.6 Percentage of TST during which CPAP Must Be Used to Reduce AHI to Below 5

Focusing on the second definition (average AHI < 5), CPAP must be used 100% of the night (when the AHI is 5 while using CPAP). In patients with moderate OSA and an AHI of 0 while using CPAP, CPAP must be worn at least 66.7 to 83.3% of the TST (▶Fig. 5.5). In patients with severe OSA, a minimum of 83.9% of nightly use is necessary when the AHI is 0 while using CPAP, but 96.2% when the AHI is 4 while using CPAP.

5.2.7 Percentage of TST during which CPAP Must Be Used to Reduce AHI by a Certain Percentage

The initial AHI must be greater than 50 to be reduced by 90%; if the initial AHI is below 50, a 90% reduction is not possible. When the AHI is 50, the patient must use

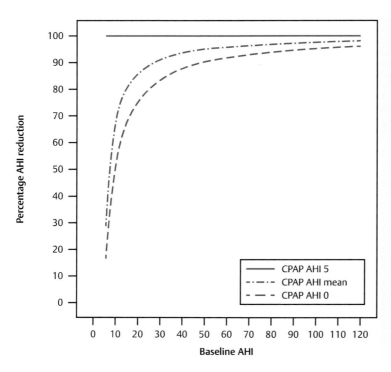

Fig. 5.5 The minimum percentage of TST during which CPAP must be used to reach a mean AHI < 5. To be *cured* of OSA, the mean AHI must be < 5. This graph represents Formula 5.2, "Percentage of TST during which CPAP must be used to reduce AHI to less than 5." AHI, apnea–hypopnea index; CPAP, continuous positive airway pressure; TST, total sleep time.

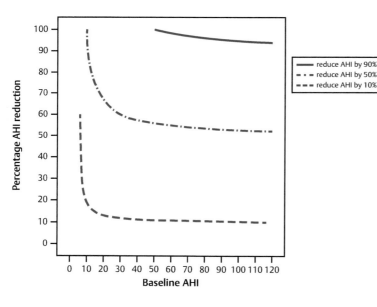

Fig. 5.6 The minimum percentage of TST during which CPAP must be used to reduce the initial AHI by a certain percentage (when the AHI is reduced to 5 while using CPAP). This graph shows the minimum percentage of TST during which CPAP must be used (when the AHI is 5 while using CPAP) to reduce the initial AHI by 10, 50, and 90%, respectively. AHI, apnea–hypopnea index; CPAP, continuous positive airway pressure; TST, total sleep time.

CPAP 100% of the TST. The percentage TST slowly dips to a maximum of 90% as the AHI increases. When trying to reduce the AHI by 10% at an AHI of 6, CPAP must be worn 60% of the TST, the percentage TST slowly decreases to 10% (▶ Fig. 5.6).

5.2.8 Discussion

Most medical devices are effective only when they are used. The effect may be 100% when always used, nil when never used, and partial when used sometimes, but not always. This is particularly true for CPAP use in OSA.

Approximately 15 to 30% of OSA patients refuse CPAP. Patients are often discouraged by the aesthetic aspect or the thought of being bound to CPAP for the rest of their lives.[55] In patients who are willing to try CPAP, pressure is titrated to reduce the individual patient's AHI to less than 5 events per hour.[56] Most patients discontinue CPAP treatment within the first few months. In spite of advances in CPAP technology, such as auto-PAP, bi-level

PAP, heated humidification, a large range of interfaces, and mask comfort improvement, as well as educational and behavioral support, patient adherence has only marginally improved in the past 23 years.[57,58,59] In a study conducted by Weaver and Grunstein, approximately 20 to 40% of patients discontinue CPAP within 3 months.[59]

On the other hand, surgery is slowly gaining momentum because of improvements in patient selection, as by means of DISE, and by applying more site-specific surgical techniques, as compared to earlier days (when the only surgical technique available was UPPP). Nevertheless, the Sher surgical success criteria might seem difficult to fulfill, especially in patients with severe or extreme OSA. It is generally easier to reach surgical success in patients with a low AHI, which is unjust. For example, a reduction of a mere 15 events per hour is needed to reach Sher's criteria in a patient with an initial AHI of 30, while a far larger reduction would be necessary in a patient with an AHI of 80 and CPAP failure. In this example, even a reduction of 60 events per hour would be insufficient to qualify for success; the gain in QoL and reduction of cardiovascular risk in this case is likely to be more dramatic than in less serious cases with a reduction of only 19 points.

The formulas given earlier in the chapter have various limitations. Assumptions were made to simplify and construct the formulas. Firstly, the authors assumed that 8 hours of sleep per night is ideal, while others would regard 7 hours of sleep per night as more realistic. The principle, however, remains the same however.

In clinical practice, it is often difficult to acquire accurate TST per night in patients using CPAP. Clinicians may want to request patients to record the hours per sleep (not hours in bed!) when applying the formula, but there is a difference between objective (estimated sleeping time by the patient) and objective sleeping time.

The authors also assumed that the AHI reverts to baseline as soon as CPAP is taken off. A washout effect cannot be ruled out when the CPAP is not in use. CPAP is thought to reduce edema of the upper airway, resulting from snoring-associated vibration and apnea-induced suction of the upper airway.

The baseline AHI may be fractionally reduced in chronic CPAP use. The authors considered this point negligible because the effect is minimal.

The authors also made the assumption that the "AHIoffCPAP" matches the AHI of the baseline PSG, and considered the AHI to be stable across the night. The question is: how good a representative is PSG of only one night? PSG has many limitations. Besides night-to-night variability, the AHI does not have a uniform distribution over the night. The AHI fluctuates because of the cyclic alternating pattern of the sleep stages, body position of the patient, medication and alcohol use, nasal congestion, and external factors influencing sleep efficiency, such as a sleep laboratory versus home recording, etc.[60] This is not only a hurdle for the present study, but a handicap for research and clinical management of OSA in general.

Some clinicians argue that other PSG variables could better be used as an outcome measure; for example, ODI as a measure of intermittent hypoxia. The ODI is also considered to be less susceptible to nightly variability.[61,62] One could generalize these formulas to other PSG outcomes such as the apnea index or ODI.

Some argue that clinical outcomes may be more appropriate metrics. There are more dimensions to consider in clinical management of OSA than AHI alone, for example, side effects, partner acceptance, cost-effectiveness, and so on.

A linear dose response between CPAP use and actual patient outcomes was assumed; the more hours a patient uses CPAP, the greater the therapeutic effect is expected. Whether the dose-response curve is linear is debatable, but unfortunately very little information is available in literature.[61] Furthermore, information can be extracted from the outcome of patients who reject CPAP completely and are left untreated.[63,64] As patients cannot "try" surgery, surgical literature does not include patients who chose not to have surgery and are left untreated.

To continue the debate initiated by Elshaug et al, who contend that "current notions of surgical 'success' are overdue for reevaluation," the authors also contend that the same holds true for CPAP compliance.[59,65] CPAP compliance rates vary greatly. Weaver and Grunstein report in their review that 29 to 83% of patients are nonadherent and use their CPAP for less than 4 hours per night.[59] Richard et al analyzed the compliance of 232 CPAP users.[56] Only 138 (59.5%) of these 232 patients were "compliant," with compliance liberally defined as CPAP use for more than 4 hours per night, for more than 5 days per week. Even in this compliant group, mean CPAP use was 6.5 hours per night (81% with a given 8 hours per night, SD 1.5), and 6.4 nights per week (91%, SD 1.4). With a CPAP use of 81% per night and 91% nights per week, compliant patients on an average used the device for 74% of TST. Patients seem to either tolerate the device well or not at all—a bimodal distribution.[51]

Stuck et al provided interesting real-life data that confirmed authors' theoretical calculations. In a large group of CPAP users, the average nightly CPAP use was 6.6 hours. While the mean AHI on CPAP was 2, the real-life AHI was 12.[66]

Elshaug et al have pointed out that when the traditional Sher's surgical definition (50% reduction in AHI and/or ≤20) is applied, the pooled success rate for Phase I procedures (soft palate) is 55%, but with AHI less than or equal to 10 as a cutoff point, success rate decreases to 31.5%; and at AHI less than or equal to 5, success rate is reduced to 13%. According to these definitions, Phase II (hard palate) success (fail) rates decreased from 86 (14%) to 45% (55%) and 43% (57%), respectively.[49,54] But, if we use the mean AHI in CPAP therapy, instead of the AHI reduction while using CPAP and aim at a mean AHI less than or equal to 5, the percentage of the TST during which CPAP should be used increases as a result.

In conclusion, a goal of a mean AHI less than or equal to 5, for both surgery and nonsurgical (CPAP) therapy, is rarely achievable. One should be aware that a cutoff point can be easily reached when surgery could be more effective in reducing the mean AHI. To "cure" OSA, the AHI should be reduced to below 5, but even with CPAP this seems to be an idealistic and nonrealistic goal. Nightly percentage use rises as one reduces the target to below 5 (see ▶Fig. 5.5). CPAP must be used at least 66.67 to 83.33% per night in patients with moderate OSA and an AHI of 0 while using CPAP. In patients with severe OSA, a minimum of 83.87% of nightly use is necessary when the AHI is 0 while using CPAP, but 100% when the AHI is 5 while using CPAP.

Each patient is unique and reacts to treatment differently; there is no guarantee of success, despite success rates and results being reported in literature. After surgery, the AHI remains relatively consistent during the night, but with CPAP it may dip below 5 during a certain percentage of TST and increase during the rest of the night when CPAP is not being used. Both may achieve the same mean AHI, but potential disparity between these treatment modalities on clinical symptoms and cardiovascular risk remains uncertain.

This chapter hopefully serves as motivation for further contemplation, debate, and discussion. Using a mean AHI in CPAP therapy is more realistic than using arbitrary compliance rates that hide insufficient reductions in AHI.

Conclusion

A goal of mean AHI less than or equal to 5 is rarely achievable, both for surgery and nonsurgical therapy (CPAP, oral device therapy). As soon as CPAP is not regularly used, one should be aware that a cutoff point is easily reached where surgery could be more effective in reducing the mean AHI.

5.3 How to Measure Clinical Success

Madeline Ravesloot and Olivier M. Vanderveken

5.3.1 Surgical Success

In 1981, Fujita et al introduced UPPP[67] as the first surgical procedure to treat OSA[68] and arbitrarily selected a postoperative decrease in AI of at least 50% from its preoperative value as the criterion for surgical response.[67] Thereafter, many authors used an RDI of 20 based on limited mortality data reported by He et al, indicating an acceleration of harm when the AHI rises above 20 to 25/h per sleep.[69] But, in surgical literature, Sher's criteria, a combination of both, is most widely cited: an AI of less than 10 or an RDI of less than 20 and at least a 50% decrease from the baseline index, postoperatively.[70]

Others have later proposed to tighten these criteria to a postoperative AHI to less than 15 (regarded as "clinically relevant" OSA), less than 10, and recently even less than 5 (as in CPAP therapy).[71,72] Some have added "response" as reduction of the AHI between 20 and 50%. The same discussion regarding success criteria has surfaced in oral device therapy. Without external validation, any arbitrary cutoff definition of success will be incorrect. Furthermore, the point at which the AHI becomes harmful remains unclear.[73]

5.3.2 Success in Conservative Treatment

CPAP and intraoral devices are regarded as successful if the AHI drops below 5 while the devices are being used; an AHI below 5 is the bar for CPAP adjustment. It is, however, common knowledge that a majority of patients are not adherent to the treatment during 100% of the TST under nonlaboratory conditions.[74] Patients seem to either tolerate the device well or not at all—a bimodal distribution, with an average of approximately 4 hours.[75] Hence the term "compliance" was introduced. Current trends define compliance as 4 hours per night as an average over all nights observed. Alternatively, Kribbs et al define criteria for regular CPAP users as the use of the treatment for at least 4 hours on 70% of the days monitored.[75]

The effectiveness of conservative treatment regarding the reduction of AHI depends both on its impact on airway obstruction and compliance.[73,76] Presently the second aspect is often overlooked.

Various articles suggest that OSA treatment effects on the AHI should no longer be reported under conditions of artificial compliance only, but in consideration of the individual compliance to the treatment. This is of particular importance when different treatment options are being compared.[73,76]

The concept of overall clinical effectiveness taking into account both therapeutic efficacy and adherence to treatment is increasingly used to report and to compare the results of different OSA treatments.[77,78,79,80]

5.3.3 AHI Defines OSA Severity

Although the AHI is only a surrogate marker for OSA, it remains the most frequently reported outcome measure in OSA. The AHI defines OSA severity, but other sleep study parameters can be more reliable (e.g., less susceptible to nightly variation) and physiologically more important (e.g., AHI, ODI, minimum oxygen saturation or percentage TST with oxygen saturation below 90%).[81]

5.3.4 Clinical Endpoints in OSA

Measures of OSA severity from PSG are important OSA treatment outcomes, yet they are intermediate outcomes.

▶ **Table 5.3** Clinical endpoints

1. Health-related consequences of OSA
   a) Primarily cardiovascular and endocrine
   b) Glaucoma

2. Behavioral consequences of OSA
   a) Excessive daytime sleepiness
      (i) Subjective sleepiness
         • Stanford Sleepiness Scale (SSS)
         • Karolinska Sleepiness Scale (KSS)
         • Epworth Sleepiness Scale (ESS)
         • Sleep-Wake Activity Inventory (SWAI)
         • Index of Daytime Sleepiness (IDS)
         • Survey Screen for Sleep Apnea (SSSA)
         • Rotterdam Daytime Sleepiness Scale (RDSS)
      (ii) Objective sleepiness
         • Multiple Sleep Latency Test (MSLT)
         • Maintenance of Wakefulness Test (MWT)
         • Oxford Sleep Resistance test (OSLER)
   b) Quality of life (health-related quality of life)
      (i) Generic instruments
         • Sickness Impact Profile (SIP) scale
         • Medical outcomes Study SF-36 (SF-36)
         • Nottingham Health Profile (NHP)
         • Functional Limitations Profile (FLP)
         • Munich Life Quality Dimension List (MLQDL)
         • WHOQOL-BREF
         • EuroQoL (EQol)
      (ii) Disease-specific instruments
         • Functional Outcome of Sleep Questionnaire (FOSQ)
         • Calgary Sleep Apnea Quality of Life Index (SAQLI)
         • OSA Patient-Oriented Severity Index (OSAPOSI)

3. Functional consequences of OSA
   a) Performance
      (i) Cognitive
         • Digit Symbol Test (DST), Letter Cancellation, block design test, Object Assembly and Picture Arrangement from the gold standard Wechsler Intelligence Scale-Revised (WAIS-R)
         • Paced Auditory Serial Addition Task (PASAT)
         • Trail Making Test (TMT) A and B
         • Wechsler Adult Intelligence Scale
         • Wechsler Memory Scale-Memory Quotient
         • Benton Visual Retention Test
         • Finger tapping test
         • Bourdon-Wiersma Test
         • Memory Distraction Tasks
         • Copying Tasks and Clock-Face Drawing
      (ii) Memory
         • Demand free-recall of words (probed recall memory task; Rey Auditory Verbal Learning Test (AVLT)
         • (Wechsler Memory Scale Story task [WMS stories]) or figure (Rey-Osterrieth Complex Figure Test: copy administration)
      (iii) Mood
         • Profile of Mood States (POMS)
         • Hospital Anxiety and Depression Scale (HADS)
         • Beck Depression Inventory (BDI)
         • Positive and Negative Affect Scale (PANAS)
         • Minnesota Multiphasic Personality Inventory (MMPI)
         • Zung Self-Rating Depression Scale Inventory (Zung)
         • Geriatric Depression Scale (GDS)
         • KDS self-rating scales for depression (KDS)
         • Symptom Distress Check List (SCL-90-R)
         • Freiburger Personality Inventory-Revised (FPI-R)
   b) Reaction time
      (i) Four Choice Reaction Time Test (FCRTT)
      (ii) Psychomotor Vigilance Test (PVT)
   c) Driving
      (i) Steer Clear
      (ii) Divided Attention Driving Tests (DADTs)
      (iii) Brake Reaction Time (BRT)
      (iv) Lateral Position Deviation (LPD)

4. Social consequences of OSA
   a) Disruptive snoring and other OSA symptoms
      (i) Snoring Severity Scale (SSS)
      (ii) Survey Screen for Sleep Apnea Index (SSSA)
      (iii) Index of Sleep Apnea
      (iv) Hawaii Sleep Questionnaire (HSQ)
      (v) Pittsburgh Sleep Quality index (PSQI)

The AHI does not capture the impact of OSA on the cardiovascular, neurological, psychological, metabolic, and emotional aspects of the disease.[81,82] Conflicting results have been published concerning the correlation between PSG indices and clinical endpoints.[83,84,85,86,87,88,89]

Kezirian et al suggested a standardized framework for presentation of surgical study results, which will enhance study interpretation, improve patient care, address fundamental unanswered questions, assist with comparison across studies, and direct future investigations. His paper can be regarded as a mandatory read for anyone reporting on results of surgical trials in patients with OSA.[81] The authors state that "OSA treatment is based not only on improving breathing patterns during sleep but also on alleviation of health-related, behavioral, functional and social consequences of the disorder." Weaver in her two-part review described patient-centered measures to evaluate many of these outcomes that are presented in ▶ Table 5.3.[90,91] She advocates that a comprehensive outcome assessment for sleep practice should include: (1) measure of subjective sleepiness; (2) disease-specific health-related quality of life (HRQoL) or functional status measures and optionally a generic instrument; (3) measure of mood; and (4) a measure of adherence to facilitate adequate interpretation of outcome responses.

Most recently, Pang and Rotenberg suggested the acronym SLEEP GOAL, a comprehensive set of success parameters: S, snoring visual analogue scale (VAS); L, latency of sleep onset; E, ESS; E, execution time; P, blood pressure; G, gross weight/BMI; O, oxygenation; A, AHI; L, life score (PSQI).[82] The authors suggest that this constellation of parameters reflect the disease burden in the OSA patient.

On the whole, the collection of these additional parameters may be labor-intensive for both research and the management of OSA, but this stands in contrast to the gross oversimplification currently taking place with the use of the AHI alone.[82]

5.3.5 Literature

The clinical endpoints, described in ▶ Table 5.3, have been studied in various publications evaluating CPAP therapy in OSA patients, as well as oral device treatment. However, in sleep surgery, literature is scarce.

The most commonly cited clinical endpoint is the ESS, a validated tool for the self-assessment of daytime sleepiness first introduced in 1991.[92] Patients are requested to answer eight questions concerning the likelihood of dozing off or falling asleep in a variety of different situations. ▶ Table 5.4 shows the effect of various single-stage upper airway surgery modalities on the ESS as reported in various review studies. Besides the Stanford Sleepiness Scale (SSS) and the Sleep-Wake Activity Inventory (SWAI) (one study) no other subjective sleepiness scales have been evaluated in patients undergoing upper airway surgery for sleep apnea. Reporting on clinical endpoints in sleep surgery is not yet common practice.

To illustrate, UPPP is one of the oldest and most widespread surgical treatments for adult OSA and an extensive body of literature is available, comparing UPPP with other surgical techniques.

Behavioral Consequences of OSA in Patients Undergoing UPPP

In a large systematic review and meta-analysis by Stuck et al, focusing on standard UPPP technique with or without tonsillectomy as a monotherapy in patients with OSA, pre- and postoperative measures of daytime sleepiness were only provided in 20 of the 53 studies (38%).[96] In eight studies, daytime sleepiness was quantified using various nonvalidated scores or by simple subjective assessment.[97,98,99,100,101,102,103,104] In 10 studies, however, the ESS was used as a validated tool for the self-assessment of daytime sleepiness.[105,106,107,108,109,110,111,112,113] While some

▶ Table 5.4 Epworth Sleepiness Scale

Surgery	N =	Mean + SD preop	Mean + SD postop	Reduction
UPPP ± TE[a]	337	11.7 (10.2–12.9)	7.3 (6.2–9.1)	
TCRFTA-BOT (book Verse)	117	10.3	6.1	
TCRFTA-palate[93]				0.85 (0.63, 1.15)[b]
TCRFTA-BOT[93]				0.59 (0.51, 0.67)[c]
HS[d94]	39	10.3 ± 4.9	7.1 ± 4.2	3.2 points
TORS BOT[e95]	335	12.9 ± 5.4	5.8 ± 3.7	7.1 points
MMA[f72]	113	13.5 ± 5.2	3.2 ± 3.2	

Abbreviations: HS, hyoid suspension; MMA, maxillomandibular advancement; TCRFTA-BOT, temperature controlled radiofrequency ablation of the base of tongue; TORS BOT, transoral robotic surgery base of tongue reduction; UPPP ± TE, uvulopalatopharyngoplasty with/without tonsillectomy.
[a]UPPP ± only. Studies of any design.
[b]Ratio of means.
[c]Ratio of means.
[d]HS only. Studies of any design.
[e]TORS BOT treatment for OSA as either a single modality or as part of multilevel treatment.
[f]MMA only. Studies of any design.

studies provided pre- and postoperative median values with ranges (including one RCT[105]) or mean changes without absolute values; mean pre- and postoperative ESS scores were reported in six studies.[106,107,108,109,110,114]

Mean preoperative ESS scores were reduced in these studies from a weighted mean of 11.7 (range 10.2–12.9) to 7.3 (range 6.2–9.1).

Four articles reported on QoL following UPPP. In an RCT setting, UPPP was found to be more effective in improving HRQoL, namely the physical and mental component score on the Short Form 36 (SF-36) questionnaire.[105] Improvement in all three dimensions of the Minor Symptoms Evaluation Profile (MSE-P) was found by Walker-Engström et al.[115] Both, Shin et al and Weaver et al found improvement on a disease-specific instrument: Calgary Sleep Apnea Quality of Life Index (SAQLI) and Functional Outcome of Sleep Questionnaire (FOSQ), respectively.[106]

Functional Consequences of OSA in Patients Undergoing UPPP

Dahlöf et al reported a significant reduction of depressive disorder after UPPP in parallel with improvement of the sleep disorder according to the DMS-III-R.[116]

One article reported on driving performance (brake reaction time [BRT] and lateral position deviation [LPD]) in 13 patients and 5 controls. Despite moderate concordance with the AI, objective results showed initial improvement in BRT, LPD, and number of off-road incidents. Moreover Haraldsson et al found that this positive effect remained even after 4 years.[97]

Health-Related Consequences of OSA in Patients Undergoing UPPP

In a small but prospective, noncontrolled study of Santamaria et al, decreased testosterone levels were found in a group of subjects with OSA compared to snorers; UPPP was performed in 12 subjects, which led to an increase in testosterone level from 13.31 ± 1.07 to 16.59 ± 0.72 and to a normalization of decreased sexual interest in all 7 affected patients.[117] Shin et al were able to demonstrate a statistically significant improvement in the International Index of Erectile Function (IIEF-5) from 15.6 ± 6.8 to 17.8 ± 5.5 in a prospective study with 30 patients receiving UPPP.[106]

With regard to cardiovascular parameters, changes in high and low frequency electrocardiogram (ECG) bands were detected in a small prospective Chinese study, while another study from Israel could not detect significant changes in the ECG after UPPP, but a statistically significant increase in right ventricular ejection fraction in a group of 18 subjects.[118,119]

Three studies assessed the survival of OSA patients after UPPP. In a retrospective study from He et al, the 5- and 8-year survival rates were assessed in nontreated patients and in patients treated with CPAP (n = 25),

tracheostomy (n = 33), or isolated UPPP (n = 60).[69] Mortality was increased in the nontreated patients with an AI more than 20. No deaths were recorded in the CPAP or tracheostomy group while mortality in the UPPP group was comparable to those in the nontreated group. However, postoperative sleep studies were only performed in part of the UPPP patients and the rate of response was low, which may be attributed to the high mean BMI in this cohort being 36.5 ± 7.4 kg/m^2.

In contrast, the survival of 149 patients receiving UPPP was compared to 208 patients receiving CPAP in another retrospective study from Keenan et al from 1994.[120] Mean follow-up was 43 ± 13 months. Patients in the CPAP group (n = 82) discontinued therapy and were excluded from the analysis, leaving 149 UPPP and 126 CPAP patients for analysis. In this cohort, 81% of patients receiving UPPP were responders according to definition (reduction in AI >50% or a reduction to <5). No difference in 5-year survival rate was detected between the two groups.

In a study conducted by Browaldh et al, no difference in the standardized mortality rate was described between the study population and the general Swedish population.[98] This study was conducted in the follow-up period of 15 years.

5.4 Combination Therapy for Sleep-Disordered Breathing

Marijke Dieltjens and Olivier M. Vanderveken

Effective treatment of OSA requires both high efficacy in terms of reduction in sleep apnea severity and high adherence to treatment.[53] This can be achieved through either invasive and noninvasive treatment options.

First-line treatment of OSA includes avoidance of aggravating factors (such as alcohol consumption before bedtime, smoking, the use of sedatives or muscle relaxants) and the treatment of overweight and obesity.[121] Weight loss should be recommended for all overweight OSA patients.[121] Often, weight loss should be combined with other treatment options.[121]

CPAP is the current gold standard therapy for patients with moderate to severe OSA.[46] However, the clinical effectiveness is often limited by relatively low patient acceptance and suboptimal adherence.[52,122] In general, about 5 to 50% of patients refuse to start CPAP therapy or discontinue in the first week.[66,123] At 1 year follow-up, 20 to 50% of patients discontinue CPAP.[124,125]

OA therapy is an alternative noninvasive treatment option for patients with mild to moderate OSA who prefer OA to CPAP, who do not respond to CPAP, who are not appropriate candidates for CPAP, or who fail treatment attempts with CPAP.[121,123] Overall, OA therapy is characterized by a lower efficacy but a higher patient compliance compared to CPAP, resulting in similar overall clinical effectiveness for CPAP and OA therapy.[77]

Overall, single treatment will be associated with an incomplete elimination of the OSA disease and/or insufficient adherence to treatment leading to an inadequate clinical effectiveness of the monotherapy for OSA. Therefore, in those cases, combination of more than one treatment modality could be promising and should be considered.

5.4.1 Combination of CPAP and Other Noninvasive Treatment Options

In literature, it is shown that CPAP therapy is characterized by a high therapeutic efficacy although compromised by a suboptimal adherence.[122] Therefore, in order to optimize CPAP therapy, the acceptance and tolerance of this treatment modality should be increased. In CPAP-intolerant patients, pressure intolerance is a frequently reported complaint.[126] Therefore, there is a need to look for additive treatment options that can reduce the required CPAP.

In a study of Lankford et al,[127] the CPAP requirements were studied in a group of patients undergoing rapid weight loss following bariatric surgery. The authors concluded that lower pressures are needed after bariatric surgery, on average a reduction of 18% in required CPAP. This lower CPAP may lead to increased tolerance and compliance.[127]

In a prospective pilot study of El-Sohl et al,[128] the feasibility of the combined use of OA therapy and CPAP was studied, as well as the additional benefits of this combination therapy on decreasing the CPAP requirements. It was concluded that the optimal CPAP could be reduced by combining OA therapy and CPAP in CPAP-intolerant patients.[128] Furthermore, this combination therapy was effective in normalizing respiratory disturbances.[128]

5.4.2 Combination of Different Types of Oral Appliance Therapy

OAs can be divided into different categories based on their mode of action. Tongue retaining devices (TRDs) use a suction pressure to hold the tongue in a forward position during sleep and thereby preventing the tongue from falling back into the pharyngeal airway.[129,130] Another category is that of mandibular advancement devices (MADs), advancing the mandible and the attached tongue during the night. The mechanism of action of MAD is usually assumed to cause enlargement of the cross-sectional upper airway dimensions by anterior displacement of the mandible and the attached tongue, resulting in improved upper airway patency.[131,132,133] It has been shown that TRD increases the velopharyngeal lateral diameter to a greater extent than the MAD, whereas the MAD produces significant anterior displacement of the tongue base muscles.[134]

In general, MAD therapy is characterized by a lower efficacy compared with CPAP therapy, but with a higher patients'acceptance and with a much lower discontinuation rate of only 10% at 1 year follow-up.[135] Therefore, for OA therapy, there is a need to look for additive treatment options that can increase the efficacy in terms of OSA severity reduction.

Based on the different expected effects on the upper airway caliber for MAD versus TRD, the combination of these OAs can be considered as a treatment option. In a study by Dort et al,[136] it was shown that a combined approach using both mandibular protrusion with an MAD and tongue retention effect through TRD can provide effective treatment in patients with moderate to severe OSA, and the addition of a tongue bulb may provide further treatment effect when mandibular protrusion was limited. However, convenient appliance designs for this combination approach are needed.

5.4.3 Combination of Oral Appliance Therapy and Surgery

UPPP is the most common surgical procedure for OSA, with an overall success rate of 41% described in literature.[48] In a study of Millman et al,[137] MAD therapy was started in patients who failed UPPP treatment. The authors concluded that OA therapy seems promising as adjuvant therapy in patients with unsuccessful upper airway surgery.

5.4.4 Combination of Positional Therapy and Other Noninvasive Treatment Options

Clinical experience indicates that in most patients with OSA, the frequency and duration of respiratory events are influenced by body position and sleep stage.[138] In approximately 50 to 60% of OSA patients, there are twice as much respiratory events in supine sleeping position when compared with the non-supine sleeping position.[139,140,141] In an additional 30% of patients, there are more respiratory disturbances in the supine position than in the other positions, although not twice as high.

The most widely used definition of POSA is proposed by Cartwright et al[142] as having a supine AHI of at least twice as high as the non-supine AHI. In general, the patients with POSA are younger, have lower BMI, and less severe OSA.[141,143,144]

Positional therapy is a treatment modality aimed at preventing sleep in the supine position.[68] The most widely used technique to avoid the supine sleeping position involves strapping a bulky object to the back of the patient thereby preventing supine positioning. Several studies have shown that such therapies have a significant positive effect on snoring and OSA severity in patients with POSA.[68,140,145,146,147,148] However, the bulky object is uncomfortable for patients and results in disturbed sleep and low long-term compliance rates.[140,145] Therefore, positional therapy has not found its way into daily OSA treatment routine to date.[149] In order to overcome such compliance problems, both a new neck-worn and a chest-worn device correcting the supine sleeping position by activating a vibration alarm were evaluated. This novel concept of positional therapy showed promising results in reducing apnea severity, together with a higher compliance.[150,151]

It has been reported previously that decreasing body weight may shift a patient with non-POSA to POSA.[152] In that opinion, in patients undergoing weight reduction and shift from a non-POSA to a POSA due to the weight loss, positional therapy can be used as adjuvant therapy.

Body position and sleep stages have been shown to significantly influence the CPAP requirements to eliminate OSA. Most studies on the effect of body position on CPAP requirements suggest that the pressure needed in the supine position is greater than that needed in the non-supine position.[153,154,155] This means that if patients can avoid the supine position, the consequent decrease in CPAP requirements can lead to a higher acceptance of the therapy.[149]

It has been reported in literature that a treatment modality for OSA that is not able to completely eliminate all breathing abnormalities leaves the patient with a residual OSA, although often less severe than the initial OSA. Therefore, the residual OSA is probably more supine-dependent since supine-dependent OSA is more frequently seen in mild OSA. In a retrospective analysis on patients undergoing MAD therapy, it was described that one-third of patients under MAD therapy have a residual POSA.[156] In a study of Cartwright et al,[68] the efficacy of combination therapy of a posture alarm giving an auditory beep when in supine position and a TRD was described. Patients were assigned to either therapy with the posture alarm, the TRD, or combination therapy with the posture alarm and the TRD. The results of that study suggested that the combination of an OA and positional therapy is better than one of the treatment modalities alone.[68]

In a more recent study by Dieltjens et al,[157] the feasibility and efficacy of adjuvant therapy with a chest-worn vibrational alarm was evaluated in patients who were unsuccessfully treated with MAD therapy due to the presence of residual POSA under MAD therapy. The results indicate that both MAD and positional therapy were individually effective in reducing the apnea severity in patients with residual POSA under MAD therapy. In addition, combination therapy of MAD and positional therapy leads to a higher therapeutic efficacy in those patients compared to one of the treatment modalities alone.[157] These findings suggest that when patients are unsuccessfully treated with MAD treatment, the presence of POSA should be checked and combination therapy could be suggested in eligible patients.

5.4.5 Combination of Positional Therapy and Surgery

In literature it is described that UPPP is most successful in reducing the OSA severity in lateral position, but the OSA severity in supine position does not change significantly after UPPP surgery.[158,159,160] So, after UPPP, the positional effect on OSA severity is more pronounced.[149] Therefore, from a theoretical approach, combination of positional therapy and upper airway surgery could increase the overall effectiveness in patients with residual POSA after surgery.[149] This idea was confirmed in a study by Benoist et al,[161] indicating that adjuvant positional therapy in patients with residual POSA after upper airway surgery can indeed increase the overall therapeutic effectiveness.

5.4.6 Conclusion

Overall, the combination of different treatment modalities in the treatment approach of patients diagnosed with OSA is underestimated and undervalued. The possible combinations are unlimited as all noninvasive and invasive therapies might be combined including so-called salvage or multilevel surgery which could be regarded as a combination in itself.

Combination therapy for OSA is promising as it is capable of increasing the acceptance and adherence of a certain single therapy by reducing the requirements of that treatment option. Furthermore, adjuvant therapy could increase the overall effectiveness by increasing the efficacy in terms of reducing the sleep apnea severity.

References

[1] Corso RM, Piraccini E, Calli M, et al. Obstructive sleep apnea is a risk factor for difficult endotracheal intubation. Minerva Anestesiol. 2011; 77(1):99–100

[2] Kim JA, Lee JJ. Preoperative predictors of difficult intubation in patients with obstructive sleep apnea syndrome. Can J Anaesth. 2006; 53(4):393–397

[3] Neligan PJ, Porter S, Max B, Malhotra G, Greenblatt EP, Ochroch EA. Obstructive sleep apnea is not a risk factor for difficult intubation in morbidly obese patients. Anesth Analg. 2009; 109(4): 1182–1186

[4] Siyam MA, Benhamou D. Difficult endotracheal intubation in patients with sleep apnea syndrome. Anesth Analg. 2002; 95(4): 1098–1102

[5] Vasu TS, Grewal R, Doghramji K. Obstructive sleep apnea syndrome and perioperative complications: a systematic review of the literature. J Clin Sleep Med. 2012; 8(2):199–207

[6] Chung F, Yegneswaran B, Liao P, et al. STOP questionnaire: a tool to screen patients for obstructive sleep apnea. Anesthesiology. 2008; 108(5):812–821

[7] Verse T. [Update on surgery for obstructive sleep apnea syndrome] HNO. 2008; 56(11):1098–1104

[8] Kezirian EJ, Hohenhorst W, de Vries N. Drug-induced sleep endoscopy: the VOTE classification. Eur Arch Otorhinolaryngol. 2011; 268(8):1233–1236

[9] Moore K. Site-specific versus diffuse treatment presenting severity of obstructive sleep apnea. Sleep Breath. 2000; 4(4):145–146

[10] Young LR, Taxin ZH, Norman RG, Walsleben JA, Rapoport DM, Ayappa I. Response to CPAP withdrawal in patients with mild versus severe obstructive sleep apnea/hypopnea syndrome. Sleep. 2013; 36(3):405–412

[11] Duchna HW. [Sleep-related breathing disorders–a second edition of the International Classification of Sleep Disorders (ICSD-2) of the American Academy of Sleep Medicine (AASM)]. Pneumologie. 2006; 60(9):568–575

[12] Kohler M, Stoewhas AC, Ayers L, et al. Effects of continuous positive airway pressure therapy withdrawal in patients with obstructive sleep apnea: a randomized controlled trial. Am J Respir Crit Care Med. 2011; 184(10):1192–1199

[13] Phillips CL, Yang Q, Williams A, et al. The effect of short-term withdrawal from continuous positive airway pressure therapy on sympathetic activity and markers of vascular inflammation in subjects with obstructive sleep apnoea. J Sleep Res. 2007; 16(2):217–225

[14] Bonsignore MR, Parati G, Insalaco G, et al. Continuous positive airway pressure treatment improves baroreflex control of heart rate during sleep in severe obstructive sleep apnea syndrome. Am J Respir Crit Care Med. 2002; 166(3):279–286

[15] Yang Q, Phillips CL, Melehan KL, Rogers NL, Seale JP, Grunstein RR. Effects of short-term CPAP withdrawal on neurobehavioral performance in patients with obstructive sleep apnea. Sleep. 2006; 29(4):545–552

[16] Pankow W, Lock S, Lies A, Becker HF, Penzel T, Lohmann FW. 24-Hour blood pressure on and off continuous positive airway pressure in patients with obstructive sleep apnoea and hypertension. Somnologie (Berl). 2004; 8(2):42–45

[17] Marrone O, Salvaggio A, Bonsignore MR, Insalaco G, Bonsignore G. Blood pressure responsiveness to obstructive events during sleep after chronic CPAP. Eur Respir J. 2003; 21(3):509–514

[18] Fiz JA, Abad J, Ruiz J, Riera M, Izquierdo J, Morera J. nCPAP treatment interruption in OSA patients. Respir Med. 1998; 92(1):28–31

[19] Boudewyns A, Sforza E, Zamagni M, Krieger J. Respiratory effort during sleep apneas after interruption of long-term CPAP treatment in patients with obstructive sleep apnea. Chest. 1996; 110(1):120–127

[20] Sforza E, Lugaresi E. Daytime sleepiness and nasal continuous positive airway pressure therapy in obstructive sleep apnea syndrome patients: effects of chronic treatment and 1-night therapy withdrawal. Sleep. 1995; 18(3):195–201

[21] Kribbs NB, Pack AI, Kline LR, et al. Effects of one night without nasal CPAP treatment on sleep and sleepiness in patients with obstructive sleep apnea. Am Rev Respir Dis. 1993; 147(5):1162–1168

[22] Leech JA, Onal E, Lopata M. Nasal CPAP continues to improve sleep-disordered breathing and daytime oxygenation over long-term follow-up of occlusive sleep apnea syndrome. Chest. 1992; 102(6):1651–1655

[23] Rauscher H, Popp W, Wanke T, Zwick H. Breathing during sleep in patients treated for obstructive sleep apnea. Nasal CPAP for only part of the night. Chest. 1991; 100(1):156–159

[24] Montplaisir J, Bédard MA, Richer F, Rouleau I. Neurobehavioral manifestations in obstructive sleep apnea syndrome before and after treatment with continuous positive airway pressure. Sleep. 1992; 15(6, Suppl):S17–S19

[25] Grunstein RR, Stewart DA, Lloyd H, Akinci M, Cheng N, Sullivan CE. Acute withdrawal of nasal CPAP in obstructive sleep apnea does not cause a rise in stress hormones. Sleep. 1996; 19(10):774–782

[26] Stradling JR, Partlett J, Davies RJO, Siegwart D, Tarassenko L. Effect of short term graded withdrawal of nasal continuous positive airway pressure on systemic blood pressure in patients with obstructive sleep apnoea. Blood Press. 1996; 5(4):234–240

[27] Sériès F, Marc I. Changes in snoring characteristics after 30 days of nasal continuous positive airway pressure in patients with non-apnoeic snoring: a controlled trial. Thorax. 1994; 49(6):562–566

[28] Filtness AJ, Reyner LA, Horne JA. One night's CPAP withdrawal in otherwise compliant OSA patients: marked driving impairment but good awareness of increased sleepiness. Sleep Breath. 2012; 16(3):865–871

[29] Turkington PM, Sircar M, Saralaya D, Elliott MW. Time course of changes in driving simulator performance with and without treatment in patients with sleep apnoea hypopnoea syndrome. Thorax. 2004; 59(1):56–59

[30] Hers V, Liistro G, Dury M, Collard P, Aubert G, Rodenstein DO. Residual effect of nCPAP applied for part of the night in patients with obstructive sleep apnoea. Eur Respir J. 1997; 10(5):973–976

[31] Gami AS, Caples SM, Somers VK. Obesity and obstructive sleep apnea. Endocrinol Metab Clin North Am. 2003; 32(4):869–894

[32] Young T, Peppard PE, Gottlieb DJ. Epidemiology of obstructive sleep apnea: a population health perspective. Am J Respir Crit Care Med. 2002; 165(9):1217–1239

[33] Schwab RJ, Pack AI, Gupta KB, et al. Upper airway and soft tissue structural changes induced by CPAP in normal subjects. Am J Respir Crit Care Med. 1996; 154(4 Pt 1):1106–1116

[34] Abbey NC, Block AJ, Green D, Mancuso A, Hellard DW. Measurement of pharyngeal volume by digitized magnetic resonance imaging. Effect of nasal continuous positive airway pressure. Am Rev Respir Dis. 1989; 140(3):717–723

[35] Ryan CF, Lowe AA, Li D, Fleetham JA. Magnetic resonance imaging of the upper airway in obstructive sleep apnea before and after chronic nasal continuous positive airway pressure therapy. Am Rev Respir Dis. 1991; 144(4):939–944

[36] Mortimore IL, Kochhar P, Douglas NJ. Effect of chronic continuous positive airway pressure (CPAP) therapy on upper airway size in patients with sleep apnoea/hypopnoea syndrome. Thorax. 1996; 51(2):190–192

[37] Collop NA, Block AJ, Hellard D. The effect of nightly nasal CPAP treatment on underlying obstructive sleep apnea and pharyngeal size. Chest. 1991; 99(4):855–860

[38] Kimoff RJ, Brooks D, Horner RL, et al. Ventilatory and arousal responses to hypoxia and hypercapnia in a canine model of obstructive sleep apnea. Am J Respir Crit Care Med. 1997; 156(3 Pt 1):886–894

[39] Weil JV, Byrne-Quinn E, Sodal IE, Filley GF, Grover RF. Acquired attenuation of chemoreceptor function in chronically hypoxic man at high altitude. J Clin Invest. 1971; 50(1):186–195

[40] White DP, Douglas NJ, Pickett CK, Zwillich CW, Weil JV. Sleep deprivation and the control of ventilation. Am Rev Respir Dis. 1983; 128(6):984–986

[41] Strollo PJ Jr, Soose RJ, Maurer JT, et al. STAR Trial Group. Upper-airway stimulation for obstructive sleep apnea. N Engl J Med. 2014; 370(2):139–149

[42] Atkins D, Best D, Briss PA, et al. GRADE Working Group. Grading quality of evidence and strength of recommendations. BMJ. 2004; 328(7454):1490

[43] Kushida CA, Littner MR, Morgenthaler T, et al. Practice parameters for the indications for polysomnography and related procedures: an update for 2005. Sleep. 2005; 28(4):499–521

[44] Kryger MH. Diagnosis and management of sleep apnea syndrome. Clin Cornerstone. 2000; 2(5):39–47

[45] Young T, Hutton R, Finn L, Badr S, Palta M. The gender bias in sleep apnea diagnosis. Are women missed because they have different symptoms? Arch Intern Med. 1996; 156(21):2445–2451

[46] Sullivan CE, Issa FG, Berthon-Jones M, Eves L. Reversal of obstructive sleep apnoea by continuous positive airway pressure applied through the nares. Lancet. 1981; 1(8225):862–865

[47] Franklin KA, Anttila H, Axelsson S, et al. Effects and side-effects of surgery for snoring and obstructive sleep apnea–a systematic review. Sleep. 2009; 32(1):27–36

[48] Sher AE, Schechtman KB, Piccirillo JF. The efficacy of surgical modifications of the upper airway in adults with obstructive sleep apnea syndrome. Sleep. 1996; 19(2):156–177

[49] Elshaug AG, Moss JR, Southcott AM, Hiller JE. Redefining success in airway surgery for obstructive sleep apnea: a meta-analysis and synthesis of the evidence. Sleep. 2007; 30(4):461–467

[50] Verse T, Baisch A, Maurer JT, Stuck BA, Hörmann K. Multilevel surgery for obstructive sleep apnea: short-term results. Otolaryngol Head Neck Surg. 2006; 134(4):571–577

[51] He J, Kryger MH, Zorick FJ, Conway W, Roth T. Mortality and apnea index in obstructive sleep apnea. Experience in 385 male patients. Chest. 1988; 94(1):9–14

[52] Kribbs NB, Pack AI, Kline LR, et al. Objective measurement of patterns of nasal CPAP use by patients with obstructive sleep apnea. Am Rev Respir Dis. 1993; 147(4):887–895

[53] Ravesloot MJ, de Vries N. Reliable calculation of the efficacy of non-surgical and surgical treatment of obstructive sleep apnea revisited. Sleep. 2011; 34(1):105–110

[54] Elshaug AG, Moss JR, Hiller JE, Maddern GJ. Upper airway surgery should not be first line treatment for obstructive sleep apnoea in adults. BMJ. 2008; 336(7634):44–45

[55] Olsen S, Smith S, Oei TP. Adherence to continuous positive airway pressure therapy in obstructive sleep apnoea sufferers: a theoretical approach to treatment adherence and intervention. Clin Psychol Rev. 2008; 28(8):1355–1371

[56] Richard W, Venker J, den Herder C, et al. Acceptance and long-term compliance of nCPAP in obstructive sleep apnea. Eur Arch Otorhinolaryngol. 2007; 264(9):1081–1086

[57] Kakkar RK, Berry RB. Positive airway pressure treatment for obstructive sleep apnea. Chest. 2007; 132(3):1057–1072

[58] Rubins JB, Kunisaki KM. Contemporary issues in the diagnosis and treatment of obstructive sleep apnea. Postgrad Med. 2008; 120(2):46–52

[59] Weaver TE, Grunstein RR. Adherence to continuous positive airway pressure therapy: the challenge to effective treatment. Proc Am Thorac Soc. 2008; 5(2):173–178

[60] Wittig RM, Romaker A, Zorick FJ, Roehrs TA, Conway WA, Roth T. Night-to-night consistency of apneas during sleep. Am Rev Respir Dis. 1984; 129(2):244–246

[61] Fietze I, Dingli K, Diefenbach K, et al. Night-to-night variation of the oxygen desaturation index in sleep apnoea syndrome. Eur Respir J. 2004; 24(6):987–993

[62] Aber WR, Block AJ, Hellard DW, Webb WB. Consistency of respiratory measurements from night to night during the sleep of elderly men. Chest. 1989; 96(4):747–751

[63] Barnes M, Houston D, Worsnop CJ, et al. A randomized controlled trial of continuous positive airway pressure in mild obstructive sleep apnea. Am J Respir Crit Care Med. 2002; 165(6):773–780

[64] Faccenda JF, Mackay TW, Boon NA, Douglas NJ. Randomized placebo-controlled trial of continuous positive airway pressure on blood pressure in the sleep apnea-hypopnea syndrome. Am J Respir Crit Care Med. 2001; 163(2):344–348

[65] Weaver TE, Maislin G, Dinges DF, et al. Relationship between hours of CPAP use and achieving normal levels of sleepiness and daily functioning. Sleep. 2007; 30(6):711–719

[66] Stuck BA, Leitzbach S, Maurer JT. Effects of continuous positive airway pressure on apnea-hypopnea index in obstructive sleep apnea based on long-term compliance. Sleep Breath. 2012; 16(2):467–471

[67] Fujita S, Conway W, Zorick F, Roth T. Surgical correction of anatomic abnormalities in obstructive sleep apnea syndrome: uvulopalatopharyngoplasty. Otolaryngology–head and neck surgery: official journal of American Academy of Otolaryngology Head Neck Surg. 1981; 89(6):923–934

[68] Cartwright R, Ristanovic R, Diaz F, Caldarelli D, Alder G. A comparative study of treatments for positional sleep apnea. Sleep. 1991; 14(6):546–552

[69] He J, Kryger MH, Zorick FJ, Conway W, Roth T. Mortality and apnea index in obstructive sleep apnea. Experience in 385 male patients. Chest. 1988; 94(1):9–14

[70] Sher AE, Schechtman KB, Piccirillo JF. The efficacy of surgical modifications of the upper airway in adults with obstructive sleep apnea syndrome. Sleep. 1996; 19(2):156–177

[71] Elshaug AG, Moss JR, Southcott AM, Hiller JE. Redefining success in airway surgery for obstructive sleep apnea: a meta-analysis and synthesis of the evidence. Sleep. 2007; 30(4):461–467

[72] Zaghi S, Holty J-EC, Certal V, et al. Maxillomandibular advancement for treatment of obstructive sleep apnea: a meta-analysis. JAMA Otolaryngol Head Neck Surg. 2016; 142(1):58–66

[73] Ravesloot MJ, de Vries N. Reliable calculation of the efficacy of non-surgical and surgical treatment of obstructive sleep apnea revisited. Sleep. 2011; 34(1):105–110

[74] Weaver TE, Grunstein RR. Adherence to continuous positive airway pressure therapy: the challenge to effective treatment. Proc Am Thorac Soc. 2008; 5(2):173–178

[75] Kribbs NB, Pack AI, Kline LR, et al. Objective measurement of patterns of nasal CPAP use by patients with obstructive sleep apnea. Am Rev Respir Dis. 1993; 147(4):887–895

[76] Ravesloot MJ, de Vries N, Stuck BA. Treatment adherence should be taken into account when reporting treatment outcomes in obstructive sleep apnea. Laryngoscope. 2014; 124(1):344–345

[77] Vanderveken OM, Dieltjens M, Wouters K, De Backer WA, Van de Heyning PH, Braem MJ. Objective measurement of compliance during oral appliance therapy for sleep-disordered breathing. Thorax. 2013; 68(1):91–96

[78] Boyd SB, Walters AS. Effectiveness of treatment apnea-hypopnea index: a mathematical estimate of the true apnea-hypopnea index in the home setting. J Oral Maxillofac Surg. 2013; 71(2):351–357

[79] Bianchi MT, Alameddine Y, Mojica J. Apnea burden: efficacy versus effectiveness in patients using positive airway pressure. Sleep Med. 2014; 15(12):1579–1581

[80] Eijsvogel MM, Ubbink R, Dekker J, et al. Sleep position trainer versus tennis ball technique in positional obstructive sleep apnea syndrome. J Clin Sleep Med. 2015; 11(2):139–147

[81] Kezirian EJ, Weaver EM, Criswell MA, de Vries N, Woodson BT, Piccirillo JF. Reporting results of obstructive sleep apnea syndrome surgery trials. Otolaryngol Head Neck Surg. 2011; 144(4):496–499

[82] Pang KP, Rotenberg BW. The SLEEP GOAL as a success criteria in obstructive sleep apnea therapy. Eur Arch Otorhinolaryngol. 2016; 273(5):1063–1065

[83] Weaver EM, Woodson BT, Steward DL. Polysomnography indexes are discordant with quality of life, symptoms, and reaction times in sleep apnea patients. Otolaryngol Head Neck Surg. 2005; 132(2):255–262

[84] Kezirian EJ, Malhotra A, Goldberg AN, White DP. Changes in obstructive sleep apnea severity, biomarkers, and quality of life after multilevel surgery. Laryngoscope. 2010; 120(7):1481–1488

[85] Moyer CA, Sonnad SS, Garetz SL, Helman JI, Chervin RD. Quality of life in obstructive sleep apnea: a systematic review of the literature. Sleep Med. 2001; 2(6):477–491

[86] Wright J, Johns R, Watt I, Melville A, Sheldon T. Health effects of obstructive sleep apnoea and the effectiveness of continuous positive airways pressure: a systematic review of the research evidence. BMJ. 1997; 314(7084):851–860

[87] Thong JF, Pang KP. Clinical parameters in obstructive sleep apnea: are there any correlations? J Otolaryngol Head Neck Surg. 2008; 37(6):894–900

[88] Piccirillo JF. Outcomes research and obstructive sleep apnea. Laryngoscope. 2000; 110(3 Pt 3):16–20

[89] Tam S, Woodson BT, Rotenberg B. Outcome measurements in obstructive sleep apnea: beyond the apnea-hypopnea index. Laryngoscope. 2014; 124(1):337–343

[90] Weaver TE. Outcome measurement in sleep medicine practice and research. Part 1: assessment of symptoms, subjective and objective daytime sleepiness, health-related quality of life and functional status. Sleep Med Rev. 2001; 5(2):103–128

[91] Weaver TE. Outcome measurement in sleep medicine practice and research. Part 2: assessment of neurobehavioral performance and mood. Sleep Med Rev. 2001; 5(3):223–236

[92] Johns MW. A new method for measuring daytime sleepiness: the Epworth Sleepiness Scale. Sleep. 1991; 14(6):540–545

[93] Baba RY, Mohan A, Metta VV, Mador MJ. Temperature controlled radiofrequency ablation at different sites for treatment of obstructive sleep apnea syndrome: a systematic review and meta-analysis. Sleep Breath. 2015; 19(3):891–910

[94] Song SA, Wei JM, Buttram J, et al. Hyoid surgery alone for obstructive sleep apnea: a systematic review and meta-analysis. Laryngoscope. 2016; 126(7):1702–1708

[95] Miller SC, Nguyen SA, Ong AA, Gillespie MB. Transoral robotic base of tongue reduction for obstructive sleep apnea: a systematic review and meta-analysis. Laryngoscope. 2017; 127(1):258–265

[96] Stuck BA, Ravesloot MJ, Eschenhagen T, de Vet HCW, Sommer JU. Uvulopalatopharyngoplasty with or without tonsillectomy in the treatment of adult obstructive sleep apnea–a systematic review. Sleep Med. 2018; 50:152–165

[97] Haraldsson PO, Carenfelt C, Lysdahl M, Törnros J. Long-term effect of uvulopalatopharyngoplasty on driving performance. Arch Otolaryngol Head Neck Surg. 1995; 121(1):90–94

[98] Browaldh N, Friberg D, Svanborg E, Nerfeldt P. 15-year efficacy of uvulopalatopharyngoplasty based on objective and subjective data. Acta Otolaryngol. 2011; 131(12):1303–1310

[99] Wilhelmsson B, Tegelberg A, Walker-Engström M-L, et al. A prospective randomized study of a dental appliance compared with uvulopalatopharyngoplasty in the treatment of obstructive sleep apnoea. Acta Otolaryngol. 1999; 119(4):503–509

[100] Larsson LH, Carlsson-Nordlander B, Svanborg E. Four-year follow-up after uvulopalatopharyngoplasty in 50 unselected patients with obstructive sleep apnea syndrome. Laryngoscope. 1994; 104(11 Pt 1):1362–1368

[101] Boot H, Poublon RML, Van Wegen R, et al. Uvulopalatopharyngoplasty for the obstructive sleep apnoea syndrome: value of polysomnography, Mueller manoeuvre and cephalometry in predicting surgical outcome. Clin Otolaryngol Allied Sci. 1997; 22(6):504–510

[102] Boot H, van Wegen R, Poublon RML, Bogaard JM, Schmitz PIM, van der Meché FGA. Long-term results of uvulopalatopharyngoplasty for obstructive sleep apnea syndrome. Laryngoscope. 2000; 110(3 Pt 1):469–475

[103] Yousuf A, Beigh Z, Khursheed RS, Jallu AS, Pampoori RA. Clinical predictors for successful uvulopalatopharyngoplasty in the management of obstructive sleep apnea. Int J Otolaryngol. 2013; 2013:290265

[104] Cadieux RJ, Manders EK, Manfredi RL, Bixler EO, Kales A. Uvulopalatopharyngoplasty as a treatment of obstructive sleep apnea precipitated by uvular prolapse. Ann Plast Surg. 1987; 19(6):566–571

[105] Browaldh N, Bring J, Friberg D. SKUP(3) RCT; continuous study: changes in sleepiness and quality of life after modified UPPP. Laryngoscope. 2016; 126(6):1484–1491

[106] Shin HW, Park JH, Park JW, et al. Effects of surgical vs. nonsurgical therapy on erectile dysfunction and quality of life in obstructive sleep apnea syndrome: a pilot study. J Sex Med. 2013; 10(8):2053–2059

[107] Sommer UJ, Heiser C, Gahleitner C, et al. Tonsillectomy with Uvulopalatopharyngoplasty in Obstructive Sleep Apnea. Dtsch Arztebl Int. 2016; 113(1–02):1–8

[108] Baradaranfar MH, Edalatkhah M, Dadgarnia MH, et al. The effect of uvulopalatopharyngoplasty with tonsillectomy in patients with obstructive sleep apnea. Indian J Otolaryngol Head Neck Surg. 2015; 67(1, Suppl 1):29–33

[109] Lundkvist K, Januszkiewicz A, Friberg D. Uvulopalatopharyngoplasty in 158 OSAS patients failing non-surgical treatment. Acta Otolaryngol. 2009; 129(11):1280–1286

[110] Boudewyns A, Mariën S, Wuyts F, De Backer W, Van de Heyning P. Short-and long-term outcomes of uvulopalatopharyngoplasty in nonapneic snorers and obstructive sleep apnea patients. Oto-Rhino-Laryngologia Nova. 2000; 10(3–4):172–179

[111] Boudewyns AN, De Backer WA, Van de Heyning PH. Pattern of upper airway obstruction during sleep before and after uvulopalatopharyngoplasty in patients with obstructive sleep apnea. Sleep Med. 2001; 2(4):309–315

[112] Bakan E, Fidan V, Alp HH, Baygutalp NK, Cokluk E. Effect of modified Fujita technique uvulopalatoplasty on oxidative DNA damage levels in patients with obstructive sleep apnea syndrome. J Craniofac Surg. 2015; 26(5):e392–e396

[113] Hsu PP, Tan AK, Tan BY, et al. Uvulopalatopharyngoplasty outcome assessment with quantitative computer-assisted videoendoscopic airway analysis. Acta Otolaryngol. 2007; 127(1):65–70

[114] Weaver EM, Woodson BT, Yueh B, et al. SLEEP Study Investigators. Studying Life Effects & Effectiveness of Palatopharyngoplasty (SLEEP) study: subjective outcomes of isolated uvulopalatopharyngoplasty. Otolaryngol Head Neck Surg. 2011; 144(4):623–631

[115] Walker-Engström ML, Wilhelmsson B, Tegelberg A, Dimenäs E, Ringqvist I. Quality of life assessment of treatment with dental appliance or UPPP in patients with mild to moderate obstructive sleep apnoea. A prospective randomized 1-year follow-up study. J Sleep Res. 2000; 9(3):303–308

[116] Dahlöf P, Ejnell H, Hällström T, Hedner J. Surgical treatment of the sleep apnea syndrome reduces associated major depression. Int J Behav Med. 2000; 7(1):73–88

[117] Santamaria JD, Prior JC, Fleetham JA. Reversible reproductive dysfunction in men with obstructive sleep apnoea. Clin Endocrinol (Oxf). 1988; 28(5):461–470

[118] Zohar Y, Talmi YP, Frenkel H, et al. Cardiac function in obstructive sleep apnea patients following uvulopalatopharyngoplasty. Otolaryngol Head Neck Surg. 1992; 107(3):390–394

[119] Jiang GF, Sun W, Li N, Sun Y, Zhang NK. Treatment effect of uvulopalatopharyngoplasty on autonomic nervous activity during sleep in patients with obstructive sleep apnea syndrome. Chin Med J (Engl). 2004; 117(5):761–763

[120] Keenan SP, Burt H, Ryan CF, Fleetham JA. Long-term survival of patients with obstructive sleep apnea treated by uvulopalatopharyngoplasty or nasal CPAP. Chest. 1994; 105(1):155–159

[121] Epstein LJ, Kristo D, Strollo PJ Jr, et al. Adult Obstructive Sleep Apnea Task Force of the American Academy of Sleep Medicine. Clinical guideline for the evaluation, management and long-term care of obstructive sleep apnea in adults. J Clin Sleep Med. 2009; 5(3):263–276

[122] Grote L, Hedner J, Grunstein R, Kraiczi H. Therapy with nCPAP: incomplete elimination of Sleep Related Breathing Disorder. Eur Respir J. 2000; 16(5):921–927

[123] Kushida CA, Littner MR, Hirshkowitz M, et al. American Academy of Sleep Medicine. Practice parameters for the use of continuous and bilevel positive airway pressure devices to treat adult patients with sleep-related breathing disorders. Sleep. 2006; 29(3):375–380

[124] McArdle N, Devereux G, Heidarnejad H, Engleman HM, Mackay TW, Douglas NJ. Long-term use of CPAP therapy for sleep apnea/hypopnea syndrome. Am J Respir Crit Care Med. 1999; 159(4 Pt 1):1108–1114

[125] Engleman HM, McDonald JP, Graham D, et al. Randomized crossover trial of two treatments for sleep apnea/hypopnea syndrome: continuous positive airway pressure and mandibular repositioning splint. Am J Respir Crit Care Med. 2002; 166(6):855–859

[126] Hudgel DW, Fung C. A long-term randomized, cross-over comparison of auto-titrating and standard nasal continuous airway pressure. Sleep. 2000; 23(5):645–648

[127] Lankford DA, Proctor CD, Richard R. Continuous positive airway pressure (CPAP) changes in bariatric surgery patients undergoing rapid weight loss. Obes Surg. 2005; 15(3):336–341

[128] El-Solh AA, Moitheennazima B, Akinnusi ME, Churder PM, Lafornara AM. Combined oral appliance and positive airway pressure therapy for obstructive sleep apnea: a pilot study. Sleep Breath. 2011; 15(2):203–208

[129] Fleetham JA, de Almeida FR. Oral appliances. In: McNicholas WT, Bonsignore MR, eds. European Respiratory Monograph. Plymouth; 2010:267–285

[130] Chan AS, Cistulli PA. Oral appliance treatment of obstructive sleep apnea: an update. Curr Opin Pulm Med. 2009; 15(6):591–596

[131] Tsuiki S, Lowe AA, Almeida FR, Kawahata N, Fleetham JA. Effects of mandibular advancement on airway curvature and obstructive sleep apnoea severity. Eur Respir J. 2004; 23(2):263–268

[132] Ng A, Gotsopoulos H, Darendeliler AM, Cistulli PA. Oral appliance therapy for obstructive sleep apnea. Treat Respir Med. 2005; 4(6):409–422

[133] Clark GT, Arand D, Chung E, Tong D. Effect of anterior mandibular positioning on obstructive sleep apnea. Am Rev Respir Dis. 1993; 147(3):624–629

[134] Sutherland K, Deane SA, Chan AS, et al. Comparative effects of two oral appliances on upper airway structure in obstructive sleep apnea. Sleep. 2011; 34(4):469–477

[135] Dieltjens M, Braem MJ, Vroegop AVMT, et al. Objectively measured vs self-reported compliance during oral appliance therapy for sleep-disordered breathing. Chest. 2013; 144(5): 1495–1502

[136] Dort L, Remmers J. A combination appliance for obstructive sleep apnea: the effectiveness of mandibular advancement and tongue retention. J Clin Sleep Med. 2012; 8(3):265–269

[137] Millman RP, Rosenberg CL, Carlisle CC, Kramer NR, Kahn DM, Bonitati AE. The efficacy of oral appliances in the treatment of persistent sleep apnea after uvulopalatopharyngoplasty. Chest. 1998; 113(4):992–996

[138] Joosten SA, Hamza K, Sands S, Turton A, Berger P, Hamilton G. Phenotypes of patients with mild to moderate obstructive sleep apnoea as confirmed by cluster analysis. Respirology. 2012; 17(1):99–107

[139] Oksenberg A, Khamaysi I, Silverberg DS, Tarasiuk A. Association of body position with severity of apneic events in patients with severe nonpositional obstructive sleep apnea. Chest. 2000; 118(4):1018–1024

[140] Oksenberg A, Silverberg D, Offenbach D, Arons E. Positional therapy for obstructive sleep apnea patients: A 6-month follow-up study. Laryngoscope. 2006; 116(11):1995–2000

[141] Oksenberg A, Silverberg DS, Arons E, Radwan H. Positional vs nonpositional obstructive sleep apnea patients: anthropomorphic, nocturnal polysomnographic, and multiple sleep latency test data. Chest. 1997; 112(3):629–639

[142] Cartwright RD. Effect of sleep position on sleep apnea severity. Sleep. 1984; 7(2):110–114

[143] Richard W, Kox D, den Herder C, Laman M, van Tinteren H, de Vries N. The role of sleep position in obstructive sleep apnea syndrome. Eur Arch Otorhinolaryngol. 2006; 263(10):946–950

[144] Mador MJ, Kufel TJ, Magalang UJ, Rajesh SK, Watwe V, Grant BJ. Prevalence of positional sleep apnea in patients undergoing polysomnography. Chest. 2005; 128(4):2130–2137

[145] Bignold JJ, Deans-Costi G, Goldsworthy MR, et al. Poor long-term patient compliance with the tennis ball technique for treating positional obstructive sleep apnea. J Clin Sleep Med. 2009; 5(5):428–430

[146] Jokic R, Klimaszewski A, Crossley M, Sridhar G, Fitzpatrick MF. Positional treatment vs continuous positive airway pressure in patients with positional obstructive sleep apnea syndrome. Chest. 1999; 115(3):771–781

[147] Permut I, Diaz-Abad M, Chatila W, et al. Comparison of positional therapy to CPAP in patients with positional obstructive sleep apnea. J Clin Sleep Med. 2010; 6(3):238–243

[148] Loord H, Hultcrantz E. Positioner–a method for preventing sleep apnea. Acta Otolaryngol. 2007; 127(8):861–868

[149] Ravesloot MJ, van Maanen JP, Dun L, de Vries N. The undervalued potential of positional therapy in position-dependent snoring and obstructive sleep apnea-a review of the literature. Sleep Breath. 2013; 17(1):39–49

[150] van Maanen JP, Meester KA, Dun LN, et al. The sleep position trainer: a new treatment for positional obstructive sleep apnoea. Sleep Breath. 2013; 17(2):771–779

[151] Bignold JJ, Mercer JD, Antic NA, McEvoy RD, Catcheside PG. Accurate position monitoring and improved supine-dependent obstructive sleep apnea with a new position recording and supine avoidance device. J Clin Sleep Med. 2011; 7(4):376–383

[152] Oksenberg A, Dynia A, Nasser K, Gadoth N. Obstructive sleep apnoea in adults: body postures and weight changes interactions. J Sleep Res. 2012; 21(4):402–409

[153] Oksenberg A, Silverberg DS, Arons E, Radwan H. The sleep supine position has a major effect on optimal nasal continuous positive airway pressure: relationship with rapid eye movements and non-rapid eye movements sleep, body mass index, respiratory disturbance index, and age. Chest. 1999; 116(4):1000–1006

[154] Pevernagie DA, Shepard JW, Jr. Relations between sleep stage, posture and effective nasal CPAP levels in OSA. Sleep. 1992; 15(2):162–167

[155] Sériès F, Marc I. Importance of sleep stage- and body position-dependence of sleep apnoea in determining benefits to auto-CPAP therapy. Eur Respir J. 2001; 18(1):170–175

[156] Dieltjens M, Braem MJ, Van de Heyning PH, Wouters K, Vanderveken OM. Prevalence and clinical significance of supine-dependent obstructive sleep apnea in patients using oral appliance therapy. J Clin Sleep Med. 2014; 10(9):959–964

[157] Dieltjens M, Vroegop AV, Verbruggen AE, et al. A promising concept of combination therapy for positional obstructive sleep apnea. Sleep Breath. 2014

[158] Katsantonis GP, Miyazaki S, Walsh JK. Effects of uvulopalatopharyngoplasty on sleep architecture and patterns of obstructed breathing. Laryngoscope. 1990; 100(10 Pt 1):1068–1072

[159] Lee CH, Shin HW, Han DH, et al. The implication of sleep position in the evaluation of surgical outcomes in obstructive sleep apnea. Otolaryngol Head Neck Surg. 2009; 140(4):531–535

[160] Lee CH, Kim SW, Han K, et al. Effect of uvulopalatopharyngoplasty on positional dependency in obstructive sleep apnea. Arch Otolaryngol Head Neck Surg. 2011; 137(7):675–679

[161] Benoist LBL, Verhagen M, Torensma B, van Maanen JP, de Vries N. Positional therapy in patients with residual positional obstructive sleep apnea after upper airway surgery. Sleep Breath. 2017; 21(2):279–288

Recommended Reading

Zorick FJ, Roehrs T, Conway W, Potts G, Roth T. Response to CPAP and UPPP in apnea. Henry Ford Hosp Med J. 1990; 38(4):223–226

6 Pediatric Obstructive Sleep Apnea

Kerstin Rohde† and Thomas Verse

Abstract

As in adults, pediatric obstructive sleep apnea (OSA) is characterized by partial or complete obstruction of the upper airway during sleep. However, definitions, prevalence, pathophysiology, and diagnostic procedures differ substantially from adult standards. Pediatric OSA is associated with multiple adverse neurodevelopmental and cardiometabolic consequences. It is common in healthy children and occurs with a higher incidence among obese children, and among kids with syndromic, neurologic, or craniofacial diseases.

Medical interventions include weight loss, nasal corticosteroids, and other allergic treatments. Oral devices and continuous positive airway pressure are also used to treat pediatric OSA. Standard surgical treatment is adenotonsillectomy (T&A). Most healthy children respond favorably to adenotonsillectomy as first-line treatment. Tonsillotomy seems to provide comparable results as tonsillectomy with decreased postoperative pain, readmissions to hospital, and complications. Persistent OSA after T&A has frequently been described in obese kids or children with underlying craniofacial deformities or syndromic or other severe comorbidities. In these children, other kinds of surgeries might be helpful.

Keywords: snoring, sleep apnea, children, definitions, prevalence, diagnosis, treatment

6.1 Diagnosis

6.1.1 Introduction

Obstructive sleep-disordered breathing (SDB) is a syndrome of upper airway dysfunction during sleep, characterized by snoring and/or increased respiratory effort secondary to increased upper airway resistance and pharyngeal collapsibility. It includes a spectrum of clinical entities such as primary snoring, upper airway resistance syndrome, obstructive hypoventilation, and obstructive sleep apnea (OSA) syndrome (▶Table 6.1).[1]

The term *obstructive sleep-disordered breathing* in children is used when symptoms of intermittent upper airway obstruction during sleep are present, but the severity of airway obstruction has not been defined by objective measurements such as polysomnography (PSG).[2]

Obstructive sleep apnea syndrome (OSAS) is characterized by repetitive episodes of upper airway obstruction that occur during sleep, usually associated with reduction in blood oxygen saturation.[3] It affects both children and adults.

In contrast, simple snoring is not associated with repetitive episodes of upper airway obstructions, (or with <5 events/hour) arousals from sleep, and low oxygen

▶ Table 6.1 Definitions of obstructive sleep-disordered breathing and its clinical entities in children

	Definition
Obstructive SDB	A syndrome of upper airway dysfunction during sleep characterized by snoring and/or increased respiratory effort that result from increased upper airway resistance and pharyngeal collapsibility
Obstructive SDB clinical entities	
Primary snoring	Habitual snoring (>3 nights/wk) without apneas, hypopneas, frequent arousals from sleep or gas exchange abnormalities
Upper airway resistance syndrome	Snoring, increased work of breathing, frequent arousals, but no recognizable obstructive events or gas exchange abnormalities
Obstructive hypoventilation	Snoring and abnormally elevated end-expiratory carbon dioxide partial pressure in the absence of recognizable obstructive events
Obstructive sleep apnea syndrome	Recurrent events of partial or complete upper airway obstruction (hypopneas, obstructive or mixed apneas) with disruption of normal oxygenation, ventilation and sleep pattern

Abbreviation: SDB, sleep-disordered breathing.
Data from Kaditis et al.[1]

saturation in arterial blood. The most common definitions of habitual snoring are: "snoring present often/frequently" for more than three or four nights per week.[4]

6.1.2 Prevalence

Primary snoring and OSA are common conditions in the pediatric population. The estimated prevalence of primary snoring in children ranges from 8 to 27%.[5] Lumeng and Chervin published a meta-analysis of studies with a prevalence of habitual snoring of 7.45% (95% CI 5.75–9.61).[4] OSAS is less common. The estimated prevalence of OSAS in children is ranging from 1 to 5%.[6]

6.1.3 Clinical Finding

The clinical symptoms of pediatric obstructive SDB during the sleep are snoring, sweating, breathing by mouth, apneas, and enforced breathing. The head is extended and the neck flexed during the sleep. The snoring is often with intermittent pauses, snorts, or gasps.

Daytime sleepiness is mostly not the leading symptom in young children. Failure to thrive, hypertension, cardiac dysfunction, and systemic inflammation are associated to OSA (▶Table 6.2).[5]

► **Table 6.2** Symptoms and signs of obstructive sleep apnea syndrome

History
Frequent snoring (≥3 nights/wk)
Labored breathing during sleep
Gasps/snorting noises/observed episodes of apnea
Sleep enuresis (especially secondary enuresis)
Sleeping in a seated position or with the neck hyperextended
Cyanosis
Headache on awaking
Daytime sleepiness
Attention deficit/hyperactivity disorder
Learning problem
Physical examination
Underweight or overweight
Tonsillar hypertrophy
Adenoidal facies
Micrognathia/retrognathia
High-arched palate
Failure to thrive
Hypertension

Data from Marcus et al.[5]

6.1.4 Physical Examination

Hypertrophy of the Tonsils and of the Adenoid Tissue

Hypertrophy of the tonsils and of the adenoid tissue seems to be the most common cause of primary snoring and OSA in children. The hypertrophy of the tonsils and adenoids causes narrowing of the airway during sleep when the muscles of the pharynx relax. This leads to partial or complete obstruction of the airway.[7] MRI studies have shown that the size of the adenoids and tonsils in children with OSA is significantly increased compared with healthy controls.[8] Children with OSA have been found to have significantly more collapsible upper airways during sleep than children without OSA.[9]

Allergic Rhinitis and Nasal Hypertrophy

Allergic rhinitis may be associated with SDB. Nasal turbinate hypertrophy increases the risk of mild OSA.[10]

Craniofacial Morphological Characteristics

In a meta-analysis, Flores-Mir et al identified that craniofacial characteristics such as steep mandibular plane, vertical direction of craniofacial growth, and retrusive

chin are related to OSA.[11] However, another meta-analysis from the same year suggested that the differences between children with SDB and controls are of marginal clinical significance.[12]

Midface Deficiency Syndrome and Mandibular Hypoplasia

Midface deficiency syndromes such as Apert syndrome, Crouzon syndrome, Pfeiffer syndrome, and unrepaired or repaired cleft palate, and marked mandibular hypoplasia (Pierre Robin sequence, Treacher Collins syndrome, Nager syndrome, Stickler syndrome, and juvenile idiopathic arthritis) are associated with increased risk of obstructive SDB.[1]

Neuromuscular disorders and uncontrolled epilepsy are related to a high risk for OSAS and nocturnal hypoventilation.[13]

Complex abnormalities (achondroplasia, Chiari malformation, Down's syndrome, Ehlers-Danlos syndrome, mucopolysaccharidoses, and Prader-Willi syndrome) have been related to OSAS and alveolar hypoventilation.[1]

Down's Syndrome

Children with Down's syndrome are predisposed to OSAS and hypoventilation because of midfacial and mandibular hypoplasia, shortened palate, relative macroglossia, narrow lumen of the nasopharynx, and pharyngeal hypotonia. Parents may not report SDB symptoms. Main risk factors for OSAS in children with Down's syndrome include age less than 8 years, male gender, and tonsillar hypertrophy.[14]

Obesity

Obesity in children is a well-established risk factor for SDB. Childhood obesity is defined as a body mass index (BMI) more than 95th percentile for age and gender.[6] Obesity is an increasing health problem in children. Since 1980, the prevalence of overweight and obesity has increased remarkably in developed countries; 23.8% of boys and 22.6% of girls were overweight or obese in 2013, compared with 16.9% of boys and 16.2% of girls in 1980.[15]

The NANO study, a cross-sectional, prospective multicenter study, assessed the contribution of obesity and adenotonsillar hypertrophy in pediatric OSA and found that 46.6% of obese children in their community had an apnea–hypopnea index (AHI) of more than 1 per hour per total sleep time.[16] The prevalence of pediatric OSAS in obese children varies in other studies from 19 to 61%.[17] In postpubertal adolescents an association between OSA and the metabolic syndrome has been shown.[18]

Blood Pressure

A greater mean blood pressure (BP) variability during wakefulness and sleep, a higher night/day BP ratio, and a reduced nocturnal dipping were observed in children with OSA as compared with normal controls.[19]

But a meta-analysis by Zintzaras and Kaditis did not demonstrate an association between OSAS and BP.[20]

Systemic Inflammation

There is emerging evidence that OSA is a disease with chronic low-grade systemic inflammation and increased oxidative stress which likely leads to end-organ morbidities.[13] Nasal nitric oxide (nNO), a marker of airway inflammation, is elevated in children with primary snoring and OSAS as compared with a healthy control group. The nNO level is not correlated with disease severity. It is probably due to the local mechanism.[21] The peripheral Th17/Treg balance is skewed toward Th17 predominance, further suggesting a systematic proinflammatory milieu in OSA. The Th17/Treg ratio correlates with severity of OSA. Adenotonsillectomy (ATE) reverses this Th17/Treg imbalance and reduces serum inflammatory cytokine levels.[22] Plasminogen activator-inhibitor 1 levels and monocyte chemoattractant protein 1 levels have been found to be significantly raised in obese children with OSA compared with obese children without OSA.[16]

Loffredo et al suggests that even children with primary snoring have significantly higher serum isoprostanes and soluble NOX2-dp levels and display evidence of endothelial dysfunction compared with healthy controls.[23]

Prematurity and Family History of Obstructive Sleep Apnea

A history of prematurity is associated with an increased risk of OSA, and there is some evidence that a family history of OSA may also be a risk factor.[1]

Behavioral and Neurocognitive Morbidities

Children with OSAS have been linked with behavioral and neurocognitive morbidities.[24] Published data from the Tucson Children's Assessment of Sleep Apnea Study (TuCASA study) showed that even mild OSA and primary snoring are associated with hyperactivity, difficulties concentrating, attention problems, and impulsivity.[25] Results of the TuCASA study revealed a significant association of SDB with behavioral problems (aggression, lower social competency, poorer communication, and/or diminished adaptive skills).

Nocturnal Enuresis

There appears to be a significant prevalence of OSAS in children with enuresis. Nocturnal enuresis is defined as urination during sleep in children older than or equal to 5 years, which is when nocturnal bladder continence is developmentally expected. Enuresis can occur in any stage of sleep and at any time of the night.[26,27] Brooks and Topol found that children referred to for suspected SDB

who had a respiratory disturbance index (RDI) of more than 1 had a higher prevalence of enuresis (47%) as compared with those who had an RDI of less than or equal to 1 (17%).[28]

The reason for the enuresis may be due to the inhibitory effects of OSA on arousal response to changes in bladder pressure, or effects of elevated brain natriuretic peptide (BNP) levels which affect the renin-angiotensin pathway, vasopressin, and excretion of sodium and water.[29]

Children with enuresis, particularly those who are obese or resistant to standard treatments, should be assessed for symptoms and physical findings suggestive of SDB, and if any symptom is present, a PSG is recommended.[27]

Quality of Life

Children with OSAS had poorer scores in the Child Health Questionnaire than healthy children. Children with OSAS had similar scores to those of patients with juvenile rheumatoid arthritis.[30]

6.1.5 Diagnostic Workup

Patient Anamnesis

The clinical practice guideline of the American Academy of Pediatrics recommends that pediatricians should ask for snoring at each health maintenance medical visit.[5] This question is a sensitive, albeit nonspecific screening measure that is quick to perform. Additional questions about the symptoms, which are listed in ▶Table 6.2, should be added to narrow this large group of snoring children. The clinical evaluation does not establish the diagnosis. Clinical signs and symptoms are unable to accurately predict pediatric OSAS. Taking patient's history has a predictive value of 65% as compared to PSG.[31]

The parent-filled questionnaire assesses symptoms of OSA, such as snoring, excessive daytime sleepiness, attention problems, and hyperactive behavior in children between ages 2 and 18 years. Its sensitivity and specificity for diagnosing OSA in otherwise healthy children are 78 and 72%, respectively. Questionnaires may be useful in predicting OSA-related neurobehavioral morbidity and its improvements after ATE.[32]

Physical examination may be normal when the child is awake, and the size of the tonsils cannot be used to predict the presence of OSAS. The predictive value is not higher than 46% with the clinical examination alone.[31]

Other clinical parameters such as demographics, physical examination, findings, and parent-reported questionnaires also do not discriminate between different levels of OSAS based on PSG parameters.[33]

Further recommendations from the American Academy of Pediatrics are as follows: If a child or adolescent snores on a regular basis and has any of the complaints or findings shown in▶Table 6.2, clinicians should either (1) obtain a PSG (Evidence Quality A, Key action strength:

Recommendation), or (2) refer the patient to a sleep specialist or otolaryngologist for a more extensive evaluation (Evidence quality D, Key Action strength: Option).[5]

Technical Measurements

Even today, the gold standard test for OSAS is the overnight, fully attended, in-laboratory PSG in a sleep facility. Despite this fact, there is a shortage of sleep laboratories with pediatric expertise. PSG is not available worldwide. Even in the high-industrial countries PSG is not available in all regions. Laboratory PSG studies of children are expensive, and parents and their young children, particularly school-aged children, are often hesitant to spend a night in the unfamiliar setting of a sleep laboratory. In an effort to simplify the diagnostic process and to make this process more accessible and convenient, a number of unattended multichannel devices have been assessed in pediatric patients (▶ Table 6.3).[34]

According to the American Academy of Sleep Medicine (AASM) guidelines, unattended devices are defined as multichannel type 2 or type 3 devices. Type 2 monitoring devices can be used to perform full PSG outside a laboratory.[35] The major difference between type 2 and 3 devices and type 1 devices is that the former two types do not require a technician. Type 3 monitoring devices (respiratory polygraphy [RP]) do not record the signals needed to determine sleep stages. Their channels include two respiratory variables (e.g., respiratory movement and airflow), a cardiac variable (e.g., heart rate or an electrocardiogram), and an arterial oxygen saturation. There is the possibility that the AHI may be underestimated due to missed hypopneas resulting in arousals, but not desaturation. Type 4 monitoring devices are also known as continuous single or dual bioparameter devices. They record one or two variables (typically arterial oxygen saturation and airflow). They can also be used without a technician. Oximetry studies have a high specificity but low sensitivity in the diagnosis of pediatric OSA. The rate of false-negative or inconclusive results is high.[36]

In a meta-analysis about unattended type 2 and type 3 devices, Certal et al described a satisfactory overall diagnostic accuracy of unattended multichannel devices as compared with the gold standard (full PSG type 1 devices). These type 2 and 3 devices are claimed as useful and valid tools for OSA screening in children.[37] The type 2 and 3 devices may theoretically be ubiquitously accessible and more cost-effective. The results may be more representative of the child's typical night's sleep at home. Ambulatory monitoring with unattended devices is considered reliable for the diagnosis of OSA in particular groups of patients.

Nevertheless, unattended type 2 and 3 diagnostic tests have been shown to have weaker positive and negative

▶ Table 6.3 Diagnostic workup

Diagnostic workup	Valence
Anamnesis	Predictive value of 65%[31]
Parent-filled questionnaire	Sensitivity 78% and specificity 72%[32]
Clinical examination	Predictive value of 46%[31]
Type 4 unattended monitoring devices (continuous single or dual bioparameter devices; e.g., arterial oxygen saturation and airflow)	High specificity but low sensitivity Rate of false-negative or inconclusive results is high[36]
Type 3 unattended monitoring devices (RP without EEG, EMG, or EOG sensors)	Advantages: • Good agreements with in-lab PSG • Less expensive • Representative of the child's typical night's sleep at home • Ubiquitously accessible Disadvantages: • Possibility that the AHI may be underestimated due to missed hypopneas resulting in arousals but not desaturation • Weaker positive and negative predictive values than PSG
Type 2 unattended monitoring devices do not (outpatient PSG without a technician)	Advantages: • Good agreements with in-lab PSG • Less expensive • Representative of the child's typical night's sleep at home • Ubiquitously accessible Disadvantages: • Weaker positive and negative predictive values than PSG
Type 1 attended monitoring devices (overnight, fully attended, in-laboratory PSG)	Advantages: • Gold standard test for diagnosing OSAS Disadvantages: • Not ubiquitously accessible • Expensive

Abbreviations: AHI, apnea–hypopnea index; EEG, electroencephalogram; EMG, electromyogram; EOG, electro-oculography; OSAS, obstructive sleep apnea syndrome; PSG, polysomnography; RP, respiratory polygraphy.

predictive values than PSG. If an alternative test fails to demonstrate OSAS in patients with high pretest probability, full PSG should be sought.[37]

The overnight, fully attended, in-laboratory PSG measurements include electroencephalography (EEG), pulse oximetry, oronasal airflow, abdominal and chest wall movements, partial pressure of carbon dioxide, and video recording (▶Table 6.4). A comprehensive list of respiratory indications for PSG in children according to the AASM is presented in ▶Table 6.5. The indications are divided into three groups: standard, guideline, and option. A standard level of recommendation has high degree of clinical certainty with use of level 1 evidence or overwhelming level 2 evidence, whereas a guideline has a moderate degree of clinical certainty. An option has uncertain clinical use.[38] The American Academy of Otolaryngology/Head and Neck Surgery (AAO/HNS) has a more selective policy for obtaining PSG (▶Table 6.6). For action statement number 1, the rationale is to avoid unnecessary interventions in children with higher surgical risk and facilitate postoperative planning. For action statement number 2, the intent is to minimize the risk of either over- or undertreatment. The AAO/HNS recommendations for postoperative monitoring were addressed in action statement number 4, but were based only on observational studies.[39]

▶ Table 6.4 Polysomnography (type 1 monitoring devices) recording specification after American Academy of Sleep Medicine

PSG recording parameters for children	Recommended level
EEG	Recommended
EOG	Recommended
Chin EMG	Recommended
ECG	Recommended
Air flow • Nasal pressure • Thermocouple/thermostat	Recommended Recommended
Oximeter	Recommended
Respiratory effort • Thoracic and abdominal respiratory inductance plethysmography • Esophageal pressure	Recommended Alternative
Body position	Recommended
Snoring sounds—microphone	Recommended
CO_2 measurement • Transcutaneous CO_2 • End-tidal CO_2	Recommended (Use at least one of these two)

Abbreviations: CO_2, Carbon dioxide; EEG, electroencephalogram; EMG, electromyogram; EOG, electro-oculography.
Data from American Academy of Sleep Medicine.[40]

▶ **Table 6.5** Respiratory indications for polysomnography in children according to the American Academy of Sleep Medicine

I. Standard

When the clinical assessment suggests the diagnosis of OSAS in children.

If there are residual symptoms of OSAS for children with mild OSA preoperatively, postoperative PSG should be performed.

Postoperative PSG is indicated to assess for residual OSAS in children with preoperative evidence for moderate-to-severe OSAS, obesity, craniofacial anomalies that obstruct the upper airway, and neurologic disorders (e.g., Down's Syndrome, Prader-Willi syndrome, and myelomeningocele).

Initiation of PAP in children with OSAS.

II. Guideline

When the clinical assessment suggests the diagnosis of congenital central alveolar hypoventilation syndrome or sleep-related hypoventilation due to neuromuscular disorders or chest wall deformities.

When there is clinical evidence of sleep-related breathing disorder in infants who have experienced an apparent life-threating event.

In children being considered for adenotonsillectomy to treat OSAS.

In children on chronic PAP support to determine whether pressure requirements have changed as a result of the child's growth and development, if symptoms recur while on PAP, or if additional or alternate treatment is instituted.

III. Option

After treatment with rapid maxillary expansion to assess for the level of residual disease and to determine whether additional treatment is necessary.

OSAS treated with an oral appliance to assess response treatment.

For noninvasive positive pressure ventilation titration in children with other sleep-related breathing disorders.

Children treated with mechanical ventilation may benefit from periodic evaluation with PSG to adjust ventilator settings.

Children treated with tracheostomy for sleep related breathing disorders as part of evaluation prior decannulation.

In the following respiratory disorders, only if there is a clinical suspicion for an accompanying sleep-related breathing disorder: chronic asthma, cystic fibrosis, pulmonary hypertension, bronchopulmonary dysplasia, or chest wall abnormality such as kyphoscoliosis.

Abbreviations: OSA, obstructive sleep apnea; OSAS, obstructive sleep apnea syndrome; PAP, positive airway pressure; PSG, polysomnography.
Data from Aurora et al.[38]

▶ **Table 6.6** Indications for polysomnography according to the American Academy of Otolaryngology/Head and Neck Surgery

Action statement no. 1

Before performing tonsillectomy, the clinician should refer children with SDB for PSG, if they exhibit any of the following: obesity, Down's syndrome, craniofacial disorders, sickle cell disease, or mucopolysaccharidoses.

Action statement no. 2

The clinician should advocate for PSG prior to tonsillectomy for SDB in children without any of the comorbidities listed in statement 1 for whom the need for surgery is uncertain or when there is discordance between tonsillar size on physical examination and the reported severity of SDB.

Action statement no. 4

Clinicians should admit children with OSA documented in results pf PSG for inpatient, overnight monitoring after tonsillectomy if they are younger than age 3 or have severe OSA (AHI of 10 or more obstructive events/h, oxygen saturation nadir < 80%, or both)

Abbreviations: AHI, apnea–hypopnea index; OSA, obstructive sleep apnea; PSG polysomnography; SDB, sleep-disordered breathing. Data from Roland et al.[39]

▶ **Table 6.7** Severity of obstructive sleep apnea: adult and pediatric

Severity of OSA	Adult AHI	Pediatric AHI
None	0–5	0
Mild OSA	6–20	1–5
Moderate OSA	21–40	6–10
Severe OSA	>40	>10

Abbreviations: AHI, apnea–hypopnea index; OSA, obstructive sleep apnea.
Data from American Society of Anesthesiologists Task Force on Perioperative Management of patients with obstructive sleep apnea.[41]

PSG in children should be performed and interpreted in accordance with the recommendations of the AASM *Manual for the Scoring of Sleep and Associated Events*.[40]

According to the latest version of the International Classification of Sleep Disorders (ICSD-3), PSG criteria for diagnosis are either (1) one or more obstructive events (obstructive or mixed apnea or obstructive hypopnea) per hour of sleep or (2) obstructive hypoventilation, as manifest by partial pressure of carbon dioxide ($PaCO_2$) more than 50 mm HG for 25% of sleep time, together with snoring, paradoxical thoracoabdominal movement, or flatting of the nasal airway pressure waveform implying flow limitation.[3] In international studies the definition of the AHI varied a lot and the AHI threshold is contested.

The cut off for AHI defining OSA ranged from 1 to 5 episodes per hour. Most studies used a criterion of more than or equal to 2 but less than or equal to 5 episodes per hour.[17] At the moment there is lack of consistency in the definition of pediatric OSA and in terminology used in the literature. Most sleep centers consider an obstructive AHI less than or equal to 1 per hour total sleeping time (TST) to be normal, AHI more than 1 but less than or equal to 5 to be mild OSA, AHI more than 5 but less than or equal to 10 to be moderate OSA, and AHI more than 10 per hour TST as severe OSA (▶Table 6.7).

There is an agreement in the international literature that an AHI more than 5 per hour requires treatment.

Drug-Induced Sleep Endoscopy

The first pediatric drug-induced sleep endoscopy (DISE) was published in 1990.[42] In the literature there is a wide variability regarding the indications and the way how it should be performed. Recently Friedman published a multi-institutional study over the current state of pediatric DISE.[43] The majority of respondents required that a PSG needs to be carried out prior to DISE. The predominant indication for DISE is residual OSA after ATE. Recent evidence has demonstrated that up to 30% of children undergoing ATE for treatment of OSA will have significant residual disease, likely due to obstruction at locations besides the tonsils or adenoids.[44] A variety of anesthetic protocols and agents are used for DISE. None of the agents adequately simulate rapid eye movement (REM) sleep.[45] During the DISE the airway sites from the nasal cavity to the glottis were regularly examined, whereas the bronchi were not.[43] Adjunctive maneuvers were frequently being performed, including a chin lift to simulate closed-mouth breathing and a jaw thrust to simulate a mandibular-repositioning device.[46] Different scoring system for DISE had been published, but a consistent scoring system is not typically used.[44,47] DISE can either be performed as an isolated procedure or in combination with sleep surgery. In the latter case, the kind of sleep surgery is selected according to DISE findings. A staged approach allows for a detailed discussion of the planned sleep surgical procedure, which improves opportunities for shared exception recovery and results.[43] Alternatively, some families prefer to have interventions performed at the time of the DISE; in these situations, the surgeon must discuss the risks and benefits of each potential sleep procedure, whereas the family must accept the uncertainty of what procedures will be performed on the day of the procedure.[43]

6.2 Treatment

6.2.1 Introduction

Different medical interventions and surgical techniques exist in the therapy of pediatric OSA. Treatment interventions are applied in a stepwise fashion until complete resolution of SDB is achieved. Depending on the severity and underlying conditions predisposing to upper airway obstruction during sleep, different treatment modalities are often combined.

6.2.2 Medical Intervention

Weight Loss

In obese adolescents with OSA, massive weight loss (>0.5 decrease in BMI z-score) is an effective treatment intervention but there is no evidence regarding the efficacy of weight loss in obese children.[48] There are no studies for the efficacy of weight loss as a treatment intervention for OSA in young children. However, weight loss will presumably be helpful.

Antibiotics

Antibiotics are not beneficial in long-term reduction of tonsillar hypertrophy, although during acuteinflammation, broad-spectrum antibiotics may provide a short-term decrease in tonsil size; one study reported that only 15% of the patients avoided surgery in long-term follow up.[49]

Nasal Corticosteroids and/or Oral Montelukast

Intranasal steroids are helpful in mild OSA if adenoid hypertrophy is the predominant etiology.[50] Beneficial effects of intranasally applied corticoids and montelukast may be due to reduction of the adenoid size.[50] If residual sleep apnea (AHI 1–5) is present after ATE, the use of intranasally applied corticosteroids and oral montelukast has been demonstrated to improve and/or normalize both respiratory and sleep disturbances.[51] The long-term efficacy and side effects of these medications have not been studied so far, and this is a limiting factor in their use.[52]

6.2.3 Oral Appliances

Oral appliances may be helpful in the treatment of children with craniofacial anomalies (e.g., retrognathia or malocclusion) that are risk factors for apnea.[53] The related complications are minor (e.g., excessive salivation).

Rapid maxillary expansion (RME) involves the use of an oral appliance that is adjusted daily to increase palatal width. RME presents another option of treatment for children with high-arched palates with associated increased nasal resistance and mild OSA. A high-arched palate may also be associated with a posterior tongue posture, which contributes to retroglossal airway narrowing. RME is most effective in prepubertal children prior to palatal suture closure. In a pilot study, Guilleminault et al showed good results with RME in combination with ATE to improve the nasal and oral airway.[54]

Continuous Positive Airway Pressure/ Noninvasive Positive-Pressure Ventilation

The usual indications for continuous positive airway pressure (CPAP) are residual OSA after ATE (AHI > 5 episodes per hour and OSA related to obesity, craniofacial abnormalities, and neuromuscular disorders).[55,56]

The use of noninvasive positive-pressure ventilation (NPPV) is indicated if nocturnal hypoventilation occurs (e.g., end-tidal carbon dioxide tension[PCO_2] > 50 mm Hg for 25% of total sleep time or peak end-tidal PCO_2 ≥ 55 mm Hg) NPPV is preferred.[56]

Marcus et al showed positive effects of CPAP and NPPV on school performance, quality of life, and neurobehavioral outcomes.[57]

Potential complications of CPAP and NPPV in children are facial skin erythema related to the mask, nasal congestion, epistaxis, rhinorrhea, and midfacial retrusion.[57]

The data about patient adherence to treatment vary in different international studies from low to quite high (>8 hours per night for 70% of patients) regardless of the use of CPAP or NPPV.[56,57]

Factors associated with better patient adherence include the degree of improvement in the AHI, overall perception of benefits from treatment, and maternal education.[58]

6.2.4 Surgical Interventions

Adenotonsillectomy

Indications, Contraindications, Patient Selection

ATE is the first-line treatment for most of children with OSA. ATE is indicated in children with OSA and adenotonsillar hypertrophy (▶Fig. 6.1, ▶Fig. 6.2).[5] Although obese children may have less satisfactory results, many can be adequately treated with ATE.[5] The recommendation of the American Academy of Pediatrics is a one-time surgical procedure. Adenoidectomy or tonsillectomy alone may not be sufficient because residual lymphoid tissue may contribute to persistent obstruction.[5] In ▶Table 6.8 the contraindications for ATE are listed.

For primary snoring the treatment indications are different. There is evidence that primary snoring is accompanied by cognitive deficits and behavioral abnormalities as well as elevated nocturnal diastolic blood pressure, but there are no studies addressing the efficacy of treatment interventions.[59] It is unclear whether or not children with primary snoring benefit from treatment interventions.

Diagnostic Workup

In authors' opinion, an otherwise healthy child does not require a sleep study prior to ATE in contrast to adults. If the medical history is typical for SDB and clinical examination shows an adenotonsillar hypertrophy, ATE is indicated. Sleep studies should be performed in patients with either syndromic disease, excessive weight, or other substantial comorbidities.

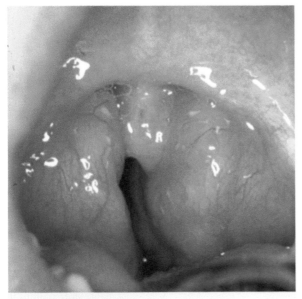

Fig. 6.1 Adenotonsillar hypertrophy.

The authors strongly recommend using a standardized protocol to record and to document the clinical findings.

The authors use a specific questionnaire that is filled in by the parents to screen for blood coagulation disorders.

For more detailed information, please refer to Chapter 6.1.

Specific Risks, Patient Information, Consent

General risks of surgery, such as pain, scarring, infection, wound healing problems, and postoperative hemorrhage need to be addressed.

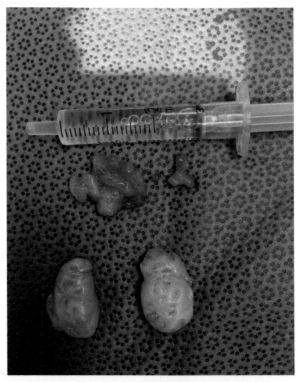

Fig. 6.2 Specimen of tonsils and adenoids directly after pediatric adenotonsillectomy (ATE).

▶ **Table 6.8** Contraindications for adenotonsillectomy

Absolute contraindications

- No adenotonsillar tissue (tissue has been surgically removed)

Relative contraindications

- Very small tonsils/adenoid
- Morbid obesity and small tonsils/adenoid
- Bleeding disorder refractory to treatment
- Submucosal cleft palate
- Other medical conditions making patient medically unstable for surgery

Data from (Marcus et al.)[5]

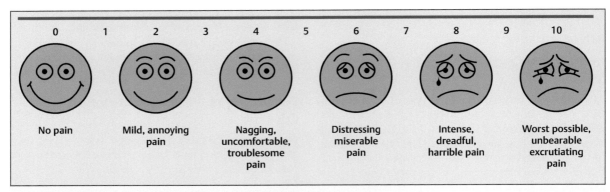

Fig. 6.3 Visual analogue scale (VAS) to evaluate postoperative pain for kids.

Apart from that, parents need to be informed that there will be a need for pain killers for a couple of days after surgery. Postoperative pain distinctively varies inter-individually, and is often difficult to rule out in children. The authors strongly recommend the use of visual analogue scale (VAS) designed for children to assess postoperative pain. This pediatric VAS (▶Fig. 6.3) uses faces instead of numbers to quantify pain. It is recommended to check for drug intolerances prior to surgery. The intensity of postoperative pain depends on the amount of thermal energy used to control blood.[60,61] This should be noted during surgery.

Postoperative hemorrhage is the most common complication after (adeno)tonsillectomy. It is recommended to check for prior bleedings and/or affinity for bleedings in the patient's history. A complete removal of the tonsils always requires a violation of the bigger blood vessels of the tonsillar capsule. Partial tonsillectomy, tonsillotomy or intracapsular tonsillectomy, avoids that risk, but removes most of the lymphatic tissue resulting in a comparable enlargement of the upper airway diameter. These surgical techniques show a significantly decreased risk for postoperative hemorrhage and pain as compared with complete tonsillectomy.[62,63,64,65,66] As postoperative hemorrhage is much more dangerous in children as compared to adults, the authors prefer tonsillotomy instead of tonsillectomy in children treated for OSA.

It is recommended to verify the child's ability to open his/her mouth and inspect the teeth. Address damage of the teeth and hematoma within the tongue and temporary loss of taste as potential complications induced by the mouth gag.

Severe wound healing deficits or intense revision surgery for blood control of postoperative bleedings may rarely result in nasopharyngeal stenosis or velopharyngeal incompetence.

6.2.5 Anesthesia and Positioning

ATE can be performed with inhalation anesthesia in children up to 25 to 30 kg. However, in children with OSA we only perform ATE under general anesthesia with the child being orally intubated and lying in supine position and the head slightly extended. Most mouth gags have a gorge to hold the intubation tube. This is why the tube needs to be placed in midline.

Equipment

Standard surgical instruments for cold steel tonsillectomies are sufficient. Modern instruments such as lasers, bovies or other monopolar instruments, the coblator system, or others can be used for dissection. For tonsillotomy we prefer the argon plasma coagulation technique as described previously and shown in the video (Video 6.1).[67] The argon plasma technique creates an oxygen-free atmosphere during the cutting process, resulting in less tissue temperature and thus less postoperative pain.

6.2.6 Operative Technique/ Operative Steps

Tonsillectomy

Multiple techniques and devices may be used to perform tonsillectomy, which may be influenced by surgeon's preference and exposure in training programs and operator's experience. Patient recovery times, postoperative morbidities, as well as cost related to the device are also important factors that may drive device choice. There is no consensus regarding the optimal technique with the lowest morbidity.[49] Most commonly used techniques include cold steel dissection and electrosurgical dissection.

During *cold steel dissection*, the tonsil is grasped, and after identification of the tonsil capsule, the tonsil is snared and removed. Electrocautery is typically used for hemostasis. *Electrosurgical dissection* uses thermal energy to dissect tissues with either a monopolar or bipolar tip. The blood loss is minimal in the electrosurgical dissection technique (▶Fig. 6.4).

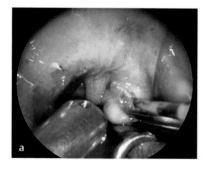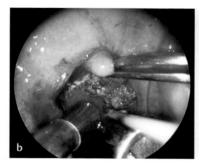

Fig. 6.4 Argon plasma-assisted intracapsular tonsillectomy in a 4-year-old girl.

All techniques have similar postoperative morbidities of hemorrhage (1.2–2.1%), dysphagia, and otalgia.[68] Plasma surgical dissection ablates and coagulates soft tissue by generating an ionized plasma layer with a radiofrequency current that breaks molecular bonds, producing a melting tissue effect. Many studies have shown this technique to cause less pain, shorten the recovery period, and requires less postoperative narcotics than other methods of tonsillectomy.[69] The Harmonic scalpel uses ultrasonic energy to vibrate its blade, providing simultaneous cutting, and coagulation of the tissue. Postoperative hemorrhage and intraoperative blood loss is low with the Harmonic scalpel. Operative times are longer compared with other techniques.[70] There are conflicting studies on post-tonsillectomy pain outcomes.[71]

Partial Tonsillectomy and Intracapsular Tonsillectomy

Partial tonsillectomy, also known as tonsillotomy or intracapsular tonsillectomy, may be performed for tonsillar hypertrophy with SDB/OSA.

The premise of partial tonsillectomy is reduction of obstructive tonsillar tissue while sparing the tonsillar capsule, thus preventing exposure of the underlying pharyngeal muscles and decreasing postoperative bleeding and pain. Technology used for partial tonsillectomy includes a microdebrider or radiofrequency device. An advantage of partial tonsillectomy is lower postoperative hemorrhage rates; however, increased intraoperative bleeding may impede visualization at times.[72] Studies on the long-term efficacy of partial tonsillectomy compared to established approaches are limited but promising.[73]

Adenoidectomy

Adenoidectomy may also be performed with a variety of devices, primarily through a transoral approach. Devices include dissection with an adenoid curette, suction monopolar cautery, microdebrider, coblation, and plasma devices. Revision adenoidectomy occurs at a rate of 1.3%.[74] Reasons for revision include persistent symptoms with adenoid re-hypertrophy, chronic adenoiditis, and recurrent otitis.

Risks, Tips, and Tricks

- Open the mouth wide enough. Separate expose of each tonsil using the mouth gag may be helpful.
- Save as much mucosa and muscle tissue as possible.
- Avoid intensive use of thermal energy in order to minimalize postoperative pain.
- Electrosurgical techniques can help reduce postoperative pain and medications.

6.2.7 Complications (Including Measures for Specific Complications)

Minor complications after ATE are dehydration, nausea, and vomiting. Local bleeding and upper airway obstruction are major complications. The most common complications of ATE are related to anesthesia risks and breathing concerns, pain, otalgia, and bleeding (▶ Table 6.9). Dehydration may occur due to poorly controlled pain, refusal of oral intake, nausea, and vomiting secondary to narcotic use.[75] The frequency of local bleeding has been reported to be 3%.[76]

Rare complications of tonsillectomy include subcutaneous emphysema, pneumomediastinum, and taste disturbance because of damage to the lingual branch of the glossopharyngeal nerve.[75] Nasopharyngeal stenosis, also an uncommon outcome, results from approximation of raw mucosal surfaces during the healing process.[75]

Children with one or more of the risk factors are recommended for hospitalization for close monitoring (▶ Table 6.10).[1,5]

6.2.8 Postoperative Care (Including Medication and Drainage)

The management of postoperative pain is crucial after tonsillectomy, but does not differ from tonsillectomy for other indications. In authors' view, a basic treatment with ibuprofen and paracetamol per os (dosage depending on body weight) works fine in children. However, there are huge inter-individual differences that require individual adaptations. As stated above, special VAS for

▶ **Table 6.9** Complications of adenotonsillectomy

Minor risks

- Pain
- Dehydration attributable to postoperative nausea (vomiting and poor oral intake)

Major risks

- Anesthetic complications
- Acute upper airway obstruction during induction or emergence from anesthesia
- Postoperative respiratory compromise
- Hemorrhage
- Velopharyngeal incompetence
- Nasopharyngeal stenosis
- Death

Data from Marcus et al.[5]

▶ **Table 6.10** Risk factors for postoperative respiratory complications in children with OSAS undergoing adenotonsillectomy

Risk factors for postoperative respiratory complications

Severe OSAS on PSG: AHI >26 episodes/h

Oximetry recording with three or more clusters of desaturation (≤4%) events and at least three desaturations to <90%

Age <3 y

Obesity
Low weight

Neuromuscular, craniofacial, or genetic disorder

Abbreviations: AHI, apnea–hypopnea index; OSAS, obstructive sleep apnea syndrome; PSG, polysomnography.
Data from Marcus et al and Kaditis et al.[1,5]

children (see ▶ Fig. 6.2) is recommended to monitor post-operative pain.

After adenoidectomy, the use of nasal decongestive drops for a couple of days is recommended by the authors. The dosage depends on age.

A follow-up visit is indicated at 6 weeks till 12 months after each treatment intervention. The clinical visit should include: symptoms, severity of SDB evaluated objectively, quality of life, morbidity from the cardiovascular and central nervous system, enuresis, and growth rate.[57,77] Polygraphy (PG) or PSG is repeated for children at risk of persistent OSA after ATE, for those with persistent syndromes of SDB postoperatively, or for patients with mild OSA who were treated with nasal corticosteroid and/or montelukast. Most studies have suggested repeating PSG or PG 6 weeks or longer after ATE or following a 12-week course with nasal corticosteroid and/or montelukast. As in the diagnostic setting PSG is the preferred objective method to detect residual OSA after treatment intervention. In case PSG is not available, alternative methods such as PG can be considered.[78]

PSG is used for the titration of CPAP or NPPV. There is limited evidence about the optimal respiratory monitoring for children who receive CPAP or NPPV.[55] The recommendation from the ERS-statement 2016 is that PSG or PG should be repeated at least annually or earlier if there are clinical indications.[1]

When persistent SDB is demonstrated based on symptoms and/or PSG further examinations such as nasopharyngoscopy, drug-induced sleep endoscopy or a MRI might be helpful to identify additional upper airway abnormalities (e.g., laryngomalacia, adenoidal tissue regrowth, tongue base obstruction, or pharyngeal collapse).[79,80]

Tagaya et al demonstrated an adenoid regrowth in 12.2% of nonobese children with OSA at 1.5 years post-ATE using the nasopharyngoscope.[81]

6.2.9 Outcome (Including EBM Data for AHI and ESS)

A recent multicenter study from the United States proved the superiority of ATE against a wait-and-see concept.[7] ▶ Table 6.11 summarizes objective PSG data before and after ATE taken only from controlled studies. Information from ▶ Table 6.11 supports ATE being the standard of choice treatment for pediatric OSA if adenotonsillar hypertrophy exists.

However, the surgical success rate for ATE in pediatric OSA depends on the definition used, and ranges about 70 to 80%, which means that a certain number of children is left with residual OSA after ATE.[96] For early detection of these cases it is important to perform follow-up sleep studies with PSG, PG, or unattended multichannel devices type 2 or 3.[37] Most improvements occur in patients with OSA and an AHI greater than 5.[97] Huang et al in a prospective cohort study provided evidence for potential OSA recurrence within 3 years after ATE.[98]

Risk factors for persistence of persisting SDB are listed in ▶ Table 6.12.

Other Improvements after Adenotonsillectomy

Children with OSA have poorer scores in quality-of-life measurements. Both generic and disease-specific health-related quality-of-life measures improve after ATE.[59]

Symptoms of SDB and SDB-associated morbidity (i.e., growth delay, frequency of enuresis, pulmonary hypertension, cor pulmonale, increased heat rate, and morbidity from the central nervous system) improve after treatment of OSA with ATE.[1]

The CHAT study presented evidence for the increase in growth rate and resolution of enuresis.[33] Gozal et al showed an improved endothelial dysfunction after treatment of OSA with ATE in majority of children; however, in children with a strong family history of cardiovascular

► **Table 6.11** Outcome of adenotonsillectomy for pediatric obstructive sleep apnea

Author	N	Follow-up (months)	Age (years)	Surgery	AHI pre	AHI post	Success (AHI < 5)	EBM grade	Control group
Stradling et al (1990)[82]	61	6	2–14	ATE	3.6	1.5	No data	3b	N = 31 no treatment
Ali et al (1996)[83]	12	3–6	6–12	ATE	3	1.4	No data	3b	N = 11 no treatment
Nieminen et al (2000)[84]	27	6	2–10	ATE	6.9	0.3	77.8%	3b	N = 30 no treatment
Montgomery-Downs et al (2005)[85]	19	4	4.4	ATE	10.1	1	100%	2b	N = 19 no treatment
Chervin et al (2006)[86]	78	12	5–13	ATE	7.3	1.1	No data	3b	N = 27 no treatment
Coticchia et al (2006)[87]	10	3	2.6–12.5	ATE	7.7	0.3	No data	2b	N = 13 RFT tonsils + AT
Tauman et al (2007)[88]	110	1–15	1–16	ATE	22	6	71.0%	3b	N = 20 no treatment
Mitchell and Kelly (2007)[89] All	72		3–17	ATE	24.1	4.1	80.6%	3b	N = 33 obese vs N = 39 nonobese
• Obese	33	5,1	3–17		31	6	69.7%		
• Nonobese	39	5,1	3.1–15.6		17.1	2.4	72.0%		
Dillon et al (2007)[90]	40	10–15	7.8	ATE	5.6	0.2	No data	3b	N = 38 ATE without OSA, N = 27 other surgeries
Gozal et al (2008)[91] All	62		3–12	ATE	16.7	4.1	75.8%	3b	N = 37 obese vs N = 25 nonobese
• Obese	37	7,9	7.9		19.2	5.5	59.5%		
• Nonobese	25	8,4	6.6		12.9	1.9	100%		
Amin et al (2008)[19]	40	12	10	ATE	9.2	1.4	50% (AHI < 3)	3b	N = 30 normal controls without treatment
Marcus et al (2013)[7]	194	7	6.5	ATE	4.8	1.3	79% (AHI < 2 + ODI < 2)	2b	N = 203 OSA, wait and see
Chiu et al (2013)[92] All	24		6.9	ATE with sutures without sutures	11.5	2.5	70.8%	3b	N =12 ATE with sutures vs. N = 12 ATE without sutures
• With sutures	12	3–4	6.9		14.6	1.6	91.6%		
• Without sutures	12	3–4	6.9		8.3	3.3	50.0%		
Villa et al (2014)[93]	25	12	5.0	ATE	17.3	1.8	No data	3b	N = 22 OSA, rapid maxillary expansion
Kuo et al (2015)[94] All	78		9.2	ATE	18.1	2.3	No data	3b	N = 39 obese vs N = 39 nonobese
• Obese	39	3	8.9		18	2.0	No data		
• Nonobese	39	3	9.4		18.1	2.5	no data		
Tang et al (2015)[95] All	70		1–18	ATE	11.8	2.0	40% (AHI < 1)	3b	ATE, different tonsillar sizes
T2+	20	<12	4.8		6.2	2.9	25% (AHI < 1)		
T3+	36	<12	5.7		10.9	1.1	50% (AHI < 1)		
T4+	40	<12	7.7		15.5	1.9	35.7% (AHI < 1)		
All	**922**	**1–15**	**1–18**	**ATE**	**12.20**	**2.38**		**A**	

Abbreviations: AHI, apnea-hypopnea-index; AT, adenoidectomy; EBM, evidence-based medicine; ODI, oxygen desaturation index; RFT, radiofrequency treatment.
Data only taken from controlled studies.

▶ **Table 6.12** Risk factors for persistence of untreated sleep-disordered breathing

Risk factors for persistence of untreated SDB
Obesity and increasing BMI percentile
Male sex
Severity of OSAS (AHI >5 episodes/h)
African-American ethnicity
Persistent tonsillar hypertrophy and narrow mandible
Retroposition of the mandibula
History of asthma
Inferior turbinate hypertrophy
Nasal septum deviation
Mallampati score 3 or 4
Prader-Willi syndrome
Syndromic craniosynostosis (midfacial hypoplasia)
Down's syndrome
Achondroplasia
Cerebral palsy

Abbreviations: AHI, apnea–hypopnea index; BMI, body mass index; OSAS, obstructive sleep apnea syndrome; SDB, sleep-disordered breathing.
Data from Marcus et al and Kaditis et al.[1,7]

disease it remained abnormal, once again suggesting the influence of genetic and environmental factors on phenotypic expression.[99] In young children, OSA has been shown to be associated with reduced insulin sensitivity in obese children, with improvements when OSA was treated.[91]

The favorable changes in sleepiness, attention deficit, behavioral problems, hyperactivity symptoms, neurocognitive skills, quality-of-life scores following ATE are not related to the preoperative severity of obstructive SDB.[33,59]

6.2.10 Other Pediatric Obstructive Sleep Apnea Surgeries

Surgery for Multilevel Obstruction

Multilevel obstruction involving any combination of the nasal, naso-, oro, and hypopharyngeal or laryngeal anatomy may be found. Certain populations are predisposed to multilevel airway collapse, including children who have obesity, nasal obstruction, neurological impairments, laryngotracheomalacia, laryngotracheal or bronchial stenosis, and craniofacial anomalies, such as Pierre Robin sequence and Down's syndrome.[100] The exact nature of dynamic airway collapse may not be appreciated by a detailed history and physical examination, therefore cine MR imaging and flexible endoscopy performed in the office and the operating room may help identify the anatomic levels of obstruction.[101] There is limited evidence available in children regarding surgical techniques for multilevel OSA. Lack of objective PSG criteria for

comparison between surgical treatment options as well as the nature of surgical intervention makes it difficult to conduct blinded studies.[49] A staged approach should be considered in children; Prager et al described an 8.2% incidence of oropharyngeal scarring and stenosis in 48 children who underwent multilevel surgery that included lingual tonsillectomy for OSA.[102]

Nasal Surgery

In children, a deviated septum is rare. It might occur after midfacial trauma. More often turbinate hypertrophy contributes to nasal airway obstruction. Septoplasty should preferably be avoided until children have stopped growing but if really needed it should be performed with careful patient selection using a limited approach. Septoplasty may be useful in improving CPAP tolerance, particularly in older children. Two main techniques exist for turbinate volume reduction: radiofrequency ablation and microdebrider-assisted reduction. A review of turbinate surgery in children comparing both techniques demonstrated that both are effective, however, maintenance of improvement at 3 years was better with the microdebrider-assisted technique.[103] Mild-to-moderate edema with subsequent nasal obstruction and thick mucus formation can be expected in the first week after the procedure.

Oropharyngeal Surgery

Surgical techniques for obstruction at oropharyngeal level such as uvulopalatopharyngoplasty (UPPP), lateral pharyngoplasty, and expansion sphincter pharyngoplasty are not commonly performed in children. UPPP has been reported to be successful in children with cerebral palsy and hypotonic upper airway muscles.[104]

Tongue Base Surgery

Surgical procedures described in children to increase the volume of the retrolingual airway are endoscopic-assisted coblation lingual tonsillectomy, glossectomy, and advancement and suspension procedures.

Lin and Koltai performed endoscopic-assisted coblation lingual tonsillectomy in 26 patients (aged 3–20 years) with PSG-proven persistent OSA after previous tonsillectomy and adenoidectomy. Statistically significant reductions in the RDI were seen when preoperative and postoperative data were compared (mean 14.7 vs 8.1). There were similar reductions in the number of apneas and hypopneas. Two patients developed adhesions between the epiglottis and tongue base; there appeared to be no consequence for airway or feeding issue. The authors concluded that the endoscopic-assisted coblation lingual tonsillectomy is a safe procedure in the treatment of retrolingual airway collapse.[105]

Wootten and Shott performed combined genioglossus advancement (Repose THS; Medtronic ENT, Jacksonville, FL, U.S.) and radiofrequency ablation in 31 children (aged

3.1–23 years) with retroglossal and base of tongue collapse and persisting OSA after ATE. Of these children 61% had Down's syndrome. Success of surgery was determined using the criteria of postoperative AHI less than 5 events per hour. The mean AHI improved significantly from 14.1 to 6.4 per hour. The success rate among patients with Down's syndrome was 58% and in patients without Down's syndrome was 66%. The authors concluded that most of the patients benefited from combined genioglossus advancement and radiofrequency ablation.[106]

Long-term effectiveness of both the procedures was unknown during the study.

Laryngeal Surgery

Laryngomalacia is primarily seen in infancy, but may present in older children. For the majority of patients, laryngomalacia may be managed expectantly without intervention. Supraglottoplasty is indicated in case of OSA where children fail to thrive or have feeding difficulties. Sharp dissection or laser techniques are used to reduce redundant mucosa or incise shortened aryepiglottic folds. Medical comorbidities are associated with worsened postoperative outcomes, although the majority of children improve after supraglottoplasty.[107]

Craniofacial Surgery

Craniofacial surgery (e.g., distraction osteogenesis) has been shown to be successful in children with syndromic craniofacial abnormalities. The aim of craniofacial surgery is to expand the dimension of the upper airway, improve respiratory complaints, PSG parameters, and quality of life. It might also be performed to facilitate decannulation or to avoid tracheotomy. Distraction osteogenesis (DOG) is a surgical technique used to expand the facial skeleton in children with congenital micrognathia or midface hypoplasia without the need for bone grafting.[108] Success rates of 95.6% have been reported in patients with micrognathia and OSA after mandibular distraction osteogenesis. In a study conducted by Tahiri et al, 82.4% of the children can be decannulated.[109] Success rates in this study were lower in the presence of other abnormalities (e.g., laryngomalacia or subglottic stenosis) or central apnea. Taylor et al showed in a systemic review of outcome following midface distraction osteogenesis for midface hypoplasia/retrusion a decannulation rate of 65.7% in children with tracheotomy.[110] Reported complications are rare but severe. They include cerebrospinal fluid leak, wound site infection, hypertrophic scarring, pseudoarthrosis, palatine perforation, apertognathia, and unilateral facial paralysis.[109,110]

Tracheostomy

Tracheostomy has the highest efficacy in the treatment of obstructive SBD, when compared with other surgical interventions. It is usually used only in severe OSA when other nonsurgical or surgical interventions have failed or are contraindicated. Early complications (e.g., wound infection, bleeding, pneumothorax, pneumomediastinum) are 3% or less.[111] Late-onset complications, in particular granulation tissue formation are reported in up to 40% of cases.[111] Inferior quality of life has been reported in children with Down's syndrome, Pierre Robin sequence, or neuromuscular disease and patients with OSA who had tracheostomy compared with those who had successful craniofacial surgery.[112]

Anesthetic Implications

Preoperative sedation should be used with caution in children with severe OSA. During induction of anesthesia, there is high risk for airway obstruction, desaturation, and laryngospasm.[113] Patients with severe OSA have an abnormal ventilator response to carbon dioxide and are likely to have greater respiratory depression in response to sedatives, narcotics, and general anesthetics, and can have significant delay in their turn to spontaneous ventilation and emergence from general anesthesia.[113] After extubation patients are at risk for postextubation obstruction, laryngospasm, desaturation, pulmonary edema, and respiratory arrest.[114] Children younger than 3 years and those with severe OSA (AHI of 10 or more, oxygen saturation nadir<80%, or both) should be observed after surgery.[115] Monitoring in an intensive care unit may be warranted in a child with very severe OSA, medical comorbidities that cannot be managed in the general ward, and those who demonstrate significant airway obstruction and desaturation in the initial postoperative period that requires interventions beyond repositioning and/or oxygen supplementation.[39]

Perioperative deaths in children with OSA occur at a low frequency. Hypoxia-induced opioid sensitivity combined with an approximate 1 to 2% incidence of rapid conversation of codeine to morphine suggest the need for new approaches for providing preoperative assessment of risk, extended postoperative observation, and the need for alternative opioids to codeine.[116]

For more information please refer to Chapter 10.

References

[1] Kaditis AG, Alonso Alvarez ML, Boudewyns A, et al. Obstructive sleep disordered breathing in 2- to 18-year-old children: diagnosis and management. Eur Respir J. 2016; 47(1):69–94

[2] Friedman NR. Pediatric sleep studies: when and how often are they necessary? Curr Opin Otolaryngol Head Neck Surg. 2013; 21(6):557–566

[3] American Academy of Sleep Medicine. International classification of sleep disorders, revised: diagnostic and coding manual. Chicago, Illinois; 2014

[4] Lumeng JC, Chervin RD. Epidemiology of pediatric obstructive sleep apnea. Proc Am Thorac Soc. 2008; 5(2):242–252

[5] Marcus CL, Brooks LJ, Draper KA, et al. American Academy of Pediatrics. Diagnosis and management of childhood obstructive sleep apnea syndrome. Pediatrics. 2012; 130(3):576–584

[6] Shine NP, Coates HL, Lannigan FJ. Obstructive sleep apnea, morbid obesity, and adenotonsillar surgery: a review of the literature. Int J Pediatr Otorhinolaryngol. 2005; 69(11): 1475–1482

[7] Marcus CL, Moore RH, Rosen CL, et al. Childhood Adenotonsillectomy Trial (CHAT). A randomized trial of adenotonsillectomy for childhood sleep apnea. N Engl J Med. 2013; 368(25):2366–2376

[8] Slaats MA, Van Hoorenbeeck K, Van Eyck A, et al. Upper airway imaging in pediatric obstructive sleep apnea syndrome. Sleep Med Rev. 2015; 21:59–71

[9] Marcus CL, McColley SA, Carroll JL, Loughlin GM, Smith PL, Schwartz AR. Upper airway collapsibility in children with obstructive sleep apnea syndrome. J Appl Physiol (1985). 1994; 77(2):918–924

[10] Lin SY, Melvin TA, Boss EF, Ishman SL. The association between allergic rhinitis and sleep-disordered breathing in children: a systematic review. Int Forum Allergy Rhinol. 2013; 3(6): 504–509

[11] Flores-Mir C, Korayem M, Heo G, Witmans M, Major MP, Major PW. Craniofacial morphological characteristics in children with obstructive sleep apnea syndrome: a systematic review and meta-analysis. J Am Dent Assoc. 2013; 144(3):269–277

[12] Katyal V, Pamula Y, Martin AJ, Daynes CN, Kennedy JD, Sampson WJ. Craniofacial and upper airway morphology in pediatric sleep-disordered breathing: Systematic review and meta-analysis. Am J Orthod Dentofacial Orthop. 2013; 143(1): 20–30.e3

[13] Dehlink E, Tan HL. Update on paediatric obstructive sleep apnoea. J Thorac Dis. 2016; 8(2):224–235

[14] de Miguel-Díez J, Villa-Asensi JR, Alvarez-Sala JL. Prevalence of sleep-disordered breathing in children with Down syndrome: polygraphic findings in 108 children. Sleep. 2003; 26(8):1006–1009

[15] Ng M, Fleming T, Robinson M, et al. Global, regional, and national prevalence of overweight and obesity in children and adults during 1980–2013: a systematic analysis for the Global Burden of Disease Study 2013. Lancet. 2014; 384(9945):766–781

[16] Alonso-Álvarez ML, Cordero-Guevara JA, Terán-Santos J, et al. Obstructive sleep apnea in obese community-dwelling children: the NANOS study. Sleep. 2014; 37(5):943–949

[17] Andersen IG, Holm JC, Homøe P. Obstructive sleep apnea in obese children and adolescents, treatment methods and outcome of treatment - A systematic review. Int J Pediatr Otorhinolaryngol. 2016; 87:190–197

[18] Redline S, Storfer-Isser A, Rosen CL, et al. Association between metabolic syndrome and sleep-disordered breathing in adolescents. Am J Respir Crit Care Med. 2007; 176(4):401–408

[19] Amin R, Somers VK, McConnell K, et al. Activity-adjusted 24-hour ambulatory blood pressure and cardiac remodeling in children with sleep disordered breathing. Hypertension. 2008; 51(1):84–91

[20] Zintzaras E, Kaditis AG. Sleep-disordered breathing and blood pressure in children: a meta-analysis. Arch Pediatr Adolesc Med. 2007; 161(2):172–178

[21] Gut G, Tauman R, Greenfeld M, Armoni-Domany K, Sivan Y. Nasal nitric oxide in sleep-disordered breathing in children. Sleep Breath. 2016; 20(1):303–308

[22] Ye J, Liu H, Li P, et al. CD4(+)T-lymphocyte subsets in nonobese children with obstructive sleep apnea syndrome. Pediatr Res. 2015; 78(2):165–173

[23] Loffredo L, Zicari AM, Occasi F, et al. Endothelial dysfunction and oxidative stress in children with sleep disordered breathing: role of NADPH oxidase. Atherosclerosis. 2015; 240(1):222–227

[24] Sedky SBD. Attention deficit hyperactivity disorders breathing in pediatric populations: a meta-analysis. Sleep Med Rev. 2014; 18(4):349–356

[25] Perfect MM, Archbold K, Goodwin JL, Levine-Donnerstein D, Quan SF. Risk of behavioral and adaptive functioning difficulties in youth with previous and current sleep disordered breathing. Sleep. 2013; 36(4):517–525B

[26] Barone JG, Hanson C, DaJusta DG, Gioia K, England SJ, Schneider D. Nocturnal enuresis and overweight are associated with obstructive sleep apnea. Pediatrics. 2009; 124(1):e53–e59

[27] Aurora RN, Lamm CI, Zak RS, et al. Practice parameters for the non-respiratory indications for polysomnography and multiple sleep latency testing for children. Sleep. 2012; 35(11): 1467–1473

[28] Brooks LJ, Topol HI. Enuresis in children with sleep apnea. J Pediatr. 2003; 142(5):515–518

[29] Sans Capdevila O, Crabtree VM, Kheirandish-Gozal L, Gozal D. Increased morning brain natriuretic peptide levels in children with nocturnal enuresis and sleep-disordered breathing: a community-based study. Pediatrics. 2008; 121(5):e1208–e1214

[30] Baldassari CM, Mitchell RB, Schubert C, Rudnick EF. Pediatric obstructive sleep apnea and quality of life: a meta-analysis. Otolaryngol Head Neck Surg. 2008; 138(3):265–273

[31] Certal V, Catumbela E, Winck JC, Azevedo I, Teixeira-Pinto A, Costa-Pereira A. Clinical assessment of pediatric obstructive sleep apnea: a systematic review and meta-analysis. Laryngoscope. 2012; 122(9):2105–2114

[32] Chervin RD, Weatherly RA, Garetz SL, et al. Pediatric sleep questionnaire: prediction of sleep apnea and outcomes. Arch Otolaryngol Head Neck Surg. 2007; 133(3):216–222

[33] Mitchell RB, Garetz S, Moore RH, et al. The use of clinical parameters to predict obstructive sleep apnea syndrome severity in children: the Childhood Adenotonsillectomy (CHAT) study randomized clinical trial. JAMA Otolaryngol Head Neck Surg. 2015; 141(2):130–136

[34] Gozal D, Kheirandish-Gozal L. New approaches to the diagnosis of sleep-disordered breathing in children. Sleep Med. 2010; 11(7):708–713

[35] Collop NA, Anderson WM, Boehlecke B, et al. Portable Monitoring Task Force of the American Academy of Sleep Medicine. Clinical guidelines for the use of unattended portable monitors in the diagnosis of obstructive sleep apnea in adult patients. J Clin Sleep Med. 2007; 3(7):737–747

[36] Nixon GM, Brouillette RT. Diagnostic techniques for obstructive sleep apnoea: is polysomnography necessary? Paediatr Respir Rev. 2002; 3(1):18–24

[37] Certal V, Camacho M, Winck JC, Capasso R, Azevedo I, Costa-Pereira A. Unattended sleep studies in pediatric OSA: a systematic review and meta-analysis. Laryngoscope. 2015; 125(1):255–262

[38] Aurora RN, Zak RS, Karippot A, et al. American Academy of Sleep Medicine. Practice parameters for the respiratory indications for polysomnography in children. Sleep. 2011; 34(3):379–388

[39] Roland PS, Rosenfeld RM, Brooks LJ, et al. American Academy of Otolaryngology—Head and Neck Surgery Foundation. Clinical practice guideline: Polysomnography for sleep-disordered breathing prior to tonsillectomy in children. Otolaryngol Head Neck Surg. 2011; 145(1 Suppl):S1–S15

[40] American Academy of Sleep Medicine. The AASM manual for the scoring of sleep and associated events: rules, terminology and technical specifications. Westchester, Ill: 2007

[41] American Society of Anesthesiologists Task Force on Perioperative Management of patients with obstructive sleep apnea. Practice guidelines for the perioperative management of patients with obstructive sleep apnea: an updated report by the American Society of Anesthesiologists Task Force on Perioperative Management of patients with obstructive sleep apnea. Anesthesiology. 2014; 120(2):268–286

[42] Croft CB, Thomson HG, Samuels MP, Southall DP. Endoscopic evaluation and treatment of sleep-associated upper airway obstruction in infants and young children. Clin Otolaryngol Allied Sci. 1990; 15(3):209–216

[43] Friedman NR, Parikh SR, Ishman SL, et al. The current state of pediatric drug-induced sleep endoscopy. Laryngoscope. 2017; 127(1):266–272

[44] Lam DJ, Weaver EM, Macarthur CJ, et al. Assessment of pediatric obstructive sleep apnea using a drug-induced sleep endoscopy rating scale. Laryngoscope. 2016; 126(6):1492–1498

[45] Ehsan Z, Mahmoud M, Shott SR, Amin RS, Ishman SL. The effects of anesthesia and opioids on the upper airway: A systematic review. Laryngoscope. 2016; 126(1):270–284

[46] Hohenhorst WRM. Drug-induced sleep endoscopy in adults with sleep-disordered breathing: Technique and the VOTE Classification system. Oper Tech Otolaryngol–Head Neck Surg. 2012; 23:11–18

[47] Chan DK, Liming BJ, Horn DL, Parikh SR. A new scoring system for upper airway pediatric sleep endoscopy. JAMA Otolaryngol Head Neck Surg. 2014; 140(7):595–602

[48] Verhulst SL, Franckx H, Van Gaal L, De Backer W, Desager K. The effect of weight loss on sleep-disordered breathing in obese teenagers. Obesity (Silver Spring). 2009; 17(6):1178–1183

[49] Sulman CG. Pediatric sleep surgery. Front Pediatr. 2014; 2:1–7

[50] Kheirandish L, Gozal D. Intranasal budesonide treatment for children with mild obstructive sleep apnea syndrome. Pediatrics. 2008; 122:149–155

[51] Kheirandish L, Goldbart AD, Gozal D. Intranasal steroids and oral leukotriene modifier therapy in residual sleep-disordered breathing after tonsillectomy and adenoidectomy in children. Pediatrics. 2006; 117(1):e61–e66

[52] Kuhle S, Urschitz MS. Anti-inflammatory medications for obstructive sleep apnea in children. Cochrane Database Syst Rev. 2011; 1(1):CD007074

[53] Carvalho FR, Lentini-Oliveira D, Machado MA, Prado GF, Prado LB, Saconato H. Oral appliances and functional orthopaedic appliances for obstructive sleep apnoea in children. Cochrane Database Syst Rev. 2007; 2(2):CD005520

[54] Guilleminault C, Monteyrol PJ, Huynh NT, Pirelli P, Quo S, Li K. Adeno-tonsillectomy and rapid maxillary distraction in pre-pubertal children, a pilot study. Sleep Breath. 2011; 15(2):173–177

[55] Amaddeo A, Caldarelli V, Fernandez-Bolanos M, et al. Polygraphic respiratory events during sleep in children treated with home continuous positive airway pressure: description and clinical consequences. Sleep Med. 2015; 16(1):107–112

[56] Ramirez A, Khirani S, Aloui S, et al. Continuous positive airway pressure and noninvasive ventilation adherence in children. Sleep Med. 2013; 14(12):1290–1294

[57] Marcus CL, Rosen G, Ward SL, et al. Adherence to and effectiveness of positive airway pressure therapy in children with obstructive sleep apnea. Pediatrics. 2006; 117(3):e442–e451

[58] DiFeo N, Meltzer LJ, Beck SE, et al. Predictors of positive airway pressure therapy adherence in children: a prospective study. J Clin Sleep Med. 2012; 8(3):279–286

[59] Garetz SL, Mitchell RB, Parker PD, et al. Quality of life and obstructive sleep apnea symptoms after pediatric adenotonsillectomy. Pediatrics. 2015; 135(2):e477–e486

[60] Cardozo AA, Hallikeri C, Lawrence H, Sankar V, Hargreaves S. Teenage and adult tonsillectomy: dose-response relationship between diathermy energy used and morbidity. Clin Otolaryngol. 2007; 32(5):366–371

[61] Habermann W, Müller W. Tissue penetration of bipolar electrosurgical currents: Joule overheating beyond the surface layer. Head Neck. 2013; 35(4):535–540

[62] Lourijsen ES, Wong Chung JE, Koopman JP, Blom HM. Postoperative morbidity and 1-year outcomes in CO_2-laser tonsillotomy versus dissection tonsillotomy. Acta Otolaryngol. 2016; 136(10):983–990

[63] Deak L, Saxton D, Johnston K, Benedek P, Katona G. Comparison of postoperative pain in children with two intracapsular tonsillotomy techniques and a standard tonsillectomy: microdebrider and radiofrequency tonsillotomies versus standard tonsillectomies. Sultan Qaboos Univ Med J. 2014; 14(4):e500–e505

[64] Acevedo JL, Shah RK, Brietzke SE. Systematic review of complications of tonsillotomy versus tonsillectomy. Otolaryngol Head Neck Surg. 2012; 146(6):871–879

[65] Walton J, Ebner Y, Stewart MG, April MM. Systematic review of randomized controlled trials comparing intracapsular tonsillectomy with total tonsillectomy in a pediatric population. Arch Otolaryngol Head Neck Surg. 2012; 138(3):243–249

[66] Windfuhr JP, Savva K, Dahm JD, Werner JA. Tonsillotomy: facts and fiction. Eur Arch Otorhinolaryngol. 2015; 272(4):949–969

[67] Bergler WF. Argon plasma coagulation (APC) surgery in otorhinolaryngology. Surg Technol Int. 2003; 11:79–84

[68] Maddern BR. Electrosurgery for tonsillectomy. Laryngoscope. 2002; 112(8 Pt 2 Suppl 100):11–13

[69] Temple RH, Timms MS. Paediatric coblation tonsillectomy. Int J Pediatr Otorhinolaryngol. 2001; 61(3):195–198

[70] Kuhle S, Urschitz MS, Eitner S, Poets CF. Interventions for obstructive sleep apnea in children: a systematic review. Sleep Med Rev. 2009; 13(2):123–131

[71] Wiatrak BJ, Willging JP. Harmonic scalpel for tonsillectomy. Laryngoscope. 2002; 112(8 Pt 2 Suppl 100):14–16

[72] Koltai PJ, Solares CA, Mascha EJ, Xu M. Intracapsular partial tonsillectomy for tonsillar hypertrophy in children. Laryngoscope. 2002; 112(8 Pt 2 Suppl 100):17–19

[73] Eviatar E, Kessler A, Shlamkovitch N, Vaiman M, Zilber D, Gavriel H. Tonsillectomy vs. partial tonsillectomy for OSAS in children–10 years post-surgery follow-up. Int J Pediatr Otorhinolaryngol. 2009; 73(5):637–640

[74] Grindle CR, Murray RC, Chennupati SK, Barth PC, Reilly JS. Incidence of revision adenoidectomy in children. Laryngoscope. 2011; 121(10):2128–2130

[75] Johnson LB, Elluru RG, Myer CM III. Complications of adenotonsillectomy. Laryngoscope. 2002; 112(8 Pt 2 Suppl 100):35–36

[76] Konstantinopoulou S, Gallagher P, Elden L, et al. Complications of adenotonsillectomy for obstructive sleep apnea in school-aged children. Int J Pediatr Otorhinolaryngol. 2015; 79(2):240–245

[77] Bonuck KA, Freeman K, Henderson J. Growth and growth biomarker changes after tonsillectomy: systematic review and meta-analysis. Arch Dis Child 2009:94:83–91.

[78] Wise MS, Nichols CD, Grigg-Damberger MM, et al. Executive summary of respiratory indications for polysomnography in children: an evidence-based review. Sleep. 2011; 34(3): 389–398

[79] Truong MT, Woo VG, Koltai PJ. Sleep endoscopy as a diagnostic tool in pediatric obstructive sleep apnea. Int J Pediatr Otorhinolaryngol. 2012; 76(5):722–727

[80] Fishman G, Zemel M, DeRowe A, Sadot E, Sivan Y, Koltai PJ. Fiberoptic sleep endoscopy in children with persistent obstructive sleep apnea: inter-observer correlation and comparison with awake endoscopy. Int J Pediatr Otorhinolaryngol. 2013; 77(5):752–755

[81] Tagaya M, Nakata S, Yasuma F, et al. Children with severe or moderate obstructive sleep apnoea syndrome show a high incidence of persistence after adenotonsillectomy. Acta Otolaryngol. 2012; 132(11):1208–1214

[82] Stradling JR, Thomas G, Warley AR, Williams P, Freeland A. Effect of adenotonsillectomy on nocturnal hypoxaemia, sleep disturbance, and symptoms in snoring children. Lancet. 1990; 335(8684):249–253

[83] Ali NJ, Pitson D, Stradling JR. Sleep disordered breathing: effects of adenotonsillectomy on behaviour and psychological functioning. Eur J Pediatr. 1996; 155(1):56–62

[84] Nieminen P, Tolonen U, Löppönen H. Snoring and obstructive sleep apnea in children: a 6-month follow-up study. Arch Otolaryngol Head Neck Surg. 2000; 126(4):481–486

[85] Montgomery-Downs HE, Crabtree VM, Gozal D. Cognition, sleep and respiration in at-risk children treated for obstructive sleep apnoea. Eur Respir J. 2005; 25(2):336–342

[86] Chervin RD, Ruzicka DL, Giordani BJ, et al. Sleep-disordered breathing, behavior, and cognition in children before and after adenotonsillectomy. Pediatrics. 2006; 117(4):e769–e778

[87] Coticchia JM, Yun RD, Nelson L, Koempel J. Temperature-controlled radiofrequency treatment of tonsillar hypertrophy for reduction of upper airway obstruction in pediatric patients. Arch Otolaryngol Head Neck Surg. 2006; 132(4):425–430

[88] Tauman R, Gulliver TE, Krishna J, et al. Persistence of obstructive sleep apnea syndrome in children after adenotonsillectomy. J Pediatr. 2006; 149(6):803–808

[89] Mitchell RB, Kelly J. Outcome of adenotonsillectomy for obstructive sleep apnea in obese and normal-weight children. Otolaryngol Head Neck Surg. 2007; 137(1):43–48

[90] Dillon JE, Blunden S, Ruzicka DL, et al. DSM-IV diagnoses and obstructive sleep apnea in children before and 1 year after adenotonsillectomy. J Am Acad Child Adolesc Psychiatry. 2007; 46(11):1425–1436

[91] Gozal D, Capdevila OS, Kheirandish-Gozal L. Metabolic alterations and systemic inflammation in obstructive sleep apnea among nonobese and obese prepubertal children. Am J Respir Crit Care Med. 2008; 177(10):1142–1149

[92] Chiu PH, Ramar K, Chen KC, et al. Can pillar suturing promote efficacy of adenotonsillectomy for pediatric OSAS? A prospective randomized controlled trial. Laryngoscope. 2013; 123(10): 2573–2577

[93] Villa MP, Castaldo R, Miano S, et al. Adenotonsillectomy and orthodontic therapy in pediatric obstructive sleep apnea. Sleep Breath. 2014; 18(3):533–539

[94] Kuo YL, Kang KT, Chiu SN, Weng WC, Lee PL, Hsu WC. Blood pressure after surgery among obese and nonobese children with obstructive sleep apnea. Otolaryngol Head Neck Surg. 2015; 152(5):931–940

[95] Tang A, Benke JR, Cohen AP, Ishman SL. Influence of tonsillar size on OSA improvement in children undergoing adenotonsillectomy. Otolaryngol Head Neck Surg. 2015; 153(2):281–285

[96] Brietzke SE, Gallagher D. The effectiveness of tonsillectomy and adenoidectomy in the treatment of pediatric obstructive sleep apnea/hypopnea syndrome: a meta-analysis. Otolaryngol Head Neck Surg. 2006; 134(6):979–984

[97] Friedman M, Wilson M, Lin HC, Chang HW. Updated systematic review of tonsillectomy and adenoidectomy for treatment of pediatric obstructive sleep apnea/hypopnea syndrome. Otolaryngol Head Neck Surg. 2009; 140(6):800–808

[98] Huang YS, Guilleminault C, Lee LA, Lin CH, Hwang FM. Treatment outcomes of adenotonsillectomy for children with obstructive sleep apnea: a prospective longitudinal study. Sleep. 2014; 37(1):71–76

[99] Gozal D, Kheirandish-Gozal L, Serpero LD, Sans Capdevila O, Dayyat E. Obstructive sleep apnea and endothelial function in school-aged nonobese children: effect of adenotonsillectomy. Circulation. 2007; 116(20):2307–2314

[100] Section on Pediatric Pulmonology, Subcommittee on Obstructive Sleep Apnea Syndrome. American Academy of Pediatrics. Clinical practice guideline: diagnosis and management of childhood obstructive sleep apnea syndrome. Pediatrics. 2002; 109(4):704–712

[101] Wooten CT, Shott SR. Evolving therapies to treat retroglossal and base-of tongue obstruction on pediatric obstructive sleep apnea. Arch Otolaryngol Head Neck Surg. 2010; 136:938–7

[102] Prager JD, Hopkins BS, Propst EJ, Shott SR, Cotton RT. Oropharyngeal stenosis: a complication of multilevel, single-stage upper airway surgery in children. Arch Otolaryngol Head Neck Surg. 2010; 136(11):1111–1115

[103] Leong SC, Kubba H, White PS. A review of outcomes following inferior turbinate reduction surgery in children for chronic nasal obstruction. Int J Pediatr Otorhinolaryngol. 2010; 74(1):1–6

[104] Seid AB, Martin PJ, Pransky SM, Kearns DB. Surgical therapy of obstructive sleep apnea in children with severe mental insufficiency. Laryngoscope. 1990; 100(5):507–510

[105] Lin AC, Koltai PJ. Persistent pediatric obstructive sleep apnea and lingual tonsillectomy. Otolaryngol Head Neck Surg. 2009; 141(1):81–85

[106] Wootten CT, Shott SR. Evolving therapies to treat retroglossal and base-of-tongue obstruction in pediatric obstructive sleep apnea. Arch Otolaryngol Head Neck Surg. 2010; 136(10):983–987

[107] Mase CA, Chen ML, Horn DL, Parikh SR. Supraglottoplasty for sleep endoscopy diagnosed sleep dependent laryngomalacia. Int J Pediatr Otorhinolaryngol. 2015; 79(4):511–515

[108] Bouchard C, Troulis MJ, Kaban LB. Management of obstructive sleep apnea: role of distraction osteogenesis. Oral Maxillofac Surg Clin North Am. 2009; 21(4):459–475

[109] Tahiri Y, Viezel-Mathieu A, Aldekhayel S, Lee J, Gilardino M. The effectiveness of mandibular distraction in improving airway obstruction in the pediatric population. Plast Reconstr Surg. 2014; 133(3):352e–359e

[110] Taylor BA, Brace M, Hong P. Upper airway outcomes following midface distraction osteogenesis: a systematic review. J Plast Reconstr Aesthet Surg. 2014; 67(7):891–899

[111] Kremer B, Botos-Kremer AI, Eckel HE, Schlöndorff G. Indications, complications, and surgical techniques for pediatric tracheostomies–an update. J Pediatr Surg. 2002; 37(11):1556–1562

[112] Cohen SR, Suzman K, Simms C, Burstein FD, Riski J, Montgomery G. Sleep apnea surgery versus tracheostomy in children: an exploratory study of the comparative effects on quality of life. Plast Reconstr Surg. 1998; 102(6):1855–1864

[113] Costa DJ, Mitchell R. Adenotonsillectomy for obstructive sleep apnea in obese children: a meta-analysis. Otolaryngol Head Neck Surg. 2009; 140(4):455–460

[114] Sanders JC, King MA, Mitchell RB, Kelly JP. Perioperative complications of adenotonsillectomy in children with obstructive sleep apnea syndrome. Anesth Analg. 2006; 103(5):1115–1121

[115] Biavati MJ, Manning SC, Phillips DL. Predictive factors for respiratory complications after tonsillectomy and adenoidectomy in children. Arch Otolaryngol Head Neck Surg. 1997; 123(5):517–521

[116] Coté CJ. Anesthesiological considerations for children with obstructive sleep apnea. Curr Opin Anaesthesiol. 2015; 28 (3):327–332

Recommended Readings

Amin R, Anthony L, Somers V, et al. Growth velocity predicts recurrence of sleep-disordered breathing 1 year after adenotonsillectomy. Am J Respir Crit Care Med. 2008; 177(6):654–659

Marcus CL, Moore RH, Rosen CL, et al. Childhood Adenotonsillectomy Trial (CHAT). A randomized trial of adenotonsillectomy for childhood sleep apnea. N Engl J Med. 2013; 368(25):2366–2376

7 Nose

Abstract

The impact of treating nasal obstruction in patients with obstructive sleep apnea (OSA) is still discussed controversially. This might be related to the ambivalent results of nasal treatments in regard to restorative sleep (very positive effect) on one hand and its influence on the severity of OSA (almost no effect) on the other hand.

Both conservative and surgical nasal treatments result in significant improvement of the quality of sleep. Patient's sleep is more restorative with huge impact on several quality-of-life parameters.

In contrast, the impact of nasal treatments on the severity of OSA is very limited. Probably, the nose does not play a significant role in the pathogenesis of OSA.

However, there are preliminary data that suggest that nasal surgeries may facilitate or enable nasal ventilation therapy.

Keywords: nose, sleep apnea, quality of life, restorative sleep, nasal surgery

7.1 Introduction

Thomas Verse

The physiological breathing route during sleep is through the nose. Less than 10% of individuals breathe through their mouths.[1,2,3] Therefore, impaired nasal breathing is accused to cause sleep-disordered breathing (SDB). In 1581, Lemnious described unquiet sleep caused by mouth breathing at night.[4] The first book dealing with the topic, *The Breath of Life*, was published by Catlin in 1861. The second edition, *Shut Your Mouth and Save Your Life*, describes the benefits of unhindered nasal breathing much better than the first one. The first case report describing an increase of daytime alertness after nasal septoplasty was already published in 1892.[5] Since that time a correlation between snoring and nasal obstruction has been reported frequently,[6,7] although this correlation does not seem to be very strong.

7.2 Pathophysiology

Thomas Verse

7.2.1 Nasal Breathing during Wakefulness

The nasal resistance (Rn) during quiet nasal breathing is about 50 to 60% of the resistance of the whole upper airway.[8] In other words, during sleep, the nose contributes the biggest part to the total resistance of the entire upper airway. This is even more essential as the nose represents the physiological breathing route in adults. In a study with 10 healthy volunteers, the oral fraction of inhaled ventilation was only 8% whereas the nasal fraction was 92%.[9]

Body posture has a substantial effect on Rn during wakefulness. Rn increases from the sitting to the lying body position, with even 10% change in body posture leading to significant changes in Rn. In patients with underlying nasal pathology such as allergic or infectious rhinitis these differences are even more distinctive.[10]

7.2.2 Nasal Breathing during Sleep

There is no difference in Rn during sleep as compared to wakefulness.[11] However, the resistance of the entire upper airway increases significantly during sleep. This indicates that the resistance of other parts of the upper airway must increase during sleep. During sleep the biggest part of the resistance of the entire upper airway is located in the pharyngeal segments. This means that relevant changes in airway patency and resistance during sleep occur within the pharynx and not within the nose.

7.2.3 Theories, How an Increase in Nasal Resistance Can Induce Airway Collapse

There are four theories concerning this question and all of them are discussed in the subsequent text.

Starling Resistor

First of all, an increase in Rn does contribute to the total resistance of the upper airway, regardless of the fact that Rn during sleep is not as important as during the awake state. Therefore, the increase in total upper airway resistance is not very strong but existing.

In contrast to the nose, the larynx and the trachea, there are no bony and cartilaginous structures in the pharynx, which can protect airway patency. This is the reason why the pharynx may act like a Starling resistor. An increased preload in terms of an increased Rn may increase the suction force, leading to pharyngeal obstruction. Trials using single-sides nasal dressings were able to induce apneas in healthy volunteers. However, the total number of induced apneas was not adequate to induce clinically relevant obstructive sleep apnea (OSA).[12,13,14]

Another study used allergic rhinitis as a more physiological model for partial nasal obstruction. Sleep studies conducted during and out of pollen season showed significantly more apneas during pollen season.[15] Again the results were statistically significant, but in absolute numbers (apnea index 0.7 vs. 1.7) the effect was too little to induce a clinical significant OSA.

Against this background partial nasal obstruction is more likely able to worsen a preexisting OSA than to trigger it by itself.

Switch to Oral Breathing

In case of complete nasal obstruction, a switch to oral breathing is necessary. As seen in healthy subjects, mouth opening increases the critical closing pressure of the upper airway and thus enables airway obstruction.[16] In other words, mouth breathing is the less stable breathing route. Besides that, upper airway resistance during sleep is higher in mouth breathing as compared to nasal breathing.[17] In a study conducted by Zwillich et al, 2 out of 10 healthy subjects developed a clinically significant OSA after nasal packing on both sides, whereas there was almost no change in the remaining 8 subjects.[18] Obviously there seems to be a subgroup of patients (20% in this study), in which the switch from nasal to oral breathing generates OSA, while in the majority of patients nothing happens. In the cited study those subjects developed OSA, who already showed a few apneas with unblocked noses.

Drop Out of Nasal Reflexes

Nasal reflexes mediated by the trigeminal nerve are assumed to maintain upper airway patency. It has been shown several times that both central and obstructive apneas occur after the use of local anesthesia within the nose.[19,20] The study of White et al describes the occurrence of severe OSA in 3 out of 10 healthy subjects after local anesthesia.[19] The other 7 subjects did not show any effect at all. Using placebo instead of local anesthesia, no patient developed OSA.

Again there seems to be a subgroup of patients in which nasal reflexes seem to play an important role in maintaining upper airway patency, whereas this correlation cannot be shown in the majority of subjects.

Nitric Oxygen

A significant amount of nitric oxygen (NO) is produced within the nose and especially within the paranasal sinuses, and from here it mixes with the inspired air depending on the intensity of nasal breathing.[21] NO is a potent bronchial dilator and increases the oxygen content of the blood.[22] In addition, NO is thought to have several functions such as keeping up the muscular tone, neuromuscular control of the pharynx, breathing stimulation, and regulation of sleep. So far, the role of NO in the pathogenesis of OSA has not been understood well enough to give a final conclusion about it.

To sum it up, nasal obstruction indeed seems to be associated with snoring and apneas. However, a distinct correlation between the severity of OSA and the amount of nasal obstruction could not have been found so far.[23] In short, the nose contributes only little or in few individuals to the pathogenesis of OSA.

7.3 Conservative Treatment of the Nose

Thomas Verse

7.3.1 Drugs

Nasal Decongestives

Two studies investigating the effects of xylometazoline[24,25] did not show any changes in apnea–hypopnea index (AHI) as compared to placebo, although Rn is significantly decreased in the xylometazoline groups. The earlier study reported a subjective improvement on the quality of sleep.[24] In contrast the more recent study did not find any effect of xylometazoline on the quality of sleep.[25]

Topical Corticosteroids

Topical corticosteroids improve both the subjective and the objective quality of sleep, and daytime performance in patients with allergic rhinitis.[26,27,28] In doing so, the improvement of subjective parameters correlates with objective nasal patency.

A randomized crossover trial included 13 patients with OSA. Each patient was treated for 4 weeks with local fluticasone and for another 4 weeks with placebo. An objective sleep study was done after each treatment section.[29] After treatment with fluticasone the AHI decreased from 30.3 ± 31.9 at baseline to 23.3 ± 21.3, whereas there was no effect after placebo treatment. Once again, a subgroup of two patients benefitted strongly from the fluticasone treatment, while the other patients showed little or no effect.

Another randomized, controlled, crossover study compared the effects of a tramazoline plus dexamethasone nasal spray versus placebo in 21 sleep apneics without subjectively impaired nasal breathing.[30] Treatment was given for 1 week each. A sleep study and a rhinoresistometry were performed at the beginning and at the end of each treatment period. The authors described a significant reduction of Rn, and several breathing parameters in the verum group as compared to placebo. In the verum group the AHI decreased from 31.1 at baseline to 25.0 after treatment. Figures for placebo were 31.1 and 29.8, respectively.

In contrast, a third randomized controlled trial (RCT) comparing fluticasone and placebo did not show any differences between the two treatments.[26]

The RCT done by Craig et al indicated that topical corticosteroids are able to reduce the AHI in adults immediately. The amount of reduction is low, and long-term data are currently not available.

Nasal Dilators

There are external and internal nasal dilators (▶Fig. 7.1). ▶Table 7.1 summarizes current data from objective polysomnographies (PSGs). Altogether there are data about

194 cases. A significant effect of nasal dilators on AHI cannot be seen so far.

Two of the studies cited in ▶ Table 7.1 also provide subjective data concerning daytime sleepiness.[31,32] In both studies the Epworth Sleepiness Score (ESS) was significantly reduced when the patients used nasal dilators as compared to baseline without dilators, although there was no change in AHI.

7.4 Nasal Surgery

Thomas Verse

Indications, Contraindications, and Patient Selection

As this book is about the specific surgical treatment of OSA and not about nasal surgery in general, this chapter will be restricted to specific sleep medical issues. For other information (i.e., diagnostic workup, specific risks, patient information, anesthesia and positioning, equipment, operative techniques, complications, and postoperative care) please refer to specialist literature.

Any surgery for SDB requires a preoperative objective sleep study to identify the severity of disease. Without preoperative sleep study, the effect of surgery on AHI cannot be determined. Sometimes surgery may even worsen the AHI. In case of a persistent OSA after surgery, the surgeon has no chance to prove the effect of his/her surgery without having the results of a preoperative sleep study. This issue may become relevant in medicolegal affairs.

Apart from this, the preoperative arrangements of nasal surgery in sleep apnea patients do not differ from nasal surgery in any other patient population.

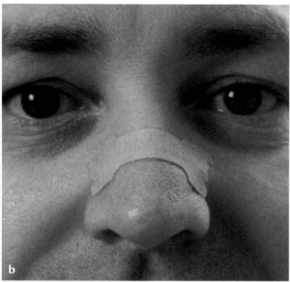

Fig. 7.1 (a) Internal and (b) external nasal dilators.

▶ Table 7.1 Influence of internal and external nasal dilators on AHI

Authors	Dilator	N	AHI with	AHI without	P value	EBM
Höijer et al (1992)[33]	Internal	10	18	6.4	0.008	3b
Metes et al (1992)[34]	Internal	10	46	44	NS	4
Kerr et al (1992)[24]	Internal + ND	10	64.9	63.2	NS	4
Hoffstein et al (1993)[35]	Internal	15	35.4	33.9	NS	4
Wenzel et al (1997)[36]	External	30	38.1	40	NS	3b
Todorova et al (1998)[37]	External	30	26.2	24.1	NS	4
Bahammam et al (1999)[38]	External	12	8.9	7.4	NS	1b
Gosepath et al (1999)[39]	External	26	26.3	31.7	0.031	4
Schönhofer et al (2000)[31]	Internal	21	37.4	36.1	NS	4
Djupesland et al (2001)[40]	External	18	12.2	9.3	<0.05	4
Amaro et al (2012)[32]	External	12	38	39	NS	3b
All		194	30.93	30.28		B

Abbreviations: AHI, apnea–hypopnea index; EBM: evidence-based medicine; ND: nasal decongestive; NS, not significant.

Postoperative Care

In case of nasal surgery the severity of OSA has significant impact on postoperative care and monitoring. This is why sleep apnea patients undergoing surgery under general anesthesia or sedation are generally at an increased risk for perioperative complications.[41,42,43] This perioperative risk is particularly increased if the OSA is treated surgically, as postoperative bleeding, swelling, and nasal packings need to be taken into account.

There are two publications dealing with specific complications after nasal surgery with nasal packings in patients with OSA.[44,45] All patients were kept in the recovery room for several hours. All complications occurred within the first few hours after surgery. This is why it is recommended to monitor all patients in the recovery room for 4 hours postoperative. If no complications are seen during this period, the patient is safe to shift to the regular ward. Vice versa, if complications occur, the patient should be monitored overnight.[46]

7.4.1 Nasal Surgery for Snoring

Thomas Verse

This book is about the treatment of OSA. However, many patients expect their simple snoring to be cured or substantially decreased after nasal surgery. This is why the issue will be covered briefly.

Outcomes

Snoring is a subjective complaint. Its disturbing character not only depends on its physical sound intensity, but also on psychoacoustic parameters such as roughness, sharpness, and loudness.[47] In addition, the perception of snoring depends on multiple parameters concerning the patient's bed-partner such as sleep quality, hearing impairment, psychological characteristics, and others. This is why the annoyance of snoring is difficult to measure in an objective way. As a consequence, there are almost no reliable data about the objective impact of nasal surgery on snoring, which could have been summarized at this point.

Considering that the nose is almost never the origin of snoring sounds, the authors made the experience, that there are much more effective surgeries in other parts of the upper airway to treat simple snoring than nasal surgeries. Actually, the majority of patients do not or only hardly benefit from nasal surgeries in terms of reduction of snoring frequency or intensity. As a consequence, authors recommend performing nasal surgeries to treat snoring without any other complaints. As stated in Chapter 7.4.2, nasal surgery has a lot of positive effects on sleep quality, recovery during sleep, and daytime symptoms in patients with nasal pathologies. Thus, we perform nasal surgery in patients with objective nasal

pathologies and/or in patients with either nonrestorative sleep and/or subjectively impaired nasal breathing.

If a patient only snores without any of the symptoms mentioned earlier, we recommend a topodiagnosis (e.g., drug-induced sleep endoscopy) to detect the site of generation of snoring sounds in order to identify a more successful kind of surgery.

7.4.2 Nasal Surgery for Obstructive Sleep Apnea

Thomas Verse

Outcomes

Altogether 30 studies have been identified, which include 772 patients with pre- and postoperative objective sleep studies before and after isolated nasal surgery in patients with OSA. Out of these studies four are case series. ►Table 7.2 summarizes the current available data. Out of these 30 studies, only 5 showed significant changes in AHI after nasal surgery. For the entire group of 772 patients the mean AHI decreased, not significantly, from 33.3 at baseline to 30.4 after nasal surgery. In other words, nasal surgery has either very limited or no effect on OSA severity. Accordingly, we did not see any effect of additional nasal surgery in our group of 70 patients (N = 52 without vs. N = 18 with additional nasal surgery), who underwent multilevel surgery for OSA.[78] In this context, the only RCT is of particular interest.[63] The study compared a surgical group (N = 27) with a placebo group (sham operation; N = 22). There were no significant changes in AHI in both groups. Significant changes were seen only in the surgical group, namely reduction of Rn seated and in supine position, reduction of the Epworth Sleepiness Scale (ESS) score, and an increase in nasal breathing.

In the vast majority of cases it does not seem possible to significantly reduce the AHI with nasal surgery alone. Accordingly, several other reviews concerning this topic report the same result.[79,80,81]

In contrast to the AHI, the respiratory disturbance index (RDI) seems to be affected by nasal surgery. The RDI is calculated as the number of apneas, hypopneas, plus respiratory-related arousals per hour of sleep. In other words, the RDI is at least as high as the AHI, but mostly higher. Two case series present RDI data.[59,76] Both studies describe a significant reduction of RDI, namely 39.0 to 29.1[59] and 28.8 to 17.1,[76] respectively. As heterogeneity between the two studies is low, the results seem reliable. In conclusion, nasal surgery may be able to reduce respiratory related arousals in patients with OSA.

Focusing on subjective outcome parameters, nasal surgeries show huge effects. All in all, 14 studies (N = 361 patients; ►Table 7.2) provide data concerning daytime sleepiness as measured with the ESS. In mean the ESS score fell from 10.9 before to 7.0 after nasal surgery,

▶ **Table 7.2** Effect of isolated nasal surgery in sleep apnea patients on AHI and ESS

Author	N	Follow-up (months)	AHI pre	AHI post	P value	ESS pre	ESS post	EBM
Rubin et al (1983)[48]	9	1–6	37.8	26.7	<0.05	No data	No data	4
Dayal and Phillipson (1985)[49]	6	4–44	46.8	28.2	NS	No data	No data	4
Caldarelli et al (1985)[50]	23	No data	44.2	41.5	NS	No data	No data	4
Aubert-T et al (1989)[51]	2	2–3	47.5	48.5	-	No data	No data	4
Sériès et al (1992)[52]	20	2–3	39.8	36.8	NS	No data	No data	4
Sériès et al (1993)[53]	14	2–3	17.8	16	NS	No data	No data	4
Utley et al (1997)[54]	4	No data	11.9	27	-	7.8	6.8	4
Verse et al (1998)[55]	2	3–4	14	57.7	-	6	12	4
Friedman et al (2000)[56]	22	>1.5	31.6	39.5	NS	No data	No data	4
Kalam (2002)[57]	21	No data	14	11	<0.05	No data	No data	4
Verse et al (2002)[58]	26	3–50	31.6	28.9	NS	11.9	7.7	4
Kim et al (2004)[59]	21	1	39[a]	29[a]	<0.0001	No data	No data	4
Balcerzak et al (2004)[60]	22	2	48.1	48.8	NS	No data	No data	4
Nakata et al (2005)[61]	12	No data	55.9	47.8	NS	11.7	3.3	4
Virkkula et al (2006)[62]	40	2–6	13.6	14.9	NS	No data	No data	4
Koutsourelakis et al (2008)[63]	27	3–4	31.5	31.5	NS	13.4	11.7	2b
Li et al (2008)[64]	51	3	37.4	38.1	NS	10.0	8.0	4
Nakata et al (2008)[65]	49	No data	49.6	42.5	NS	10.6	4.5	4
Morinaga et al (2009)[66]	35	No data	43.5	38.6	NS	No data	No data	4
Tosun et al (2009)[67]	27	3	6.7	5.6	NS	9.4	4.1	4
Li et al (2009)[68]	44	3	36.4	37.5	NS	10.6	7.6	3b
Bican et al (2010)[69]	20	3	43.1	24.6	<0.05	17.1	11.1	4
Choi et al (2011)[70]	22	3	28.9	26.1	NS	8.8	6.3	4
Sufioğlu et al (2012)[71]	28	3	32.5	32.4	NS	9.3	5.9	4
Victores and Takashima (2012)[72]	24	3	23.6	20.4	NS	12.3	6.6	4
Hu B et al (2013)[73]	79	6	27.7	26.3	NS	No data	No data	3b
Poirier et al (2014)[74]	11	6	33.2	29.4	NS	No data	No data	4
Yalamanchali et al (2014)[75]	56	1.5	33.5	29.4	NS	No data	No data	4
Park et al (2014)[76]	25	2	23.9	12.2	<0.05	9.7	5.8	4
Xiao Y et al (2016)[77]	30	3	49.7	43.1	<0.05	No data	No data	3b
All	772	1–44	33.34	30.42		10.91	6.95	B

Abbreviations: AHI, apnea–hypopnea index; EBM, evidence-based medicine; ESS, Epworth Sleepiness Scale; NS, not significant; RDI, respiratory disturbance index.
[a]In the study of Kim et al (2004) only RDI data are given.

indicating a significant reduction of daytime sleepiness in these patients. A review published by Li and colleagues described similar data.[79]

Other publications report a highly significant improvement of quality-of-life parameters after isolated nasal surgery in sleep apnea patients, using the "Snore Outcome Survey"[64] or the "SF-36."[82] A recent study investigated 61 sleep apneics before, and 3 months after nasal surgery using the NOSE-questionnaire, the Pittsburgh Sleep Quality Index, and other questionnaires.[83] The patients benefited in all dimensions measured.

To sum it up, isolated nasal surgery has various measurably subjective benefits in sleep apnea patients resulting in a more restorative sleep. However, the severity of OSA as defined in AHI can only be reduced in single cases.

7.4.3 Nasal Surgery to Improve Positive Airway Pressure Treatments

Annemieke Beelen, Linda B.L. Benoist, and Nico de Vries

Nasal surgery is an accepted treatment among sleep medical scientists to enable or facilitate nasal positive airway pressure (PAP) treatments in patients with nasal pathology.[84] Preliminary data show a decrease in effective continuous positive airway pressure (CPAP) after nasal surgery of approximately 2 mbar (▶Table 7.3). Unfortunately, data in ▶Table 7.3 are taken from uncontrolled case series. This means that data of higher evidence might change this assessment in future.

Introduction

PAP is a generally accepted treatment for patients with moderate to severe OSA. PAP was introduced in 1981 by Sullivan and has since been proven as the most effective treatment for patients with OSA in reducing the AHI. PAP is also effective in improving quality of life and reducing daytime sleepiness.[95,107] See also Chapter 4 for PAP treatments.

PAP creates a pneumatic splint in the upper airway, preventing it from collapsing during sleep. The effectiveness of this therapy is dependent upon its ability to overcome airway collapse (efficacy) as well as the time over which a patient uses it during sleep (compliance).[95,108]

These two components, efficacy and compliance, are used to calculate the mean disease alleviation (MDA) which serves as a measure of the overall therapeutic effectiveness.[109]

The MDA for PAP treatments shows that a lack of compliance results in a reduced therapeutic effectiveness.

Compliance in Positive Airway Pressure Treatments

It is a clinical reality that the compliance rate is poor in PAP treatment for OSA. Crawford et al described that about 25% of patients do not take up CPAP or discontinue in the first 2 weeks. Furthermore, for long-term use (longer than 1 month), adequate compliance can vary from 46 to 89%. Adequate compliance can be defined as more than 4 hours of use on 70% of the nights.[92,103,110] In short, PAP is a treatment with high efficacy, but with low compliance. This is in contrast with oral appliances with moderate efficacy and high compliance. Sutherland et al showed that CPAP (high efficacy and low compliance) and oral appliances (moderate efficacy and high compliance) could, in theory, result in similar profiles of treatment effectiveness.[108] It can be stated that compliance in the PAP treatment is a significant component of the overall treatment effectiveness.

There are various reasons for discontinuing the treatment or poor compliance. These include nasal congestion, rhinorrhea, epistaxis, dryness of the mouth and nose, aerophagia, and skin irritation. Other problems reported include mask discomfort, mask leakage, claustrophobia, the inconvenience of being connected to a machine, less intimacy with the bed partner, difficulty in falling asleep, frequent nocturnal awakenings, lack of symptomatic benefit, intolerance of high expiratory pressure, costs not covered by health insurance, and the noise of the device.[99,102,103,110]

Pressure Levels in Positive Airway Pressure

In patients who are willing to try CPAP, pressure is titrated to reduce the individual patient's AHI to fewer than 5 events per hour. Pressure level requirements for CPAP may vary over time due to several factors such as nasal congestion, change in weight, use of medication or alcohol, changes in jaw position, the cyclic alternating pattern of sleep stages, or body position. Also of influence is the duration of the CPAP treatment.[98,99,100,102,106]

To sum up, we can state that a properly functioning nasal passage is important for both treatment compliance and lowering the pressure levels needed. A reduced nasal passage, due to hypertrophy of the inferior nasal turbinates is generally taken to be one of the common reasons for poor compliance in PAP treatment. Nasal decongestives and topical corticosteroids are indicated to enhance a poor nasal passage caused by hypertrophy of the inferior nasal turbinates (see Chapter 7.1). In patients with nasal obstruction due to allergic rhinitis, studies have shown that topical corticosteroids improved both subjective and objective quality of sleep and performance during the day.[26,27,28] However, in cases where topical corticosteroids are not sufficiently effective, alternative treatments to reduce the swelling of the inferior turbinates are indicated.

Nasal Surgery to Improve Positive Airway Pressure

Although nasal surgery is not first-line treatment of OSA itself, it is widely accepted as adjunctive measure in case of problems with CPAP due to impaired nasal passage.[84] Preliminary data show a decrease in effective CPAP after nasal surgery of approximately 2 mbar (▶Table 7.3). Unfortunately, the data in ▶Table 7.3 are taken from uncontrolled case series. This means that data of higher evidence might change this assessment in the future.

Invasive nasal surgery is not the treatment of choice, as in most cases it is performed under general anesthesia with its associated risks. Furthermore, invasive nasal surgeries are associated with more serious complications and often require the use of nasal packs postoperatively. The ideal treatment would be a patient-friendly procedure that can be performed on an outpatient basis under local anesthesia, does not involve nasal packs, has no serious complications, and has a continued long-term effect.

▶ Table 7.3 Effect of isolated nasal surgery on effective CPAP

Author	N	CPAP pre (cm H$_2$O)	CPAP post (cm H$_2$O)	P value	EBM
Mayer-Brix et al (1989)[85]	3	9.7	6	No data	4
Friedman et al (2000)[56]	6	9.3	6.7	<0.05	4
Dorn et al (2001)[86]	5	11.8	8.6	<0.05	4
Masdon et al (2004)[87]	35	9.7	8.9	NS	4
Nakata et al (2005)[61]	5	16.8	12	<0.05	4
Zonato et al (2006)[88]	17	12.4	10.2	<0.001	4
Sufioğlu et al (2012)[71]	28	11.2	10.4	NS	4
Poirier et al (2014)[74]	18	11.9	9.2	NS	4
All	117	11.2	9.4		C

Abbreviations: CPAP, continuous positive airway pressure; EBM, evidence-based medicine; NS, not significant.

Radiofrequency-Induced Thermotherapy

Submucosal radiofrequency-induced thermotherapy (RFITT) is a treatment that can be used to improve nasal passage using a minimally invasive procedure to shrink turbinate volume. Several studies have shown that mucociliary function also remains intact with RFITT.[90,93,97,105] In contrast to more invasive surgical turbinate reduction methods, RFITT can be performed in an outpatient setting under local anesthesia and without nasal packing, therefore reducing the burden of nasal packs, adverse side-effects, and the risks associated with general anesthesia.[91] Besides the technical feasibility of the treatment, when using it in clinical practice it is important to also consider the tolerance and experience of the patient. A number of studies have already reported on the long-term effects of RFITT.[94,101,104] Radiofrequency ablation has been shown to be an efficient, easy to use technique which does not lead to serious complications in the treatment of the nasal obstruction caused by inferior turbinate hypertrophy.[93,96]

The Surgical Procedure

Before the procedure, the nose is anesthetized with cotton pads moistened with xylometazoline/tetracaine (10%). After 30 minutes, the cottons pads should be removed and this is followed by a local injection of lidocaine 1%/adrenaline (1:200,000) in the inferior turbinates. The bipolar coagulation applicator (Celon ProBreath*; see ▶Fig 7.1) is inserted via the anterior side of the inferior turbinate until the mucous membrane at the posterior end. The applicator is activated in the posterior part at a power setting of 15 W. To obtain coagulation over the entire length of the inferior turbinate, the applicator is retracted about 1 cm in posterior-anterior direction and the procedure is repeated four times. The end of each coagulation is indicated by a high-pitched audio signal. The procedure is repeated on the other side. Following the procedure, patients are observed for about 1 hour and are discharged if no side effects such as bleeding occurred.

*For this procedure, the authors used a Celon ProBreath Olympus applicator and the associated radiofrequency generator (Celon LabENT).

Key Points

- Sleep does not affect the nose but the pharynx, leading to an enormous increase in collapsibility of the pharyngeal segments of the upper airway. In other words, the nose is neither the site of obstruction during an apnea nor the site of generation of snoring sounds, and therefore PSG parameters hardly correlate with nasal parameters.[89]
- Neither conservative nor surgical improvement of nasal breathing has significant impact on AHI. Preliminary data indicate that nasal surgery may reduce the frequency of respiratory-related arousals in OSA patients.
- In contrast, improvement of nasal breathing has significant impact on quality-of-life parameters as it improves sleep quality and its restorative function.
- Nasal treatments seem justified, if a patient is subjectively suffering from his/her disturbed nasal breathing and/or if daytime sleepiness is present that cannot be treated otherwise.
- In addition, nasal surgery can enable or facilitate PAP treatments.

References

[1] Niinimaa V, Cole P, Mintz S, Shephard RJ. Oronasal distribution of respiratory airflow. Respir Physiol. 1981; 43(1):69–75

[2] Ogura JH. Presidential address. Fundamental understanding of nasal obstruction. Laryngoscope. 1977; 87(8):1225–1232

[3] Rodenstein DO, Stănescu DC. The soft palate and breathing. Am Rev Respir Dis. 1986; 134(2):311–325

[4] Lemnious L. The touchstone of complexions. London; 1581

[5] Catlin CL. The effects of intra-nasal obstruction on the general health. Med Surg Rep. 1892; 67:259–260

[6] Stradling JR, Crosby JH. Predictors and prevalence of obstructive sleep apnoea and snoring in 1001 middle aged men. Thorax. 1991; 46(2):85–90

[7] Deegan PC, McNicholas WT. Predictive value of clinical features for the obstructive sleep apnoea syndrome. Eur Respir J. 1996; 9(1):117–124

[8] Ferris BG, Jr, Mead J, Opie LH. Partitioning of respiratory flow resistance in man. J Appl Physiol. 1964; 19:653–658

[9] Fitzpatrick MF, Driver HS, Chatha N, Voduc N, Girard AM. Partitioning of inhaled ventilation between the nasal and oral routes during sleep in normal subjects. J Appl Physiol (1985). 2003; 94(3):883–890

[10] Rundcrantz H. Postural variations of nasal patency. Acta Otolaryngol. 1969; 68(5):435–443

[11] Douglas NJ, White DP, Pickett CK, Weil JV, Zwillich CW. Respiration during sleep in normal man. Thorax. 1982; 37(11):840–844

[12] Lavie P, Fischel N, Zomer J, Eliaschar I. The effects of partial and complete mechanical occlusion of the nasal passages on sleep structure and breathing in sleep. Acta Otolaryngol. 1983; 95(1–2):161–166

[13] Suratt PM, Turner BL, Wilhoit SC. Effect of intranasal obstruction on breathing during sleep. Chest. 1986; 90(3):324–329

[14] Miljeteig H, Hoffstein V, Cole P. The effect of unilateral and bilateral nasal obstruction on snoring and sleep apnea. Laryngoscope. 1992; 102(10):1150–1152

[15] McNicholas WT, Tarlo S, Cole P, et al. Obstructive apneas during sleep in patients with seasonal allergic rhinitis. Am Rev Respir Dis. 1982; 126(4):625–628

[16] Meurice JC, Marc I, Carrier G, Sériès F. Effects of mouth opening on upper airway collapsibility in normal sleeping subjects. Am J Respir Crit Care Med. 1996; 153(1):255–259

[17] Fitzpatrick MF, McLean H, Urton AM, Tan A, O'Donnell D, Driver HS. Effect of nasal or oral breathing route on upper airway resistance during sleep. Eur Respir J. 2003; 22(5):827–832

[18] Zwillich CW, Pickett C, Hanson FN, Weil JV. Disturbed sleep and prolonged apnea during nasal obstruction in normal men. Am Rev Respir Dis. 1981; 124(2):158–160

[19] White DP, Cadieux RJ, Lombard RM, Bixler EO, Kales A, Zwillich CW. The effects of nasal anesthesia on breathing during sleep. Am Rev Respir Dis. 1985; 132(5):972–975

[20] McNicholas WT, Coffey M, McDonnell T, O'Regan R, Fitzgerald MX. Upper airway obstruction during sleep in normal subjects after selective topical oropharyngeal anesthesia. Am Rev Respir Dis. 1987; 135(6):1316–1319

[21] Djupesland PG, Chatkin JM, Qian W, et al. Aerodynamic influences on nasal nitric oxide output measurements. Acta Otolaryngol. 1999; 119(4):479–485

[22] Blitzer ML, Lee SD, Creager MA. Endothelium-derived nitric oxide mediates hypoxic vasodilation of resistance vessels in humans. Am J Physiol. 1996; 271(3 Pt 2):H1182–H1185

[23] Leitzen KP, Brietzke SE, Lindsay RW. Correlation between nasal anatomy and objective obstructive sleep apnea severity. Otolaryngol Head Neck Surg. 2014; 150(2):325–331

[24] Kerr P, Millar T, Buckle P, Kryger M. The importance of nasal resistance in obstructive sleep apnea syndrome. J Otolaryngol. 1992; 21(3):189–195

[25] Clarenbach CF, Kohler M, Senn O, Thurnheer R, Bloch KE. Does nasal decongestion improve obstructive sleep apnea? J Sleep Res. 2008; 17(4):444–449

[26] Craig TJ, Mende C, Hughes K, Kakumanu S, Lehman EB, Chinchilli V. The effect of topical nasal fluticasone on objective sleep testing and the symptoms of rhinitis, sleep, and daytime somnolence in perennial allergic rhinitis. Allergy Asthma Proc. 2003; 24(1):53–58

[27] Hughes K, Glass C, Ripchinski M, et al. Efficacy of the topical nasal steroid budesonide on improving sleep and daytime somnolence in patients with perennial allergic rhinitis. Allergy. 2003; 58(5):380–385

[28] Stuck BA, Czajkowski J, Hagner AE, et al. Changes in daytime sleepiness, quality of life, and objective sleep patterns in seasonal allergic rhinitis: a controlled clinical trial. J Allergy Clin Immunol. 2004; 113(4):663–668

[29] Kiely JL, Nolan P, McNicholas WT. Intranasal corticosteroid therapy for obstructive sleep apnoea in patients with co-existing rhinitis. Thorax. 2004; 59(1):50–55

[30] Koutsourelakis I, Minaritzoglou A, Zakynthinos G, Vagiakis E, Zakynthinos S. The effect of nasal tramazoline with dexamethasone in obstructive sleep apnoea patients. Eur Respir J. 2013; 42(4):1055–1063

[31] Schönhofer B, Franklin KA, Brünig H, Wehde H, Köhler D. Effect of nasal-valve dilation on obstructive sleep apnea. Chest. 2000; 118(3):587–590

[32] Amaro ACS, Duarte FHG, Jallad RS, Bronstein MD, Redline S, Lorenzi-Filho G. The use of nasal dilator strips as a placebo for trials evaluating continuous positive airway pressure. Clinics (Sao Paulo). 2012; 67(5):469–474

[33] Höijer U, Ejnell H, Hedner J, Petruson B, Eng LB. The effects of nasal dilation on snoring and obstructive sleep apnea. Arch Otolaryngol Head Neck Surg. 1992; 118(3):281–284

[34] Metes A, Cole P, Hoffstein V, Miljeteig H. Nasal airway dilation and obstructed breathing in sleep. Laryngoscope. 1992; 102(9):1053–1055

[35] Hoffstein V, Mateika S, Metes A. Effect of nasal dilation on snoring and apneas during different stages of sleep. Sleep. 1993; 16(4):360–365

[36] Wenzel M, Schönhofer B, Siemon K, Köhler D. [Nasal strips without effect on obstructive sleep apnea and snoring] Pneumologie. 1997; 51(12):1108–1110

[37] Todorova A, Schellenberg R, Hofmann HC, Dimpfel W. Effect of the external nasal dilator Breathe Right on snoring. Eur J Med Res. 1998; 3(8):367–379

[38] Bahammam AS, Tate R, Manfreda J, Kryger MH. Upper airway resistance syndrome: effect of nasal dilation, sleep stage, and sleep position. Sleep. 1999; 22(5):592–598

[39] Gosepath J, Amedee RG, Romantschuck S, Mann WJ. Breathe Right nasal strips and the respiratory disturbance index in sleep related breathing disorders. Am J Rhinol. 1999; 13(5):385–389

[40] Djupesland PG, Skatvedt O, Borgersen AK. Dichotomous physiological effects of nocturnal external nasal dilation in heavy snorers: the answer to a rhinologic controversy? Am J Rhinol. 2001; 15(2):95–103

[41] Vasu TS, Grewal R, Doghramji K. Obstructive sleep apnea syndrome and perioperative complications: a systematic review of the literature. J Clin Sleep Med. 2012; 8(2):199–207

[42] Bahammam A, Delaive K, Ronald J, Manfreda J, Roos L, Kryger MH. Health care utilization in males with obstructive sleep apnea syndrome two years after diagnosis and treatment. Sleep. 1999; 22(6):740–747

[43] McNicholas WT, Ryan S. Obstructive sleep apnoea syndrome: translating science to clinical practice. Respirology. 2006; 11(2):136–144

[44] Kezirian EJ, Weaver EM, Yueh B, Khuri SF, Daley J, Henderson WG. Risk factors for serious complication after uvulopalatopharyngoplasty. Arch Otolaryngol Head Neck Surg. 2006; 132(10):1091–1098

[45] Regli A, von Ungern-Sternberg BS, Strobel WM, Pargger H, Welge-Luessen A, Reber A. The impact of postoperative nasal packing on sleep-disordered breathing and nocturnal oxygen saturation in patients with obstructive sleep apnea syndrome. Anesth Analg. 2006; 102(2):615–620

[46] Rösslein M, Bürkle H, Walther A, Stuck BA, Verse T. [Position Paper: perioperative management of adult patients with obstructive sleep apnea in ENT surgery] Laryngorhinootologie. 2015; 94(8):516–523

[47] Rohrmeier C, Herzog M, Haubner F, Kuehnel TS. The annoyance of snoring and psychoacoustic parameters: a step towards an objective measurement. Eur Arch Otorhinolaryngol. 2012; 269(5):1537–1543

[48] Rubin AHE, Eliaschar I, Joachim Z, Alroy G, Lavie P. Effects of nasal surgery and tonsillectomy on sleep apnea. Bull Eur Physiopathol Respir. 1983; 19(6):612–615

[49] Dayal VS, Phillipson EA. Nasal surgery in the management of sleep apnea. Ann Otol Rhinol Laryngol. 1985; 94(6 Pt 1):550–554

[50] Caldarelli DD, Cartwright RD, Lilie JK. Obstructive sleep apnea: variations in surgical management. Laryngoscope. 1985; 95(9 Pt 1):1070–1073

[51] Aubert-Tulkens G, Hamoir M, Van den Eeckhaut J, Rodenstein DO. Failure of tonsil and nose surgery in adults with long-standing severe sleep apnea syndrome. Arch Intern Med. 1989; 149(9):2118–2121

[52] Sériès F, St Pierre S, Carrier G. Effects of surgical correction of nasal obstruction in the treatment of obstructive sleep apnea. Am Rev Respir Dis. 1992; 146(5 Pt 1):1261–1265

[53] Sériès F, St Pierre S, Carrier G. Surgical correction of nasal obstruction in the treatment of mild sleep apnoea: importance of cephalometry in predicting outcome. Thorax. 1993; 48(4):360–363

[54] Utley DS, Shin EJ, Clerk AA, Terris DJ. A cost-effective and rational surgical approach to patients with snoring, upper airway resistance syndrome, or obstructive sleep apnea syndrome. Laryngoscope. 1997; 107(6):726–734

[55] Verse T, Pirsig W, Kroker B. Obstruktive Schlafapnoe und verlegende Polyposis nasi. Laryngorhinootologie. 1998; 77(3): 150–152

[56] Friedman M, Tanyeri H, Lim JW, Landsberg R, Vaidyanathan K, Caldarelli D. Effect of improved nasal breathing on obstructive sleep apnea. Otolaryngol Head Neck Surg. 2000; 122(1): 71–74

[57] Kalam I. Objective assessment of nasal obstruction in snoring and obstructive sleep apnea patients: experience of a Police Authority Hospital. Ann Saudi Med. 2002; 22(3–4):158–162

[58] Verse T, Maurer JT, Pirsig W. Effect of nasal surgery on sleep-related breathing disorders. Laryngoscope. 2002; 112(1):64–68

[59] Kim ST, Choi JH, Jeon HG, Cha HE, Kim DY, Chung YS. Polysomnographic effects of nasal surgery for snoring and obstructive sleep apnea. Acta Otolaryngol. 2004; 124(3):297–300

[60] Balcerzak J, Przybyłowski T, Bielicki P, Korczyński P, Chazan R. [Functional nasal surgery in the treatment of obstructive sleep apnea]. [in Polish] Pneumonol Alergol Pol. 2004; 72(1–2):4–8

[61] Nakata S, Noda A, Yagi H, et al. Nasal resistance for determinant factor of nasal surgery in CPAP failure patients with obstructive sleep apnea syndrome. Rhinology. 2005; 43(4):296–299

[62] Virkkula P, Bachour A, Hytönen M, et al. Snoring is not relieved by nasal surgery despite improvement in nasal resistance. Chest. 2006; 129(1):81–87

[63] Koutsourelakis I, Georgoulopoulos G, Perraki E, Vagiakis E, Roussos C, Zakynthinos SG. Randomised trial of nasal surgery for fixed nasal obstruction in obstructive sleep apnoea. Eur Respir J. 2008; 31(1):110–117

[64] Li HY, Lee LA, Wang PC, Chen NH, Lin Y, Fang TJ. Nasal surgery for snoring in patients with obstructive sleep apnea. Laryngoscope. 2008; 118(2):354–359

[65] Nakata S, Noda A, Yasuma F, et al. Effects of nasal surgery on sleep quality in obstructive sleep apnea syndrome with nasal obstruction. Am J Rhinol. 2008; 22(1):59–63

[66] Morinaga M, Nakata S, Yasuma F, et al. Pharyngeal morphology: a determinant of successful nasal surgery for sleep apnea. Laryngoscope. 2009; 119(5):1011–1016

[67] Tosun F, Kemikli K, Yetkin S, Ozgen F, Durmaz A, Gerek M. Impact of endoscopic sinus surgery on sleep quality in patients with chronic nasal obstruction due to nasal polyposis. J Craniofac Surg. 2009; 20(2):446–449

[68] Li HY, Lee LA, Wang PC, Fang TJ, Chen NH. Can nasal surgery improve obstructive sleep apnea: subjective or objective? Am J Rhinol Allergy. 2009; 23(6):e51–e55

[69] Bican A, Kahraman A, Bora I, Kahveci R, Hakyemez B. What is the efficacy of nasal surgery in patients with obstructive sleep apnea syndrome? J Craniofac Surg. 2010; 21(6):1801–1806

[70] Choi JH, Kim EJ, Kim YS, et al. Effectiveness of nasal surgery alone on sleep quality, architecture, position, and sleep-disordered breathing in obstructive sleep apnea syndrome with nasal obstruction. Am J Rhinol Allergy. 2011; 25(5):338–341

[71] Sufioğlu M, Ozmen OA, Kasapoglu F, et al. The efficacy of nasal surgery in obstructive sleep apnea syndrome: a prospective clinical study. Eur Arch Otorhinolaryngol. 2012; 269(2):487–494

[72] Victores AJ, Takashima M. Effects of nasal surgery on the upper airway: a drug-induced sleep endoscopy study. Laryngoscope. 2012; 122(11):2606–2610

[73] Hu B, Han D, Li Y, Ye J, Zang H, Wang T. Polysomnographic effect of nasal surgery on positional and non-positional obstructive sleep apnea/hypopnea patients. Acta Otolaryngol. 2013; 133(8):858–865

[74] Poirier J, George C, Rotenberg B. The effect of nasal surgery on nasal continuous positive airway pressure compliance. Laryngoscope. 2014; 124(1):317–319

[75] Yalamanchali S, Cipta S, Waxman J, Pott T, Joseph N, Friedman M. Effects of endoscopic sinus surgery and nasal surgery in patients with obstructive sleep apnea. Otolaryngol Head Neck Surg. 2014; 151(1):171–175

[76] Park CY, Hong JH, Lee JH, et al. Clinical effect of surgical correction for nasal pathology on the treatment of obstructive sleep apnea syndrome. PLoS One. 2014; 9(6):e98765

[77] Xiao Y, Han D, Zang H, Wang D. The effectiveness of nasal surgery on psychological symptoms in patients with obstructive sleep apnea and nasal obstruction. Acta Otolaryngol. 2016; 136(6):626–632

[78] Verse T, Baisch A, Maurer JT, Stuck BA, Hörmann K. Multilevel surgery for obstructive sleep apnea: short-term results. Otolaryngol Head Neck Surg. 2006; 134(4):571–577

[79] Li HY, Wang PC, Chen YP, Lee LA, Fang TJ, Lin HC. Critical appraisal and meta-analysis of nasal surgery for obstructive sleep apnea. Am J Rhinol Allergy. 2011; 25(1):45–49

[80] Rombaux P, Liistro G, Hamoir M, et al. Nasal obstruction and its impact on sleep-related breathing disorders. Rhinology. 2005; 43(4):242–250

[81] Georgalas C. The role of the nose in snoring and obstructive sleep apnoea: an update. Eur Arch Otorhinolaryngol. 2011; 268(9):1365–1373

[82] Li HY, Lin Y, Chen NH, Lee LA, Fang TJ, Wang PC. Improvement in quality of life after nasal surgery alone for patients with obstructive sleep apnea and nasal obstruction. Arch Otolaryngol Head Neck Surg. 2008; 134(4):429–433

[83] Stapleton AL, Chang YF, Soose RJ, Gillman GS. The impact of nasal surgery on sleep quality: a prospective outcomes study. Otolaryngol Head Neck Surg. 2014; 151(5):868–873

[84] Verse T, Hörmann K. The surgical treatment of sleep-related upper airway obstruction. Dtsch Arztebl Int. 2011; 108(13):216–221

[85] Mayer-Brix J, Müller-Marschhausen U, Becker H, Peter JH. Wie häufig sind pathologische HNO-Befunde bei Patienten mit obstruktivem Schlaf-Apnoe-Syndrom? HNO. 1989; 37(12):511–516

[86] Dorn M, Pirsig W, Verse T. Postoperatives Management nach rhinochirurgischen Eingriffen bei schwerer obstruktiver Schlafapnoe. Eine Pilotstudie. HNO. 2001; 49(8):642–645

[87] Masdon JL, Magnuson JS, Youngblood G. The effects of upper airway surgery for obstructive sleep apnea on nasal continuous positive airway pressure settings. Laryngoscope. 2004; 114(2):205–207

[88] Zonato AI, Bittencourt LR, Martinho FL, Gregório LC, Tufik S. Upper airway surgery: the effect on nasal continuous positive airway pressure titration on obstructive sleep apnea patients. Eur Arch Otorhinolaryngol. 2006; 263(5):481–486

[89] Hoffstein V, Chaban R, Cole P, Rubinstein I. Snoring and upper airway properties. Chest. 1988; 94(1):87–89

[90] Bäck LJ, Hytönen ML, Malmberg HO, Ylikoski JS. Submucosal bipolar radiofrequency thermal ablation of inferior turbinates: a long-term follow-up with subjective and objective assessment. Laryngoscope. 2002; 112(10):1806–1812

[91] Cavaliere M, Mottola G, Iemma M. Comparison of the effectiveness and safety of radiofrequency turbinoplasty and traditional surgical technique in treatment of inferior turbinate hypertrophy. Otolaryngol Head Neck Surg. 2005; 133(6): 972–978

[92] Crawford MR, Espie CA, Bartlett DJ, Grunstein RR. Integrating psychology and medicine in CPAP adherence–new concepts? Sleep Med Rev. 2014; 18(2):123–139

[93] Coste A, Yona L, Blumen M, et al. Radiofrequency is a safe and effective treatment of turbinate hypertrophy. Laryngoscope. 2001; 111(5):894–899

[94] Cukurova I, Demirhan E, Cetinkaya EA, Yigitbasi OG. Long-term clinical results of radiofrequency tissue volume reduction for inferior turbinate hypertrophy. J Laryngol Otol. 2011; 125(11):1148–1151

[95] Giles TL, Lasserson TJ, Smith BJ, White J, Wright J, Cates CJ. Continuous positive airways pressure for obstructive sleep apnoea in adults. Cochrane Database Syst Rev. 2006(1):CD001106

[96] Kezirian EJ, Powell NB, Riley RW, Hester JE. Incidence of complications in radiofrequency treatment of the upper airway. Laryngoscope. 2005; 115(7):1298–1304

[97] Means C, Camacho M, Capasso R. Long-term outcomes of radiofrequency ablation of the inferior turbinates. Indian J Otolaryngol Head Neck Surg. 2016; 68(4):424–428

[98] Oksenberg A, Silverberg DS, Arons E, Radwan H. The sleep supine position has a major effect on optimal nasal continuous positive airway pressure: relationship with rapid eye movements and non-rapid eye movements sleep, body mass index, respiratory disturbance index, and age. Chest. 1999; 116(4):1000–1006

[99] Olsen S, Smith S, Oei TPS. Adherence to continuous positive airway pressure therapy in obstructive sleep apnoea sufferers: a theoretical approach to treatment adherence and intervention. Clin Psychol Rev. 2008; 28(8):1355–1371

[100] Pevernagie DA, Shepard JW, Jr. Relations between sleep stage, posture and effective nasal CPAP levels in OSA. Sleep. 1992; 15(2):162–167

[101] Porter MW, Hales NW, Nease CJ, Krempl GA. Long-term results of inferior turbinate hypertrophy with radiofrequency treatment: a new standard of care? Laryngoscope. 2006; 116(4):554–557

[102] Ravesloot MJ, de Vries N. Reliable calculation of the efficacy of non-surgical and surgical treatment of obstructive sleep apnea revisited. Sleep. 2011; 34(1):105–110

[103] Richard W, Venker J, den Herder C, et al. Acceptance and long-term compliance of nCPAP in obstructive sleep apnea. Eur Arch Otorhinolaryngol. 2007; 264(9):1081–1086

[104] Safiruddin F, Vroegop AV, Ravesloot MJ, de Vries N. Long-term self-reported treatment effects and experience of radiofrequency-induced thermotherapy of the inferior turbinates performed under local anesthesia: a retrospective analysis. Eur Arch Otorhinolaryngol. 2012

[105] Sapçi T, Sahin B, Karavus A, Akbulut UG. Comparison of the effects of radiofrequency tissue ablation, CO_2 laser ablation, and partial turbinectomy applications on nasal mucociliary functions. Laryngoscope. 2003; 113(3):514–519

[106] Sériès F, Marc I. Importance of sleep stage- and body position-dependence of sleep apnoea in determining benefits to auto-CPAP therapy. Eur Respir J. 2001; 18(1):170–175

[107] Sullivan CE, Issa FG, Berthon-Jones M, Eves L. Reversal of obstructive sleep apnoea by continuous positive airway pressure applied through the nares. Lancet. 1981; 1(8225):862–865

[108] Sutherland K, Phillips CL, Cistulli PA. Efficacy versus effectiveness in the treatment of obstructive sleep apnea: CPAP and oral appliances. Journal of Dental Sleep Medicine. 2015; 2(4):175–181

[109] Vanderveken OM, Dieltjens M, Wouters K, De Backer WA, Van de Heyning PH, Braem MJ. Objective measurement of compliance during oral appliance therapy for sleep-disordered breathing. Thorax. 2013; 68(1):91–96

[110] Weaver Terri E, Ronald R. Grunstein, Adherence to Continuous Positive Airway Pressure Therapy the Challenge to Effective Treatment, Proceedings of the American Thoracic Society Vol 5 2008

Recommended Reading

Verse T, Wenzel S. [Treating nasal obstruction in obstructive sleep apnea patients] HNO. 2016:64

8 Surgery in Adults

Abstract

This chapter starts with minimally invasive surgery of the palate, palatal implants, and stiffening procedures. Then the various current invasive palatal procedures, including tonsils, are presented. Thereafter, current techniques for the base of tongue, including implants and transoral robotic surgery, are discussed. Subsequently, hyoid bone surgeries, genioglossal advancement, hypoglossal nerve stimulation, surgery for larynx and trachea, maxillofacial surgery, distraction osteogenesis maxillary expansion, and multilevel surgery are discussed in detail. Indications and contraindications, patient selection, diagnostic workup, risks, patient information, consent, anesthesia and positioning, surgical technique, complications, and postoperative care are discussed for each technique.

Keywords: palalal surgery, base of tongue surgery, hypoglossal nerve stimulation, maxillofacial surgery

8.1 Minimally Invasive Surgery

8.1.1 Interstitial Radiofrequency in the Soft Palate

Marc Blumen

Definition and Principle

Interstitial radiofrequency is a minimally invasive technique that was introduced in sleep surgery by the Stanford team in 1996. Powell and Riley were looking for a safe technique to treat the tongue and possibly reduce the tongue volume. They met the CEO of a company that commercialized radiofrequency tissue ablation applied to other tissues than pharyngeal, in particular prostatic tissues. This meeting sets the point for radiofrequency development in sleep surgery. They first experienced radiofrequency ablation in vitro on a beef tongue then in vivo on porcine tongues. As the results were satisfactory in terms of safety and efficacy, experience went on humans quite fast thereafter.

Interstitial radiofrequency uses the same principle as electrocautery but with different frequency waves. It uses low-frequency waves, between 300 and 4,000 KHz delivered by a generator through an electrode. These waves induce two types of lesion, mainly thermal but also electrical.

Low-frequency waves produce a molecular agitation, responsible for a heating around the electrode. The heat is going to induce lesions at the level of the cellular membrane, the cytoskeleton, the cellular metabolism, and the nucleus. All these phenomenons create a coagulative necrotic lesion which has an elliptic circumscribed submucosal shape. This lesion leads to scar formation.

Several studies evaluated the effects of interstitial radiofrequency on pharyngeal tissue, especially the soft palate and the tongue.

The first study on the effects of radiofrequency was on porcine tongues which evaluated the treatment effects by piezoelectric sensors placed around the treatment area. The authors observed after 10 days a 26.3% reduction in tongue volume.[1] The effects of radiofrequency on human tissues remain controversial. The volume reduction is not always found in the studies. Stuck et al did not find any volume reduction[2] and Blumen et al did find a reduction but only in some patients.[3] Powell et al in the first study in mankind on soft palate showed that there was retraction of the uvula on lateral cephalometry.[4]

The main action seems to be linked to the scaring process with rigidification and some kind of retraction of the treated tissue.

Radiofrequency to treat snoring or sleep apnea is used in different sites: soft palate, tongue base, inferior turbinates, and tonsils.

Indications, Contraindications, and Patient Selection

Indications are mainly as follows:
- Simple snoring when the soft palate is believed to be the vibrating site.
- Mild, and in some cases, moderate obstructive sleep apnea syndrome (OSAS) in case the soft palate is believed to be the obstruction site mostly due to excessive compliance.

There are no absolute contraindications. A pacemaker is a relative contraindication when the system uses a monopolar electrode.

In simple snoring, nasal obstruction or a long uvula may hinder good results.

In obstructive sleep apnea (OSA) vibration or obstruction of other sites than the ones treated, high body mass index (BMI) and high apnea–hypopnea index (AHI) (>30/h) are not good indications.

Diagnostic Workup

Radiofrequency does not need a specific preoperative workup.

In order to have good results in simple snoring, there is a need to carefully select the patient: evaluate the bed partner's quality of sleep and the reality of the burden caused by the snoring, try to determine the site of vibration by awake clinical examination and eventually during a drug-induced sleep endoscopy (DISE), and rule out a nasal obstruction possibly responsible for the snoring. It is of course mandatory to have a sleep study to rule out severe OSA, quantify the amount of snoring and determine if it is positional.

Specific Risks, Patient Information, and Consent

There are no specific risks.

The patient needs to be informed of a slight discomfort during 4 to 5 days after the procedure. The level of discomfort is far less than the postlaser or postsurgery pains[5] applied on the soft palate. Snoring is more pronounced during approximatively 10 days, but the maximum level is during the 48 first hours after the procedure; this is linked to the edematous tissue response. A foreign body sensation could be felt by the patient during the following weeks, generally due to a long uvula touching the tongue base. Pharyngeal dryness can occur but is rare.

Anesthesia and Positioning

The procedure is performed under local anesthesia, generally in a sitting position.

Equipment

Radiofrequency waves are delivered by a radiofrequency generator. There are several radiofrequency generators that deliver waves at different wave lengths. A study compared four different radiofrequency generators, which did not show any significant differences in terms of efficacy on snoring.[6]

The electrode through which the radiofrequency waves are delivered to the tissues can be either monopolar or bipolar. Some systems have a temperature retro control that controls the temperature at the tip of the electrode and the impedance in order to progressively deliver the energy, enabling the lesion to grow and widen as wished.

The electrode can be single use or resterilizable.

Operative Technique/Steps

The treatment is performed in a consultation room or in ambulatory operating room in a sitting position.

A local anesthesia is performed within the soft palate with norepinephrine and xylocaine 1%. Some practitioners ask their patients to gargle with contact anesthetics.

Doses injected depend on the soft palate thickness. It is recommended to blow up thin soft palate in order to increase the palate thickness to avoid heat diffusion at the surface of the soft palate, which induces mucosal lesions.

Local injections should be made first at the level of entry of the neurovascular bundles penetrating the soft palate (▶Fig. 8.1). After a couple of minutes, injections should be made to cover only the treated areas. There is no need to inject the uvula. The velar webs, if treated, should be injected at the top.

A tongue depressor should be used to isolate the soft palate from the tongue. It is preferable to have the patient breathe partially through his nose (if possible) in order to verticalize the soft palate.

The electrode is introduced perpendicularly to the surface of the soft palate, and then when the electrode is inside the soft palate, it should be tilted 45% to try to follow the soft palate curvature.

Before delivering the energy with a pedal, it is recommended to tilt back and forth the tip of the electrode to check it is still within the tissue.

If the tip is seen just underneath the mucosa, it is preferable to take it back a little and try to replace midway between the anterior and posterior surfaces of the soft palate. During energy delivery, if pain is felt in the neck, it means that the tip of the electrode has gone through the posterior surface of the soft palate into the posterior pharyngeal wall; this occurs when the posterior airway space (PAS) is small and when the patient is breathing through the mouth.

Several protocols have been described for the electrode placement. The original technique consists of three puncture deliveries:[4] one vertical and median and two high, slightly oblique laterally (▶Fig. 8.2). For each puncture, one lesion was created. The punctures are created high at the junction between the hard and soft palate. It is recommended not to make a puncture within the uvula (not make the tip of the electrode go further than 1 or 2 mm below the base of the uvula) because of a risk of major edema the following night and possible respiratory distress and/or uvula necrosis in the following weeks.

Other protocols were described using more punctures or more lesions per puncture (▶Fig. 8.3). Some articles

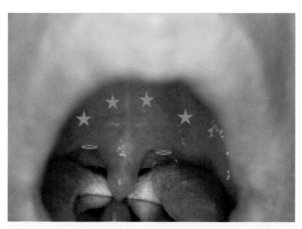

Fig. 8.1 Points of entry of local anesthesia injections.

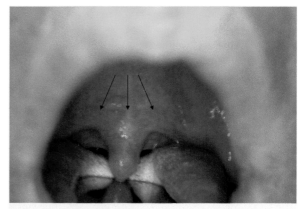

Fig. 8.2 Original technique: One (vertical) puncture in the midline and one puncture (oblique end outwards) on each side.

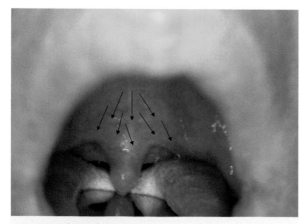
Fig. 8.3 Other technique: More punctures or more lesions per puncture. The goal is to treat the entire soft palate.

describe higher energy levels per puncture to try to increase the size of the lesion, and thus the scaring area. It seems logical to create as much scarring as possible to cover the entire soft palate, or at least theoretically cover the areas that vibrate and/or obstruct. It is difficult to know in practice what these areas are on an awake clinical examination. These areas are probably better assessed during a DISE.

Snoring vibrations are most often generated at the level of the soft palate, especially at its inferior border. Obstructions seem to occur along a median and vertical width of tissue but can also involve the entire soft palate starting at the hard–soft palate junction down to the inferior border of the soft palate. Hence, it seems logical to cover this region with radiofrequency lesions. If these regions are not well determined, it seems compulsory to cover the entire soft palate. According to the soft palate anatomy (long/short/wide/narrow), the number of punctures and lesions per puncture can be more or less.

Most often, three to five punctures and several lesions per puncture are necessary, taking great care not to overlap the lesions to avoid mucosal lesions.

The delay between two sessions is generally 6 to 8 weeks. This is to enable the scaring to take place and obtain a stiffer tissue.

Shorter delays may induce overtreatment in some patients. Longer delays between sessions do not seem to be problematic.

The inferior part of the soft palate is involved in palatal flutter and sometimes low velopharyngeal obstruction, thus section of the velar webbing and a significant shortening of the uvula with radiofrequency in the cutting mode could be added to interstitial radiofrequency with better results than interstitial radiofrequency alone.[7]

The number of treatment sessions is variable in the studies. In the earlier times, the authors would perform three or more sessions. With time, the surgeons tried to reduce the number of sessions. One study tried to determine the number of sessions required to reach

a satisfactory result. A minimum of three sessions were needed.[8]

Each puncture was followed by three lesions. The three sessions could probably cover the entire surface of the soft palate, but it could be covered in less than three sessions using more punctures or with a smaller soft palate.

One study[9] was published to determine if the results on snoring after the first session was predictive of the final results in two to three sessions with or without a uvula shortening, depending on the anatomy—after the first session, when the snoring volume reduced significantly, adding sessions enabled to satisfy 58% of the bed partners, whereas if the snoring volume did not decrease significantly only 38% of the bed partners were satisfied.

Risks, Tips, and Tricks

- When the technique is not performed well, or in case of a thin soft palate, it is visible on follow-up superficial mucosal lesions (erosions) or deep lesions (ulcerations and even perforations).
- In the earlier times, occurrence of mucosal lesions was high. Terris and Chen found an incidence of up to 60% of lesions.[10] More recently, these rates decreased drastically. Farrar et al,[11] in their meta-analysis, calculated a 2.4% of mucosal erosions, a 1.2% of perforations, and a 0.3% abscess occurrence—the local complication rate was 3.9%.
- To avoid lesions, one can treat the entire surface of the soft palate in two or three sessions to avoid puncture overlapping.
- Similarly, it is compulsory not to be too close to the anterior surface of the soft palate and to blow up the thickness of the soft palate, especially when it is thin, with local anesthetics.
- When the surgeon delivers the energy to the tissues, he/she must look for the occurrence of mucosal blanchening. If this is the case, energy delivery should be stopped and the electrode should not be withdrawn and placed at the same level and deeper—the risk being to create a deeper lesion and increase the risk of perforation.
- Superficial mucosal lesions heal in approximately 15 days and are associated with pain or great discomfort. Local care and analgesics can be given. Perforations on thick soft palate usually heal without a residual perforation, without having to put stiches. On thin soft palates, perforation can persist if nothing is done.

Complications

No persistent side effects regarding swallowing, voice, or speech were observed after performing interstitial radiofrequency.[12] No velar insufficiency, bleeding, or significant infections,[13] or pharyngeal stenosis were described.

Postoperative Care

Postoperative treatment is not compulsory. Analgesics can be prescribed. If a physician wants to make the patient comfortable, he/she could prescribe oral steroids on the first night.

Outcomes

Snoring

Radiofrequency of the soft palate was proven superior to placebo.[14] On a short-term basis (3 months), snoring intensity decreased significantly in all studies.[15,16] Adding UPP to radiofrequency increases the efficacy of radiofrequency[17] on snoring.

Radiofrequency efficacy decreases with time. Relapse occurs early: after 19 months, patients' snoring increased by more than twofold.[18] After 3 years, snoring relapsed from a postoperative score of 3.6 at 6 months to 5.6 (preoperative score 8.1). Only 25% of the patients were satisfied. After 6 years, there was a 92% relapse of the snoring sound but with a level inferior to preoperative (8.1 ± 2.9 to 3.5 ± 2.2 cm on a short term then increased to 5.7 ± 2.9 cm).[19]

Epworth score decreased significantly in 69% of the studies on radiofrequency on a short-term basis.[16]

Radiofrequency on the soft palate alone can decrease RDI in some patients with mild to moderate OSA.[20] A meta-analysis[21] showed a nonsignificant trend toward improvement of short-term mean RDI (RoM 0.67, 95%, CI 0.43–1.03, p = 0.07, I2 = 83%).

BMI is the most important general factor that influences results of radiofrequency on snoring.[16] Best results are obtained in patients with BMI less than 25 kg/m² and worst in those with BMI 30 kg/m².[22,23] A large or long uvula is a negative factor to treat snoring with radiofrequency alone.[24] On a long-term basis, sectioning the uvula preserves to a certain degree relapse.[19]

Among all factors studied (AHI, BMI, sex, age, snoring score, Epworth) that could influence results of radiofrequency on mild to moderate OSA, initial AHI is the one that could influence the greatest postoperative AHI in a normal weight population.[25]

Key Points

- Interstitial radiofrequency probably reduces tissue compliance but probably gives little volume reduction as well.
- If the surgeon thinks that the factor that induces airway collapse is an excessive compliance (no retrovelar narrow space during wakefulness, not a long palate, no other obstacles), without obesity nor severe sleep apnea, radiofrequency can be indicated, especially since it has low morbidity.
- Technically, there is a learning curve. One should pay attention to introduce the electrode at equal distance of the anterior and posterior surface of the soft palate. If the soft palate is thin, the surgeon should increase its thickness with infiltration. He/she should also be careful not to overlap the punctures to avoid mucosal lesions.
- Results on snoring are good. Nevertheless, long-term follow-up should have a high rate of relapse, which needs to be explained to the patient beforehand. Adding an uvulectomy increases the success rate.
- Results on mild and moderate OSA are acceptable if the patients are properly selected.

8.1.2 Palatal Implants and Other Stiffening Procedures

Marina Carrasco-Llatas

Introduction

As discussed in previous chapters of the book, in most patients, the main source of vibration of the upper airway, producing loud snoring, is the palate. This is why the idea of stiffening the palate, so it becomes more rigid and the vibration reduces, is so appealing. Nevertheless, one should always keep in mind that snoring could also originate at lateral pharyngeal walls (LPWs), tongue base, epiglottis, and even the posterior wall.[26] There are several procedures that aim at stiffening the palate, such as interstitial radiofrequency treatment (RFT) (see Section 8.1.1), but in this chapter we will cover various other options that have the same objective, so the reader can choose between them.

Along this chapter, injection snoreplasty (IS) and palatal implants (PIs) will be discussed. There is another technique called cautery-assisted palatal stiffening operation (CAPSO) that apparently has the same result. With CAPSO, a strip of palatal mucosa is removed and the palate is left to heal on secondary intention.[27] Nevertheless, the author believes that CAPSO is more painful and does not provide any benefit to PIs or IS, so CAPSO will not be discussed in detail in this section. In general, PIs and IS can help to reduce snoring but they are not as useful as conventional surgery in reducing AHI. Therefore, they should not be considered first-line therapy for patients with moderate to severe OSAS.

Injection Snoreplasty

Definition

IS means to inject, submucosally, a sclerosant agent that produces an aseptic inflammation with subsequent fibrosis, with the aim to stiffen the palate. It was first introduced by Brietzke and Mair in 2001 as an inexpensive and painless way to treat snoring.[28]

Brietzke and Mair used 3% sodium tetradecyl sulfate as sclerosant agent.[28] This drug is not easily available in some European countries. Thus, other agents have also been used. The agents that have proven efficacy in animal studies were ethanol 50% (mixing 1 mL of ethanol 99% and 1 mL of lidocaine)[29] and polidocanol 3%.[30] Its injection produces a submucosal fibrosis similar to the one obtained by radiofrequency[28,30] or CAPSO.[31]

Indications, Contraindications, and Patient Selection

This technique can be performed in patients with snoring, without OSAS, or in patients with mild OSAS, not obese, tonsil grade 0 or 1 with no evidence of tongue base obstruction in awake clinical exploration or DISE. Some authors have suggested to use IS as a treatment method previous to classical palatal surgery, arguing that if snoring is better after the injection, one can assume that the origin of the sound is the palate.[32]

It should not be performed in patients with moderate to severe OSAS or in patients with big tongues (modified Mallampati index 4). If the patient has a strong gag reflex, it might be difficult to perform the procedure under local anesthesia.

Although it has not been described in the literature, probably it is not useful in patients with long and thick uvulas. In such patients, it makes more sense to opt for techniques that shorten the uvula.

Diagnostic Workup

Previous diagnostic workup to perform IS includes a complete history and awake examination of the patient, or DISE, as well as a diagnostic sleep study.

Specific Risks, Patient Information, and Consent

This technique is performed in an outpatient basis, in the consulting room.

The procedure itself is easy, quick, and with little discomfort.

The most common complication is an ulceration of the mucosa at the injection point that, as a rule, heals within a week.

Patients should be warned that during the first few days snoring will get worse due to the inflammation of the palate. After the first week, it should be better. If snoring improves but not enough to achieve patient and bed partner satisfaction, the treatment can be repeated after 4 to 6 weeks.

Although there are no publications reporting results longer than 18 months, snoring can be expected to deteriorate over time, as it happens with other techniques such as RFT. Patient should be informed about this potential relapse of snoring.

Anesthesia and Positioning

To perform IS at least a topical anesthesia of the palate is necessary. The author also suggests local anesthesia of the palate so the sclerosant agent does not cause pain during the injection. The patient is seated, similar to the usual upper airway exploration.

Equipment

The only equipment needed is an insulin or tuberculin syringe with its needle. ▶ Fig. 8.4 shows the syringe used

by the author; as the syringe is slim, it can reach the palate, allowing a proper visualization. Nevertheless, it can contain only 1 mL of the sclerosant agent, so it has to be charged twice. Brietzke and Mair used a syringe with bent ¾-inch 27-gauge needle.

Operative Technique/Steps

1. Topical anesthesia of the palate with lidocaine 10 or 14% benzocaine sprays.
2. Local anesthesia (lidocaine or mepivacaine) of the soft palate at the hard–soft palate junction, so it does not mix with the sclerosant agent. Usually 1.5 to 2 mL of anesthetic agent is used, divided in three injection points. The first one is at the center of the hard–soft palate junction, and two more laterally in order to block the palatine nerves (▶ Fig. 8.5). Brietzke and Mair do not use local anesthesia instead they apply benzocaine gel (200 mg/gm) at the palate for 5 to 10 minutes.
3. Injection of 1 mL of the sclerosant agent at the center of the soft palate (submucosally), 1 cm above the uvula root (▶ Fig. 8.6). The sclerosant agent must form a blister under the mucosa. Muscular injection should not be performed.
4. Injection of 0.5 mL of the sclerosant agent at the sides of the palate, also submucosally. These lateral injections were originally described as the injection points in a second step, but they can be performed in the first injection day as well.

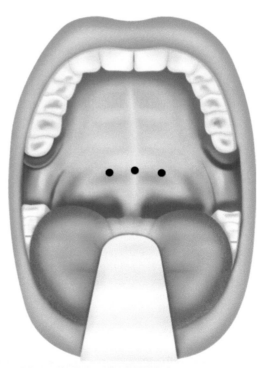

Fig. 8.5 Points of anesthesia injection.

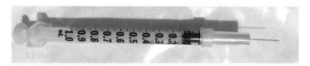

Fig. 8.4 Syringe used by the author for injection snoreplasty.

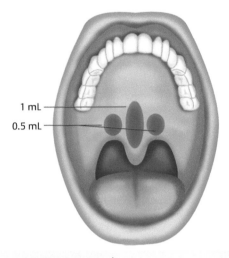
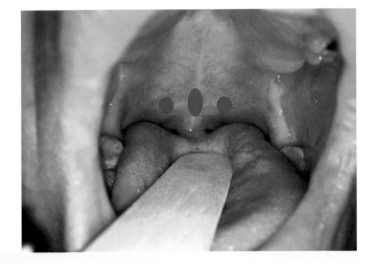

Fig. 8.6 Injection snoreplasty.

Complications

The most common complication is ulceration of the mucosa at the injection point that, if occurs, will heal without any specific care, in a short time. This ulceration can cause some pain and discomfort, but it is usually not a painful event (▶Fig. 8.7).[33]

Although it is not a complication, the patient should be informed that, due to the infiltration and the inflammation that will follow, snoring might be worse during the first few days (usually for 2–4 days). The patient will encounter more swelling if the injection is started closer to the base of the uvula, as the sclerosant agent will reach it. It is therefore important to inject 1 cm above the base of the uvula. This edema of the palate can cause some discomfort, but it does not cause any breathing problems.

The occurrence of an asymptomatic palatal fistula has been described. It also heals spontaneously in less than 6 weeks. It mostly occurs in patients with thin palates, usually women, with a frequency of 2.6%.[33]

Other possible secondary effects, due to the rigidity of the palate, can be a weird sensation when swallowing or pronouncing letters that elevate the palate. These effects are rare and more commonly observed if the procedure is performed in patients that had a previous palatal surgery to treat snoring or OSA.

Postoperative Care

The patient is advised to use painkillers such us ibuprofen, metamizol, or paracetamol in case of pain or discomfort.

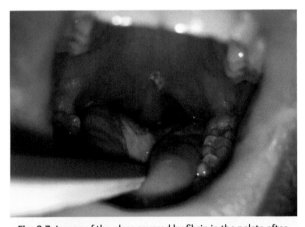

Fig. 8.7 Image of the ulcer covered by fibrin in the palate after injection snoreplasty, some edema of the posterior pillar can be seen too, despite the injection was not performed there, as the sclerosant agent moves down due to gravity. The ulcer heals without pain.

The level of pain is usually low, reaching a mean of 3.5 on a visual analog scale (VAS).[33] Antibiotics are not needed.

Outcomes

▶Fig. 8.8 shows outcome after IS. The fibrosis produced by the sclerosant agent can be seen over the uvula.

There are few articles published on IS; all of them are case series. One study compared IS with radiofrequency of the soft palate.[34] There are a few studies and it is not easy to merge them in a table because they use different objective and subjective scales. Therefore, the author will just comment on the main results.

The longest follow-up period was 19 months in 22 patients in the study by Brietzke and Mair.[33] There were no objective changes in mean AHI index (7.5/h pre to

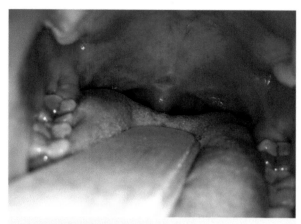

Fig. 8.8 Results after injection snoreplasty.

8.5/h post). No data about effect on the ESS were provided. Subjective improvement of snoring was 75%.

Olszewska et al followed up 21 patients for 6 months. Mean AHI did not change (4.6/h to 3.6/h). Sleepiness (e.g., ESS) decreased from 9 to 5 and snoring time decreased from a mean of 110 to 22 minutes during the polysomnography (PSG).[35]

Al-Jassim and Lesser found a subjective improvement on snoring in 62% of 60 patients after 1 year.[32]

Labra et al achieved a decrease in mean AHI from 14.5 to 4.1. The snoring index improved as well (14.9 to 20.4), ESS changed significantly from 9.6 to 8.2, in 11 patients after 6 months.[36]

Iseri and Balcioglu followed up 30 patients for 6 months; in VAS, snoring was reduced from 7.8 to 2.9. Subjective satisfaction with the procedure was 76.7%, comparable to radiofrequency.[34]

> ### Key Points
>
> Injecting submucosally in the center of the palate can be considered in simple snorers or patients with mild OSA (AHI < 15), nonobese patients who had tonsillectomy previously, or small tonsils and low Mallampati index.

Palatal Implants

Definition

PIs were first described in 2004 by Nordgard et al.[37] The implant itself is a segment of braided, polyethylene terephthalate (PET) woven yarns around 18-mm long with an outer diameter of 1.5 mm. Notable biological characteristics of PET include biostability, promotion of tissue ingrowth, and a well-characterized fibrotic response with fibrous capsule formation typically being complete by 4 weeks.[37] PIs were presented as a minimally invasive single-stage treatment without any need of specific or expensive equipment. The commercial name is Pillar, distributed by Medtronic.

Indications, Contraindications, and Patient Selection

PIs can be offered to simple snorers and patients with mild OSAS. Some authors use it as a second surgery to improve palatal snoring after failed uvulopalatopharyngoplasty (UPPP).[38]

There are anatomical factors to considerate before PIs. The soft palate length measured from the hard–soft palate junction to the base of the uvula is an important patient-selection criterion for implant insertion. A length of less than 24 mm is not recommended for 18-mm implant insertion, as more extrusions can be expected. Extrusion rate is higher in thin palates too. The uvular length, defined as the distance between the uvular base and tip, is another feature to consider, as the results in patients with a uvula longer than 15 mm are not as good compared to patients with shorter ones.[39] Tonsils should be grade 0, 1, or 2.

BMI is also important; patients should not be obese (BMI < 30).

Diagnostic Workup

As with IS, the previous diagnostic workup includes a complete history and awake examination of the patient (or DISE), as well as a diagnostic sleep study.

Specific Risks, Patient Information, and Consent

Although palatal infection has been described, the procedure is safe and the complication rate is low. The most frequent complication is partial extrusion of the implant(s) that forces to remove it. As in all procedures that address snoring, with time there is a relapse of snoring: the mean (standard deviation [SD]) preoperative score was 9.5 (0.5), mean week-52 score was 5.0 (1.6), and mean 4-year score was 7.0 (1.8).[40] Therefore, patients can expect relief from snoring, but it might recur over the years.

Although voice onset time for the letter "k" is shorter before implantation, no important changes on voice are to be expected.[41] Expected changes in patient's compliance to continuous positive airway pressure (CPAP) or in the CPAP pressure[42] or in swallowing function are not longer than 1 week.[43]

Pillar implantation induced changes in middle ear function up to 26.7% of the patients. Patients complained of otalgia or pressure feeling in the ear, however, the changes were temporary and not significant 1 week after surgery.[44]

Anesthesia and Positioning

The procedure is usually performed under local anesthesia. It can be performed under general anesthesia in case it is combined with other upper airway procedures (e.g., nasal surgery). Local anesthesia of the palate will produce swelling that will facilitate the implant insertion. To reduce the risk of bleeding, a mix of lidocaine or bupivacaine with adrenaline is recommended. Palatal local infiltration with anesthesia will reduce discomfort if performed after the topical one.

Equipment

The implants are provided by the manufacturer with the instrument designed for its insertion (▶Fig. 8.9). It is recommended to use fiberscope in order to check the correct position of the implants and that they do not extrude at the posterior part of the palate.

Operative Technique/Steps

1. Rinse the mouth with an antiseptic solution such as chlorhexidine.
2. Use topical and local anesthesia.
3. The mucosa of the soft palate is perforated in the midline about 5 mm distal to the trailing edge of the hard palate.
4. The insertion of the cannula must be through the muscular layer toward the base of the uvula until the insertion depth marker on the delivery tool reaches the insertion point.
5. A thumb slider on the handle is pulled down to retract the needle tip while an obturator housed within the needle maintains the position of the implant, leaving it in place when the delivery device is withdrawn from the tissue.
6. Two more implants are inserted on each side of the first one, approximately 2 mm away in order to create fibrosis bridges between them in order to obtain the best results (▶Fig. 8.10).
7. Check the correct insertion of the implants with the fiberscope and adjust the implant if it is not completely inside the muscular layer of the palate, or extrudes at the posterior side of the palate.

Complications

The most frequent complication is extrusion, which occurs approximately in 9.3% of the patients (range 0–25%).[43] Once a Pillar implant is extruding, it should be removed and a new one should be implanted. Extrusion rate is the highest during the first year, but has also been described during the second year.

Pain and foreign body sensation disappear, usually within the first week, and these symptoms are self-limiting. Pain level is very low; patients can return to normal life the next day. Mucosal ulcerations, fistulas, or infections have been rarely reported.[43] If any infection occurs, the implant should be removed.

Approximately 25% of the patients complain of otalgia or pressure feeling in the ear after implantation but these symptoms typically do not last longer than 1 week.[44]

Postoperative Care

Antibiotics are needed peri and postoperatively. Most of the authors recommend starting the same day as the surgery and continue for 4 more days (5 days of antibiotics).

Painkillers are prescribed in case of pain. Steroids are not needed and should be avoided to prevent infection.

Outcomes

Choi et al published a meta-analysis in which the articles published until March 2011 were reviewed. They included 363 OSA patients and 174 snorers. The meta-analysis showed that PIs reduced snoring, sleepiness, and AHI. Standardized mean difference (SMD) was –0.591 for snoring, –0.481 for sleepiness, and –0.378 for AHI. The common representation of the SMD is Cohen's d, which suggests that bigger size is more effective in clinically meaningful terms. An effect size (SMD) between two means within a range closely encompassing 0.20± is considered small (possibly clinically nonsignificant), 0.50± is considered a medium effect, and 0.80± or greater is considered large (and clinically significant).

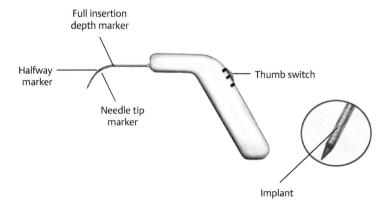

Fig. 8.9 Instrument to insert the palatal implants.

Full insertion depth marker

Halfway marker

Needle tip marker

Thumb switch

Implant

All these SMD are closer to 0.5, which is a moderate effect, but statistically significant. Therefore, we should consider that patients might still have loud snoring, daytime sleepiness, or high AHI after receiving the Pillar implants.[43]

Rotenberg and Luu reported subjective improvement, which deteriorated significantly over time, and was only minimally sustained at 4 years postoperatively.[40]

The results of different studies are summarized in ►Table 8.1.

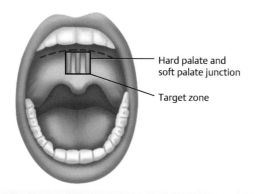

Fig. 8.10 Placement of the palatal implants.

Hard palate and soft palate junction

Target zone

Key Points
Select the patient properly—the patient should not be obese and should not have big uvula, large tonsils, short or thin palate, and moderate to severe OSA. Insert the implant 5 mm away from the junction of the hard–soft palate, in the middle of the palate, inside the muscular layer, and insert the instrument completely straight toward the uvula. The next two implants should be 2 mm apart on each side.

►**Table 8.1** Results of different articles on palatal implants

Author	N	Follow-up (months)	AHI (pre)	AHI (post)	Success (%)	ESS (pre)	ESS (post)	ESS (p)	EBM
Friedman et al[38]	23	6	33	26	21.7	13.2	8.7	< 0.0001	4
Friedman et al. 2006 Oto HNS	29	7.5	12.7	11.5	24.1	No data	No data	No data	3b
Walker et al. 2006 Oto HNS	53	3.0	25.0	22.0	20.8	11.0	6.9	< 0.001	4
Nordgard et al. 2006 Oto HNS, 565	25	3.0	16.2	12.1	36.0	9.7	5.5	< 0.001	4
Nordgard et al. 2007 Oto HNS	26	12.0	16.2	12.5	50.0	8.3	5.4	< 0.001	4
Goessler et al. 2007 Acta	16	3.0	16.5	11.2	37.5	7.2	4.6	<0.05	4
Walker et al. 2007 Oto HNS, 137: 822–7	22	14.5	19.7	18.3	59.1	11.7	8.4	No data	4
Friedman et al. 2008 Oto HNS	29	3.0	23.8	15.9	41.9	12.7	10.2	<0.001	2b
Steward et al. 2008 Oto HNS	47	3.0	16.8	19.7	26.0	10.6	8.7	<0.01	2b
Neruntarat 2011 Eur Arch Oto	92	26–32	21.7	10.8	52.2	12.3	7.9	<0.001	4
Huang et al. 2011 Laryngoscope	21	6.0	14.1	9.0	63.8	No data	No data		3b
Maurer 2012 Eur Arch Otorhinolaryngol 2012; 269:1851–1856	10	3.0	19.1	8.4	No data	7.1	6.9	n.s.	2b
Choi JH et al. Laryngoscope 2015; 125:1239–1243	11	4–6	8.4	6.3	No data	9.1	7.1	0.031	4
All	404	4.6	19.9	14.9	37.7	11.3	7.8		B

Abbreviations: AHI, apnea–hypopnea index; ESS, Epworth sleepiness scale.
Note: EBM = level of evidence-based medicine.

8.1.3 Uvulopalatoplasty

Ullrich Sommer

Definition

After its first description by Fujita in 1981, UPPP found its way in to the routine therapeutic arsenal of surgery for sleep disordered breathing.[45] Due to its widespread use and—at least in numerous case series—well-documented effect, further research was undertaken to help diminish the possible side effects like postoperative pain or swallowing problems.

Therefore, in 1986 Carenfelt introduced a technique called "laser uvulopalatoplasty" (LUPP). Contrary to UPPP, LUPP was a modification to the conventional technique as for the first time it used a laser to reshape the velum.[46] Briefly, in LUPP, the tonsils are removed and a palatal mucosal incision is made along the line of the crease created by gently lifting the uvula upward. Afterward, the reshaped pharynx is sutured much like in the original Fujita UPPP. According to the original publication, the use of a laser should help decrease the abovementioned side effects. Nevertheless, general anesthesia is mostly still needed for the LUPP procedure.

Another technique to treat the soft palate was introduced by Kamami in 1980 called "laser-assisted uvulopalatoplasty" (LAUP). LAUP consists of placing bilateral vertical incisions or trenches directly along both sides of the uvula followed by laser ablation of the uvula.[47,48] After publication, the procedure was widely used in Europe and by the end of 1990s, this became popular in the United States as well.[49] LAUP was carried out under local anesthesia and did not require conventional sutures for reshaping of the soft palate. Until now, more than 120 articles on LAUP have been published in peer-reviewed magazines. Due to the significant postoperative pain and the specific safety issues associated with LAUP, different methods for tissue cutting were sought after. The upcoming cutting devices based on radiofrequency energy seemed to be ideal for that purpose. Therefore, the term "radiofrequency-assisted uvulopalatoplasty" (RAUP)[50,51] was introduced for these types of procedures where parts of the soft palate were resected using radiofrequency-powered cutting devices. This resection of the soft palate was often combined with interstitial RFT and was then called RF-UPP.[52]

Indications, Contraindications, and Patient Selection

With respect to RAUP, clear data related to indication, contraindication, and patient selection are missing, as consistency regarding the device for electrocautery is low. As the basic surgical concept is identical with LAUP, we also assume there is no difference regarding the abovementioned parameters.

As the effect regarding AHI-lowering is limited, and even increases in AHI have been described in case of LAUP, the only acceptable indication for these kinds of surgery is simple snoring.[53] With limited clinical efficacy of interstitial radiofrequency surgery of the soft palate in primary snoring in patients with excessive soft tissue at the palatal arches (webbing) and with uvula hyperplasia, these patients tend to be suitable for UPP.[52] The following conditions are known contraindications for LAUP and thereby for RAUP as well.

Overweight, arterial hypertension, mental irregularities or lack of cooperation,[54] and being a professional speaker, singer, or wind instrument player are known relative contraindications.[55] A solely retrolingual site of formation of snoring sounds, tonsillar hypertrophy, trismus, craniofacial malformation and cleft palate, macroglossia, prominent plication of the rear oropharyngeal wall, heavy retching, previously existing velopharyngeal incompetence, floppy epiglottis, and neuromuscular diseases of the pharynx are local factors that should lead to rejection of LAUP or RAUP.[54]

Diagnostic Workup

In line with the "Standards of Practice Committee" of the AASM "[...] surgical candidates for LAUP as a treatment for snoring should undergo a preoperative clinical evaluation and a PSG or a cardiorespiratory study to determine if the candidate has a sleep-related breathing disorder (SRBD) including OSA (standard) [...]."[47] Furthermore the patients complaints should be recorded pre- and postoperatively. A questionnaire regarding snoring using a VAS seems appropriate.[56]

Specific Risks, Patient Information, and Consent

An informed consent should include severe postoperative pain, foreign body sensation (which is reported by 8–25% of the patients), voice changes (in 0–17.2%), and an increase in the incidence of dry mouth between 16 and 42%.[57,58,59,60] Additionlly, general risks of sedation and local anesthesia should be taken into account.

Anesthesia and Positioning

LAUP and RAUP are commonly performed under local anesthesia with the patient being seated comfortably in either a clinical chair or on a surgical table. As sedation is not ultimately needed for this procedure it depends on the patients' needs and may be done by titration of midazolam or propofol intravenously up to the desired sedation level. Local anesthesia may be administered using 5 mL 2% prilocaine with 0.01% adrenaline directly at the site of surgery.

Equipment

For LAUP, the CO_2 laser is used most often, yet some authors described successful procedures using a NdYAG or the KTP laser.[61,62] No comparative information pointing to differences between various laser types has been found in the literature yet.[63] For RAUP, a radiofrequency generator with an output frequency in the range of MHz, such as the Sutter Curis or Olympus Celon ProCut Series, is needed for minimizing thermal damages to the surrounding tissue, yet achieving adequate coagulation. As a cutting device, a coagulation needle electrode with a diameter between 0.2 and 0.4 mm should be used (▶Fig. 8.11). Argon shielding is not needed for this procedure.

Operative Technique/Steps

LAUP

After insertion of a suitable mouth gag (may not be needed, mostly depends on the sedation level) and the depression of the tongue, a backstop has to be inserted to protect the posterior pharyngeal wall from the laser beam. The CO_2 laser is set to 8 W, continuous wave, and superpulse mode. To avoid velopharyngeal incompetence and increased postoperative complications, the original one-stage technique after Kamami should be modified in a way that by directing of the laser beam, an inverse V-shaped incision is made bilaterally to the uvula, cutting about only 5 mm into the anterior pillar of the soft palate (▶Fig. 8.12).

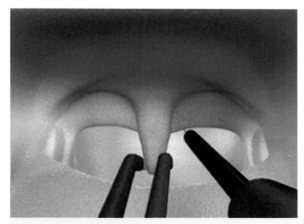

Fig. 8.11 Tissue cutting system used for radiofrequency-assisted uvulopalatoplasty procedures.

Afterward, the uvula is pulled downward by grabbing the excessive tissue with a forceps. This way, the uvula muscle becomes apparent and should be preserved by any means. After removing redundant mucosa from the muscular tissue, special care is taken to coagulate any bleeding that might occur. This procedure may be repeated multiple times in a 6 to 8 weeks interval until the desired effect is achieved. ▶Fig. 8.13 shows a typical intraoperative setting with the lines to cut marked in yellow.

RAUP

In the case of using the Olympus Celon ProCut electrode, the radiofrequency generator is set to 20 W. For other devices, the wattage has to be adjusted accordingly. A triangular incision is then cut bilaterally through the uvula, only extending about 5 mm into the anterior pillar of the soft palate. Any hypertrophic mucosa of the posterior arch of soft palate and the uvula is thereupon also resected with the ProCut electrode (▶Fig. 8.14). The palatal muscles should be left intact in any case. Also, the RAUP procedure may be repeated multiple times until the desired effect is achieved.

> ### Risks, Tips, and Tricks
>
> - UPP is an unsuitable treatment for OSA.
> - For treatment of snoring, RAUP should be preferred over LAUP because of its better safety profile.
> - Do not extend cuts deep into the muscular tissue of the soft palate.
> - Take small steps. It's generally better to repeat surgery multiple times than to cause complications.
> - LAUP appears comparable to UPPP in relieving subjective snoring.

Complications

As written in the specific risk section, one of the most common complication of this type of surgery is foreign body sensation, which is also the hardest to treat and most annoying for the patient.[57,58,59,60] To prevent this type of complications, it's most important not to extend the vertical velar incisions into muscle tissue of the soft palate and therefore treat the patient in repeated sessions. The same

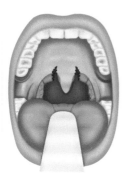
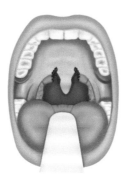
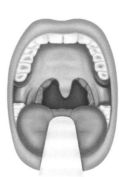

Fig. 8.12 Surgical technique of laser-assisted uvulopalatoplasty.

applies to nasopharyngeal stenosis, which most likely is also caused by extended circular resection of the soft palate. These complications are usually hard to treat with a huge impact on patient's quality of life. Disturbed sensation and postnasal secretion most likely are of temporary nature. For patients using, or going to use, nasal CPAP there are some cases where extended surgery of the soft palate made it impossible to further use the CPAP device. Yet, according to the author's own experience, if resection of the soft palate is taken with carefulness and in multiple sessions, this complication is likely never to appear.

Postoperative Care

After sedation with midazolam, the patient needs to be under supervision of a medical professional or a designated supervisor for at least 12 hours. During this time, the patient will not be able to drive in public road traffic. Surgical or postoperative antibiotic prophylaxis is usually not necessary.[64] Due to the high amount of postoperative pain the procedure is usually associated with adequate

management of postoperative pain, which is crucial after soft palate surgery. In our experience, medication with ibuprofen (four times 400–600 mg) in addition with metamizole (four times 0.5–1 g) is sufficient for most of the patients. Opioids for pain management are only needed in rare occasions. For the judgment of an adequate healing process, ▶ Fig. 8.15 shows a typical postsurgery state after 2 weeks and ▶ Fig. 8.16 shows the same after 3 months.

Outcomes

Until now, two high-quality studies regarding LAUP are published. One of them was published by Ferguson in 2003.[65] Forty-six patients with an AHI between 10 and 27 were randomized in two groups. The active group was treated with LAUP; the control group did not receive any surgical intervention. After 7 months, the AHI in the active group dropped from 19 to 15; the AHI in the control group rose from 16 to 23. The second publication from Larrosa in 2004 randomized 28 patients with an AHI < 30/h in an active and a sham-surgery group.[66] There

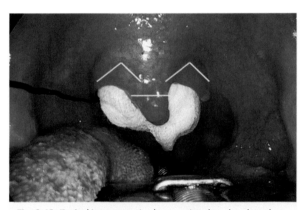

Fig. 8.13 Typical intraoperative laser-assisted uvulopalatoplasty setting with the lines to cut marked in yellow.

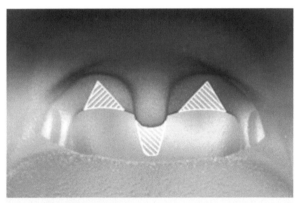

Fig. 8.14 Amount of tissue resected in radiofrequency-assisted uvulopalatoplasty.

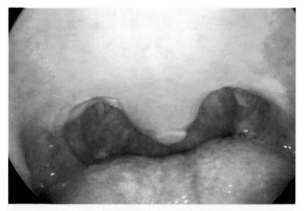

Fig. 8.15 Laser-assisted uvulopalatoplasty 2 weeks postoperatively.

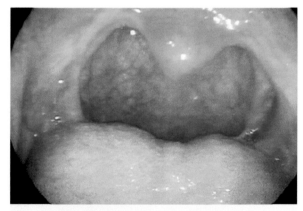

Fig. 8.16 Laser-assisted uvulopalatoplasty 3 months postoperatively.

▶Table 8.2 Studies available for LAUP

Author	Design	Year	N	Age	BMI	Pre-OP AHI	Post-OP AHI	AHI change
Larrosa	RCT	2004	13	—	27 ± 2	14 ± 8	15 ± 18	11%
Ferguson	RCT	2003	21	—	—	19 ± 4	15 ± 8	−21%
Goktas	RCS	2014	23	63	30 ± 4	28 ± 17	25 ± 20	−12%
Peng	RCS	2009	96	49	—	7–89	5–42	—
Abdullah	RCS	2008	1	—	—	67	41	−39%
Kern	RCS	2003	64	43 ± 11	27 ± 4	51 ± 31	26 ± 21	−49%
Walker	RCS	1999	40	53 ± 2	31 ± 1	25 ± 3	15 ± 3	−39%
Chisholm	PCS	2007	20	—	32 (28–38)	48 ± 20	13 ± 11	−73%
Pavelec	PCS	2006	63	20–67	—	7 ± 6	5 ± 4	−32%
Atef	PCS	2005	62	—	—	26 ± 10	11 ± 10	−58%
Berger	PCS	2003	25	50 ± 10	28 ± 3	25 ± 14	33 ± 23	31%
Finkelstein	PCS	2002	26	53 ± 10	28 ± 3	30 ± 22	25 ± 19	−16%
Lin	PCS	2002	25	41 ± 6	28 ± 2	40 ± 7	32 ± 14	−21%
Seemann	PCS	2002	10	49	35	52 ± 25	45 ± 28	−13%
Berger	PCS	2001	7	54 ± 7	26 ± 3	5 ± 0	7 ± 5	29%
Ryan	PCS	2000	44	49 ± 11	30 ± 4	29 ± 17	19 ± 15	−34%
Berger	PCS	1999	10	49 (25–71)	29	13 ± 10	24 ± 10	83%
Mickelson	PCS	1999	36	52 ± 11	31 ± 8	28 ± 17	18 ± 14	−36%
Lauretano	PCS	1997	17	—	—	27 ± 10	29 ± 10	7%
Hanada	PCS	1996	64	54 ± 10	—	14 ± 11[a]	9 ± 10[a]	−39%
Skatvedt	PCS	1996	13	48 (26–63)	27 (21–37)	22 ± 24	8 ± 11	−75%
Terris	PCS	1996	7	41 ± 13	—	11 ± 11	22 ± 10	92%
Petri	PCS	1994	30	47 (31–63)	28 (20–37)	26 (15–48)[a]	7 (2–23)[a]	−70%

[a]Only apnea index is given.
Abbreviations: post-OP AHI, postoperative apnea–hypopnea index; pre-OP AHI, preoperative apnea–hypopnea index; PCS, prospective case series; RCS, retrospective case series.
Modified from Camacho et al.[53]

was no difference between the two groups. ▶Table 8.2 gives an overview regarding available studies.[53] The two aforementioned randomized controlled trials (RCTs) are listed at the top of the table. Beside these, studies like retrospective or prospective case series (RCS/PCS) only were published (see ▶Table 8.2).

Due to these indifferent outcome parameters in laser-assisted surgery of the soft palate, the American Academy of Sleep Medicine (AASM) Guidelines (2001) issued the following recommendations for patient selection[47]:

- LAUP is not recommended for the treatment of the SRBDs including OSA.
- LAUP is not recommended as a substitute for UPPP in the treatment of SRBDs including OSA.
- LAUP appears comparable to UPPP in relieving subjective snoring.

These recommendations to not perform LAUP in OSA patients nowadays receives ample consensus between authors.[63,67]

Nevertheless, LAUP seems to be an adequate treatment modality for simple snoring. In a recent meta-analysis, patients demonstrated decreased snoring intensity after LAUP, which, as the authors state, is likely secondary to scar tissue causing the soft palate to stiffen.[53] Snoring outcomes were quantified for 14 studies with 429 patients. There was significant heterogeneity in the manner in which the data were presented, with the highest number of studies reporting the VAS in which a 0 to 10 scale was used. The pre- and post-LAUP VAS for 158 patients was 8.4 ± 1.2 and 5.2 + 2.2, respectively. For most studies, snoring decreased.[53] The AASM's practice parameters for LAUP, therefore, note that LAUP and UPPP are comparable with respect to relieving snoring.[47]

Due to the slightly better long-term complications, for treatment of snoring, RAUP may be favorable.[58,68] Results for treatment of simple snoring for RAUP are depicted in ▶Table 8.3.

► Table 8.3 Results for treatment of simple snoring for RAUP

Author	Design	Year	N	Follow-up (months)	VAS	VAS (pre)	VAS (post)
Wedman	PCS	2002	40	3	0–10	8.4	2.3
Cincik	RCT	2006	18	1.5	0–4	3.1	0.4
Belloso	RCT	2006	17	12	1–10	7.1	4
Lim	PCS	2007	24	6	1–10	7.9	3.3

Abbreviations: PCS, prospective case series; RCS, retrospective case series; VAS, visual analog scale.
Data modified after Hörmann and Verse.[63]

8.2 Invasive Procedures

8.2.1 Palate and Tonsils

Tonsillectomy and Tonsillotomy

Thomas Verse

Tonsillectomy

Definition

Tonsillectomy means the complete removal of all lymphatic tissue of the palatine tonsil. This surgery is often called "extracapsular tonsillectomy." While performing this surgery, the bigger blood vessels at the outside of the tonsilar capsule need to be severed and closed by sutures or electrosurgery afterward.[69] "Hot tonsillectomy" means the use of lasers or radiofrequency instruments. The deapth of tissue damage and postoperative pain depend on the amount of energy applied to the tissue. "Cold tonsillectomy" disclaims the use of electrical or thermal energy for blood control.

Indications, Contraindications, and Patient Selection

In children with sleep disordered breathing and enlarged tonsils, we perform a tonsillotomy (see the next section). Partial tonsillectomy techniques that do not touch the tonsilar capsule with its bigger blood vessels are able to substantially reduce postoperative pain and hemorrhage in children.[70,71,72,73,74] Since postoperative hemorrhage is much more dangerous in children as compared to adults, we only perform tonsillectomies in children with frequently recurrent acute tonsillitis. To treat SRBDs we prefer tonsillotomies (synonym: partial tonsillectomy, intracapsular tonsillectomy).

In adults, we only perform tonsillectomy in patients with OSA. In case of adult simple snoring, there are less-invasive techniques that are also effective in reducing snoring. Interstitial RFTs of tonsils combined with treatments (RFT) of the soft palate and/or tongue base work well, at least in our hands. RFT treatments are less invasive and have much less complications.[13,75] In order to minimize complications as much as possible, we prefer less-invasive techniques instead of complete tonsillectomies in patients with simple snoring.

In contrast, the sleep apnea patient is at risk for several health impairments like stroke, heart attack, other vascular damages, systemic inflammation, metabolic dysregulation, and other health impairments.[76,77,78,79] Therefore, the pretreatment situation for sleep apnea patients is different from that of primary snorers (who are otherwise healthy) and this difference allows more invasive surgeries.

The complete removal of the tonsils results in bigger gain of airway volume than a partial tonsillectomy. This is why we always recommend a tonsillectomy to our sleep apnea patients, if the tonsils are still left within the pharynx, and secondly the site of obstruction is located at the oropharyngeal level, and thirdly a surgical treatment is desired by the patient.

UPPP surgeries in order to treat OSA should always be combined with tonsillectomies, as tonsillectomy has been shown to double the success rate of UPPP procedures.[80] Since an additional UPPP does not add much inconvenience to a patient that undergoes tonsillectomy we rarely perform isolated tonsillectomy, but mostly perform UPPP and tonsillectomy. Apart from the UPPP sutures, that might need to be taken out some days after surgery, the postoperative morbidity seems to be the same. Apparently, most sleep surgeons feel the same because the available data on isolated tonsillectomy to treat OSA are both rare and mostly a bit outdated (see ► Table 8.4).

In our material, we were able to show a significant correlation between tonsil size (as measured in milliliter) and severity of OSA (unpublished own data).[94] In other words, the bigger the tonsils, the more likely they contribute to the severity of OSA, and the more likely a tonsillectomy will have a significant impact on the reduction of the AHI. The same correlation has been shown for UPPP surgery with tonsillectomy.[95,96] This makes us think that a complete tonsillectomy should provide superior results as compared to partial tonsillectomies. However, the superiority of tonsillectomy against partial tonsillectomy has not been presented so far in adults.

Naturally, the patients need to be able to open the mouth wide enough to insert the mouth gag and the surgical instruments. Sometimes dental pathologies exist that might interfere with the insertion of the mouth gag.

▶Table 8.4 Influence of isolated tonsillectomy on AHI

Author	N	Follow-up (months)	AHI (pre)	AHI (post)	Success (%)	ESS (pre)	ESS (post)	EBM
Orr and Martin[81]	3	1–30	55.5	9.8	100.0	No data	No data	4
Rubin et al[82]	5	2–6	50.9	26.6	40.0	No data	No data	4
Moser et al[83]	4	2–43	20.1	7.5	75.0	No data	No data	4
Aubert-Tulkens et al[84]	2	1–15	31.1	18.9	50.0	No data	No data	4
Houghton et al[85]	5	1–3	54.6	3.6	100.0	No data	No data	4
Miyazaki et al[86]	10	No data	14.0	3.0	No data	No data	No data	4
Verse et al[87]	9	3–14	46.6	10.1	88.9	No data	No data	4
Martinho et al[88]	7	3	81.0	23.0	85.7	No data	No data	4
Nakata et al[89]	30	6	69.0	30.1	60.0	12.1	4.8	4
Nakata et al[90]	20	6	55.7	21.2	No data	11.5	5.4	4
Stow et al[91]	13	2	31.7	5.5	92.3	No data	No data	4
Tan et al[92]	34	3	42.2	13.1	73.5	No data	No data	4
Senchak et al[93]	19	2–6	18	3.2	94.7	12	9	4
All	161	1–43	45.56	15.12	77.09	11.90	6.13	C

Abbreviations: AHI, apnea–hypopnea index; ESS, Epworth sleepiness scale.
Note: EBM = level of evidence-based medicine.

Please check preoperatively and address this issue in the informed consent.

As in any sleep apnea case, severe comorbidities need to be excluded. The patient must be suitable for surgery under general anaesthesia.

As tonsillectomy is affected with the risk of postoperative hemorrhage in—depending on the definition used—up to 11% of the cases,[97] we do not perform surgery in patients with blood coagulation disorders, and in patients in need for anticoagulative medications that cannot be paused during the perioperative period. We recommend the preoperative use of a questionnaire asking for blood coagulation disturbances.

Like UPPP, tonsillectomy may affect the fundamental frequency of the voice.[98] Therefore, we are very cautious with the indication of tonsillectomies in professional singers and speakers. We remember a case of a radio moderator who had undergone tonsillectomy; after surgery some of his listeners were not able to recognize his voice again!

Rare complications of tonsillectomy are taste disturbances, in particular the persisting perception of a bitter taste. This issue needs to be discussed with professional chefs or ambitious cooks.

Diagnostic Workup

Any kind of sleep apnea surgery requires objective preoperative sleep studies. Without a preoperative sleep study, the effect of the surgery on the AHI cannot be determined after surgery. Apart from that subjective complaints need to be recorded pre- and postoperatively. Please refer to Chapter 5 to find the instruments that are available for this purpose.

We strongly recommend to use a standardized protocol to record and to document the clinical findings. Concerning the tonsils, we use the clinical staging system by Friedman[99] that provides five different tonsil sizes from 0 to 4 (▶Fig. 8.17).

To screen for blood coagulation disorders we use a specific questionnaire. In addition, we routinely test for olfactory and taste functions to identify preexisting taste disorders.

Specific Risks, Patient Information, and Consent

The general risks of surgery (i.e., pain, scarring, infection, wound healing problems, and postoperative hemorrhage) need to be addressed. Edema of the uvula occurs frequently and may induce globus sensation or even dyspnea. Such edema usually responds well to corticosteroids.

Apart from this, patients need to be informed that there will be a need for painkillers for 12 days in mean after surgery. Postoperative pain distinctively varies interindividually. Please check for intolerances prior to surgery. The intensity of postoperative pain depends on the amount of thermal energy used for blood control.[100,101] Please take a note of this during surgery.

Postoperative hemorrhage is the most common complication after tonsillectomy. The method of tonsillectomy used does not seem to have a substantial effect on the incidence of postoperative hemorrhage.[102,103] Please check for prior bleedings and/or affinity for bleedings in the patient's history. Prebulged or pulsatile tonsils may indicate an aberrant course of one of the branches of the external carotic artery.

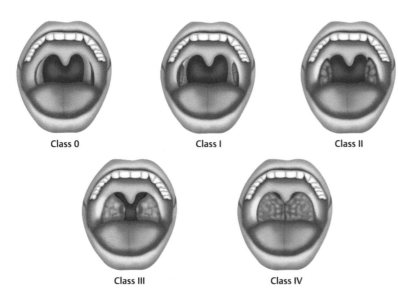

Fig. 8.17 Friedman tonsil size.

Class 0   Class I   Class II

Class III   Class IV

Please verify the patient's ability to open his/her mouth and have a look at the teeth. Address damages of the teeth and hematoma within the tongue as potential complications induced by the mouth gag. Sometimes, even hypaesthesia of parts of the tongue may occur as a consequence of the pressure induced by the mouth gag. Fortunately, hypaesthesia is mostly temporary.

As mentioned above, the patients need to be informed about potential taste and voice disturbances.

Severe wound healing deficits or intense revision surgery for blood control of postoperative bleedings may rarely result in nasopharyngeal stenosis or velopharyngeal incompetence.

Anesthesia and Positioning

We routinely perform tonsillectomies under general anesthesia with the patient being orally intubated and lying in supine position with the head slightly extended. Most mouth gags have a gorge to hold the intubation tube. This is why the tube needs to be placed in midline.

Tonsillectomy under local anesthesia is still possible, but is associated with a lot of discomfort for the patient and much more sportive for the surgeon. Therefore, in my department, tonsillectomy is only performed under local anesthesia, if the patient is an adult and either does not want and/or cannot undergo tonsillectomy under general anesthesia.

Equipement

Standard surgical instruments for cold steel tonsillectomies are sufficient. Modern instruments can be used for dissection like lasers, bovies or other monopolar instruments, the coblator system, or others.

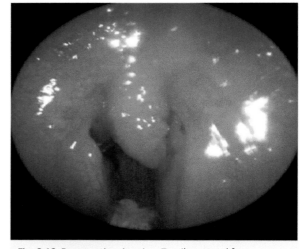

Fig. 8.18 Preoperative situation. Tonsils exposed for tonsillectomy.

Operative Technique/Steps

Transoral Approach

Insert the mouth gag. Often, it is helpful to fully expose one tonsil by pushing the tongue to the opposite side. The tongue is held in that position by the adequate tongue blade (▶ Fig. 8.18). Incision is made around the upper pole of the tonsil.

Exposure of the Tonsilar Capsule

After grasping the upper tonsilar pole with the surgical forceps or a clamp, the tonsil is pulled medially and dissected along its capsule while damaging the pharyngeal muscles as little as possible. In case of scarring, sharp instead of blunt dissection is recommended in order to save the peritonsilar tissue.

For blood control, we recommend compression with a swab for up to 5 minutes. Afterward, we carefully use cautery. Ligation sutures are only used in case of severe bleedings, as sutures intend to increase the level of postoperative pain.

Risks, Tips, and Tricks

- Open the mouth wide enough. Separate exposition of each tonsil using the mouth gag maybe helpful.
- Save as much mucosa and muscle tissue as possible.
- Avoid intensive use of thermal energy in order to minimalize postoperative pain.
- Use sharp instruments for the dissection in case of intensive scar tissue.
- Long-lasting local anesthesia can help to reduce pain within the first 1 to 3 days after tonsillectomy.
- Maybe intraoperative cooling of the wounds helps to reduce postoperative pain as well.
- A very careful resection of mucosa at the tip of the uvular reduces uvular edema after surgery.
- Edema of the uvula responds well to cortiocosteroids.
- Hot tonsillectomy techniques can help to reduce intraoperative blood loss.

Complications

Postoperative Pain

According to our own data, postoperative need for analgetic drug intake is 12 days in mean. Under medication, patients should be free of pain unless during swallowing. Use VASs, separately for swallowing and no swallowing, to record treatment success. In childen, faces pain scales instead of numbered scales should be used to get the information.[104]

Hot, spicy, and sour foods and drinks are not recommended during the first 1 to 2 weeks after surgery.

Hemorrhage

As stated earlier, postoperative hemorrhage is the most common and potentially dangerous complication. Patients should be advised to avoid physical effort, sauna, hot showering or baths, and other activities that potentially increase blood flow in the head and neck region.

Wound Infection

Although the mouth is always contaminated with various microorganisms, wound infections do not occur very frequently. This is why we do not subscribe antibiotics as a general role, but only in case of infection. We allow our patients to brush their front teeth. In addition, we provide a local antiseptic mouth solution to improve mouth hygiene.

Some surgeons reduce the fibrin films by carefully brushing the tonsillar wounds with myrrh solution or other agents.

Postoperative Care

As in any other sleep apnea surgery, the severity of OSA has a significant impact on postoperative care and monitoring. This is why sleep apnea patients undergoing surgery under general anesthesia or under sedation, in general, are at an increased risk for perioperative complications.[105,106,107]

This perioperative risk is particularly increased if OSA is treated surgically, as postoperative bleeding and swellings within the pharynx need to be taken into account. According to a review,[108] postoperative complications are rare and occur within the first 4 hours after extubation. This result is in accordance to our own experience. As a result, we keep our sleep apnea patients in the recovery room for 4 hours after extubation. If there are no complications, the patients are regarded to be safe and will be discharged to the regular ward. In case of complications, the patients are monitored overnight.[109]

The management of postoperative pain is crucial after tonsillectomy, but does not differ from tonsillectomies for other indications. A basic treatment with ibuprofen (four times 400–600 mg) in addition with metamizole (four times 0.5–1 g) works fine in adults. However, there are huge interindividual differences that require individual adaptations. If the basic treatment is not sufficient, we in time add opioids (e.g., three times 10 mg oxycodone). Please refer to Chapter 10.2 for further information about the postoperative care and medication.

Some authors recommend the intraoperative use of long-lasting local anaesthesia (like bupivacaine). We did not achieve a substantial benefit. Other authors recommend the use of ice cubes to cool the wound intraoperatively.[110] Unfortunately, this trick did not show us any significant effect in our patients. For this reason, we stopped intraoperative ice cooling.

Antibiotics are not mandatory for the perioperative period and perioperative antibiotic prophylaxis is not applied routinely.

Corticosteroids are used to protect airway compromise that may occur in the immediate postoperative phase, especially in OSA patients. At least in a pediatric population, the use of corticosteroids did not show an increase of postoperative bleedings.[111] Therefore, steroids can be used if necessary.

Outcomes

Tonsillectomies are rarely performed as isolated procedures to treat OSA. This is why objective outcome data are limited. There are 13 case series including 161 patients providing PSG data pre- and postoperatively (see ▶ Table 8.4). Data about tonsil size are inconsistent, as there is no standard instrument to describe tonsilar size. Having read the articles, I can say that most but not all patients were chosen as they had enlarged tonsils prior to surgery. This means that there may be a bias in the patient population, as the patient might have had bigger tonsils as compared to the general population.

The follow-up varies from 1 to 43 months with mainly short-term follow-up periods. The AHI decreased in mean from 45.6 at baseline to 15.1 (–66.9%) after surgery. Surgical success rates a given between 40 and 100%. More recent studies used the Sher criteria (reduction of AHI by at least 50% below 20).

Only three series (69 patients) provide data about daytime sleepiness as measured with the ESS. The ESS score decreased from 11.9 (presurgery) to 6.1 (–48.7%) after surgery.

In conclusion, data are difficult to compare. The level of evidence is low, as the data were taken from case series only, and the total number of patients is limited. However, the data show a huge impact of tonsillectomy on AHI and ESS at least in the short-time run (see ▶ Table 8.5).

In addition, there are some studies that show a superior effect of UPPP if combined with a tonsillectomy as compared to patients without a concomitant tonsillectomy, as they had undergone a tonsillectomy prior to UPPP.[80]

Tonsillotomy

Definition

Tonsillotomy means the partial removal of lymphatic tissue of the palatine tonsils without touching the bigger blood vessels at the outside of the tonsilar capsule. Synonyma are: intracapsular tonsillectomy or partial tonsillectomy. Usually only minor bleedings are observed that do not need closure by sutures or electrosurgery.

Indications, Contraindications, and Patient Selection

As mentioned above, in children with sleep disordered breathing we always perform a tonsillotomy instead of a tonsillectomy due to the decreased risk for postoperative hemorrhage and pain.[70,71,72,73,74] As postoperative hemorrhage is much more dangerous in children as compared to adults, we only perform tonsillectomies in children with frequently recurrent acute tonsillitis.

In adults suffering from simple snoring we prefer less-invasive surgeries like interstitial RFTs of tonsils maybe combined with RFT of the soft palate and/or tongue base or UPPs. These surgeries can be done under local anaesthesia and on an outpatient basis. We do neither perform tonsillectomies nor tonsillotomies in adults with simple snoring.

In adults there is no sufficient data available so far to prove the efficiency of tonsillectomy in treating OSA. It can be estimated that the subtotal removal of the lymphatic tissue will have a similar effect as the complete removal. However, this has not been shown yet.

Therefore, tonsillotomy is a surgical procedure reserved for children only. Please refer to Chapter 6 for more detailed information about the treatment of pediatric OSA.

Key Points

In children (adeno)tonsillectomy still is the standard procedure to treat pediatric OSA. Due to the reduced risk for postoperative hemorrhage and significantly reduced postoperative pain, a subtotal tonsillectomy (tonsillotomy, intracapsular tonsillectomy) that does not touch the tonsilar capsule with its bigger blood vessels should be preferred. For further information concerning pediatric OSA, refer to Chapter 6.

In adults tonsillectomy is rarely performed as an isolated procedure. Therefore, scientific data are limited. However, the effect of tonsillectomy on AHI and on daytime sleepiness is significant with the bigger the tonsilar size the bigger the effect on AHI. In UPPP surgery a concomitant tonsillectomy doubles the success rate of palatal surgery.

Concerning the surgery itself, and its complications tonsillectomy in OSA patients does not differ from tonsillectomy for other indications apart from the generally increased risk for airway compromise in OSA patients. Due to this fact OSA patients undergoing surgery need a special perioperative management (refer to Chapter 10 for detailed information).

Uvulopalatopharyngoplasty

Boris A. Stuck and Madeline Ravesloot

Definition

In all likelihood, the most commonly performed surgical procedure for OSA is UPPP in combination with tonsillectomy. It was first introduced in 1979 by Fujita et al and, apart from tracheostomy, it was the only available treatment option for adult OSA until the introduction of CPAP therapy. The technique was a modification of a similar procedure introduced by Ikematsu in 1963 to treat snoring

▶Table 8.5 Effect of isolated nasal surgery in sleep apnea patients on AHI and ESS

Author	N	Criterion of success	Success rate without TE (%)	Succes rate with TE (%)
Stevenson et al[100]	84	AI-Red. > 50%	21/48	24/36
Schwartz et al[112]	13	AI < 10 during nREM	2/7	4/6
McGuirt et al[113]	79	AI < 5 + Red. > 50%	2/27	27/52
Boot et al[114]	38	ODI-Red. > 50%	2/14	11/24
Hessel and de Vries[115]	55	AHI < 20 + Red. > 50%	7/18	25/37
All	269		30%	59%

Abbreviations: AHI, apnea–hyponea index; ESS, Epworth sleepiness scale; TE, tonsillectomy.

and it is still the most commonly performed surgical procedure for OSA.[116,117,118] Aim of the procedure is to increase the retropalatal (RP) airway and reduce the collapsibility of the pharynx, by resection of excessive mucosa at the free edge of the uvula and soft palate followed by suturing of the anterior and posterior pillar after tonsillectomy.[119,120]

The technique of UPPP was subject to change over time and still lacks standardization. In general, however, there is a tendency toward less-radical procedures with preservation of at least part of the uvula and the musculature of the anterior and posterior pillar. This development toward less-aggressive techniques was initiated as it became evident that complete soft-tissue resections at the soft palate performed in the 1980s and 1990s were associated with significant long-term morbidity and the outcome was not superior to muscle sparing techniques.

When referring to UPPP in general, it is performed with concomitant tonsillectomy. Nevertheless, UPPP can be performed without tonsillectomy, in particular in patients who have undergone tonsillectomy previously. Especially in the early literature, it often remains unclear whether UPPP was performed with our without tonsillectomy. In the more recent literature and in the subsequent chapter, however, UPPP is defined as UPPP with tonsillectomy unless otherwise specified.

Indications, Contraindications, and Patient Selection

UPPP can be considered in patients with OSA of any degree, as long as the individual anatomy appears suitable. In selected cases, UPPP may also be considered from snoring, although the invasiveness of the procedure should be weighed against the relative inoffensive nature of primary snoring.

UPPP has often been misused as the first-line surgical treatment for OSA, without adequate assessment of obstruction site(s) and regardless of predictive factors.[121] Assessment of the site(s) of obstruction, however, is paramount to surgical success. With regard to upper airway anatomy, a relevant obstruction at the velum and/or the oropharyngeal level should be present, which typically appears as a thickened uvula, excessive mucosa at the posterior pillar of the soft palate, and tonsillar hypertrophy (▶Fig. 8.19).

In the current literature, there is some evidence that the outcome of UPPP is related to tonsil size, leading to superior outcome in patients with larger tonsils.[95,96,100,122,124,125] As long as UPPP is considered as an isolated procedure, relevant obstruction at other levels of the upper airway should be ruled out, although UPPP can be combined with other surgical approaches and is an essential part of multilevel upper airway surgery.

As with other surgical approaches, surgical outcome is associated with the severity of the disease and individual BMI; patients with mild to moderate OSA and limited obesity being superior candidates.[126,127,128] In this regard, treatment effects are usually limited in patients with a

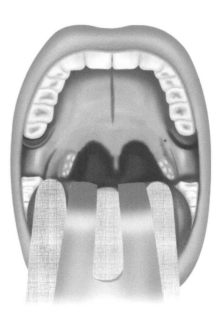

Fig. 8.19 UPPP, preoperative view.

BMI above 32. A maximum AHI, however, can hardly be defined in patients with very large tonsils, resulting in near total oropharyngeal obstruction; UPPP often leads to dramatic improvement regardless of baseline AHI.

UPPP should be indicated with care in professional speakers and singers, as voice changes may occur along with the procedure. In addition, potential changes in the sound of selected consonants have to be kept in mind. In addition, changes in taste perception may occur along with tonsillectomy, although this is usually temporary and resolves over time.[129] Nevertheless, professional "tasters" (chefs) should be consulted accordingly. Preexisting velopharyngeal dysfunction/insufficiency is a contraindication for UPPP. As with other surgical procedures, general contraindications for surgery need to be considered. With regard to bleeding being the major complication associated with tonsillectomy, special care should be taken to rule out relevant coagulation disorders with medical history and/or targeted coagulation tests.

As the anatomy at the level of the soft palate and the oropharynx can directly be assessed with clinical examination, several clinical staging systems have been suggested for treatment selection, mostly based on tonsil size and position of the soft palate.[95,96,100,122,127,125] Superior outcome was demonstrated in patients in whom upper airway obstruction was defined according to these clinical criteria. Furthermore, upper airway pressure measurements and DISE were suggested for upper airway assessment to identify patients with upper airway obstruction.[115,130,131,132,133] A superior outcome was described in patients with upper airway obstruction compared to mixed or lower airway obstruction as defined with pressure measurements or

DISE. Whether these additional diagnostic measures are superior to clinical staging/clinical assessment, however, remains unclear.

Diagnostic Workup

For the assessment of the severity of OSA, PSG or out-of-center sleep testing (OCST) is required. Clinical assessment is essential for treatment selection and an obstruction at the level of the soft palate and the tonsils should be present. Standardized protocols for clinical assessment and staging systems (e.g., for tonsil size and tongue position) may be used for documentation purposes and to improve treatment selection. Further testing such as upper airway pressure measurements or DISE is not mandatory in cases of obvious obstruction at this level but may be considered in unclear cases or to rule out other relevant levels of obstruction. Medical history should identify professional voice users or tasters and patients with preexisting velopharyngeal dysfunction/insufficiency. BMI should be assessed to consult patients regarding the expected surgical outcome and the potential necessity for weight reduction.

With regard to the risk of transient postoperative changes in taste perception, preoperative testing of gustatory function (e.g., with the help of taste strips etc.) may be considered.

General medical history is important to identify perioperative risk factors and should include clinical signs of coagulopathy and current medication to identify potential medication interfering with blood coagulation. Coagulation tests should be performed, especially in patients with known or suspected coagulopathies or corresponding medication.

Specific Risks, Patient Information, and Consent

As with other surgical techniques, patients should be informed that surgical success cannot be guaranteed and that individual success is hard to predict. Velopharyngeal dysfunction including nasal regurgitation of fluids can occur in the early postoperative period, although with muscle-sparing, less-radical surgical techniques velopharyngeal function can be preserved in almost every case. Persisting velopharyngeal insufficiency (VPI) or postoperative velopharyngeal stenosis has been reported but is usually a result of aggressive surgery with muscle resection, which should be avoided. Patients have to be informed about the expected success rate of approximately 60 to 70%.[134]

Postoperative pain is usually significant and exceeds typical post-tonsillectomy pain. Pain management is essential especially in the early postoperative period. The most relevant early postoperative complication, however, is bleeding at the site of tonsillectomy (see Complications under this section).

Patients need to be informed that, due to postoperative edema, snoring and obstructive events may persist in the early postoperative period and that the postoperative outcome cannot be assessed before 4 to 6 weeks. If patients are receiving CPAP treatment before surgery, the ongoing use of CPAP is recommended during this period, until control PSG or OCST has assessed surgical outcome.

Anesthesia and Positioning

UPPP requires general anesthesia. Head positioning is in slight hyperextension and is equivalent to standard tonsillectomy with midline position of the tube in a downward direction.

Equipment

A standard tonsillectomy set is sufficient for UPPP. For the resorbable palate sutures, Vicryl 2.0 or comparable material is used.

Procedural Steps

Surgery is performed in general anesthesia, with an oral endotracheally placed tube in the midline. The patient lies in supine position with the head slightly extended. A mouth gag with adequate tonsil blade is put in place for optimal exposure of the oropharynx. If no previous tonsillectomy has been performed, UPPP starts with tonsillectomy. There is no preferred surgical technique for tonsillectomy with regard to UPPP and the selection of the technique is at the surgeons' discretion. Particular care however should be taken to achieve proper haemostasis at the end of tonsillectomy. If electrocautery is used, it should be applied with care to avoid major thermal damage to the surrounding tissue.

An incision at the free edge of the mucosa of the posterior pillar is done approximately 5 mm laterally to the uvula at both sides. The posterior pillar is then mobilized and pulled anteriorly and laterally for reconfiguration of the oropharynx with resorbable sutures. We recommend three to four sutures on both sides. For these sutures, the needle is passed through the anterior pillar and the tonsillar fossa and then through the posterior pillar (right side). Passing the suture two times through all the three structures helps to prevent loss of this suture during the postoperative period. Loss of sutures with unintended disintegration of the two pillars may occur in the postoperative period. To prevent suture loss, it should be ensured that enough soft tissue is included in the sutures (not only mucosal approximation, but also soft-tissue relocation). For the left side, starting with the posterior pillar is usually preferred (for right-handed surgeons). It is advised to avoid sutures that are too tight, due to risk of stenosis. After reconfiguration of the pillars, the uvula is shortened by excising excessive soft tissue. We recommend to not completely resect the uvula to preserve its paramount function in velopharyngeal closure.

The stump of the uvula and the mucosa of the pillars at the parauvular area are closed with sutures. One may also start with the trimming of the uvula followed by reconfiguration of the pillars.

Pre- and postoperative views are provided in ▶ Fig. 8.19 and ▶ Fig. 8.20.

Risks, Tips, and Tricks

- Use an appropriately sized mouth gag for optimal exposure.
- Tonsillectomy should be performed with care to avoid damage to the surrounding structures.
- Minimize the use of electrocautery.
- Avoid resection or incision of palatine musculature.
- For the incision of the mucosa of the posterior pillar, keep a distance of 2 to 3 mm from the uvula to avoid excessive swelling of the uvula.
- Ensure to grab enough soft tissue when suturing the palate, otherwise the sutures will cut through the wound edges.
- Be careful with suturing the pillars for approximation, the sutures will cut through the pillar if the knots are too tight.

Complications

The most relevant complication is postoperative bleeding associated with tonsillectomy and comparable complication rates with regard to postoperative hemorrhage

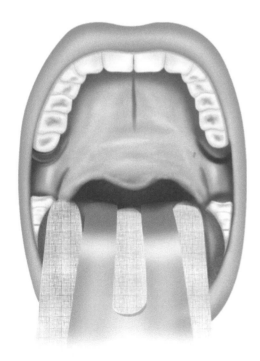

Fig. 8.20 UPPP, postoperative view.

have to be expected. Another relevant complication is velopharyngeal dysfunction that may occur in the early postoperative phase in up to 8% of patients,[114,116] although even persistent VPI has been reported. In addition, airway compromise has been described due to postoperative edema. In general, postoperative complication rates however are relatively low. In studies with larger sample sizes (>50), complication rates for postoperative bleeding, airway compromise, or velopharyngeal dysfunction of about 2% were reported.[124,135,136] In the largest sample of Kezirian et al including 1,570 patients with isolated UPPP, the overall postoperative complication rate was 1.3%.[137]

In addition, complications related to the use of a mouth gag (teeth damage, numbness of the tongue, hematoma) should be mentioned (also see section on Tonsillectomy earlier in this chapter). Transient taste disturbances are not infrequent but usually disappear over time. Persistent taste changes however are a rarity.

Postoperative Care

Most patients can be discharged at the third postoperative day, although the duration of hospital stay varies significantly within different health care systems, especially for tonsillectomy. Resorbable sutures may be removed after some weeks, but are usually left in place until spontaneous resorption. Antibiotics are not mandatory for the perioperative period and perioperative antibiotic prophylaxis is not applied routinely. Corticosteroids may be administered during the early postoperative period in cases of significant edema. Sufficient pain medication is required and is usually based on oral anti-inflammatory drugs, such as ibuprofen or metamizol. According to individual needs, oral treatment with opioids may be necessary, but should be administered with caution in patients with severe OSA.

Outcomes

Being one of the earliest surgical techniques for OSA, an extensive body of literature regarding UPPP is available and it can be assumed that UPPP is one of the best studied surgical approaches in sleep medicine. With regard to the treatment of OSA, more than 1,000 articles on UPPP have been published. The assessment of surgical outcome however is compromised by the fact that the majority of these studies do not provide objective data on isolated UPPP for OSA. Especially in the early publications, patients with OSA were mixed with snoring subjects or combined surgical procedure were described, often lacking sufficient diagnostic measures for OSA.[134]

The published literature contains retrospective case series and prospective studies, including a limited number of controlled and randomized controlled trials. Although the majority of trials reported short- and medium-term follow-up, studies with long-term follow-up of up to 10 years were published. Among the RCTs, three studies were presented comparing UPPP with an untreated control group,[138,139,140] two of them reported on the same cohort but with different outcome data.[138,139] In a most recent systematic review, two meta-analyses were performed using data of the available RCT (▶ Fig. 8.21).[134]

With regard to objective outcome measures (respiratory events/AHI), these meta-analyses demonstrate that UPPP was significantly more effective in reducing the AHI than no other treatment (large effect)[139,140] or compared to baseline (large effect).[139,140,141] Various studies provide success or response rates, although various definitions for success were used. Success/response rates range from 31.3 to 96.0%. Studies reporting on long-term outcome demonstrated a tendency toward a weakening of the initial effect over time, but the study results are conflicting.

In addition, UPPP has a significant effect on daytime sleepiness and daytime performance. Again, a meta-analysis was presented in the systematic review by Stuck et al,[134] which demonstrated that UPPP is significantly more effective in reducing the ESS in comparison to no treatment. Moreover, several other beneficial effects were described regarding UPPP. In the study of Santamaria et al[142] baseline testosterone levels could be increased with UPPP and Shin et al[143] were able to demonstrate a statistically significant improvement in the International Index of Erectile Function (FIEF 5). With regard to sleep stages, an improvement was demonstrated in selected trials.[126,144] Finally, the survival of 149 patients receiving UPPP was compared to 208 patients receiving CPAP in a retrospective study from 1994[145] with a mean follow-up of 43 ± 13 months. No difference in 5-year survival was detected between the two groups. In the study from Browaldh et al from Sweden with the longest follow-up period of about 15 years,[146] the standardized mortality rate of the study population was compared to the general Swedish population and no difference in the standardized mortality rate was described.

Key Points

In all likelihood, UPPP is still the most commonly performed surgical procedure for OSA. The technique of UPPP was subject to change over time and still lacks standardization; in this chapter, UPPP was defined as UPPP with tonsillectomy. UPPP can be combined with other surgical approaches and is an essential part of multilevel upper airway surgery. It can be considered in patients with OSA of any degree, as long as the individual anatomy appears suitable. The outcome of UPPP is related to tonsil size, severity of the disease, and BMI, patients with mild to moderate OSA and limited obesity being superior candidates. UPPP should be indicated with care in professional speakers and singers; it contraindicated in patients with preexisting velopharyngeal dysfunction. Several clinical staging systems were suggested for treatment selection, mostly based on tonsil size and position of the soft palate. Upper airway pressure measurements and DISE were also suggested for upper airway assessment to identify patients with upper airway obstruction, whether these additional diagnostic measures are superior to clinical staging/clinical assessment however remains unclear. The most relevant complications are postoperative bleeding associated with tonsillectomy and velopharyngeal dysfunction. In addition, airway compromise has been described due to postoperative edema. In general, postoperative complication rates however are relatively low; in studies with larger sample sizes they range about 2%. Regarding postoperative outcome, an extensive body of literature regarding UPPP is available, the published literature containing retrospective case series and prospective studies, including a limited number of controlled and RCTs. With regard to objective outcome measures (respiratory events/AHI), current meta-analyses demonstrate that UPPP is significantly more effective in reducing the AHI in comparison to no treatment. Success/response rates range from 31.3 to 96.0% with various definitions used for these criteria. In addition, UPPP has a significant effect on daytime sleepiness and various aspects of daytime performance.

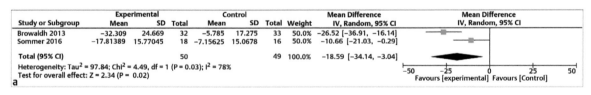

Fig. 8.21 Meta-analysis for apnea–hypopnea index (AHI). (a) Meta-analysis demonstrating mean difference of AHI in the two randomized controlled trials (RCTs) comparing uvulopalatopharyngoplasty (UPPP) with an untreated control group. (b) Meta-analysis demonstrating mean difference of AHI in the three RCTs comparing results before and after UPPP. CI, confidence interval; SD, standard deviation. According to Stuck et al.[134]

Modifications of UPPP

Uvulopalatal Flap Techniques

Thomas Verse

Definition

The "uvulopalatal flap" (UPF) has first been described by Powell et al in 1996 as a reversible alternative to conventional UPPP.[147] The basic idea was to remove a rhomb of mucosa, fat, and salivatory glands only at the oral side of the palate without resecting the muscles. The lower edge of the rhomb is surged upward, and by folding the rhomb the defect is closed with sutures. This original version of the UPF was performed without a tonsillectomy. The authors claimed this surgery to be reversible; however, it turned out it was not.

Other authors refined the technique by adding a tonsillectomy. This new development was called extended uvulopalatal flap (EUPF) and was first described by Li et al in 2003.[148]

All flap techniques do not leave a visible uvula, a fact that is associated with increased xerostomia after surgery.

Indications, Contraindications, and Patient Selection

The UPF is a technique that addresses soft palate obstruction (anterioposteriorly, and in combination with a tonsillectomy also laterally) in patients with simple snoring and OSA. UPF surgery can easily be done in patients who had undergone tonsillectomy earlier in their life. In this patient group we favored UPF over conventional UPPP, as in UPF surgery it is not necessary to reopen the tonsillar beds. In fact, it reduces surgery time and morbidity after surgery.

Naturally, the patients need to be able to open their mouth wide enough to insert the mouth gag and the surgical instruments. Sometimes dental pathologies exist that might interfere with insertion of the mouth gag. Please check preoperatively and address this issue in the informed consent.

As in any sleep apnea case, severe comorbidities need to be excluded. The patient must be suitable for surgery under general anesthesia.

As tonsillectomy is affected with the risk of postoperative hemorrhage in—depending on the definition used—up to 11% of the cases we do not perform surgery in patients with blood coagulation disorders, and in patients in need for anticoagulative medications that cannot be paused during the perioperative period.[97] We recommend the preoperative use of a questionnaire, asking for blood coagulation disturbances (refer to the section on Tonsillectomy and Tonsillotomy earlier in this chapter).

Like any kind of soft palate surgery, UPS may affect the fundamental frequency of the voice. Therefore, we are very cautious with the indication oftonsillectomy in professional singers and speakers.

Rare complications of tonsillectomy are taste disturbances, in particular the persisting perception of a bitter taste. This issue needs to be discussed with professional chefs or ambitious cooks.

In addition, neuromuscular diseases, neurological or psychiatric illnesses in need of treatment, cleft palates, chronic alcoholism, soporific drug abuse, severe bite misalignments, preexisting velopharyngeal stenosis or incompetences, and severe certain craniofacial deformities are regarded as contraindications.

Diagnostic Workup

As any kind of sleep apnea surgery, UPF requires objective preoperative sleep studies. Without a preoperative sleep study the effect of the surgery on the AHI and other objective parameters cannot be determined after surgery. Apart from this, subjective complaints need to be recorded pre- and postoperatively. Please refer to Chapter 5 to find the instruments that are available for this purpose.

Please screen for dysphagia and taste and speech disorders prior to surgery. To screen for blood coagulation disorders we use a specific questionnaire. In addition, we routinely test for olfactory and taste functions to identify preexisting taste disorders.

Specific Risks, Patient Information, and Consent

The general risks of surgery (i.e., pain, scarring, infection, wound healing problems, and postoperative hemorrhage) need to be addressed. Edema or hematoma of the soft palate may occur and may induce foreign body sensation or even dyspnea. Such an edema usually responds well to corticosteroids.

As mentioned earlier, xerostomia is a frequent problem after UPS surgery. As no visible uvula remains after the procedure, moisturing of the throat will be disturbed. This might be a significant impairment in patients who need to talk a lot or for a longer time. Please explain your patients that this might happen.

Apart from this, patients need to be informed that there will be a need for painkillers for up to 12 days in mean after surgery. Postoperative pain distinctively varies interindividually. Please check for intolerances prior to surgery. The intensity of postoperative pain depends on the amount of thermal energy used for blood control.[100,101] Please take a note of this during surgery.

Postoperative hemorrhage is the most common complication after tonsillectomy. In its original version without tonsillectomy we have hardly ever seen a relevant postoperative bleeding.

Please verify the patient's ability to open his/her mouth and have a look at the teeth. Address damages of the teeth and hematoma within the tongue as potential complications induced by the mouth gag. Sometimes, even hypoesthesia of parts of the tongue may occur as a consequence of the pressure induced by the mouth gag. Fortunately, hypoesthesia is mostly temporary.

As mentioned above, the patient needs to be informed about potential swallowing, taste, and voice disturbances.

We use absorbable sutures. These sutures last a couple of weeks. In order to reduce discomfort, we remove these in 10 to 12 days after surgery.

Anesthesia and Positioning

We routinely perform UPS under general anesthesia with the patient being orally intubated and lying in supine position with the head slightly extended. Most mouth gags have a gorge to hold the intubation tube. This is why the tube needs to be placed in midline.

However, there are some reports in the literature that UPF surgery can be done under local anaesthesia.[149]

Equipement

Standard surgical instruments for cold steel tonsillectomies are sufficient. Modern instruments can be used for dissection like lasers, bovies or other monopolar instruments, the coblator system, or others.

Operative Technique/Steps

Transoral Approach

Insert the mouth gag. We always start with topical disinfection of the oral mucosa by using a chlorhexidine solution (0.2%).

For original UPF resect the redundant mucosa at the tip of the uvula first. Then grasp the remaining tip of the uvula and pull it upward to determine the size of the rhomb, where the oral mucosa needs to be resected (▶Fig. 8.22). Sometimes a lateral incision through the webbing is necessary to rotate the UPF upward. We recommend marking the rhomb with a marker.

Using a bovie resect the mucosa and all fat and glands on the oral side of the rhomb without injuring the underlying mucosa. Careful blood control is strongly recommended to avoid postoperative infections and suture insufficiencies.

Now, rotate the inferior margin of the flap into the defect and close the wound with 2–0 resorbable sutures (▶Fig. 8.23).

In case of concomitant tonsillectomy, we recommend to perform the tonsillectomy first (for tonsillectomy, please refer to the section on Tonsillectomy and Tonsillotomy earlier in this chapter). This technique results in an opening of the velopharyngeal valve both anteriorly and laterally (▶Fig. 8.24).

Risks, Tips, and Tricks

- Open the mouth wide enough.
- Initially, resect the uvular tip carefully.
- Use a pen to mark the amount of mucosa resected from the anterior soft palate.
- Sometimes a lateral cut through the webbing is needed to sufficiently surge up the flap.
- Use strong enough suture material (2–0) and enough sutures (≥ 7).
- Remove sutures after 10 to 12 days.
- See section on Tonsillectomy earlier in this chapter.

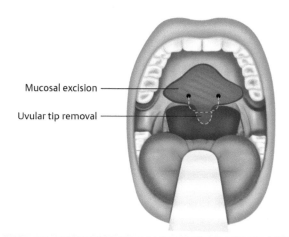

Fig. 8.22 Amount of tissue resected for uvulopalatal flap at the oral side of the soft palate.

Mucosal excision

Uvular tip removal

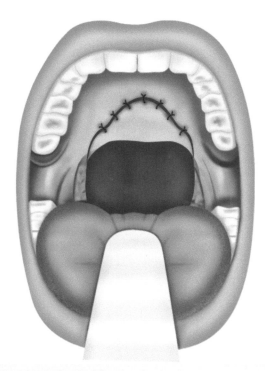

Fig. 8.23 Uvulopalatal flap closed with at least seven sutures (2–0 absorbable threats).

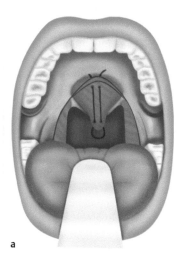 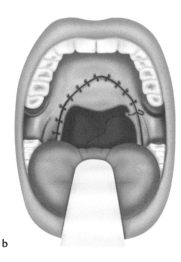

Fig. 8.24 Extended uvulopalatal flap. **(a)** Amount of tissue resected. **(b)** Surgery completed.

a   b

Complications

Postoperative Pain

As any kind of soft palate surgery, UPF can induce significant postoperative pain. According to our own data, postoperative need for analgetic drug intake is 12 days in mean with high interindividual variability. Under medication patients should be free of pain unless during swallowing. Use VASs separately for swallowing and no swallowing to record treatment success.

Hot, spicy, and sour foods and drinks are not recommended during the first 1 to 2 weeks after surgery.

Hemorrhage

As stated earlier, postoperative hemorrhage is not a frequent problem in UPF surgery as long as the tonsils are not removed within the same surgery.

In tonsillectomy, however, it is the most common and potential dangerous complication. Patients should be advised to avoid physical effort, sauna, hot showering or bathing, and other activities that potentially increase blood flow in the head and neck region.

Wound Infection

Although the mouth is always contaminated with various microorganisms wound infections do not occur very frequently. This is why we do not subscribe antibiotics as a general rule, but only in case of infection. We allow our patients to brush their front teeth. In addition, we provide a local antiseptic mouth solution (e.g., chlorhexidine solution) to improve patient's mouth hygiene.

As we use absorbable, braided threads, we need to remove these in 10 to 12 days after surgery.

Postoperative Care

As in any other sleep apnea surgery the severity of OSA has a significant impact on postoperative care and monitoring. This is why sleep apnea patients undergoing surgery under general anaesthesia or under sedation are at an increased risk for perioperative complications.[105,106,107]

This perioperative risk is particularly increased if OSA is treated surgically, as postoperative bleeding and swellings within the pharynx need to be taken into account. According to a review, postoperative complications are rare and occur within the first 4 hours after extubation.[108] This result is in accordance with our own experience. As a result, we keep our sleep apnea patients in the recovery room for 4 hours after extubation. If there are no complications, the patients are regarded to be safe and will be discharged to the regular ward. In case of complications, the patients are monitored overnight.[109]

As stated earlier, management of postoperative pain is crucial after soft palate surgery. A basic treatment with ibuprofen (four times 400–600 mg) in addition with metamizole (four times 0.5–1 g) works fine in adults. However, there are huge interindividual differences that require individual adaptations. If the basic treatment is not sufficient in time add opioids might be added (e.g., three times 10 mg oxycodone). Please refer to Chapter 10.2 for further information about the postoperative care and medication.

Antibiotics are not mandatory for the perioperative period and perioperative antibiotic prophylaxis is not applied routinely.

Outcomes

So far, there are only two case series that published objective data about the isolated use of the UPF without tonsillectomies in OSA patients.[150,151] The prior study reports about 30 patients. The mean AHI significantly decreased in this group from 19.2 at baseline to 8.2 2 months after surgery. The more recent series included 83 OSA patients.[151] The follow-up period was 54 months in mean. The AHI decreased from 45.6 to 19.4. In both studies, patients benefitted in terms of daytime fatigue. The ESS score decreased from 5.5 to 3.0 in the study by Hörmann, and from 16.4 to 7.7 in the study by Nerunturat, respectively.

There is more data available for UPF plus tonsillectomy (e.g., EUPF). However, all but one study is published by the same working group. ▶ Table 8.6 summarizes the latest available objective PSG data about the effectiveness of UPF and EUPF.[152] According to ▶ Table 8.6, data about EUPF show very homogenous results with a success rate of more than 75%. This is much more as for any other kind of soft palate surgery. We were not able to reproduce these favorable results.

> ## Key Points
>
> The UPF is an easy and quick to perform technique to address palatal obstruction. We used this technique frequently in patient after prior tonsillectomy. However, frequent and disturbing postoperative xerostomia after UPF lead to decreasing numbers of patients that are treated with this technique.
>
> In combination with tonsillectomy, the UPF enlarges the oropharynx both in anterioposterior and in lateral dimension.

Z-palatopharyngoplasty

Hsin-Ching Lin and Michael Friedman

Definition

Clinically, numerous amounts of OSA/hypopnea syndrome (HS) individuals who could not tolerate or were not willing to accept CPAP therapy as a long-term treatment will consider alternatives, including upper airway surgery. For this group of patients, the benefits of OSA surgery have been demonstrated.[159] The traditional method of UPPP remains the most common surgical procedure performed as treatment for OSA but has demonstrated frequent technical failure. Systematic review of reported success rate for UPPP was however around 40.7% in nonselected OSA patients.[160] In view of its limited success in treating OSA, many adjunctive or modified procedures have been proposed or performed concurrently or sequentially to alleviate upper airway obstructions. Several advances have been made in the surgical treatment of OSA, and considerable interest has increased with the recent refinements in the last decade.[147,161,162,163]

The concept of Z-palatopharyngoplasty (ZPPP) was first introduced by Friedman et al as a modification of classic UPPP in 2004 and modified from the Z-palatoplasty procedure and pharyngoplasty.[3] The initial publication described its use for OSA patients without tonsils. The key of this technique is to not remove velopharyngeal musculature to widen the velopharyngeal space; instead, the zeta-flaps will create the necessary superoanterolateral tension to widen the pharynx and also ameliorate some of the possible complications of traditional UPPP. The theory behind ZPPP, which represents a double Z-plasty, is to change scar contraction tension lines to an anterior-transverse vector (as compared with an anterior-medial pull in classic UPPP). This change serves to widen the anteroposterior and lateral oropharyngeal air apace at the level of the velopharynx. The technique of ZPPP also has incorporated

▶ Table 8.6 Objective results of modified UPPP surgeries without additional tongue base surgeries

Author	N	Technique	Follow-up (months)	AHI (pre)	AHI (post)	Success rate (%)	ESS (pre)	ESS (post)	EBM
Hörmann et al[150]	30	Flap	2	19.2	8.2	46.7	5.5	3	4
Neruntarat[151]	83	Flap	54	45.6	19.4	51.8	16.4	7.7	4
Elbassiouny[153]	28	SPWF	6	46	11	No data	No data	No data	4
Li et al[148]	33	EUPF	6	41.6	12.5	81.8	No data	No data	4
Li et al[154]	105	EUPF	12	43.8	15	80	No data	No data	4
Li et al[155]	55	EUPF	6	43.6	21.1	82	11.8	7.5	4
Li et al[156]	84	EUPF	6	46.5	14.6	No data	11	7.2	4
Li et al[157]	50	EUPF	6	44.5	13.4	84	No data	No data	4
Li et al[122]	110	EUPF	6	44.4	15	78.2	No data	No data	3b
Lin et al[158]	55	EUPF	6	43.6	12.1	No data	11.8	7.3	3b
All	1,070		10.14	43.07	15.55	70.92	11.52	6.09	B

Abbreviations: AHI, apnea–hypopnea index; ESP, expansion sphincter pharyngoplasty; ESS, Epworth sleepiness scale; EUPF, extended uvulopalatal flap; LP, lateral pharyngoplasty; MEUP, microdebrider-assisted uvulopalatoplasty; rPP, relocation pharyngoplasty; SPWF, soft palate webbing flap; UPPP, uvulopalatopharyngoplasty.
Notes: EBM = level of evidence-based medicine; flap = uvulopalatal flap.

this concept by removing the bulky, LPWs and maintaining the adequate tension to prevent its collapse in selected OSA patients.

The results from the initial study showed more successes with acceptable morbidity for OSA patients using ZPPP rather than UPPP. Subsequential publications have discussed further modification for patients with OSA.[164,165,166,167,168,169] These articles described ZPPP as a relatively aggressive surgical procedure; however, it resulted in improved success rates for those patients studied.

Any new surgical technique must be performed by multiple surgeons, accumulating more experience, in order to validate its safety and efficacy. The safety and efficacy of ZPPP combined with tongue base tissue voulme reduction for treating moderate/severe OSA with unfavorable airway anatomy has been reported.[165,169,170]

Indications, Contraindications, and Patient Selection

Indications include the following:
1. Age ≥ 20 years old.
2. Significant symptoms of habitual snoring and/or excessive daytime somnolence.
3. Moderate/Severe OSA.
4. Failure or refusal of attempts at conservative treatments, such as oral appliances or CPAP.
5. Friedman Tongue Position (FTP) ≥ III[96,99].
6. RP and/or LPW obstructions identified by fibroscopic examination with/without Mueller's maneuver or DISE.
7. Selected revision palate surgery.
8. BMI < 35 kg/m².

Contraindications of ZPPP include the following:
1. No palatal obstruction during DISE.
2. Professional voice users and patients not willing to accept risk of VPI.
3. Previous palatal defect reconstruction surgery.
4. OSA patients with Friedman's stage I disease.

Because ZPPP is a relatively aggressive soft palate procedure for OSA, it is usually applied to moderate/severe OSA patients who frequently had multilevel obstructions of the upper airway. Therefore, additional septoplasty or endoscopic sinus surgery without nasal packing and/or tongue base procedure, such as radiofrequency reduction of the tongue base (RFBOT) or transoral endoscopic Coblator open tongue base resection (Eco-TBR), can be simultaneously performed during the same-staged surgery to treat the additional obstruction site(s).

Diagnostic Workup

Overnight, attended comprehensive diagnostic sleep studies (e.g., PSG) should be performed in a temperature-controlled and sound attenuated room. The patient(s) should be evaluated for the risk of regular general anesthesia. The severity of upper airway collapse/obstruction(s) is examined based on Friedman's OSA staging system and identified by fibroscopic examination with/without Mueller's maneuver or DISE.

Specific Risks, Patient Information, and Consent

Patients have to be informed about the expected success rate (approximately 60%) and the possibility of a combination of other surgical procedures such as nasal and/or hypopharyngeal surgery. Swallowing problems may last for several days, most typically in the initial 3 to 5 days. Frequently drinking water may help speed up the recovery process. Voice changes may initially occur but usually will not persist. Taste disturbance and VPI might also occur initially.

Pain

In the case of ZPPP as the only procedure or combined with other procedures, pain must be anticipated. A combination of multiple oral and/or local narcotics may help reduce the severity of pain.

Anesthesia and Positioning

The author (H-C. L.) prefers that the procedure is performed under general anesthesia with regular orotracheal intubation. The neck should be in slight hyperextension (pillow under shoulders) with an armed tube diverted upward, exposure is obtained using a standard mouth retractor.

Equipment

Standard tonsillectomy/UPPP net.

Operative Technique/Steps

The surgical techniques (see ►Fig. 8.25, ►Fig. 8.26, ►Fig. 8.27, ►Fig. 8.28, ►Fig. 8.29, ►Fig. 8.30, ►Fig. 8.31, ►Fig. 8.32; Video 8.1) are as follows: (1) the procedure starts with a bilateral tonsillectomy preserving as much mucosa as possible; (2) after the tonsillectomy, a subtotal uvulectomy is done (if necessary); (3) two adjacent flaps are outlined on the palate; (4) only mucosa of the anterior aspect of the two zetaplasty (ZPP) flaps is removed; (5) the two flaps are separated from each other by splitting the palatal segment down the midline; (6) the palatoglossus muscle is cut, if necessary, to allow for lateral expansion of the air-space; (7) a very meticulous two-layer closure (with Vicryl suture 2–0 and 3–0) bringing the midline all the way to the anterolateral margin of the palate, and tonsillar fossa is accomplished. The goal is to increase the nasopharyngeal and

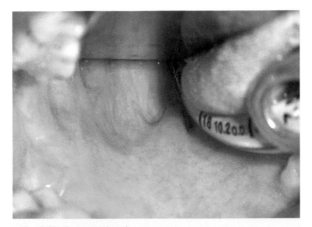

Fig. 8.25 Preoperative view.

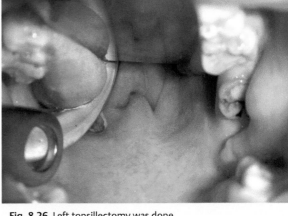

Fig. 8.26 Left tonsillectomy was done.

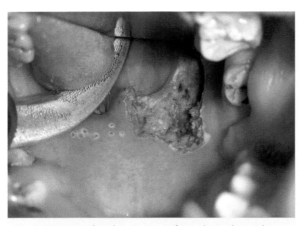

Fig. 8.27 A partial uvulectomy is performed together with this procedure, if the uvula is greater than 1 cm. The incision of the palatopharyngeal flap is marked. The mucosa over right palatopharyngeal flap is removed, exposing the palatal musculature. The soft palate and shorten uvula are split in the midline. Cut the palatoglossus muscle if necessary.

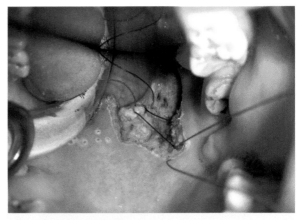

Fig. 8.28 Submucosal closure is very important.

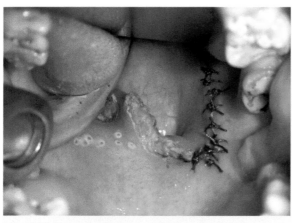

Fig. 8.29 The uvular flaps along with the soft palate are reflected back laterally over the soft palate. Two-layered submucosal closure of the palatopharyngeal flaps and lateral pharyngeal wound.

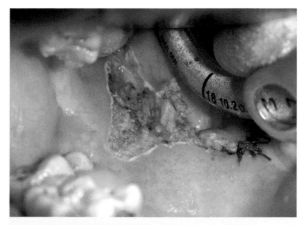

Fig. 8.30 The mucosa over left palatopharyngeal flap is removed, exposing the palatal musculature.

oropharyngeal airway in both the anterior posterior dimension with minimum tissue resection, and to preserve the soft palate shape. In addition, the ZPPP procedure often corrects significant nasopharyngeal stenosis when present. On the basis of severity of

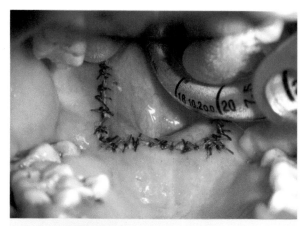

Fig. 8.31 Two-layered mucosal closure of the palatopharyngeal flaps and lateral pharyngeal wound.

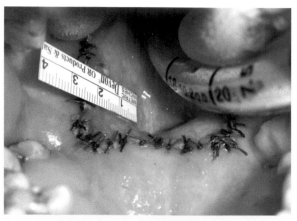

Fig. 8.32 Z-palatopharyngoplasty could widen the anteroposterior and lateral oropharyngeal air space at the level of the velopharynx.

disease and anatomy, tongue base tissue volume reduction or tongue base suspension procedure could also be performed at the same time.

Risks, Tips, and Tricks

- Encourage oral hygiene before the surgery.
- Select the adequate OSA patients for ZPPP, such as a wide open mouth and good dentition.
- Use cold or low-temperature instruments during the surgery.
- Avoid damaging too much palatal and oropharyngeal mucosa.
- Achieve good hemostasis and ensure a very meticulous two-layer closure of the ZPPP wound.
- Raise the systolic blood pressure of the patient to over 100 mm Hg to check the wound status before finalizing the procedure.
- Prepare the surgical and anesthesia team to gently wake the patient in the operating room.

Complications

There were no perioperative complications or cases of immediate postoperative airway obstruction in our experience. The number of days of narcotic pain medication (ibuprofen 400 mg, qid) used ranged from 4 to 16 days. Difflam Spray (benzydamine hydrochloride, 3 mg/mL) could be used to spray two to four puffs directly to the sore area every 2 to 4 hours for local pain and inflammation. We did not have any patients who had serious postoperative bleeding from an oropharyngeal wound and needed to return to the operating room for hemostasis.

Temporary postoperative VPI was noted, in our experience, in around 40% of the patients. The VPI lasted between 3 days to 1 month and appeared to bother the patients most significantly during the first week after surgery. As per our patients' reports, the severity of the VPI usually decreased after the first week and was thereafter only noted occasionally when drinking quickly or when attempting to swallow food or liquid while talking. None of the cases had permanent VPI, which bothered the patient's daily life. Some patients, around 30%, reported temporary ear fullness or pressure postoperatively, but none had this discomfort for more than 2 weeks. The majority of minor complications encountered were related to postoperative throat discomfort such as sensation of a lump in the throat, dry throat, and frequent throat clearing. However, typical complaints included inability to clear phlegm, swallowing changes, and tightness in the throat. Patients must be willing to accept these possible changes while choosing this surgical treatment. None of the patients had palatal fistula or infection after ZPPP that required additional surgery.

Since ZPPP had created anterior and lateral forces to increase the oropharyngeal space, this might induce secondary tongue base collapse in some patients due to loss of some support from original soft palate or oropharyngeal framework in sleep. The patients should be well informed about this potential risk preoperatively.

Other complications and risks associated with surgery and anesthesia are presented as well.

Postoperative Care

The patients were extubated after fully recovering from the anesthesia in the operating room. We did not encounter the complication of immediate acute airway obstruction that needed to be reintubated or noticed any acute surgical wound bleeding after extubation.

The patient was in a head-up position with a backrest elevation of around 30 to 45 degrees, especially in the first night after surgery. Intravenous antibiotics (cefazolin) were given postoperatively and oral antibiotics (cefadroxil) were used for 5 days after surgery. Low-dose steroids were prescribed for 5 days. Nonsteroidal anti-inflammatory drugs (NSAIDs, ibuprofen,

400 mg per 6 hours), proton-pump inhibitor or H2-receptor antagonists, and chlorhexidine-diluted povidone-iodine mouth rinses were prescribed for 1 week. A cool liquid or soft diet started 4 to 6 hours after surgery. Soft foods, such as ice cream, sherbet, yogurt, pudding, apple sauce, and Jell-O, should be encouraged. However, similar to most palatal surgeries, complaints of obviously postoperative pain in the throat and dysphagia are to be expected after ZPPP. Pain is often worse at night and may prompt the need for additional pain medication. An ice collar can also be helpful for postoperative sore throats. Oral narcotics are used after discharge for 5 to 14 days. Patients generally are able to return to a normal diet after 14 days.

Strenuous physical activity following surgery is not encouraged till 10 to 14 days after surgery.

Outcomes

So far, there is not much information about the effect of isolated ZPPP procedure in the literature. There were nine articles,[164,165,166,167,168,169,171,172] which reported the issue related to ZPP(P) and only seven case series[164,165,166,167,168,169] with a total of 203 patients could be identified to summarize the surgical outcomes (see ▶ Table 8.7).

The follow-up periods were short and lasted not longer than 6 months. The objective and subjective data both show a significant improvement of OSA severity as well as its daytime symptoms. This should have an extended study to observe the possible long-term success rate after ZPPP and/or adding a tongue base procedure. Additionally, controlled trials are still missing.

There are two additional large reviews which overlap with the data in ▶ Table 8.7. One is from Friedman et al[171]

in 2015 and the other is our unpublished data. Friedman reported his 5 years experience and suggested that ZPP(P) might serve as a potential alternative to traditional UPPP in treating palatal-level obstruction in patients with and without tonsils. In our experience of 220 patients with OSA who underwent ZPPP and/or simultaneous nasal and tongue base surgery (unpublished data, up to December 2016), we did not have any cases of massive wound bleeding peri- and postoperatively, or severe permanent VPI after ZPPP.

Key Points

ZPPP is a reasonably effective alternative treatment for OSA patients with palatal obstruction who refuse of cannot tolerate CPAP therapy as a long-term treatment. It can be performed as a primary treatment in case of isolated RP obstruction, revised surgery for previous conservative UPPP or as part of multilevel surgery when nasal, RP, and/or retrolingual obstruction are present in OSA patients. Indications are AHI > 15/h, BMI < 35 kg/m², and obvious obstruction on palatal level during DISE.

Success rates as part of multilevel surgery have been reported and vary between 46 and 68%. ZPPP has a low morbidity and literature shows it is one of the most effective treatment options for patients with OSA.

In conclusion, the reported literature shows reasonable surgical outcomes and relative safety of ZPPP combined with/without tongue base surgery in selected OSA patients with unfavorable upper airway anatomy. Our experience has been encouraging overall, and the procedure could be one of our surgical treatments of choice for OSA patients.

▶ Table 8.7 Surgical success is defined as having a postoperative apnea–hypopnea index (per hour, AHI) of 20 or less and at least a 50% reduction in the number of respiratory events

Author	N	Adjunctive procedure	Follow-up (months)	AHI (pre)	AHI (post)	Success (%)	ESS (pre)	ESS (post)	EBM
Friedman et al (2004)[149] (for patients without tonsil)	25	RFBOT	6	41.8	20.9	68	12.5	8.3	4
Friedman et al (2007)[152] (revised UPPP failure)	31	Nil	6	No data	No data	67.7	14.3	7.3	4
Lin et al (2010)[153]	43	RFBOT	6	51.5	23.4	60.5	12.8	10	4
Yi et al (2011)[154]	26	GAHM	6	65.6	30.1	46.2	13.5	6.9	4
Xiong et al (2004)[155]	23	Nil	6	No data	No data	65.2	No data	No data	4
Liu et al (2013)[156]	20	Nil	6	No data	No data	60	No data	No data	4
Lin et al (2014)[157]	35	Eco-TBR	> 3	50.6	26.5	62.9	11	8.7	4
All	203	—	3–6	—	—	—	—	—	4

Abbreviations: Eco-TBR: transoral endoscopic coblation open tongue base resection; ESS, Epworth sleepiness scale; GAHM, genioglossus advancement and hyoid suspension; RFBOT, radiofrequency reduction of the tongue base; UPPP, uvulopalatopharyngoplasty.
Note: EBM = level of evidence-based medicine.

Declaration of Interest

The authors report no conflicts of interest. The authors are responsible for the content and writing of this section.

Relocation—UPPP

Thomas Verse

Definition

The "relocation pharyngoplasty (rPP)" has first been described in 2009 by Li and Lee.[173] It is a further development of Li's "EUPF" described in 2003.[148] The latter technique is a palatopharyngeal flap combined with resection of the supratonsillar fat tissue, covering mucosa. The suturing is done in a double layer in order to achieve a widening of the velopharyngeal valve anteriorly but also laterally (▶Fig. 8.33; Video 8.2).

The rPP is a comparable technique that instead of a palatopharyngeal flap only gets along with a careful shortening of the uvula. As a result, the remaining uvula secures lumbrification of the throat after surgery. This is an important fact, as xerostomia is a frequent and severe problem after palatopharyngeal flap surgeries.

Indications, Contraindications, and Patient Selection

The rPP is a technique that addresses soft palate obstruction (anterioposteriorly and laterally) in patients with simple snoring and OSA. If tonsils are still in place, they should be removed within the same sitting. However, rPP can be performed in patients who have had undergone tonsillectomy earlier in their life.

Naturally, the patients need to be able to open their mouth wide enough to insert the mouth gag and the surgical instruments. Sometimes dental pathologies exist that might interfere with insertion of the mouth gag. Please check preoperatively and address this issue in the informed consent.

As in any sleep apnea case, severe comorbidities need to be excluded. The patient must be suitable for surgery under general anesthesia.

As tonsillectomy is affected with the risk of postoperative hemorrhage in—depending on the definition used—up to 11% of the cases we do not perform surgery in patients with blood coagulation disorders, and in patients in need for anticoagulative medications that cannot be paused during the perioperative period.[97] We recommend the preoperative use of a questionnaire asking for blood coagulation disturbances (refer to section on Tonsillectomy and Tonsillotomy earlier in this chapter).

Like any kind of soft palate surgery, rPP may affect the fundamental frequency of the voice. Therefore, we are very cautious with the indication of tonsillectomy in professional singers and speakers.

Rare complications of tonsillectomy are taste disturbances, in particular the persisting perception of a bitter taste. This issue needs to be discussed with professional chefs or ambitious cooks.

In addition, neuromuscular diseases, neurological or psychiatric illnesses in need of treatment, cleft palates, chronic alcoholism, soporific drug abuse, severe bite misalignments, preexisting velopharyngeal stenosis or incompetences, and certain severe craniofacial deformities are regarded as contraindications.

Diagnostic Workup

Any kind of sleep apnea surgery requires objective preoperative sleep studies. Without a preoperative sleep study the effect of the surgery on the AHI and other objective parameters cannot be determined after surgery. Apart from this, subjective complaints need to be recorded pre- and postoperatively. Please refer to Chapter 5 to find the instruments that are available for this purpose.

Please screen for dysphagia and taste and speech disorders prior to surgery. To screen for blood coagulation

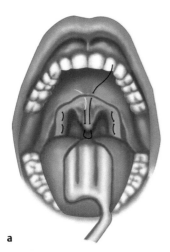 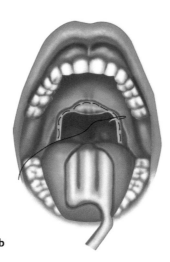

Fig. 8.33 (a, b) Extended uvulopalatal flap.

a   b

disorders we use a specific questionnaire. In addition, we routinely test for olfactory and taste functions to identify preexisting taste disorders.

Specific Risks, Patient Information, and Consent

The general risks of surgery (i.e., pain, scarring, infection, wound healing problems, and postoperative hemorrhage) need to be addressed. Edema of the uvula occurs frequently and may induce foreign body sensation or even dyspnea. Such an edema usually responds well to corticosteroids.

Apart from this, patients need to be informed that there will be a need for painkillers for up to 12 days in mean after surgery. Postoperative pain distinctively varies interindividually. Please check for intolerances prior to surgery. The intensity of postoperative pain depends on the amount of thermal energy used for blood control.[100,101] Please take a note of this during surgery.

Postoperative hemorrhage is the most common complication after tonsillectomy. The method of tonsillectomy used does not seem to have a substantial effect on the incidence of postoperative hemorrhage.[102,103] Please check for prior bleedings and/or affinity for bleedings in the patient's history. Prebulged or pulsatile tonsils may indicate an aberrant course of one of the branches of the external carotid artery.

Please verify the patient's ability to open his/her mouth and have a look on the teeth. Address damages of the teeth and hematoma within the tongue as potential complications induced by the mouth gag. Sometimes, even hypoesthesia of parts of the tongue may occur as a consequence of the pressure induced by the mouth gag. Fortunately, hypoesthesia is mostly temporary.

As mentioned earlier, the patient needs to be informed about potential swallowing, taste, and voice disturbances.

Severe wound healing deficits or intense revision surgery for blood control of postoperative bleedings may rarely result in nasopharyngeal stenosis or velopharyngeal incompetence.

We use absorbable sutures. These sutures last a couple of weeks. In order to reduce discomfort, we remove these in 10 to 12 days after surgery.

Anesthesia and Positioning

We routinely perform rPP under general anesthesia with the patient being orally intubated and lying in supine position with the head slightly extended. Most mouth gags have a gorge to hold the intubation tube. This is why the tube needs to be placed in midline.

Equipment

Standard surgical instruments for cold steel tonsillectomies are sufficient. Modern instruments can be used for dissection like lasers, bovies or other monopolar instruments, the coblator system, or others.

Operative Technique/Steps

Transoral Approach

Insert the mouth gag. Often, it is helpful to fully expose one tonsil by pushing the tongue to the opposite side. The tongue is held in that position by the adequate tongue blade.

We always start with topical disinfection of the oral mucosa by using a chlorhexidine solution (0.2%).

If still in place, remove the tonsils first. By doing this it is crucial to save the surrounding muscle tissue as carefully as possible.

Now, the posterior pillar is grasped with a forceps and pulled anteriorly, laterally, and cranially. While doing this we perform an incision very caudally through the posterior pillar (in contrast to the originally published technique by HY Li) in order to reduce the tension (▶ Fig. 8.34). Now, the posterior pillar can easily be moved craniolaterally overlapping the anterior pillar. Mark this position of the posterior pillar with a sterile pen on the mucosa of the anterior pillar. Once the overlapping part of the anterior pillar is plotted, it can be resected. Include the underlying

Fig. 8.34 (a, b) Relocation pharyngoplasty (Hamburg technique).

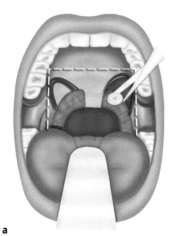
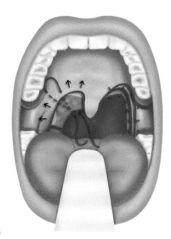

a   b

supratonsillar fat tissue in your resection. After careful blood control (use a little energy as possible to avoid postoperative pain) the posterior pillar is sutured into the newly created defect. We strongly recommend two layers of sutures. We use 2–0 Polysorb (company: Covidien) absorbable, braided material to suture the muscle tissue. Please use at least three sutures per side. Afterward, we close the mucosa with 3–0 absorbable, braided threads. Please use at least six mucosal sutures per side. ▶ Fig. 8.35 shows the patient's left side is done. As the right side has not been touched, the image nicely illustrates the opening of the velopharyngeal valve anterolaterally.

After having done the same steps to the other side, we carefully reduce the redundant mucosa of the uvula (▶ Fig. 8.36). It is crucial to keep a clearly visible uvula to avoid postoperative xerostomia. Depending on the amount of mucosa taken out we close the wound with the same 3–0 absorbable, braided thread.

Risks, Tips, and Tricks

- Open the mouth wide enough. Separate exposition of each side using the mouth gag maybe helpful.
- While performing the tonsillectomy, save as much mucosa and muscle tissue as possible.
- Avoid intensive use of thermal energy in order to minimize postoperative pain.
- Use sharp instruments for the dissection in case of intensive scar tissue.
- The caudal incision through the posterior palatal pillar reduces the tension of the flap.
- Use a pen to mark the amount of mucosa resected from the anterior pillar.
- Use two layers of sutures (2–0 for muscle tissue, 3–0 for mucosa).
- Remove sutures after 10 to 12 days.
- A very careful resection of mucosa at the tip of the uvula reduces uvular edema after surgery.
- Edema of the uvula responds well to corticosteroids.

Complications

Postoperative Pain

As any kind of soft palate surgery, rPP can induce significant postoperative pain. According to our own data, postoperative need for analgetic drug intake is 12 days in mean with high interindividual variability. Under medication patients should be free of pain unless during swallowing. Use VASs. separately for swallowing and no swallowing to record treatment success.

Hot, spicy, and sour foods and drinks are not recommended during the first 1 to 2 weeks after surgery.

Hemorrhage

As stated earlier, postoperative hemorrhage is the most common and potential dangerous complication. Patients should be advised to avoid physical effort, sauna, hot showering or bathing, and other activities that potentially increase blood flow in the head and neck region.

Wound Infection

Although the mouth is always contaminated with various microorganisms wound infections do not occur very frequently. This is why we do not subscribe antibiotics as a general rule, but only in case of infection. We allow our patients to brush their front teeth. In addition, we provide a local antiseptic mouth solution (e.g., chlorhexidine solution) to improve patient's mouth hygiene.

As we use absorbable, braided threads, we need to remove these in 10 to 12 days after surgery.

Postoperative Care

As in any other sleep apnea surgery the severity of OSA has a significant impact on postoperative care and monitoring. This is why sleep apnea patients undergoing surgery under general anaesthesia or under sedation are at an increased risk for perioperative complications.[105,106,107]

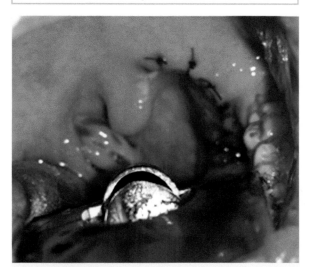

Fig. 8.35 Relocation pharyngoplasty (Hamburg technique). Left side done, right side untouched.

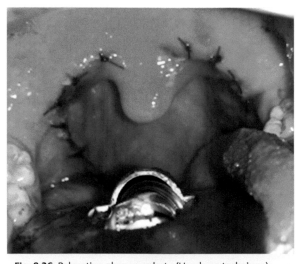

Fig. 8.36 Relocation pharyngoplasty (Hamburg technique). Surgery completed.

This perioperative risk is particularly increased if OSA is treated surgically, as postoperative bleeding and swellings within the pharynx need to be taken into account. According to a review, postoperative complications are rare and occur within the first 4 hours after extubation.[108] This result is in accordance with our own experience. As a result, we keep our sleep apnea patients in the recovery room for 4 hours after extubation. If there are no complications, the patients are regarded to be safe and will be discharged to the regular ward. In case of complications, the patients are monitored overnight.[109]

As stated earlier, management of postoperative pain is crucial after soft palate surgery. A basic treatment with ibuprofen (four times 400–600 mg) in addition with metamizole (four times 0.5–1 g) works fine in adults. However, there are huge interindividual differences that require individual adaptations. If the basic treatment is not sufficient in time add opioids might be added (e.g., three times 10 mg oxycodone). Please refer to Chapter 10.2 for further information about the postoperative care and medication.

Some authors recommend the intraoperative use of long-lasting local anesthesia (like bupivacaine). We did not achieve any substantial benefit. Other authors recommend the use of ice cubes to cool the wound intraoperatively.[110] Unfortunately, this trick did also not show any significant effect in our own patients. For this reason, we stopped intraoperative ice cooling again.

Antibiotics are not mandatory for the perioperative period and perioperative antibiotic prophylaxis is not applied routinely.

Outcomes

So far, there are two case series that published objective data about the isolated use of rPP in OSA patients.[173] The prior study reports about 10 patients. The mean AHI significantly decreased in this group from 43.4 at baseline to 15.1 6 months after surgery. The more recent series included 47 OSA patients.[174] The follow-up period was 6 months as well. The AHI decreased from 59.5 to 22.6. Patients with positional obstructive sleep apnea (POSA) benefitted significantly better as compared to those patients without POSA.

▶ Table 8.8 summarizes the latest available objective PSG data about the effectiveness of modern modifications of UPPP.[175] According to ▶ Table 8.8, data about the different surgical techniques seem to be very similar. However, apart from lateral pharyngoplasty, data still need to be regarded as preliminary. This means, data are presently not sufficient to tell which technique might be superior. Probably this question will depend on the surgeon's skills and preferences anyway.

By now, we performed more than 200 rPP surgeries in our department. We mostly combine it with hypopharyngeal surgeries. This is why we are not able to add substantial new data about the isolated use of rPP. Clinical experience is promising with no increased complication rates or postoperative discomfort so far as compared to conventional UPPP. Having tried most of the techniques summarized in ▶ Table 8.8, we currently prefer the rPP, as it shows good results in out hands.

Key Points

The rPP nicely opens the velopharyngeal valve anterolaterally without the risk of velopharyngeal incompetence. We gained superior results as compared to conventional UPPP. Due to this fact rPP is our standard procedure to treat velopharyngeal collapse in OSA patients.

As compared to the original technique published by HY Li,[173] we perform an additional incision through the caudal part of the posterior pillar in order to reduce the tension of the posterior pillar while it is rotated superolaterally.

Two layers of absorbable, braided sutures work fine in our hands. However, the superficial mucosal sutures need to be taken out after 10 to 12 days.

Lateral Wall Addressing Pharyngoplasties

Claudio Vicini, Mohamed Salah El-Rashwan, Giuseppe Meccariello, Chiara Bellini, and Andrea Marzetti

Introduction

Since the last century, generations of ear, nose, and throat (ENT) specialists have performed thousands of pharyngeal procedures removing tonsils and adenoids for recurrent infections or breathing problems. We may consider all of them as "not aware" sleep surgeons. In the area of simple snoring, Ikematsu (1964), as a real pioneer, designed the first surgical solution offering an anatomy-customized palate procedure.[183] In the area of sleep apnea a German team introduced tracheostomy as cure for severe obstructive disease, demonstrating at the same time the crucial role of upper airway collapse in producing OSA, and introducing us to a new treatment modality.[184] Deeply inspired by the previous work of Ikematsu, Fujita (1981) was the first surgeon who described an original palatal procedure in order to fix snoring and obstructive sleep apnea hypopnea syndrome (OSAHS) at the same time.[45] After its introduction in 1981, UPPP was intensively applied all over the world, receiving in all but a few countries a high degree of appreciation. UPPP was so frequently modified and adapted by so many different surgeons and opinions that a list of the entire span of individual versions is probably impossible to complete. In a very rough and schematic way, two different lines of development and improvement of UPPP may be described:

1. The first line of development includes all the techniques related to UPPP designed with the goal to *increase the ratio between outcomes and costs/ complications rate* reducing the invasiveness and on the other hand improving efficacy, or both. It

▶ Table 8.8 Objective results of modified UPPP surgeries without additional tongue base surgeries

Author	N	Technique	Follow-up (months)	AHI (pre)	AHI (post)	Success rate (%)	ESS (pre)	ESS (post)	EBM
Hörmann et al[150]	30	Flap	2	19.2	8.2	46.7	5.5	3	4
Neruntarat[151]	83	Flap	54	45.6	19.4	51.8	16.4	7.7	4
Elbassiouny[153]	28	SPWF	6	46	11	No data	No data	No data	4
Li et al[148]	33	EUPF	6	41.6	12.5	81.8	No data	No data	4
Li et al[154]	105	EUPF	12	43.8	15	80	No data	No data	4
Li et al[155]	55	EUPF	6	43.6	21.1	82	11.8	7.5	4
Li et al[156]	84	EUPF	6	46.5	14.6	no data	11	7.2	4
Li et al[157]	50	EUPF	6	44.5	13.4	84	No data	No data	4
Li et al[122]	110	EUPF	6	44.4	15	78.2	No data	No data	3b
Lin et al[158]	55	EUPF	6	43.6	12.1	No data	11.8	7.3	3b
Li and Lee[173]	10	rPP	6	43.4	15.7	50	9.6	6.3	4
Li et al[174]	47	rPP	6	59.5	22.6	49	12.2	7.5	4
Pang and Woodson[163]	23	ESP	7	44.2	12	82.6	No data	No data	2b
Hsu et al[176]	35	EUPF+LP	3	47.6	23.4	43	10.2	4.3	2b
Cahali[162]	10	LP	8.2	41.2	9.5	60	13	5	4
Cahali et al[177]	15	LP	7.9	41.6	15.5	53.3	14	4	2b
de Paula Soares et al[178]	18	LP	6	33.5	20.9	50	No data	No data	4
Sorrenti and Piccin[179]	85	LP	6	33.3	11.7	89.2	No data	No data	4
Chi et al[180]	25	LP	5	34.1	17.3	No data	10.5	7.7	2b
Han et al[181]	68	Han-UPPP	6	32.1	12.7	69.1	10.1	4.5	4
Liu et al[168]	51	Han-UPPP oder ZPPP	6		65.6	45.1	12.8	5.5	3b
	31	Han-UPPP				35.5			
	20	ZPPP				60			
Huang and Cheng[182]	50	MEUP	6	37.9	6.1	80	9.8	5.2	4
All	1,070		10.14	43.07	15.55	70.92	11.52	6.09	B

Abbreviations: AHI, apnea–hypopnea index; ESP, expansion shincter pharyngoplasty; ESS, Epworth sleepiness scale; EUPF, extended uvulopalatal flap; LP, lateral pharyngoplasty; MEUP, microdebrider-assisted uvulopalatoplasty; rPP, relocation pharyngoplasty; SPWF, soft palate webbing flap; UPPP, uvulopalatopharyngoplasty; ZPPP, z-palatopharyngoplasty.
Notes: EBM = level of evidence-based medicine; Flap = uvulopalatal flap.

includes different geometries of section (parasagittal vs. circular), the use of reversible flaps, the application of manipulations of the bony palate plate, the introduction of many different minimally invasive technologies (lasers, radiofrequency, coblation, implants, sclerosant agents, conventional or barbed sutures, etc.).

2. The second line of development in the story of the sleep surgery was the attempt to *address concurrent collapsing area(s) contributing to apnea but different from palate* (e.g., tongue base, LPW), which includes tongue base surgery, facial bone framework procedures, multilevel procedures, etc.

In recent years, a special group of modifications has gained increasing diffusion and popularity. The common feature of this group of surgeries is the special attention to lateral displacement and splinting of the LPW. It means that this type of procedures fit to both the lines of development outlined above. Herein we will include all those techniques as *lateral wall addressing pharyngoplasties* (or simply LWAPs).

Definitions

It is somehow hard to give a precise and comprehensive definition of LWAP. First of all to some extent the most classic UP3s included some action in the area of the lateral walls inside the palatine tonsil bed. Tonsillectomy and sutures between anterior and posterior pillar had some effect in gaining space in the lateral pharyngeal area, and some tightening of the same wall was observed. In some conservative modifications of the classic UPPP the transversal enlarging effect was particularly evident. On the other hand, many common palate procedures for snoring and OSA are very clearly far from this LWAP philosophy: laser-assisted UPPPs (LAUPS) and UPFs, transpalatal advancement and interstitial procedures (snoreplasty, RFVR, Pillar) may be excluded. All the so called LWAPs share a common aim to be particularly in addressing the LPW, but basically all the LWAPs increase the anteroposterior diameters as well and at the same time.

The prototypic lateral pharyngoplasty by Cahali "consists of a microdissection of the superior pharyngeal constrictor muscle within the tonsillar fossa, sectioning of this muscle, and suturing of the created laterally based flap of that muscle to the same-side palatoglossus muscle. In addition, a palatopharyngeal ZPP is performed to prevent RP collapse. The created vector pulls the pharyngeal constrictor laterally toward the palatoglossus muscle.

In Woodson and Pang (2007) expansion sphincter pharyngoplasty (ESP), the tip of a posterior pillar/palatopharyngeal muscle superiorly based flap is pulled up and laterally toward the pterygoid hamulus (three-dimensional vector lateral, anterior, and superior; ▶ Fig. 8.37; Video 8.3).[163]

In Li and Lee's rPP, an intact posterior pillar is laterally suspended to the anterior pillar/palatoglossus muscle (anterolateral vector).[173]

In Vicini et al's barbed reposition pharyngoplasty (BRP, 2015), an inferiorly weakened intact posterior pillar is superolateral suspended by a fan of superolateral pulling vectors created by means of a running barbed suture.[185]

A very elegant application of the basic Z-plasty (technique to increase soft-tissue length along a selected axis) was introduced by Friedman (2004), sculpturing a couple of Z-flaps in the soft palate which produce a couple of superolateral directed enlarging vectors.[161]

Finally, the best definition including all the published variations in LWAPs probably is a group of pharyngeal surgical procedure for sleep disordered breathing which share a common prevalent superolateral enlarging vector of force devised for enlarging the pharyngeal airway and, more important, for splinting lateral wall and prevent its inward collapse (see ▶ Table 8.9).

Historical Perspective: The First Steps

The first series of 10 lateral pharyngoplasties was published by Michel Cahali, San Paolo (Brasil) in 2003 as a prospective randomized pilot study performed in an academic tertiary center as part of a doctoral thesis.[162] In a next study, the authors stated, "lateral pharyngoplasty produces better clinical and PSG outcomes in the treatment of OSAHS than does UPPP, without resultant differences in the cross-sectional measurements of the pharyngeal airway between these treatments."[177] More recently, a new article introduced a more conservative modification of the original technique in preserving stylopharyngeal muscle, with very interesting results in reducing long-term dysphagia.[186]

In 2014, in a small case series, the authors affirmed, "lateral pharyngoplasty proved to reduce the values obtained in the 24-hour ABPM due to a significant reduction of blood pressures during sleep in patients with OSA 6 months after surgery.[178] Although the patients presented with reductions in AHI, arousals, and desaturation time, this was not correlated with the improvement in arterial blood pressure."

Lateral Wall Anatomy

The LPW anatomy is generally divided into two levels: RP and RG (retroglossal). This division has importance from an anatomical rather than physiological point of view as the LPW works as a single unit. Here the important

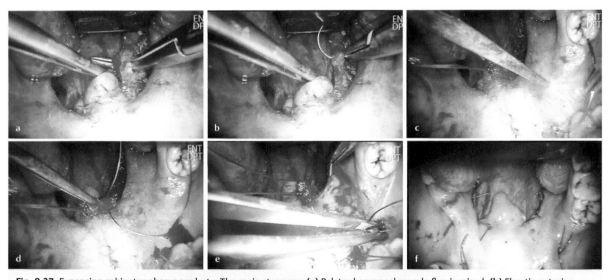

Fig. 8.37 Expansion sphincter pharyngoplasty. The main steps are: **(a)** Palatopharyngeal muscle flap is raised. **(b)** Flap tip suturing. **(c)** Palate tunneling. **(d)** Flap repositioning. **(e)** Flap tip suture to the Hamulus. **(f)** Final view.

► **Table 8.9** Comparative synopsis of the main features of five LWATs

LWAT	Lateral pharyngo-plasty	Expansion sphincter pharyngoplasty	Relocation pharyngoplasty	Barbed reposition pharyngoplasty	Zetaplasty	LWAT	Lateral pharyngo-plasty	Expansion sphincter pharyngoplasty
Author	Cahali[162]	Woodson and Pang[163]	Li[173]	Vicini[185]	Friedman[161]	Author	Cahali[162]	Woodson and Pang[151]
Vector tail	Superior constrictor	Dissected posterior pillar	Intact posterior pillar	Released, posterior pillar	Full thickness palate flap	Vector tail	Superior constrictor	Dissected posterior pillar
Vector tip	Anterior pillar	Hamulus	Anterior pillar	Pterygo man-dibular Raphe	Lateral soft palate	Vector tip	Anterior pillar	Hamulus
Suture	Reabsorbable, separate, traditional	Reabsorbable, flap tip suture	Reabsorbable, separate, traditional	Reabsorbable, running, barbed	Reabsorbable, separate, traditional	Suture	Reabsorbable, separate, traditional	Reabsorbable, flap tip suture
Uvula	spared	Removed/Spared	trimmed	Anteriorized	split	Uvula	spared	Removed/Spared

Note: The enlarging action is described as a vector with a tail in the mobilized structure and a tip where the mobilized structure is suspended by different types of sutures.

structures are described from medial to lateral regarding the RP LPW: the lining mucous membrane, the palatine tonsils (a mass of lymphoid tissue incompletely surrounded by capsule) bounded by the palatoglossus muscle anteriorly, the palatopharyngeal muscle posteriorly and the superior constrictor pharyngeal muscle laterally, a group of small muscles including the tensor veli palatini, levator veli palatini, salpingopharyngeus, styloglossus, and stylopharyngeus muscles. The ptery-gomandibular raphe arising from the pterygoid hamulus, attached in the posterior end of the mylohyoid line of the mandible giving origin to the superior constrictor muscle of the pharynx. This raphe has a very important clinical importance in LPW surgeries.

The supratonsillar fossa is the region above the upper pole of the palatine tonsil occupied by a fat pad and Weber's minor salivary glands. This area is of particular importance while performing different types of LPW addressing techniques.

Moving down to the RG level, the most important anatomical structure is the hyoid bone which consists of a body, two lesser horns, and two greater horns. It plays a central role in the upper aerodigestive tract as it is the only bone not articulating with other bones. The stylo-hyoid ligament has a stabilizing role to the hyoid bone, suspended through posterosuperior vector to the styloid process. The middle constrictor muscle of the pharynx makes the hyoid bone fixed to the pharynx. It arises from the greater horn of the hyoid bone and any movement causes tension in the LPW at the RG level.

The parapharyngeal fat pad is very important in the pathophysiology of the LPW collapse in patients with OSA. It is directly related to obesity, especially central. We have to realize that obesity is not the only determinant for the volume of the parapharyngeal fat, but other factors such as age, sex, craniofacial size, and ethnicity have to be considered as well.

Lateral Wall Pathophysiology

In the last few years, an increasing number of articles have emerged that define in a comprehensive way the central role of the LPW in the determination of the pharyngeal obstruction related to OSA.

The pathophysiological mechanisms for OSA are multifactorial by nature. The most important risk factors include increased anatomic compromise, increased pharyngeal dilator muscle dysfunction, lowered arousal threshold, increased ventilatory control instability, and/or reduced lung volume.

The two most important mechanisms with direct effect on LPW collapse include[1] anatomic theory: parapharyngeal fat deposition and thickening of soft tissue of pharyngeal wall and[2] a neural hypothesis: decreased neural output to pharyngeal dilator muscles during sleep, leading to muscle hypotonia.[187]

Obesity is a direct risk factor for OSA and LPW collapse, as the parapharyngeal fat pads cause collapse and narrowing of upper airway during sleep. Larger neck circumference has been associated with greater severity of OSA.[188]

Welch et al investigated fat tissue and upper airway volume in the neck during a weight-loss program and found that there is an increase in the upper airway volume in both the RP and RG regions after weight loss. Larger fat tissue volume in the RP area may be associated with positive segmental closing pressures. Also, fat tissues deposited in the lateral wall a the RG area may add to the volume of total collapsible soft tissues in the corresponding segment of airway, which predisposes to increased RG collapsibility.[189]

Schwab et al (2003) were the first to use magnetic resonance imaging (MRI) to assess upper airway in OSA.[190] They found that the volume of the soft-tissue structures surrounding the upper airway is enlarged in patients with sleep apnea and that this enlargement is a significant risk factor for OSA, particularly at the LPW.

Huon et al (2016) used dynamic MRI in proving that increased LPW collapsibility is a major determinant of airway obstruction in (severe) OSA.[191] Increased collapsibility of the LPW may reflect inadequate neuromechanical response to airway obstruction in patients with severe OSA, while in the matched patients with mild OSA, coordinated airway dilation mechanism during sleep is preserved.

There is a strong association between LPW collapse and severity of oxygen desaturation during DISE.[192]

Soares et al (2016) linked failure of surgery with the presence of severe LPW collapse in the preoperative DISE.[193]

In 2015, Liu et al used static measures and dynamic sleep MRI to observe patterns of dynamic airway collapse in patients with mild and severe OSA.[194] They found that longer upper airway lengths and more inferior and posterior position of the hyoid are associated with severe OSA. They noticed the cut-off to be approximately between 8 and 9 cm for upper airway length, as measured from the level of the posterior nasal spine to the hyoid bone. They also linked the severity of the disease with the presence of LPW collapse.

In the same year, Liu et al also showed that maxillomandibular advancement (MMA) increases LPW stability, as based on VOTE scoring from DISE.[195] Based on the above mentioned information regarding the pathophysiology of LPW collapse, preoperative assessment using DISE is crucial in order to be able to know the pattern of pharyngeal collapse. In case of LPW collapse during DISE, the subsequent surgical technique has to address this specific collapse pattern.

Dynamic MRI might also be a tool, to add to the information obtained from DISE, and might be of use to assess soft-tissue thickness, either at pharyngeal or parapharyngeal level.

Lateral Wall Expanding/Stenting Mechanism

The various LWAP techniques work in a different way, but basically share the same goal: lateralizing and stenting the LPW. All techniques share a common biophysical background—to create an enlarging vector directed mainly laterally, and at the same time anteriorly and cranially in a different degree. For didactic purposes we will describe the main vector for each different technique, with special reference to the basic features of each vector: the tail, the head, the direction, and the force. In some techniques, additional effects must be considered.

In lateral pharyngoplasty as originally described by Cahali, the tail of the vector is located in a surgically developed, lateral based, superior constrictor flap and the head of the vector points to the adjacent palatoglossus muscle inside the anterior pillar. The anterolateral pulling force is produced by 3 to 4 separate sutures. It must be stressed that in the Cahali technique the combination of the superior constrictor lateral blunt dissection, the muscle interruption, and the possible posterior wall splitting in the midline allows an easy mobilization of the posterior pillar toward the anterior pillar, without significant tension. In addition, a palatopharyngeal elongating Z-plasty is performed to prevent RP collapse.

In Li's technique the vectorial analysis is quite similar to the Cahali technique (tail in palatopharyngeal muscle, head in palatoglossus), as well the separate sutures array. In addiction, a careful supratonsillar fossa defatting is described. Due to the lack of manipulation in the posterior pillar area, the tensile strength of the separate sutures is slightly superior to lateral pharyngoplasty.

In ESP, the vectorial analysis is particularly interesting. A single, very effective vector connects the tail in the tip of a posterior pillar raised muscle flap to the head, located precisely at the ipsilateral hamulus. The required tension may differ according to the different oropharyngeal anatomy, but the complete transsection of the palatopharyngeal muscle makes a significant flap transposition possible with a limited amount of tension.

In BRP, the vector analysis may be summarized as a fan-like array of multiple small vectors connecting the palatopharyngeal muscle at different levels to the pterygomandibular raphe at different levels as well. The raphe is lateral, anterior, and superior to the posterior pillar, and this strategic location provides the lucky relationship that explains the efficacy of the technique.

In addition, the palatopharyngeal muscle is weakened in order to allow an easier lateralization and anteriorization, without high levels of tensile tension for the suture. Furthermore, the barbed running suture tends to distribute the overall required tension in a significant number of suture loops. Inside any loop the tension is not concentrated in the single knot, but widely dispersed in hundred of barbs, which implies a higher level of stability. It was experimentally measured an average tension for the main loops of the running barbed suture of 1.9 N.

Indications, Contraindications, and Patient Selection

By definition, a prevalent LPW collapse is the logic application for all the different options of LWATs. It is worth mentioning that all LWATs share a different degree of anterior palate displacement/stenting, which is an additional useful way of action.

Diagnostic Workup

The diagnostic workup is not different from the basic approach to any other sleep surgical procedure.

Specific Risks, Patient Information, and Consent

Any different LWATs may register a different percentage of common complications, including intra and postoperative bleeding, VPI, dysphagia, late scarring, as summarized in ▶Table 8.10. In LP, the risk of intrusion into the parapharyngeal space seems to be a little higher. In ESP,

▶ Table 8.10 Results of studies on lateral wall addressing pharyngoplasties

Study	N	Age	BMI	Palatoplasty	Pre-OP AHI	Post-OP AHI	Success rate[a] (%)	F/U
Pang, 2007[163]	45	42.1	28.7	ESP	44.2 ± 10.2	12.0 ± 6.6	82.6	6
				UPPP	38.1 ± 6.46	19.6 ± 7.9	68.1	
Sorrenti and Piccin[179]	85	42.7	—	FEP	33.3	11.7	89.2	36
Vicini et al[196]	24	54.2	27.2	ESP	38.5 ± 14.3	9.9 ± 8.6	91.7	9
				UPPP	38.3 ± 19.6	19.8 ± 14.1	50	
Ulualp[197]	50	8	32	MESP	60.5 ± 38.5	2.4 ± 3.9	80	6
				TA	59.8 ± 33.6	6.2 ± 6.0	60	
Carrasco et al[198]	53	43.9	27.5	ESP	27.7 ± 7.5	6.5 ± 5.2	90	6.9
				PPR	47.2 ± 21.4	18.4 ± 17.4	72.7	
				ZP	22.5 ± 4.4	13.9 ± 9.0	25	
				LP	48.0 ± 35.5	15.2 ± 12.3	70	
				UPPP	47.3 ± 27.1	12.0 ± 7.1	71.4	

Abbreviations: FEP, functional expansion pharyngoplasty; LP, lateral pharyngoplasty; MESP, modified expansion sphincter pharyngoplasty; PPR, partial palate resection; pre-OP AHI, preoperative apnea–hypopnea index; post-OP AHI, postoperative apnea–hypopnea index; TA, adenotonsillectomy; UPPP, uvulopalatopharyngoplasty; ZP, Z-palatoplasty.

Notes: N = total number of patients enrolled; Age = mean age; BMI = mean of body mass index; ESP = expansion sphincter pharyngoplasty; F/U = mean follow-up in months.

[a]Success rate is defined as 50% reduction of preoperative AHI and AHI < 20, except in Ulualp:[197] postoperative AHI < 5.

bleeding during the soft palate tunneling may be an issue. If this happens during surgery, in general, the bleeding can be stopped by applying local pressure. In BRP, a late suture extrusion may be encountered. Generally speaking, the reported rate of significant complications seems to be reasonably low.

Anesthesia and Positioning

Anesthesia and positioning is not different for LWATs from classic UP3 or UPF.

Equipment

No special equipment is required, besides a proper set of barbed sutures for BRP.

Operative Technique/Steps

A detailed description of all the different techniques is beyond the purpose of this chapter. As an example, we will describe a basic BRP as we previously described in our pilot study. All the procedures are performed with patients under general anesthesia and orally intubated, exposed by a Boyle–Davis mouth gag together with lateral cheek retractors to provide wide access to the surgical field. The patient is positioned in supine position with under the shoulders an inflatable bag to keep the head extended. The first step is bilateral tonsillectomy with identification and meticulous preservation of the palatoglossus and palatopharyngeus muscles. The most important trick is to preserve as much mucosa as possible, covering both anterior and posterior pillars.

Two releasing partial incisions was carried out using a pinpoint bowie (Colorado) at the inferior (caudal) part of the palatopharyngeal muscle, but the muscle is not dissected from the posterior pillar flap. A full thickness (mucosa and muscle) triangle is removed at the superolateral corner of the tonsil ogiva, in order to obtain a wider and most squared oropharyngeal inlet. At the same time, a careful debulking of the supratonsillar fat pad is carried out.

The center of the palate is marked at palatal spine. The pterygomandibular raphe in both sides is located by digital palpation and marked as well. We use a single barbed suture, bidirectional polydioxanone absorbable Monofilament, size 0, with transition zone in the middle. One needle is introduced at the center point then passed submucosally, turning around the pterygomandibular raphe till it comes out at the most superior part of the raphe at one side; the thread is pulled until it hangs at the central transition zone which is a free zone present between the two directions of the thread (▶Fig. 8.38b). The needle is again introduced close to the point of exit through the pterygomandibular raphe till it comes out in the upper pole, then through the upper part of the palatopharyngeus muscle and comes out near the mucosa of the posterior pillar but not through it (▶Fig. 8.38c).

The needle is then again passed through the upper pole, wherein the suture will be suspended around the raphe. Traction is applied only on the thread and no knots are needed (▶Fig. 8.38d). This leads to repositioning of the posterior pillar to a more lateral and anterior location. The stitch is repeated at least three times between raphe

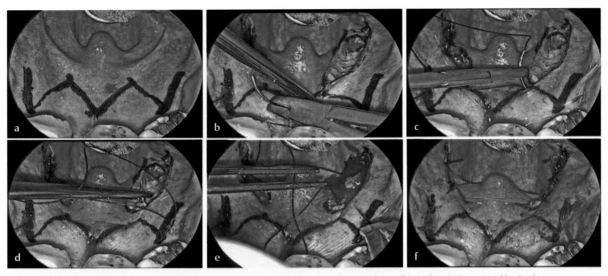

Fig. 8.38 Barbed reposition pharyngoplasty. **(a)** Landmarks and preplanned suture lines. **(b)** Midline bidirectional barbed suture (first step). **(c)** Second leg is lateral to pterygomandibular raphe. **(d)** Needle passing into the tonsil fossa. **(e)** Suture around the posterior pillar. **(f)** Final view.

and muscle till the lower pole of the muscle is reached. The opposite side is done by the same way till the lower pole is reached. Finally, each thread comes out at the raphe of the same side, for locking of the stitches and looseness prevention; a superficial stitch in the opposite direction is taken, then the thread is cut while pushing the tissue downward for more traction (▶ Fig. 8.38).

• Marking the center of the palate, pterygomandibular raphe, and squaring of anterior pillars.
• The barbed suture is around the upper part of the right raphe and it hangs at the central transition zone.
• The needle is passed through the upper part of the palatopharyngeus muscle and it comes out near the mucosa of posterior pillar and not through it.
• The needle is passed through the upper pole and is suspended around the raphe, pulling the barbed suture without taking down the knots.

The tip of uvula is not removed if it is short, instead a small island of the mucosa is removed from its anterior aspect by monopolar diathermy, and then coagulation of the submucosal tissue is done by bipolar diathermy. Once suturing this mucosal gap, the uvula will bend forward. If the uvula is too long, remove its tip, and then the same technique is carried out. At the end, ordinary stitches are done between the mucosa of both pillars for their closure.

Comparative Results

Literature reports a long list of comparative studies comparing any new described technique with UPPP as classic reference. Generally speaking, all the new LWATs proved to be superior to the basic UPPP (see ▶ Table 8.9). The preliminary data of an ongoing multicenter study on outcome of barbed relocation pharyngoplasty are shown in ▶ Fig. 8.39.

Limits and Complications

In ▶ Table 8.11, a list of complications of the LWATs is summarized.

Future Perspectives

Year by year, the new generation of LWATs is replacing the classic UPPP with its endless number of minor variations. In the near future, we expect that UPPP will be just a historical surgical procedure, in the same way in which laryngeal surgery transcervical thyrotomy was almost totally deserted.

Secondly, to imagine the possibility to avoid the need of an additional hyoid procedure in a multilevel setting, if LWATs proves to be sufficient for stenting the inferior lateral wall at the retrolingual level. This special concept is still under evaluation by means of ongoing comparative studies.

Anterior Palatoplasty

Kenny P. Pang, Edward B. Pang, and Kathleen A. Pang

Definition

Collapse of the upper airway is often multilevel—at the level of the palate/velopharynx, the base of tongue, and/or the LPWs. Many patients with OSA have either a thick redundant soft palate or bulky LPWs that contribute to the collapse and obstruction of the upper airway. These areas of collapse should be addressed, if one is aiming to relieve the patient of the apneas.[200,201]

Many techniques that have been introduced to treat snoring and OSA are mainly aimed to create scar tissue, in order to incite fibrosis and stiffen the palate. With the stiffened palate, the vibration of the palate diminishes. Hence, the snoring would reduce. The palatal stiffening

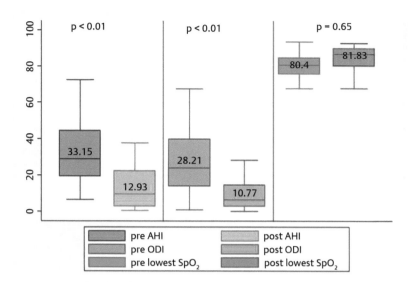

► Table 8.11 Reported complication after pharyngoplasties

Study	Number of patients	Type of procedure	Complication rate (%)	Type of complications
Pang et al[199]	487	UPPP ESP	7.1	Negative-pressure pulmonary edema (0.4%) Tongue edema (1.8%) Bleeding (3.1%) Hypertension (3.1%) Oxygen desaturation (1.2%) Airway obstruction (0.2%)
Vicini et al[196]	24	UPPP ESP	12.5	Pneumonia (4.2%) Subcutaneous emphysema (4.2%) Severe edema (4.2%)
Lundkvist et al[136]	158	UPPP	2.5	Bleeding (1.2%) Severe pharyngeal edema (1.2%)
Kezirian et al[137]	3,130	UPPP	1.6	Reintubation, pneumonia, prolonged ventilation (>48 h), emergent tracheotomy, pulmonary edema, cardiac arrest, myocardial infarction, cerebrovascular accident, pulmonary embolism, hemorrhage of more than 4 U of packed red blood cells, coma, wound infection, deep venous thrombosis, renal failure, or systemic sepsis

Abbreviations: ESP, expansion sphincter pharyngoplasty; UPPP, uvulopalatopharyngoplasty.

surgery was first introduced by Ellis in 1994[202] (involving stripping of a small area of uvular and palatal mucosa) and modified by Mair in 2000.[203] Both techniques showed encouraging results, although it produced a stellate and puckered scar on the soft palate that resulted in tenting and pulling of the LPWs medially, and therefore narrowing of the lateral distance between the tonsillar pillars laterally. These anatomic manifestations might explain why some patients did not have much benefit from the procedure. Pang et al described the modified CAPSO technique done under local anesthesia.[204] This technique showed encouraging results for patients with snoring and mild OSA.[204] The modified CAPSO technique was renamed as the anterior palatoplasty in 2009, as the technique involved the anterior surface of the soft palate primarily.[205]

Indications, Contraindications, and Patient Selection

The anterior palatoplasty can be performed as an isolated procedure in patients with mild to moderate OSA, without tongue base obstruction noted on Mueller's maneuver and/or DISE. Studies have showed better results when BMI was <32 kg/m². The anterior palatoplasty can be part of multilevel surgery in patients with moderate to severe OSA, with tongue base obstruction noted noted on Mueller's maneuver and/or DISE. The anterior palatoplasty is best performed in patients with anteroposterior velopharyngeal collapse, small tonsils, lower BMI, and with no retrolingual collapse. However, patients with big tonsils may also have anteroposterior velopharyngeal collapse noted; these patients may have an anterior palatoplasty and a tonsillectomy performed at the same sitting. The anterior palatoplasty may be performed under local anesthesia in the office/clinic (as an outpatient setting) or performed under general anesthesia.

The following OSA patients should not have the anterior palatoplasty performed as a single procedure: patients with AHI > 40, BMI > 32, patients with LPW collapse (should have a combined ESP), and patients with total tongue base collapse.

Diagnostic Workup

PSG (overnight PSG or WatchPAT device) or related measures are used to assess the severity of OSA, followed by DISE to gather information of the level(s) of obstruction.

Specific Risks, Patient Information, and Consent

Risks are related to anesthesia and are specific to surgery.

General risks of surgery, including postoperative pain, infection, and secondary hemorrhage, are to be addressed.

Patients may have odynophagia for 7 to 10 days postoperative; the pain on swallowing usually subsides by day 10 or 11 postoperative.

Analgesics are given for 10 to 14 days, with 1-week course of prophylactic antibiotics (e.g., Augmentin). Pain varies from patient to patient, but, in general, the pain from this procedure is typically not excruciating.

Postoperative secondary hemorrhage rate is similar to that of tonsillectomy.

Anesthesia and Positioning

Most of the articles had the anterior palatoplasty technique done under general anesthesia; however, the anterior palatoplasty technique can be done under local anesthesia in the office as well. General anesthesia would be the standard choice if the patient had relatively larger sized tonsils (tonsil size 2, 3, or 4) and a tonsillectomy was needed.

Equipment

There is no specific specialized or expensive equipment required; the electrocautery would suffice, although some surgeons might prefer to use the coblation technology.

Vicryl 4–0 sutures would be preferable but may vary based on the surgeon's preference.

Operative Technique/Steps

The procedure may be done under local anesthesia in the office as an outpatient. The patient is seated in an examination chair with the mouth open. Topical lignocaine (10%) is used to anesthetize the palatal region. A total of 2 to 4 mL of 1:80.000 adrenaline and 2% xylocaine is injected into three sites of the soft palate (▶Fig. 8.40). A partial uvulectomy (usually using diathermy/radiofrequency/coblation) may be performe (▶Fig. 8.41),

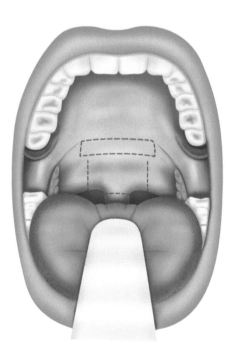

Fig. 8.40 Typical anterior palatoplasty markings.

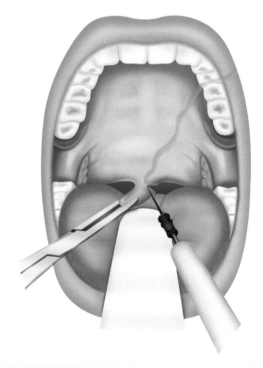

Fig. 8.41 Partial uvulectomy.

followed by superolateral cuts (parauvular cuts) on either side of the uvula (▶Fig. 8.42), especially if there is very prominent posterior and/or anterior palatal arch webbing

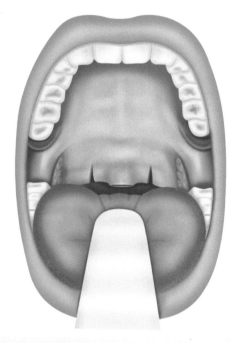

Fig. 8.42 Lateral cuts made on the palatal posterior arches.

through both soft palatal arches. A horizontal rectangular strip of mucosa is removed from the soft palate (about 40–50 mm in length by 7–10 mm in width) down to the muscle layer (▶Fig. 8.43). Hemostasis is achieved with electrocautery. The horizontal stripped area on the soft palate is sutured with Vicryl 4–0 round body curved needle. A minimum of 10 to 20 sutures are used to appose the wound edges (while suturing, the entire soft palate is transposed anteriorly and superiorly; ▶Fig. 8.44).

The same procedure may be carried out under general anesthesia with the patient in supine position using the Boyle–Davis mouth gag with an oral intubation. Tonsillectomy is first performed followed by the anterior palatoplasty (in the same fashion as described earlier). The anterior and posterior tonsillar pillars may or may not be sutured together, depending on the author/surgeon's preference.

The barbed anterior palatoplasty is a variant or evolved technique of the anterior palatoplasty.[206] This technique is similar to the anterior palatoplasty, the barbed thread would be the addition, in order to allow the suture to suspend the different mucosa and muscular planes without the need to tie knots. The authors use the double needle QUILL knotless tissue closure device, Angiotech Pharmaceutical Inc., Vancouver, Canada.[206] The barbed suture is passed from the pterygoid hamulus, pterygomandibular raphe from both sides, and passed through the rectangle box superiorly and inferiorly in a zig-zag fashion. The authors conclude their description of the procedure

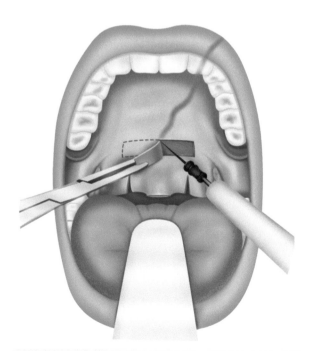

Fig. 8.43 The horizontal strip of mucosa being removed.

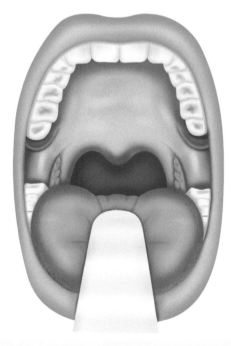

Fig. 8.44 Typical superior upward scarring of the palatal tissue from the anterior palatoplasty.

by including the Roman Blind technique proposed by Mantovani et al.[207,208]

Complications

Postoperative Pain

The anterior palatoplasty technique is typically less painful than the traditional UPPP; the pain from the anterior palatoplasty is usually from the combined tonsillectomy procedure (if any). Generous analgesics are recommended. Soft diet with avoidance of hot and spicy food would be prudent.

Hemorrhage

Secondary hemorrhage is not common but similar to tonsillectomy surgery. Bleeding from the anterior palatoplasty procedure per se is fairly rare.

Postoperative Care

All patients are prescribed with anesthetic gargles (Difflam) and lozenges (Difflam), NSAIDs (naproxen sodium), narcotics (such as codeine), and/or cyclooxygenase–2 inhibitors.

Outcomes

We performed a systematic literature search using Medline, Google Scholar, Cochrane Library, and Evidence-Based Reviews (up to June 30, 2016) databases for procedures that included the anterior palatoplasty and its variants, mainly the modified CAPSO and the barbed anterior palatoplasty.[206]

The primary efficacy outcome was preoperative and postoperative AHI values, following the anterior palatoplasty with or without any comparison with the traditional UPPP and/or other surgical method like the UPF. The secondary outcome was surgical success rate defined as a reduction of postoperative AHI by 50% (compared to preoperative AHI) and an AHI value below 20. Means with SD were summarized for the major outcome and the AHI change before and after surgical intervention was evaluated as for the treatment effect. Other outcomes taken into consideration include, snoring VAS reduction, ESS, snoring reduction (as a percentage), pain levels (as a VAS), pain duration (number of days) and 2-year satisfaction (based on patient and bed partner reports).

The database search identified six studies potentially eligible for review and analysis (see ▶ Table 8.12 and ▶ Table 8.13).[204,205,206,209,210,211] Two studies had compared the anterior palatoplasty with either the UPF[209] or the modified UPPP[210] (illustrated separately in ▶ Table 8.3). All these studies had reported the various result outcomes in terms of AHI, lowest oxygen desaturation, ESS, snore VAS, snoring reduction, and/or pain score and pain duration (see ▶ Table 8.12 and ▶ Table 8.13). Five of these studies reported the ages, BMI, and pre/postoperative AHI; however, only two articles reported their pre/postoperative

▶ Table 8.12 Illustrating the pre- and postoperative AHI, LSAT, and success rates of the six articles included

	N	Age	BMI	AHI		LSAT		Success (%)	F/U	EBM
				Pre	Post	Pre	Post			
Pang[204]	13	35.7	28.4	12.3	5.2	88.3	92.5	75	3	4
Pang et al[205]	77	39.3	24.9	25.3	11.0	81.4	92.0	71.8	33.3	4
Marzetti[209]	38	>20	26.7	22.0	8.6			86	2	3b
Ugur[210]	50	43	28.8						24	3b
Ugur[211]	42	39.2	35.3	13.2	7.3			57.1	24	4
Salamanca[206]	24	46	28.6	8.9	3.8					4
Overall	278		28.6	16.3	7.1	84.5	92.0	72.5	17.3	B

Abbreviations: AHI, apnea–hypopnea index; LSAT, lowest oxygen saturation.
Notes: Success rates (in all chapters) are defined as 50% reduction of preoperative AHI and an AHI < 20. Success rate is in percentage (N = total number in study; age = mean age of patients; BMI = mean body mass index of patients; F/U = mean follow-up in months); EBM = level of evidence-based medicine.

lowest oxygen values, while four articles reported their overall postoperative success rates, defined as a reduction of postoperative AHI by 50% (compared to preoperative AHI) and an AHI value below 20.[204,205,206,209,210,211]

The numbers of patients in each article ranged from 13 to 77 (total = 278), and mean age ranged from 21 to 51 years. Their mean BMI was 28.6. Substantial and consistent improvement in PSG outcomes were observed in patients after anterior palatoplasty. The results showed that the anterior palatoplasty technique had significant improvement in the AHI postoperatively. The calculated pooled mean preoperative AHI (in six articles) improved from 16.3 to 7.1; the lowest oxygen saturation (in two articles) improved from a mean of 84.5% to 92%; and the snore VAS (in five articles) improved from 7.5 to 3.1, while the Epworth score (in five articles) reduced from 11.3 to 7.3, postoperatively (see ▶ Table 8.12 and ▶ Table 8.13). One study by Marzetti et al revealed that the overall snoring reduction as 80% in their 38 patient pool. The overall prorated pooled success rate for the patients (in the four studies that reported, $n = 170$) was 72.5%, mean follow up of 17.3 months (see ▶ Table 8.12).

Two of these six articles had included a comparison group, comparing with the anterior palatoplasty technique[209,210] (see ▶ Table 8.14). Marzetti et al had compared the anterior palatoplasty technique with the traditional UPF technique.[209] They found that the respective AHI and ESS had significant improvement in the anterior palatoplasty group compared to the UPF group ($p < 0.05$) (see ▶ Table 8.14). Interestingly, Marzetti et al reported that both the pain intensity and duration were lesser in the anterior palatoplasty compared to the traditional UPF group. Ugur et al also had similar results with the anterior palatoplasty group having better improvements in both ESS and snoring reduction compared to the modified UPPP group[210] (see ▶ Table 8.13). Ugur et al showed that the 2-year overall satisfaction rate was significantly better in the anterior palatoplasty group compared to the modified UPPP group (85% compared to 70%, respectively) (see ▶ Table 8.14).

▶ **Table 8.13** Illustrating the preoperative and postoperative ESS, snore VAS, and pain scores of the six articles included

	N	Age	BMI	ESS		Snore VAS		Pain Score	Pain Duration	EBM
				pre	post	pre	post			
Pang[204]	13	35.7	28.4	12.2	8.9	8.3	3.3	Mild	10 days	4
Pang[205]	77	39.3	24.9	16.0	7.9	8.4	2.5	Mild	10 days	4
Marzetti[209]	38	>20	26.7	8.5	4.9		80% ↓	5.1	7 days	3b
Ugur[210]	50	43	28.8	8.4	6.5	5.3	3.4	6		3b
Ugur[211]	42	39.2	35.3	11.5	8.3	6.2	3.4			4
Salamanca[206]	24	46	28.6			9.2	2.9	Mild-mod		4
Overall	278		28.6	11.3	7.3	7.5	3.1			B

Abbreviations: ESS, Epworth sleepiness scale; VAS, visual analog scale.
Notes: N = total number in study; age = mean age of patients; BMI = mean body mass index of patients; EBM = level of evidence-based medicine.

▶ **Table 8.14** Demonstrating the comparative results between the AP with the respective traditional techniques of the UPF and the mod. UPPP

		N	Age	BMI	ESS		AHI		Snore VAS		Success (%)	F/U	Pain VAS	Pain (d)	2 y satisfaction
					pre	post	pre	post	pre	post					
Marzetti[209]	AP	15	48.3	26.5	8.5	4.9	22.0	8.6		80% ↓	86	2	5.1	7	
	UPF	19	46.3	26.6	8.1	5.2	23.0	9.6		70% ↓	84	2	6.8	10.8	
Ugur[210]	AP	26	43.2	28.1	8.4	6.5			5.3	3.4		24	6.0		85%
	mod. UPPP	24	42.1	29.8	9.8	7.3			6.8	4.6		24	8.0		70%

Abbreviations: AHI, apnea–hypopnea index; AP, anterior palatoplasty; ESS, Epworth sleepiness scale; LSAT, lowest oxygen saturation; UPF, uvulopalatal flap; mod. UPPP, modified uvulopalatopharyngoplasty; VAS, visual analog scale.
Notes: Success rates (in all chapters) are defined as 50% reduction of preoperative AHI and an AHI < 20. Success rate is in percentage. (N = total number in study; age = mean age of patients; BMI = mean body mass index of patients; pain (d) = duration of pain in days; F/U = mean follow-up in months).

8.2.2 Tongue Base

Tongue Suspensions and Tongue Implants

Evert Hamans

Definition

OSA is a multilevel disease. Determining the anatomical and physiological site of obstruction is critical for matching a patient to the appropriate surgical intervention(s). At this time, there is no consensus for which procedure is best used to address the soft tissue of the tongue in OSA.[212] However, the practice of a patient-specific operative approach to level of obstruction is gaining acceptance among sleep apnea surgeons.

The tongue base is involved in sleep-disordered breathing in up to 46.6% of the cases in mild to moderate OSA as part of multilevel collapse. In 9.4% of the cases, the tongue base is causing single-level collapse.[213] For patients with clinical signs of tongue base obstruction and without typical findings at the soft palate, tongue base surgery may be beneficial.

Tongue base procedures that do not remove tissue aim to tether the tongue via sutures/ribbons/barbs to the mandible or to compress the tongue from within in order to stabilize it.

Currently, two tongue suspension systems are FDA (Food and Drug Administration) and/or CE approved: Airvance (formerly Repose) from Metronic and Encore from Siesta Medical. The Airvance is a minimally invasive procedure that involves stabilizing the tongue base using a triangular suture configuration anchored to a titanium screw embedded in the mandibular cortex and was first approved in 1998. The Encore system is a similar procedure but creates a suture loop within the tongue without creating penetrations through the mucosal surface of the tongue.

Currently, there is one tongue implant approved in Europe. The ReVENT system (Revent Medical) consists of spring-like implants covered with bioabsorbable material that creates a spring-like force in the tongue in order to keep the airway open.

Experimental work has been done with several implants: magnets, adjustable tongue anchor 202, and piezoelectric tongue anchor. These procedures are either stopped because of failure or extrusion or are still in a phase of optimization by the company.

Indications, Contraindications, and Patient Selection

Tongue suspension and tongue implants can be used as stand-alone procedures, although in a systematic review it is recommended not to do so.[215] In general, these procedures are indicated in patients with mild to moderate OSA with tongue base involvement, and CPAP and/or MAD failure/intolerance or not reimbursed. Absolute contraindications are radiotherapy of the head and neck region in the past, macroglossia, and lingual tonsil hypertrophy. Relative contraindications are earlier RFT of the tongue base, patients with dysphagia, or speech disorders, BMI > 32. Patient selection is performed by clinical examination and DISE. The presence of complete tongue base collapse and the absence of complete circular collapse of the soft palate during DISE are a prerequisite for these procedures.

Diagnostic Workup

Every patient who is considered for tongue suspension or tongue implants should have a clinical ENT examination, a PSG test, and a drug-induced sedated endoscopy. A thorough history is important to exclude contraindications for these procedures.

Risks, Patient Information, and Consent

Since the neurovascular bundles enters in the lateral tongue base on both sides, bleeding and tongue paralysis are the most important risks of performing tongue base suspension or using implants. The surgeon needs to be well aware of the course of these bundles. Other adverse events include hematoma, infection, and granulation tissue formation. Temporarily postoperative complaints like pain, dysphagia, and speech difficulties may occur. Long-term adverse events including erosion or migration of the implant or suspension tetherline or implant failure may occur. Patients need to be informed about the procedure itself, about postoperative complaints and about adverse events in the short and long term. According to most safety accreditations, a written and signed informed consent is required for such procedures.

Anesthesia and Positioning

In general, tongue suspension and tongue implant procedures are performed under general anesthesia for the comfort of both patient and surgeon. Depending on the preference of the surgeon and the patient and on the learning curve and skills of the surgeon, these procedures might be performed under local anesthesia.

In case of general anesthesia, nasal intubation is preferable in order to have better access to the surgical field. Prophylactic antibiotics (1 g cefazoline) are given intravenously.

For both the looping systems and the tongue implant system, the patient is positioned in supine position on the operating table. The mouth and tongue mucosa are desinfected with a local disinfectant. The submental region (from chin till thyroid notch) needs to be sterile and draped in a way that the mouth can still be approached by a nonsterile hand of the surgeon.

Equipment

For both the tongue base loops and the tongue implants, more or less the same surgical instruments are needed: surgical blade, surgical forceps, scissors, needle holder, and bipolar coagulation. The help of an assistant can be very useful.

Operative Technique/Steps

Airvance System

Via a submental incision, a titanium bonescrew is placed at the inner rim of the mandible. The nonresorbable tetherline, which is attached to this bonescrew, is looped through the tongue base by first bringing it to one side of the tongue base with a large needle, puncturing through the tongue surface and picking it up in the mouth, and second looping the tetherline with a curved needle through the tongue base to the other side of the tongue base, and then back to the bonescrew. In this way a triangular loop is created with its top on the midline of the mandible and its base at the tongue base (▶ Fig. 8.45). The correct positioning of the loop on both sides of the tongue base needs to be controlled by a nonsterile hand of the surgeon in the patient's mouth. The amount of tongue advancement that is clinically required (at the discretion of the surgeon) is executed by pulling the loop and knotting it. Once the loop is knotted, no more adaptation is possible. The skin is closed in two layers.

Encore System

Via a submental incision, a nonresorbable loop is positioned in the tongue base with the use of a special designed suture passer. This suture passer allows the loop to be positioned in the tongue base (▶ Fig. 8.46) without puncturing the mucosa of the mouth, keeping the implanted loop sterile. The correct position of the loop needs to be controlled by a nonsterile hand of the surgeon in the patient's mouth. A bonescrew is attached on the midline at the inner side of the mandible. Both ends of the suture loop are now entered in the titratable system of the bonescrew. The amount of tongue advancement that is clinically required is defined by the surgeon by pulling the ends of the loop through the screwsystem and securing it at the proper tension. When clinically required, a second loop can be implanted in a lower position of the tongue base, always controlled by the nonsterile hand of the surgeon in the patient's mouth. The advantage of this system is the titratability during the procedure. If the amount of tongue advancement is clinically not sufficient, more advancement can be achieved in a second stage. Via the same submental approach, the loop and the bonescrew need to be explored, the titratable screw within the bonescrew is disengaged and the loop is tightened a bit more and secured again. This procedure can be executed in the other direction also. The skin is closed in two layers.

This procedure is reversible. If necessary, the loop and the bonescrew can be removed. This should be a simple procedure in most patients; however, some bony overgrowth on the bonescrew can complicate this procedure.

ReVENT System

This system was introduced as a multilevel implant combining the use of both PIs and tongue base implants.[216] The use of the PIs was stopped by the company because of lack of efficacy and the rate of extrusion of these PIs. The company came with a new concept of implantation focusing on the tongue base implants.

Via a submental incision, four guide wires are punctured in the tongue on the midline. Each guide wire should be

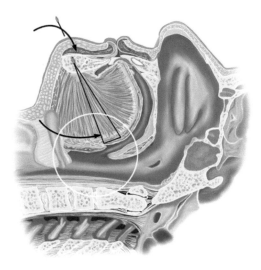

Fig. 8.45 Triangular loop through the tongue base.

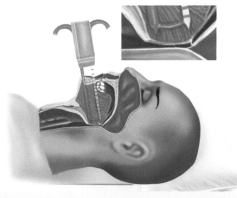

Fig. 8.46 Suture passer introduces the loop in the tongue base.

inserted as deep as possible, until the end of the wire is palpable with the nonsterile hand of the surgeon in the patient's mouth at the surface of the tongue base (▶Fig. 8.47). A special tool is developed in order to insert the guide wires correctly on the midline and in the correct angle. It is important that the loop heals close to the surface of the tongue base. The length of the implants is variable, according to the patient's anatomy (55, 65, or 75 mm).

The tongue implant is a silicone elastomer with loops at each end. The loops are designed to allow tissue healing to anchor the implant in place. The loops also include radiopaque markers for locating the implants postimplementation, if required. The implant body contains segment of bioabsorbable polymer (▶Fig. 8.48) that are absorbed by the body during healing, initiating the dynamic system. The implant is intended for permanent implantation in the tongue base and dynamically supports the tissue after healing.

This procedure is reversible. The implants can be removed via the same submental access. The healing process might create strong fibrosis around the two loops, resulting in possible difficult removal.

Complications

Overall, postoperative complication rates associated with tongue suspension have been reported in the range of 12.5 to 18%.[217,218] Complications may include suture breakage, bleeding, floor of mouth edema, infection (more commonly sialadenitis or very rarely mandibular osteomyelitis), and hypoglossal nerve injury (which are rare). Transient velopharyngeal dysfunction is reported in 25% of patients undergoing tongue suspension and limited anterior excursion in 10 to 15%.[217] Disproportionate pain relative to wound size and suture extrusion is reported in

3 of 28 cases.[218] In recent years, the surgical access site for tongue suspension has switched from the floor of mouth to a submental incision. With this change, complications of floor of mouth edema and suture extrusion can be expected to be reduced.

Every procedure on the tongue (base) with the use of implants or loops can be complicated due to pre-or postoperative bleeding. Good knowledge of the vascular anatomy of the tongue can help in avoiding such complications. The risk of postoperative infection is imminent when using foreign bodies, but it can be avoided by the use of prophylactic antibiotics, proper sterile preparation of the surgical field, and respecting the separation between the sterile and the nonsterile field while performing the procedure. Infection is more likely in the procedures where the mucosa of the mouth is punctured. In case of infection, the implant(s) or loop(s) need to be removed.

Damage to the hypoglossal nerve is unlikely since these procedures address only the posterior tongue (base) and the tongue midline.

Postoperative Care

All procedures discussed here are considered minimally invasive procedures. Postoperative drainage is not required. Postoperative pain might require painkillers (e.g., NSAIDs). In case of postoperative oedema, oral corticosteroids can be considered. Temporary dysfagia might require a proper diet, and temporary speech difficulties might require a few days of work disability. The patient should be instructed that any form of increase in pain and/or local swelling should be reported as soon as possible. The operative wound is protected with a bandage for a week.

Outcomes

In a 2006 systematic review, Kezirian and Goldberg examined six articles on the treatment of hypopharyngeal obstruction with tongue-base suspension (five articles of

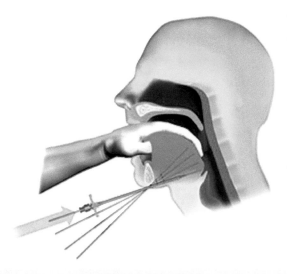

Fig. 8.47 Four guide wires introduced in the tongue base prior to implant placement. Used with permission from Siesta Medical, Inc.

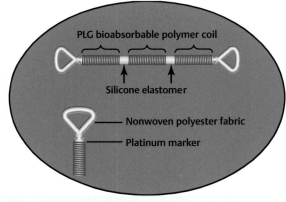

Fig. 8.48 Silicon elastomer surrounded by bioabsorbable polymer of a tongue implant.

EBM level 4; one article of EBM level 2).[219] Each individual study reported significant improvements in AHI and daytime somnolence; however, cure rates were 20 to 57% with overall success in 22 of 77 cases (35%). All patients evaluated had moderate to severe OSAHS. In four of the studies (totaling 49 patients), patients underwent multilevel surgery involving a palatal reconstruction. In two of the studies (totaling 28 patients), tongue suspension was performed as a stand-alone procedure. Since that time, a number of studies have evaluated the use of tongue suspension in conjunction with UPPP[215] with 116 patients studied and an improved average cure rate of 71% (range of 50–81%) in contrast to the classical UPPP success rate of 40%.[160] Outcome data (AHI, ESS) are not published on the ReVENT system yet, although good feasibility and low morbidity are reported.[219]

Key Points

Tongue suspension is a reasonable effective treatment for patients with tongue base obstruction who are CPAP and/or MAD intolerant/ineligible. Indications are mild to moderate OSA, complete tongue base collapse during DISE, and BMI < 32. It can be performed as a stand-alone procedure for isolated tongue base obstruction or as part of a multilevel treatment. The procedure is performed preferably under general anaesthesia, although it is possible under local anaesthesia as well. Data on tongue implants are limited to good feasibility and low morbidity. Both procedures are minimally invasive and can be performed in day care. Tongue suspension has poor results as a stand-alone procedure but has good results when combined with UPPP.

Lingual Tonsillectomy

Thomas Verse

Definition

The lingual tonsils consist of lymphatic tissue that is located at the back of the tongue base. If hyperplastic, usually two lingual tonsils can be seen, one on each side. Hyperplasia of the lingual tonsils most often occurs in patients who have had undergone a tonsillectomy prior in their life. Lingual tonsils are covered externally by stratified squamous nonkeratinized epithelium. The epithelium invaginates inward to form a single crypt. Beneath the epithelium is a layer of lymphoid nodules containing lymphocytes. These tonsils are surrounded by thin capsule of connective tissue which separates them from adjacent structures. Mucous glands located at the root of tongue are drained through several ducts into the crypt of lingual tonsils. Secretions of these mucous glands keep the crypt clean and free of any debris. Therefore, the lingual tonsils are less prone to infection.

Since DISE is routinely used for airway evaluation prior to sleep surgery, hypopharyngeal obstruction is diagnosed much more frequently.[220,221,222] One of the pathological findings that has been found to cause hypopharyngeal obstruction is enlarged lingual tonsils.

This is why LT is performed more frequently within the last few years. LT means the (sub)total resection of the lymphatic tissue at the back of the tongue base without resection of muscle tissue.

Indications, Contraindications, and Patient Selection

LT is a technique that addresses retrolingual obstruction (mainly anteroposteriorly) in patients with OSA. To my knowledge, there are no reports about the use of LT in simple snoring so far. If the lingual tonsils are substantially enlarged, and an anteroposterior obstruction pattern has been observed during DISE, LT might be a useful part of sleep apnea surgery.

As LT is performed transorally, patients need to be able to open their mouths wide enough to insert the surgical instruments. To a certain extend a limited mouth opening can be managed by the use of the CO_2-laser and a distending operationg laryngoscope.

Dental pathologies might interfere with insertion of the mouth gag or laryngoscope and need to be taken into account. Please check preoperatively and address this issue in the informed consent.

As in any sleep apnea case, severe comorbidities need to be excluded. The patient must be suitable for surgery under general anesthesia.

LT will affect swallowing, taste, and speaking within the first couple of days. Swallowing problems may last even longer. This potential complication needs to be mentioned in the informed consent. Long-lasting taste disturbances are rare. However, the possibility of its occurrence needs to be discussed with professional chefs or ambitious cooks.

In addition, neuromuscular diseases, neurological or psychiatric illnesses in need of treatment, cleft palate, chronic alcoholism, soporific drug abuse, severe bite misalignments, preexisting swallowing disturbances, and severe craniofacial deformities are regarded as contraindications.

Diagnostic Workup

Any kind of sleep apnea surgery requires objective preoperative sleep studies. Without a preoperative sleep study the effect of the surgery on the AHI and other objective parameters cannot be determined after surgery. Apart from this, subjective complaints need to be recorded pre- and postoperatively. Please refer to Chapter 5 to find the instruments that are available for this purpose.

Please screen for dysphagia and taste and speech disorders prior to surgery. To screen for blood coagulation disorders we use a specific questionnaire. In addition, we routinely test for olfactory and taste functions to identify preexisting taste disorders.

Specific Risks, Patient Information, and Consent

The general risks of surgery (i.e., pain, scarring, infection, wound healing problems, and postoperative hemorrhage) need to be addressed.

Patients usually develop swallowing problems for a couple of days. Usually, patients can return to normal diet after 3 days. Corticosteroids can help to improve swallowing.

Painkillers will be necessary for up to 12 days after surgery. Postoperative pain distinctively varies interindividually. Please check for intolerances prior to surgery. Patients report less pain after coblation-assisted LT as compared to laser-assisted surgery. Probably this is due to the fact that thermal damage in the surrounding tissue is less with coblation surgery.

Some patients report a different sensation while swallowing. Some people feel that they gained space behind the tongue. Some patients report that they need to concentrate on swallowing. Severe aspiration or dysphagia has not been reported so far.

Postoperative hemorrhage occurs less frequent as compared to tonsillectomy. Blood supply comes through the dorsal lingual artery, tonsillar branches of the facial artery, and the ascending pharyngeal artery. Theses vessels have smaller diameters as compared to tonsillar blood vessels. However, postoperative bleeding is possible and if it occurs, mostly it requires revision surgery. This is why we only perform LT as an inpatient procedure.

Please verify the patient's ability to open his/her mouth and inspect the dental status. Address damages of the teeth and hematoma within the tongue as potential complications induced by the mouth gag. Sometimes, even hypesthesia of parts of the tongue may occur as a consequence of the pressure induced by the mouth gag. Fortunately, hypoesthesia is mostly temporary.

As mentioned earlier, the patient needs to be informed about potential swallowing, taste, and voice disturbances.

Anesthesia and Positioning

We routinely perform LT under general anesthesia with the patient being orally intubated and lying in supine position with the head slightly extended.

In patients with limited mouth opening we perform laser surgery via a distending operating laryngoscope. In patients who are able to open their mouths wide enough we prefer coblation surgery due to reduced postoperative pain. For both kinds of LT good relaxation is required.

Some authors prefer nasal intubation. Oral intubation works fine and saves nasal trauma.

Equipement

For coblation assisted surgery we use a FK retractor (▶ Fig. 8.49). Precondition for successful surgery is a wide mouth opening of the patient. The FK retractor provides a couple of spatulas that allow excellent exposure of the lingual tonsils (▶ Fig. 8.50). We use the Coblator technique for both tissue resection and coagulation. However, more intense bleedings often require additional electrocautery, either monopolar or bipolar. A surgical suction system is necessary as well.

For laser surgery we use a distending operating laryngoscope (▶ Fig. 8.51). We prefer the CO_2-laser (AcuPulse, Lumenis) with a power setting of 8 W (continuous mode). For blood control a monopolar electrocautery system is strongly recommended.

In both surgeries a toothed rack helps to avoid damage of the teeth.

Operative Technique/Steps

Coblation Surgery

Transoral Approach

Insert the FK retractor and expose each lingual tonsil separately. Mind the teeth and the lip. Both can easily be damaged when inserting the retractor.

We always start surgery with topical disinfection of the oral mucosa by using a chlorhexidine solution (0.2%). Preferred power setting of the coblation II ENT system (Smith–Nephew) is 9:4 W. We use the Procise XP wand (▶ Fig. 8.52).

The head of the probe is moved over the surface of the lingual tonsil with little pressure on the tissue. By doing so the tissue is reduced to a fluid state and extracted by suction. Smaller bleedings can be coagulated by the coagulation mode of the Coblator system.

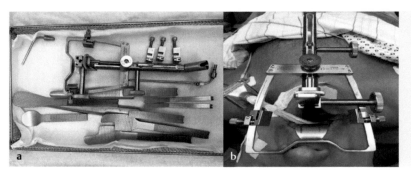

Fig. 8.49 FK retractor. **(a)** Retractor with its different spatulas. **(b)** Retracter in situ.

More severe bleedings require monopolar or bipolar electrocautery.

The resection is carried out until the epiglottis can be seen, and the vallecula is completely free of lymphatic tissue (▸Fig. 8.53, ▸Fig. 8.54). If needed, an assistant can help to make the whole vallecula visible by pressing the tissue from the outside of the neck manually.

If LT is combined with soft palate surgery, we always perform the LT first. After LT we insert a moist compress in the hypopharynx as a temporary tamponade to achieve blood control without electrocautery, while the soft palate surgery is done.

Laser Surgery

We prefer laser surgery if the patient's mouth opening is limited. In these cases exposure of the lingual tonsils is easier when using the distending operating laryngoscope. Unfortunately, the laryngoscope does not provide enough space to insert the coblation probe. Therefore, we use the CO_2-laser. Power setting is 8 W (continuous mode). Needless to say that you need to include laser precaution measures, as mentioned earlier. The cutting of lymphatic and muscle tissue is different and is easily recognized by the surgeon. As in coblation surgery electrocautery is needed for blood control. We use monopolar cautery due to the narrowness in the distending laryngoscope.

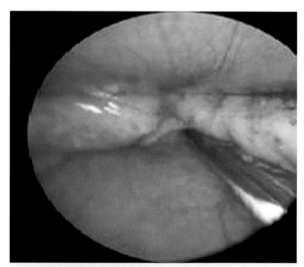

Fig. 8.50 Exposure of lingual tonsils.

> ### Risks, Tips, and Tricks
>
> - Use either coblation or laser surgery depending on the patient's ability to open his/her mouth.
> - coblation surgery is less painful after surgery, but difficult to perform in narrow throats.
> - Mind the upper teeth, and lower lip while inserting the retractor.
> - You might need electrocautery for blood control in addition.
> - Temporary tamponade of the hypopharynx (maybe while performing additional soft palate surgery) helps to reduce electrocautery, reducing postoperative pain levels.

Complications

Postoperative Pain

As most OSA surgeries, LT can induce significant postoperative pain. According to our own data, postoperative need for analgetic drug intake is up to 12 days in mean with high interindividual variability. Under medication, patients are free of pain unless during swallowing. Use VAS separately for swallowing and no swallowing to record treatment success.

Hot, spicy, and sour foods and drinks are not recommended during the first 1 to 2 weeks after surgery.

Hemorrhage

As stated earlier, postoperative hemorrhage is much less frequent as compared to pharyngeal tonsillectomy. An

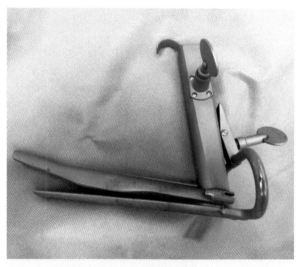

Fig. 8.51 Distending operating laryngoscope.

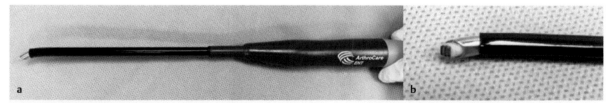

Fig. 8.52 Coblation Procise XP wand. (a) Probe. (b) Tip of the wand.

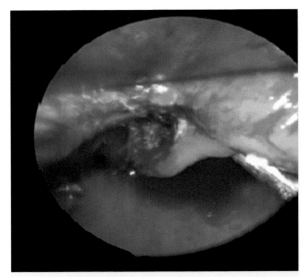

Fig. 8.53 Coblation LT (Harburg technique). Left side done, right side still untouched.

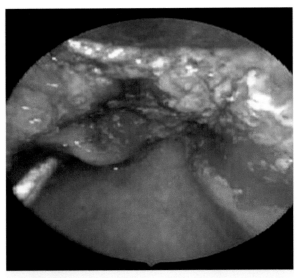

Fig. 8.54 Coblation LT (Harburg technique), same patient as in ▶Fig. 8.53. Right side done as well.

avascular plane was revealed deep to the lingual tonsils that might explain this fact.[223] However, postoperative haemorrhage was observed in 2.8% in a group of 108 OSA patients after LT with the Coblator technique.[224] Therefore, patients should be advised to avoid physical effort, sauna, hot showering or bathing, and other activities that potentially increase blood flow in the head and neck region.

Dysphagia

Most people suffer from severe dysphagia for the first 3 days. Corticosteroids may be helpful in some cases. Please make sure that the patient gets sufficient fluid intravenously until he/she returns to normal fluid intake.

Wound Infection

In contrast to palatal surgery, we recommend antibiotic prophylaxis during perioperative phase. We administer three times 1.5 g cefuroxime for 5 days intravenously. In addition, we provide a local antiseptic mouth solution (e.g., chlorhexidine solution, 0.2%) to improve patient's mouth hygiene.

Postoperative Care

As in any other sleep apnea surgery, the severity of OSA has a significant impact on postoperative care and monitoring. Thus, sleep apnea patients undergoing surgery under general anaesthesia or under sedation are at an increased risk for perioperative complications.[105,106,107]

This perioperative risk is particularly increased if OSA is treated surgically, as postoperative bleeding and swellings within the pharynx need to be taken into account. According to a review,[108] postoperative complications are rare and occur within the first 4 hours after extubation. This result is in accordance with our own experience. As a result, we keep our sleep apnea patients in the recovery room for 4 hours after extubation. If there are no complications, the patients are regarded to be safe and will be discharged to the regular ward. In case of complications, the patients are monitored overnight.[109]

As stated earlier, management of postoperative pain is crucial after soft palate surgery. A basic treatment with ibuprofen (four times 400–600 mg) in addition with metamizole (four times 0.5–1 g) works well in adults. However, there are huge interindividual differences that require individual adaptations. If the basic treatment is not sufficient in time, opioids might be added (e.g., three times 10 mg oxycodone). Please refer to Section 10.2 for further information about the postoperative care and medication.

As stated earlier, we recommend an antibiotic prophylaxis perioperatively for 5 days.

Outcomes

Presently, there is only one article reporting objective data from sleep studies before and after isolated LT in adult patients.[225] The authors performed isolated LT with the Coblator technique in 27 patients with OSA, as described in this chapter. Follow-up in this case series (EBM level 4) was 6 months. The mean AHI decreased significantly from 33.7 at baseline to 18.7 after surgery. The surgical success rate (reduction of AHI by 50% and below 20) was 55.6%. By comparing responders and nonresponders baseline AHI turned out to be the only significant parameter that differed between the two groups, with nonresponders presenting with higher AHI values before surgery.

Apart from that two other studies investigated the objective effect of LT on AHI measured as by PSG. A case series of 20 patients underwent UPPP with tonsillectomy plus LT. The latter was performed with a robot.[226] The AHI decreased significantly by 56.7% in three months, from

55.6 at baseline to 24.1 after surgery. Daytime sleepiness measured with the ESS improved significantly as well (13.4 before vs. 5.9 after surgery).

The only controlled study was published by our working group.[227] We compared two groups of patients. Group A underwent UPPP with tonsillectomy plus LT (n = 58), and group B underwent UPPP with tonsillectomy plus hyoid suspension plus interstitial RFTs of the base of tongue. Follow-up was 3.3 months in mean. Both AHI (34.5 before vs. 17.4 after surgery, reduction by 49.6%) and ESS (10.4 before vs. 6.3 after surgery) decreased significantly. Patients in group A benefitted more than those in group B, indicating that LT is an effective treatment in OSA surgery if enlarged lingual tonsils are present.

▶ Table 8.15 summarizes the present data.

LT is used in children as well, mainly as a second-line treatment in kids with persisting OSA after adenotonsillectomy. A recent meta-analysis[228] included four studies with a total of 73 children (mean age, 8.3 years). LT was performed for persistent OSA due to lingual hypertrophy after adenotonsillectomy in all cases. The AHI decreased from 12.6 at baseline to 5.2 after LT. The overall success rate was 17% (95% CI: 7–35%) for a postoperative AHI less than 1 and 51% (95% CI: 25–76%) for a postoperative AHI less than 5.

Another article describes the results of LT in 92 children with a syndromic diagnosis. For 18 children, PSG data were provided. The median AHI decreased significantly from 8.5 to 3.8. After surgery, the percentage of patients with an AHI < 5 increased from 27.8 to 61.1% (p = 0.08).[229]

Key Points

LT is an effective treatment in patients with enlarged lingual tonsils. Severe complications are rare. Postoperative haemorrhage is the most frequent complication, if that occurs in up to 3% of the cases.

In our center, we perform LT under general anesthesia as an inpatient procedure. Dysphagia and postoperative pain require medical treatment.

We prefer the coblation technique, unless the patient is unable to open his/her mouth wide enough. In these cases, we perform laser surgery. Nasal intubation is a good option but not a necessary one. In order to avoid nasal trauma, we usually have our patients orally intubated.

Transoral Robotic Surgery

Claudio Vicini, Filippo Montevecchi, and Khai Beng Chong

Definition

Transoral robotic surgery (TORS) refers to a variety of procedures utilizing the da Vinci Surgical System produced by Intuitive Surgical Inc., Sunnyvale, CA. TORS involves precise endoscopic excision of oral, orohypopharyngeal, and laryngeal tissue with a variety of articulated, wristed instruments placed alongside a three-dimensional, high-definition endoscopic camera, all controlled by the surgeon from a remote O.R. console. TORS was pioneered by Weinstein and O'Malley at Penn University as a minimally invasive technique for treatment of oropharyngeal cancers[230] and was FDA approved for adult head and neck surgery in December 2009.[231] It has since been adopted worldwide and is considered by many practitioners to be the most effective and reproducible minimally invasive surgical technique available. The experience with TORS between 2010 and 2014 led to the FDA approval (September 2014) of TORS for "removal of benign tissue from the base of tongue." Traditional TBR is generally done either via a transcervical technique or transorally with an endoscope for visualization.[3,231,232,233,234,235,236,2367,238,239] Each of these approaches has significant potential limitations. The open techniques are technically difficult and morbid, and the transoral endoscopic approaches are hampered by relatively poor exposure and limited, nonarticulated instrumentation. By using TORS the advantages of the magnified three-dimensional high-definition visualization, and the precision and dexterity afforded by two-handed, articulating robotic instrumentation, are obvious and "intuitive." Additionally, peer-reviewed articles and books have shown that TORS for OSA allows the surgeon to address the base of tongue obstruction with several advantages.[240,241]

TBR refers to the primary focus of this targeted TORS for OSA; a robotic-assisted resection of a part of the tongue base from roughly the foramen cecum to the vallecula. Note that in the context of sleep disordered breathing, the term "reduction" is preferred to "resection," a term usually associated with cancer applications. TBR can include removal of lingual tonsillar tissue, tongue base musculature, or both. The amount of resection can vary from several cc to more than 50 cc as needed, based upon the patient's anatomy and

▶ **Table 8.15** Objective results of LT in adults

Author	Technique	N	Add. proc.	Follow-up (months)	AHI (pre)	AHI (post)	Success (%)	ESS (pre)	ESS (post)	ESS (p)	EBM
Lee et al[226]	TORS	20	UPPP	3	55.6	24.1	45.0	13.4	5.9	0.003	4
Verse et al[227]	Laser	58	UPPP	3.3	34.5	17.4	58.6	10.4	6.3	< 0.001	3b
Wee et al[225]	Coblator	27	None	6	37.7	18.7	55.6	no data	no data		4
All		105			39.34	19.01	55.24	11.17	6.20		

Abbreviations: Add. proc, additional procedure; AHI, apnea–hypopnea index; ESS, Epworth sleepiness scale; UPPP, uvulopalatopharyngoplasty.
Note: EBM = level of evidence-based medicine.

degree of prolapse during sleep. Irrespective of histology or volume of the resected tissue, the goal is to clear the airway. After TBR, it is possible to continue to perform supraglotto-plasty (SGP) (see section on   later in this chapter).

Indications, Contraindications, and Patient Selection

TORS TBR can be used for appropriate cases of clinically significant OSA.[242] Most patients treated with this surgery have PSG evidence of at least moderate to severe OSA (respiratory disturbance index [RDI] ≥ 20) and excessive daytime somnolence (as documented by an ESS score >10). Ideal candidates have significant obstruction at the tongue base (with a Cormack and Lehane grade of >2) and/or prolapse of adjacent supraglottic tissue, as determined by awake supine endoscopic examination or by DISE. It is important for the surgeon to avoid patients with unfavorable anatomy, which do not allow sufficient exposure (significant retrognathia, inability to hyperextend the neck, trismus, or an interincisive distance <2.5 cm).

It is well accepted that OSA surgery should not be offered to patients who are tolerant of and compliant with CPAP therapy.[243] TORS tongue base surgery can be offered to CPAP nonadherent patients as a primary procedure or after previous surgery failure when the anatomy is appropriate. Associated nasal obstruction and disproportionate palate and tonsil tissue may be treated concurrently with TORS as per the surgeon's judgment, although it has been reported that simultaneous multilevel surgery can increase potential postoperative morbidity.[120] Concurrent surgical procedures that have been performed with TORS TBR SGP include septal and turbinate surgery, as well as a number of variations of palatal surgery, such as traditional UPPP, expansion sphincteroplasty, barbed pharyngo-plasty, Z-palatoplasty, and others.[177,185,196] Such pharyngeal surgery may be carried out conventionally or robotically according to surgeon's preference and/or experience.

There are several important contraindications to TORS TBR. Surgery should not be offered to patients who are successfully treated without surgery. Other contraindications include conditions that increase the perioperative risks or reduce the success rate of sleep surgery, such as comorbidities that result in an ASA score >2, significant or unstable cardiovascular disease, progressive neuromuscular disease, need for anticoagulation, significant psychological instability, etc. Local contraindications to the procedure include the oral and neck anatomic constraints enumerated previously. Significant micrognathia and macroglossia (with high modified Mallampati–Friedman scores) can limit exposure for TORS procedures, although we still managed to operate on many of such patients successfully. Caution should also be undertaken in cases presenting with significant post-UPPP dysphagia, as it is possible that TBR could worsen the dysphagia.

Diagnostic Workup

The preoperative workup is the same as what has been described for OSA surgery in general. This includes a thorough sleep history, assessment of general medical condition, comprehensive upper airway examination with awake fiberoptic endoscopy, and a PSG. In addition to the usual ENT examination, this assessment should include BMI, neck circumference, tonsil size (grade 0 to IV), modified Mallampati–Friedman Scoring (I to IV), and Cormack and Lehane Scoring. Documentation of somnolence and sleep quality can include the ESS score and results of any of the standardized subjective quality of life questionnaires (SF36, Stanford sleepiness scale, Beck depression index, etc.). Radiographic imaging is not essential, but when indicated it can include panoramic radiography, lateral cephalometry, CT, and/or MRI.[244] Although not routinely utilized by most surgeons before OSA surgery, CT or MRI of the neck can help in selected cases to better define the pattern of soft-tissue collapse in relation to the mass of obstructive lingual tissue, as well as determining whether the tissue is primarily lymphatic (lingual tonsillar tissue), muscular, or both. In addition, fiberoptic DISE has been found to be helpful in determining the site of obstruction.[245,246,247,248]

Anesthesia and Positi\oning

TORS TBR is performed under general anesthesia.[249] The surgical team must be prepared for a difficult intubation, which could require the use of specialized instrumentation, such as a fiberoptic endoscope, GlideScope, light wand, etc. Extended anesthesia respiratory circuitry is necessary, as the anesthesiologist is stationed at the foot of the bed. This allows for the surgical assistant to sit at the head of the bed without interference, and allows for the da Vinci Vision cart and patient cart to be positioned along the sides of the patient's head as described for other TORS procedures. In Europe it is more customary to perform a tracheostomy immediately after intubation for lingual TORS surgery.[250,251] This is not routinely advocated in the United States and the surgery is done either via orotracheal or nasotracheal intubation with a small caliber endotracheal tube. If a tracheotomy is thought to be indicated at the conclusion of the TORS procedure because of potential bleeding or airway edema, then it can be performed at that time. Intravenous steroids are given to minimize lingual edema and nausea prevention, and intravenous broad spectrum antibiotics are infused preoperatively as per hospital protocol or the surgeon's preference.

Equipment

This surgery is performed with the da Vinci Surgical System manufactured by Intuitive Surgical, Sunnyvale, CA, USA. TORS requires either the S HD or the Si da Vinci models; the Standard (or S) system is not sufficient for these procedures. This robotic equipment include:
- High definition camera. A 0- and 30-degree camera is available with the robotic system. Both 12 mm and 8 mm diameter scope have excellent optics and allow for adequate working space in the mouth. They provide magnification up to 10 times, resulting in a clear

three-dimensional image, with easy identification of vessels and nerves.

- Two 5-mm articulated Endo Wrist instrument arms, one placed on either side of the camera. These instrument arms provide all degrees of freedom, 180 degree of articulation and 540 degree of rotation, with tremor filtration and amplitude scaling, and allow for bimanual tissue manipulation in multiple planes. A grasper is placed on one arm—usually a 5 mm Maryland forceps (cat. no. 420143) can be used—and a spatula tip monopolar cautery (cat. no. 400160) on the other for dissection and coagulation. A compatible laser fiber can be used in lieu of the cautery and is preferred by some surgeons.
- Control of the robotic arms and camera is managed from the surgeon's console, which is placed within close proximity and direct visualization of the operating table. These controls include a patented Intuitive Motion algorithm which digitally reproduces the surgeon's hand and wrist movements.
- High-definition two-dimensional video observation of the surgery for the surgical assistant and room personnel via a monitor attached to the robot (SHD model) or the control tower/Vision Cart (Si model).

Although TORS does not require much additional equipment beyond the robotic tools listed above, there are several other important instruments which should be readily available on the operating room back table. It is best to have all of these instruments open and readily accessible. These include:

- *Mouth gags:* Two commonly used mouth gags include the Davis–Meyer gag (Karl Storz America) and the FKWO retractor (Olympus, Japan). The Davis–Meyer system includes a multiple tongue blades of different lengths (▶ Fig. 8.55), each with integrated suction tubes for smoke evacuation, and is usually sufficient for the procedure. A small sized blade is usually best, especially in the initial TBR dissection. The FKWO retractor has integrated adjustable cheek retractors but no suction ports on its various sized tongue blades; this retractor is sometimes superior to the Davis–Meyer system for the SGP portion of the surgery.

- *Headlight:* A headlight is used when placing the mouth gag to ensure adequate exposure.
- The robotic monopolar cautery is usually sufficient for hemostasis, though a vessel clip applier and an insulated bipolar forceps should be readily available. A tonsillectomy type suction cautery device is also sometimes needed.
- The bedside assistant may use small diameter suction devices (Lawton suction Cat. 160274 and/or Medicon suction Cat. 098508) to suction blood and smoke from the surgical field (▶ Fig. 8.56). The suction device can also be used as a retractor to improve the primary surgeon's visualization.

Surgical Team

The bedside TORS team is comprised of:
- A primary surgeon seated at the robotic console. This console is situated in close proximity to the operating table, usually off to one side but within view of the operative site. This console affords a three-dimensional view of the surgical field and houses the controls for the two robotic arms and the camera.
- An assistant (who may be a second surgeon) seated at the head of the patient. The assistant retracts tissue and evacuates blood and smoke, adjusts the robotic arms and camera as needed to avoid arm collisions, and assists with hemostasis via bipolar electrocoagulation or with vessel clips. A speaker system with built-in microphone is manufactured inside the robotic system to improve communication between the primary surgeon and the assistant.
- A surgical scrub technician, who aids in passing instruments and providing equipment as needed.

Surgical Steps
Exposure

The intubated patient is positioned supine, with the neck flexed and head hyperextended in the "sniffing position." If a planned tracheotomy is to be performed, it is done at this point. The upper dental arch is protected to prevent

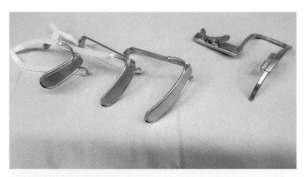

Fig. 8.55 Complete set of tongue blades of different sizes with integrated suction tubes for smoke.

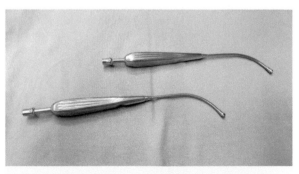

Fig. 8.56 Bedside assistant's suction devices (Lawton suction Cat. 160274 and/or Medicon suction Cat. 098508), which can be used for retraction and the evacuation of smoke and blood.

trauma by the robotic camera and instrument arms. The tongue is pulled anteriorly with stay sutures and pushed forward by using one of the two mouth gags listed previously. As this can result in the compression of the ventral tongue against the lower incisors, usage of a lower tooth guard for protection can be considered. The tongue base is then exposed as described above with the appropriate mouth gag. The length of tongue blade and amount of tongue retraction is adjusted so that the distal end of the blade should be just rostral to the superior aspect of the planned resection in the midline (usually around the foramen cecum). It is not unusual at this point for the epiglottis to be obscured by the mounded up tongue base. If this is the case, it will come in to view as the tongue reduction progresses. The robot is docked as per normal TORS protocol.

Tongue Base Reduction

TBR is based on the principles of TORS TBR described in 2006 by O'Malley et al, and enlarges the anteroposterior airway dimension at the level of the tongue base. This reduction usually extends rostrally from the foramen cecum level to the vallecula; the SGP extension of the procedure can include vallecular mucosa and/or part of the epiglottis as necessary (see section on Skin-Lined Tracheostomy later in this chapter). The lateral oropharyngeal dimensions are not augmented with this surgery, and are better addressed by tonsillectomy with one of the variations of UPPP or lateral pharyngoplasty. As there can be considerable variation in anatomy between patients, the goal is not to remove a predetermined volume of tongue base but to improve the Cormack and Lehane grade from III or IV to grade II or better.[252] Although it is safest to limit the tissue resection to the superficial layer of lingual lymphoid tissue, most cases require extension of the dissection into the lingual musculature. This deeper dissection

can lead to exposure of the lingual artery and its dorsal branches, the hypoglossal nerve, and the lingual nerve. Although the volume of excised tissue is generally in the 14 to 20 cc range, this can vary from as little as 7 cc to as much as 50 cc. The procedure is divided into several standardized steps, outlined below, and usually takes about 30 minutes to complete.[253,254,255]

Right-Side Lingual Tonsillectomy
Instruments: Maryland Forceps Left Arm, Spatula Tip Cautery Right Arm

The 30 degree up facing robotic camera is set at relatively low magnification and wide angle view to give a panoramic view of the tongue base at this point, and can be set to higher magnification as the case progresses. The incision begins in the midline from the rostral end of the planned resection to the vallecular (▶Fig. 8.57). The foramen cecum is a good landmark for the upper extent of this incision, as it is distal to the circumvallate papillae and is in the midline. This incision splits the lingual tonsillar tissue in the midline and extends deeply to the junction between lymphoid tissue and the underlying muscle.

The borders of the right lingual tonsil are identified and marked with cautery to outline the resection margins (▶Fig. 8.58). This extends superiorly from the sulcus terminalis, laterally from the amygdaloglossal sulcus, and inferiorly to the glossoepiglottic sulcus. If the lingual tonsillar tissue is bulky enough that these landmarks are not visible, the central tongue base can first be debulked at this point.

The target tissue is then resected, with the deep plane at the lymphomuscular junction (▶Fig. 8.59). This can usually be done in an en bloc fashion with minimal blood loss. The bedside assistant can facilitate this resection by using a suction or retracting device for counter traction

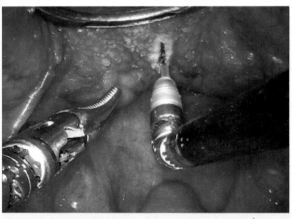

Fig. 8.57 The procedure starts with a midline split of the two lingual tonsils from foramen caecum in order to identify the tip of epiglottis and vallecular.

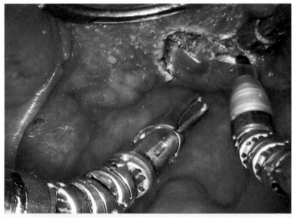

Fig. 8.58 Initial dissection of the right tongue base posteriorly to the circumvallate papilla.

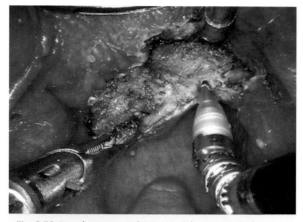

Fig. 8.59 In order to grasp the tissue, a deep cut must be created to allow the Maryland forceps to gain adequate purchase of the tissue.

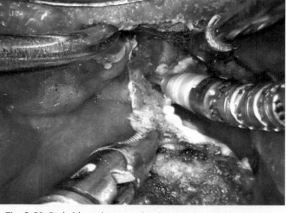

Fig. 8.60 Bed-side assistant maintains counter traction in order to assist the surgeon during dissection; increased tension allows more precise and quicker dissection.

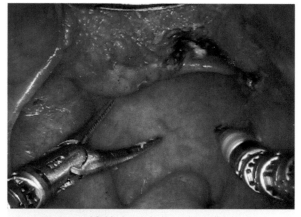

Fig. 8.61 Surgical field after right lingual tonsillectomy.

of the tissue (▶Fig. 8.60). The inferior limit of the surgical bed can be recognized by a bluish color of the vallecular mucosa. A number of small vessel branches from the lingual artery will be encountered and usually are taken care of easily with cautery. Larger vessels may be clipped as needed. Visualization of these vessels is improved by increasing the scope magnification. At the end of the right side tongue base reduction a portion of epiglottis is visible (▶Fig. 8.61).

Left-Side Lingual Tonsillectomy

Instruments: Maryland Forceps Right Arm, Spatula Tip Cautery Left Arm

The left LT is completed in the same fashion as was done on the right, after swapping the instruments (▶Fig. 8.62). The spatula tip monopolar cautery is now in the left instrument arm and the grasping forceps is in the right (▶Fig. 8.63). At the end of this step all the epiglottis is visible (▶Fig. 8.64).

Risks, Tips, and Tricks

At the end of these steps, additional tissue is removed as needed to ensure a Cormack and Lehane grade of II or better. A minimum overall volume of 7 cc is recommended for fixing obstruction. When entering the muscular layer it is important to avoid injury to the neurovascular structures including the dorsal branches of the lingual arteries and hypoglossal nerves. It is usually safe to remove a layer of muscle ≤10 mm within the entire tongue base surgical site. An additional 5-mm thick strip of muscle may generally be safely removed in the tongue base within 5 mm (may be more at the superior aspect of the resection) of either side of the midline without encountering the hypoglossal nerves. This additional midline muscle resection should be done carefully and under sufficiently high magnification. It is of paramount importance to use the tongue base midline as the point of reference to minimize the risk to the hypoglossal nerve, lingual artery, and lingual neural branches. Because of inherent anatomical variability, and tissue distortion from tongue retraction and mouth gag placement, precise localization of these structures is not possible.

In our experience, two additional points must be noted:
a) The relationship of the lingual artery and hyoid bone is a reliable landmark and is described in other articles or books.[241,256,257]
b) The three-dimensional HD Da Vinci camera allows the identification of the crucial structures before damaging them, working carefully step by step, with a mix of blunt and sharp dissection.

Complications

The largest series of patients to undergo TORS for OSA was described in the multicentric study published by Vicini et al.[240] There were no complications recorded in 79.5% of the cases, with no deaths in the cohort. The most

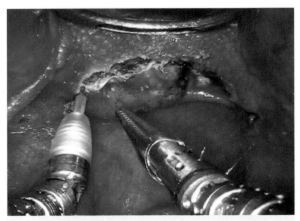

Fig. 8.62 Left lingual tonsillectomy is completed in the same way as the right lingual tonsillectomy, after side inversion of the robotic arms and tools. Initial mucosa dissection.

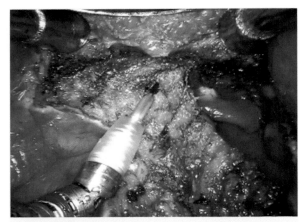

Fig. 8.63 Left lingual tonsillectomy is completed in the same way of the right after side inversion of the robotic arms and tools. Dissection of deeper layers.

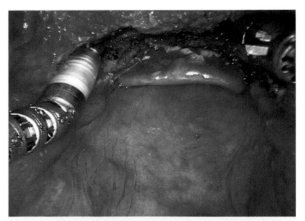

Fig. 8.64 Surgical field at the end of the lingual tonsillectomy. At this step, a view of the epiglottis is possible.

common patient complaint was a transient mild hypogeusia (14.2%), which recovered within 8 months in all patients. Bleeding was the second most common complication (5% of the procedures). In most of the cases (2.9%), late postoperative bleeding was self-limiting and did not require surgical intervention. Only 1.7% of the patients required an additional surgical procedure to control the bleeding. Finally, in 0.4% of the surgeries, a significant intraoperative hemorrhage was reported. Pharyngeal scarring with minimal-to-mild stenosis was a late complication in 0.4% of the procedures. Transient pharyngeal edema was observed in 0.4% of the patients. More severe complications (teeth injury, pharyngeal wall penetration, intraoperative bleeding requiring open control of vessels, and death) have not been reported.

Postoperative Care

The wound is inspected carefully for hemostasis, with cautery or vessel clips being used as needed for persistent bleeding. A thin layer of hemostatic agent can be applied on the tissue surface, as some clinicians feel that it may help with postoperative discomfort.

The tongue and airway are inspected for edema. If no prior tracheotomy was done, the patient is then assessed for possible extubation under observation in the operating room. Patient can also be kept intubated overnight in the ICU if necessary, based on the surgeon's preference.

Placement of a nasogastric feeding tube should be considered, and some centers routinely use NG tubes for all TORS patients in the immediate postoperative period. This is again based on the surgeon's preference.

As these patients are undergoing surgery for obstructive airway problems (i.e., OSA), they may develop bleeding and/or airway edema after TORS tongue base surgery. The initial postoperative observation should be done in a closely monitored setting. In most institutions this would be the ICU or PCU rather than the typical postoperative hospital ward. Continuous pulse oximetry is recommended.

There should be suction apparatus available at all times at the patient's bedside. The patient should be watched closely for bleeding, as there is a large area of exposed tissue at the surgical site which must undergo healing by secondary intention. As with all cases of similar pharyngeal surgical wound, such as "simple" tonsillectomy, the risk of postoperative bleeding has a bimodal distribution, with one peak within hours of surgery and the second within 7 to 10 days of surgery.

Postoperative intravenous steroids can help with nausea, airway edema, and pain from the inflammatory response. It is advisable to continue oral steroids postdischarge on a tapering dose, as some patients may experience a significant crescendo of pain up to a week postoperatively. This is likely due to hyperinflammation or dissolution of the protective fibrinous exudative coating over the surgical site. In addition to steroids, narcotics are used as needed, with close observation of the respiratory rate and level of consciousness, as recommended postoperatively for any OSA procedures.

The length of stay can vary considerably depending on a number of variables and the surgeon's comfort level. Tracheotomy by itself necessitates a multiday hospital stay. Other determinants include the presence of other concurrent OSA procedures (e.g., UPPP), general patient health, other comorbidities, pain control, and swallowing ability.

Patients are followed up closely after discharge. Diet is normalized as healing progresses, and a formal therapist-directed swallowing therapy is rarely needed (<10% of cases). Postoperative PSG is performed once healing is complete, usually at least 3 to 6 months later.

Outcomes

The multicentric study series reported by Vicini et al[240] showed an improvement from a mean preoperative AHI of 43.21 to a postoperative AHI of 17.54. In this article 66.9% of the outcomes were successful, with the remaining 33.1% unsuccessful with different degrees of severity. In a few cases, the postoperative AHI worsened. Improvements were also seen in ESS and lowest oxygen saturation. All improvements were found to be statistically significant.

Key Points

Traditional surgery to address base of tongue obstruction during sleep has significant limitations. While many patients benefit from the use of CPAP therapy, noncompliant patients require a surgical procedure to eliminate the obstruction. TORS for OSA allows the surgeon to address the base of tongue obstruction with several advantages. The minimally invasive procedure is well tolerated by patients. Currently, all the series published have shown clinical benefit to patients.

Hyoid Bone Surgeries

Nico de Vries

Definition

The concept of hyoid surgery was first introduced by Riley et al in 1984.[258] They reported on a patient with OSA whom after UPPP had persistent symptoms and underwent inferior sagittal mandibular osteotomy combined with hyoid myotomy and suspension (ISO). The latter is a surgical procedure where the hyoid bone was advanced and suspended to the inferior border of the anterior mandible using fascia lata[258,259,260] (so-called hyoid suspension type 1). Although Riley's technique had good results (positive surgical outcome) it also had some disadvantages, mainly due to its morbidity associated with fascia lata harvesting. Another possible downside was the unfavorable cosmetic change as a result of the anterior and upward displacement of the hyoid bone.

A modified HS was presented by Riley et al in 1994 in which the hyoid was pulled down and attached to the thyroid lamina rather than being suspended to the mandible (hyoid suspension type 2).[261]

Hörmann and Baisch presented a different approach (modified HS according to Hörmann) in 2004, which was simple, less invasive, and could be performed under local anesthesia. The surgery was part of the Mannheim multilevel surgery protocol. In this procedure, the hyoid is stabilized anteriorly and inferiorly using a single-steel wire which is sutured through the thyroid cartilage and slung around the hyoid body, preserving the strap muscles and stylohyoid ligaments.[262,263]

Two modifications of this technique have been described in the literature.[264,265] These authors[265] found a thyroid cartilage fracture in some patients possibly caused by traction of the steel wire. They revised the Hörmann technique and added fixation of a titanium miniplate with screws into the thyroid cartilage to the procedure. The other article[264] presented a modification to avoid exposure of the steel wire to the pharyngeal mucosa. This option was based on computed tomography (CT) imaging. They drilled a hole in the middle third of the body of the hyoid bone and inserted a steel wire through that hole.

The modified technique introduced by Riley et al is also known as hyoidthyroidpexia and currently commonly performed as part of multilevel surgery.[261,266,267,268,269]

Indications, Contraindications, and Patient Selection

Hyoidthyroidpexia as an isolated procedure can be considered in patients with moderate to severe OSA, with total tongue base obstruction on DISE. Ideally, the BMI is <32 kg/m². Hyoidthyroidpexia as a component of multilevel surgery can also be considered in patients with moderate to severe OSA, with total tongue base obstruction on DISE. In case of partial tongue base obstruction on DISE, we feel that a less-invasive tongue base procedure, such as radiofrequent ablation of the tongue base should be considered first. In our experience, hyoidthyroidpexia is less effective in very high AHIs. As a rule, an upper limit of 55 to 60 is advised. In higher AHIs, more aggressive procedures, for example, bimaxillary osteotomies or TORS should be considered upfront.

In sum, hyoidthyroidpexia can be considered in patients with an AHI 20 to 60, BMI < 32, and during DISE total tongue base obstruction. In case of hypertrophic lingual tonsils these should be removed. We have the feeling that the larynx needs to be prominent to achieve a good result. This is why HS type 2 is mainly used in men. Only if the hyoid's position is behind the thyroid (in the sagittal dimension), HS can bring the hyoid anteriorly.

Contraindications are listed below:
- AHI < 20
- AHI > 60

- BMI > 32
- No or partial tongue base collapse
- Previous removal of the hyoid because of a thyroglossal cyst (Sistrunk procedure)

In our experience, during microlaryngoscopy it might be difficult to visualize the anterior part of the true vocal cords after HS type 2. In case microlaryngoscopy is envisioned, this should be mentioned.

A relative contraindication is professional speakers and singers.

Diagnostic Workup

PSG or related measures are used to assess the severity of OSA, followed by DISE to gather information of the level(s) of obstruction.

Hyoidthyroidpexia can be considered in patients with a BMI < 32, combined with a total anteroposterior tongue base obstruction during DISE.

Ultrasound or other imaging of the neck and hyoid can be considered: We have encountered several patients with an unexpected thyroglossal cyst during surgery. In those patients, the decision had to be made to remove the cyst while leaving the hyoid in (with increased risk for recurrence of the cyst) or to remove the cyst and the medial part of the hyoid (Sistrunk procedure), which excludes further execution of hyoidthyroidpexia.

Specific Risks, Patient Information, and Consent

Patients have to be informed about the expected success rate (approximately 60%).

Swallowing problems might occur, mostly in hyoidthyroidpexia as part of multilevel surgery, and are rare in hyoidthyroidpexia as the only procedure or combined with radiofrequent ablation of the tongue. Voice changes are not to be expected.

Pain: In case of hyoidthyroidpexia as the only procedure or combined with radiofrequent ablation of the tongue, the pain is usually limited. In case of hyoidthyroidpexia as part of multilevel surgery, intense pain must be anticipated. The most feared is postoperative hemorrhage (see Complications under this section). We use Mercilene 0. In case one uses steel wires, however, it should be mentioned that MRA is possible, but difficult in the hyoid region. The scar, the incision is usually in a skin line, and the change in the lateral aspect of the neck should be mentioned. Very rarely, abscesses and wound healing problems occur, which might lead to a more disfiguring scar on the neck.

Anesthesia and Positioning

Although hyoidthyroidpexia under local anesthesia has been reported, we prefer to perform hyoidthyroidpexia, even as the only procedure, under general anesthesia. The head should be in slight hyperextension (pillow under shoulders) with an armed tube diverted upward.

In case of hyoidthyroidpexia as component of multilevel surgery, it might be needed to reposition the tube onece or twice. A common combination is radiofrequent ablation of the tongue, followed by a palatal procedure, and finally hyoidthyroidpexia. In this situation, in case one starts with radiofrequent ablation of the tongue base, the tube is first placed in the corner of the mouth. For the subsequent palatal procedure, the tube is repositioned to the midline in a downward direction. A second repositioning is needed in an upward direction for the neck procedure.

Equipment

Standard oncology net.

Procedural Steps

General anesthesia, with an oral endotracheally placed tube. The patient lies in supine position with the head slightly extended. The operating area is rinsed with chlorhexidine 0.5% in alcohol 70%. A horizontal skin incision of approximately 5 cm is then made in a relaxed skin tension line at the level of the thyrohyoid membrane, between the hyoid and thyroid cartilage. There is no need to go further laterally than the medial border of the sternocleidomastoid muscle. And when applicable, excessive fat tissue is excised for better visualization.

Ligation of large anterior jugular veins is performed if needed. The three strap muscles, hyoidthyroid, sternothyroid and omohyoid, are dissected inferiorly as close to the hyoid as possible, using cautery. After release of the strap muscles mobilization of the hyoid is tested. When mobilization has found to be insufficient the tendon of the stylohyoid muscle is cut in addition, but this is, in our experience, hardly ever necessary. The hyoid bone is then mobilized in anterocaudal direction and permanently fixated to the thyroid cartilage with two nonresorbable sutures on each side (▶ Fig. 8.65). We use Mercilene 0. A sharp cutting needle is used to pierce the thyroid cartilage. The two permanent sutures per side are brought through the cartilage of the thyroid and around the bone of the hyoid. After approximation, the hyoid should be against or slightly on top the thyroid. The more anterocaudally fixated hyoidthyroid complex improves the PAS and neutralizes retrolingual obstruction.[270]

Meticulous hemostasis is of utmost importance, a drain in inserted, closure in layers, with intracutaneous stitches. Tracheostomy is *not* indicated.

Complications

In general, the morbidity associated with hyoidthyroidpexia is low. Complications and patient acceptance were previously shown by our group by Richard et al in 2011. Using charts and patients questionnaires we reported on

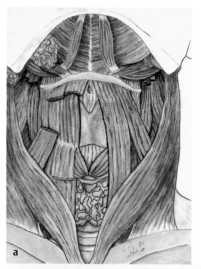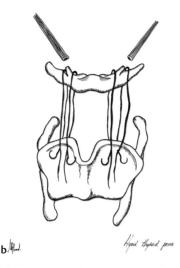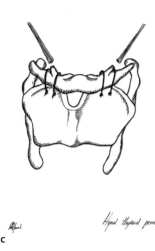

Fig. 8.65 (a–c) Hyoid bone surgeries.

adverse events and no major complications were seen. Minor complications (infection, wound abscess, fistula) occurred in 6 of 39 patients in the period from March 2000 to April 2006. Mean admission time was 3.3 days. It was concluded that hyoidthyroidpexia is a well-tolerated procedure with a low complication rate for moderate to severe OSA patients with tongue base obstruction.[271] Finally, in a case report by Safiruddin et al, we presented cases were an association with OSA and thyroglossal duct cysts were shown. One should be aware that a previous Sistrunk procedure is a contraindication for hyoidthyroidpexia and in hyoidthyroidpexia, preoperative imaging can be considered to rule out thyroglossal duct cysts.[270]

The most feared direct postoperative complication is a bleeding. This should be considered an absolute emergency. Because of the swelling in the neck, reintubation might be extremely difficult, or impossible. In such a case, reopening of the neck before new general anesthesia, or even tracheostomy, should be considered.

Postoperative Care

Most patients are discharged after two nights.

A drain is inserted, and removed after the drain production is less than 10 cc/24 h. This is often on the second day after surgery. Sutures can be removed after 1 week.

In case of hyoidthyroidpexia as the only procedure, we do not routinely administer antibiotics. In case hyoidthyroidpexia is combined with radiofrequent ablation of the tongue base, we give amoxicillin 2.4 g during surgery and continue with amoxicillin orally for 1 week. Corticosteroids should not be given, since tongue base abscesses have been reported after application of steroids after radiofrequency of the tongue base. In hyoidthyroidpexia as the only procedure, the pain is usually very limited, and paracetamol is often sufficient. In case of

hyoidthyroidpexia as component of multilevel surgery the pain can be considerable and stronger painkillers might be indicated—opioids should however be avoided. In case of hyoidthyroidpexia as the only procedure, there is no need to adjust the diet; in case of hyoidthyroidpexia as part of multilevel surgery, a tonsillectomy dietary scheme is prescribed.

As an alternative, cefuroxime for 5 days can be considered. According to the recent literature, an intraoperative dosage could be sufficient.

Outcomes

Hyoidthyroidpexia offers a simple surgical solution in patients with moderate to severe OSA and a complete retrolingual obstruction during DISE compared to the more radical alternatives like maxillomandibular osteotomies and tracheostomy. Hyoid surgery can be performed as the only procedure or in combination with other procedures, such as the minimally invasive surgical options as radiofrequent ablation of the tongue base. We presently, as a routine, add radiofrequent ablation of the tongue base to hyoidthyroidpexia, when hyoidthyroidpexia is performed. In case of multilevel obstruction as assessed during DISE, multilevel surgery combining the hypopharynx procedure with a palatal procedure—for example, UPPP or z-palatoplasty—in patients who previously underwent/had a tonsillectomy, ESP, or uvula flap is also often executed.[272]

So far, there is not much information about the effect of isolated hyoid suspension procedures in the literature. Only four case series with all 85 patients could be identified (see ▶Table 8.16).

All the authors performed type 2 hyoid suspensions in their patients. The follow-up periods were short and lasted not longer than 6 months. Both, objective and

▶ **Table 8.16** Surgical succes is defined as having a postoperative RDI of 20 or less and at least a 50% reduction in the number of respiratory events

Author	N	Type	Follow-up (months)	AHI (pre)	AHI (post)	Success (%)	ESS (pre)	ESS (post)	EBM
Riley et al[260]	15	2	3–6	44.7	12.8	53.3	No data	No data	4
den Herder et al[267]	31	2	6	32.1	22.2	52	7.6	4.3	4
Stuck et al[270]	14	2	2	35.2	27.4	40	9.1	6.1	4
Piccin et al[264]	25	2	4–10	43.1	10.9	76	16	7.4	4
All	85		2–6	38.1	18.1	57.3	10.9	5.8	C

Abbreviations: AHI, apnea–hypopnea index; ESS, Epworth sleepiness scale; RDI, respiratory disturbance index.

Notes: N = total number of patients enrolled; EBM = level of evidence-based medicine.

subjective data show a significant improvement of OSA severity and its daytime symptoms. However, controlled trial is still missing.

Success of the ISO performed by Riley et al was evaluated in 55 patients. Responders were defined as having a postoperative RDI of 20 or less and at least a 50% reduction in the number of respiratory events.

They found an overall surgical success of 67.0% (37 patients).[259] Later Riley et al performed a review of 306 consecutively treated surgical patients. Outcome was evaluated after phase I surgery, which consisted of an UPPP for palatal obstruction and genioglossal advancement (GA) with hyoid myotomy and suspension for hypopharyngeal obstruction. Patient who had an unsuccessful phase I surgery were offered a phase II reconstruction, which consisted of MMA. Results based on polygraphic recordings showed an overall success rate of 76.5%.[160]

In 1994, results of the isolated modified HS were presented in 15 consecutive patients. Fourteen patients previously had undergone GA and UPPP. In 12 out of 15 patients there was a subjective improvement in excessive daytime sleepiness (EDS). Overall the mean RDI improved from 65.7 ± 18.3/h to 21.3 ± 23.6/h.[261] Additional studies have demonstrated the efficacy of the modified HS, or hyoidthyroidpexia.[261,266,267,268,269] In 2002, Vilaseca et al evaluated the effect of UPPP in combination with mandibular osteotomy with genioglossus and hyoid advancement. Mean AHI significantly decreased from 60.5 ± 16.5/h to 44.6 ± 27/h. They found an overall success of 35%. The relatively low percentage of success was related to the severity of the studied OSA subjects. When the AHI was lower the success rate increased to 57% in moderate OSA patients (n = 7) and to 100% in mild OSA (n = 2).[267] Neruntarat presented results of the revised hyoid suspension in 32 patients. The mean RDI significantly improved from 44.4 ± 8.7/h to 15.2 ± 5.6/h and the mean baseline BMI was 29.4 ± 2.4 kg/m² and did not change following surgery. Based on Sher's criteria,[273] surgical success was achieved in 78% of the patients.[266] Contrasting with the previously mentioned studies, a study in 2005 by Bowden et al reported a relative poor surgical outcome in a group of

29 patients who underwent hyoid suspension combined with UPPP when this had not been done previously. The mean preoperative AHI (36.5 ± 27.6/h) and BMI (34.1 ± 6.4 kg/m²) values did not change significantly following surgery. Only 17% of patients met the criteria for surgical success.[274] When comparing studies and their designs, results are strikingly different.[266,274] Both studies use the same criteria for surgical success. However, the demographic parameters were significantly different, with clearly higher AHI and BMI baseline values in the latter study, with less favorable outcome.

For our group, Den Herder et al evaluated the effect of HS as a single procedure and later we also reported on the outcome of multilevel surgery, including HS.[268,272] In the first study, the effect of primary and secondary HS (in patients who previously had undergone UPPP) was evaluated in a total of 31 patients. The mean AHI significantly decreased from 32.1 ± 10.2/h to 22.2 ± 15.2/h, with a surgical success rate of 52%.[268] The second study showed similar results of one-stage multilevel surgery (i.e., UPPP, RFTB, HS with or without GA) in 22 patients with both RP and retrolingual obstruction. The mean AHI significantly decreased from 48.7 to 28.8/h, surgical success rate was 45%, and the BMI did not change following surgery.[272] A retrospective chart review of 109 patients reported the effect of HS as part of multilevel surgery (septoplasty and turbinate reduction and UPPP) and showed that the median AHI dropped from 35.0 to 14.0/h. Different criteria for surgical success were used, where nonresponders were defined as having a postoperative AHI > 20/h or having an unchanged or increased AHI. They found an overall success rate of 61.5% and showed that nonresponders had a significantly higher average BMI compared with responders (29.1 ± 3.1 vs. 27.7 ± 2.8 kg/m²).[269]

Results of the Hörmann and Baisch modification of the HS, in which the hyoid was suspended using a single steel wire, were reported in 2006. Eighty-three patients had undergone multilevel surgery, of which 67 patients had undergone HS. The mean AHI in the HS group decreased from 38.3 ± 21.1/h to 18.9 ± 19.5/h and the success rate was found to be 59.7%.[262,275]

Key Points

There are two types of Hyoid suspension: type 1 and type 2. We only have information on type 2. Hyoidthyroidpexia is a reasonably effective alternative treatment for OSA patients with tongue base obstruction who cannot tolerate CPAP. It can be performed as primary treatment in case of isolated retrolingual obstruction, or as part of multilevel surgery when both RP and retrolingual obstruction is present in moderate to severe OSA patients. Indications are AHI 20 to 60, BMI <32 kg/m², and total obstruction on tongue base level during DISE. So far, it is not clear if BMI is a strong indication parameter. The individual pathoanatomical findings and DISE findings might be more important than BMI, although—generally speaking—success rates decrease with rising BMI values.

Success rates of isolated hyoidthyroidpexia or as part of multilevel surgery have been extensively reported and vary between 17 and 78%, depending on variables such as baseline AHI, baseline BMI, level and configuration of obstruction during DISE, and on the definition of surgical success used. Increasing BMI negatively affects treatment outcome. Hyoidthyroidpexia has low morbidity, and literature shows it is a well-accepted treatment option.

Genioglossal Advancement

José Enrique Barrera

Definition

OSA is the leading cause of cardiovascular diseases, cognitive derangement, and overall increased healthcare utilization.[258] Multilevel surgery has been established as the mainstay of treatment for the surgical management of OSA, combined with a UPPP, genioglossus advancement (GA), also known as geniotubercle advancement, which has been developed to target hypopharyngeal obstruction.

Depending on patient anatomy, GA can obtain a goal of 8 to 14 mm of advancement thus increasing tension on the genioglossus and geniohyoid muscles with the goal of reducing the severity of sleep apnea.[258,259,276,277] Patients are traditionally selected for surgery based on the level of obstruction, which often occurs at the level of the base of tongue, although most patients demonstrate retropalatal obstruction as well. Since the introduction of GA to advance the genioglossus muscle along with UPPP as described by Riley et al, multilevel reconstruction surgery has demonstrated improved outcomes in relieving OSA in patients who demonstrate multilevel obstruction.[258,259,277]

Indications, Contraindications, and Patient Selection

All patients considered for skeletal surgery are first diagnosed by PSG, Epworth evaluation, and fiberoptic laryngoscopy.

Candidates for surgery present with an AHI > 5 events per hour, and/or a RDI > 5 with an ESS > 8, who either did not tolerate or refused a trial of CPAP. Presurgical patients present with evidence of obstruction as demonstrated by awake physical examination, documenting Friedman II or III classification. Exclusion criteria for skeletal surgery include age <12 years, chronic pulmonary disease on oxygen, and those affected with an untreated sleep disorder other than OSA that represents their primary sleep disorder. Preoperative assessment included documentation of history; ESS evaluation; complete physical examination; and PSG. Outcomes are defined by success, cure, and responder criteria. Success is defined as an AHI < 20 and/or a 50% decrease in AHI of the preoperative value. Cure is defined as an AHI < 5 events per hour. Responder is defined as significant improvement in the AHI and/or RDI after surgical intervention.

Obstruction can occur at a number of points in the airway. Physical examination of these patients may reveal hypertrophy of the adenoids and tonsils, retrognathia, micrognathia, macroglossia, deviation of the nasal septum, turbinate hypertrophy, a thick short neck, or tumors in the nasopharynx or hypopharynx. Both primary and secondary medical conditions are associated with OSA, owing to their effects on the upper airway anatomy. These may include temporomandibular joint disorders, myxedema, goiter, acromegaly, and lymphoma.

Fiberoptic nasopharyngoscopy is utilized to identify obstruction at the nasopharynx, oropharynx, and hypopharynx and to rule out laryngeal anomalies. It can help estimate the degree of lateral wall collapse, palatal narrowing, and tongue base obstruction. The site of obstruction can be classified by Fujita classification with type I being palatal obstruction only, type II presenting as a combined palatal and tongue base obstruction, and type III being a tongue base obstruction pattern only. Without performing fiberoptic evaluation, the site of obstruction may not be discernable.

Cephalometric evaluation is a simple way to evaluate individual patient's upper airway site of obstruction. Cephalometric evaluation has long been used in evaluation of the airway in OSA. The metrics used for evaluation are SNA, SNB, PNS, mandibular angle, PAS, and mandibular plane hyoid (MP-H) (▶ Fig. 8.66). These metrics are used to evaluate preoperative obstruction and follow postoperative results. It is recommended that this two-dimensional X-ray be supplemented with a 3D fiberoptic to evaluate the airway.

Contraindications to GA surgery include significant microgenia whereby the mandibular height precludes a 1-cm advancement due to insufficient bone, inability to capture the geniotubercle in the advanced segment, or adverse risk to dentition.

Diagnostic Workup

The definitive objective test is a study during sleep. The gold standard at present is an attended PSG evaluation. This level I study assesses the cardiorespiratory system,

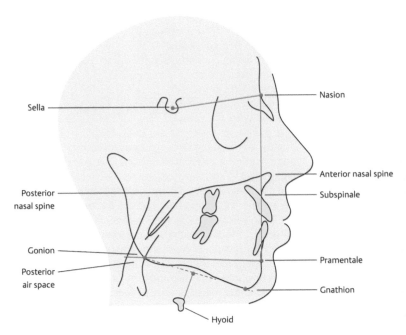

Fig. 8.66 Cephalometric figure.

Sella

Nasion

Posterior
nasal spine

Anterior nasal spine

Subspinale

Gonion

Pramentale

Posterior
air space

Gnathion

Hyoid

revealing oxygenation information, and records EEG, EOG, EMG. It reveals sleep stage information and estimates the percentage of apnea, hypopneas, and respiratory-related events during sleep. Ambulatory studies are estimated as level III and do not determine sleep stage data.

A CT of the maxillofacial skeleton may assist the surgeon in determining the height and width of the mandibular segment, identifying the position of the geniotubercle, and assessing dentition prior to surgery. Panoramic X-ray and a lateral cephalogram can be used as an alternative to assess predictive skeletal markers associated with skeletal dental abnormalities as well as evaluate boney and skeletal anatomy.

DISE[278,279] and sleep MRI[280,281] have emerged as modalities to diagnose the site of airway obstruction prior to surgery. At our institution, the most consistent finding is a narrowed PAS and low hyoid position.[282]

Specific Risks, Patient Information, and Consent

Specific risks associated with GA surgery include those related with skeletal surgery of the craniofacial skeleton. Paresthesia of the mandibular incisors, hardware failure, tooth injury, tooth loss, malunion, and nonunion of the mandible should be considered. The most common risk is paresthesia of the mandibular incisors, which is due to injury to the periapical nerves with osteotomy. Patients should be aware of these risks prior to considering the surgery.

Anesthesia and Positioning

General anesthesia is considered for all patients undergoing GA. A nasal or oral intubation can both be performed in preparation for the surgery. Positioning is supine.

Equipment

A maxillofacial instrument set is needed for GA surgery. In addition, a high-powered drill and sagittal saw are necessary to perform the osteotomies.

Operative Technique

General anesthesia is performed with either a nasal or oral intubation. The operating area is rinsed with chlorohexidine gluconate 0.12% mouth rinse. RP obstruction is addressed with UPPP. Fujita et al introduced UPPP with tonsillectomy in 1979.[45] Many modifications have been published, the basic procedure involves palate shortening with closure mucosal incisions, tonsillectomy, and lateral pharyngoplasty.

GA is performed as described by Riley et al.[283] Furthermore, after local anesthetic with a concentration of 1:100,000 epinephrine is injected at the lower gingivolabial sulcus, an incision is created along the anterior mandible. Subperiosteal dissection is then achieved exposing the anterior face of the mandible along its inferior border and then laterally identifying the mental neurovascular bundles. A horizontal window osteotomy is then created using a sagittal saw approximately 5 mm below the roots of the canine and approximately 10 mm above the inferior border of the mandible. The bone cut is then connected with two vertical osteotomies completing the rectangular window. Making a bicortical anterior osteotomy performs the GA. The width of the mandible, which had been pulled forward via the window osteotomy, is measured. The facial cortex and medullary bone is then removed and the lingual cortex holding the origin of the genioglossus muscle is rotated perpendicular to the window osteotomy. The osteotomized segment is then secured inferiorly with a single bicortical titanium screw (▸Fig. 8.67). Closure is performed with a 3–0 chromic with closure of the mentalis muscle and gingiva-buccal sulcus. Although named GA, the aforementioned operative technique advances both genioglossus and geniohyoid muscles (▸Fig. 8.68).

Risks, Tips, and Tricks

- An incision should be made in the gingivabuccal sulcus with adequate cuff on the detached gingiva.
- Dissection proceeds in the subperiosteal layer.
- The osteotomy is made with an oscillating saw. Care must be taken to avoid injury to the tooth roots.
- Osteotomy should be performed at least 20 mm from the tooth crown. A CT scan can be used to confirm proper placement of the bony cuts.
- Identify the root of the canine and do not cut bone above this level.
- Preserve at least 10 mm of inferior border of mandible.
- Distract the boney segment anteriorly and ensure hemostasis.
- Hemostasis is obtain by using small telfa packs in the medullary cavity. Avoid cautery at the anterior segment of the manbible as this could lead to paresthesia.
- Use a 2.0 mm lag screw to secure the mandible segment.
- Copiously irrigate throughout the surgery.
- Close the incision with a 3–0 chromic on a UR-6 needle to reattach the mentalis muscle and the detached gingiva.

Complications

Potential complications associated with GA include tooth injury or loss, paresthesias, mandibular fracture, difficulty in swallowing, wound infection, nonunion, and malunion of the mandible (▸Fig. 8.69). Detachment of hardware after GA can also occur in cases of poor osteosynthesis (▸Fig. 8.70). Evaluation of swallow before and after GA has shown no increase in incidence of swallow or speech dysfunction.[284]

Postoperative Care

Most patients are discharged after two nights. In patients with severe OSA and evidence of hypoxemia, a monitored bed is recommended. Patients with unstable blood pressure or hypertension may require an arterial line to monitor pressures continuously as well as intravenous antihypertensive medications.

Routine preoperative antibiotics are helpful due to oral incisions, which are exposed to mouth flora. Our practice recommends Clindamycin 900 mg intravenously every 8 hours for three doses. Corticosteroids are helpful to decrease jaw swelling, but not more than three doses are necessary. A soft diet is recommended for the first week, as patients may experience tooth hypesthesia.

Outcomes

GA is a simple technique that does not move the teeth or jaw and therefore does not affect the dental bite. The

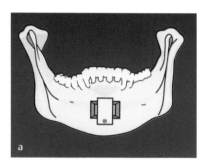
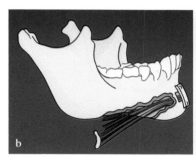

Fig. 8.67 Genioglossus advancement. **(a)** Anterior-inferior osteotomy shown with 2.0 mm screw fixation. **(b)** Anterior-inferior osteotomy's lateral view.

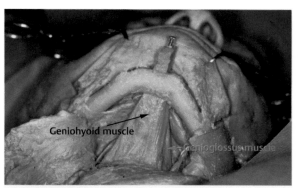

Fig. 8.68 Cadaveric dissection, showing advancement of both genioglossus and geniohyoid muscles.

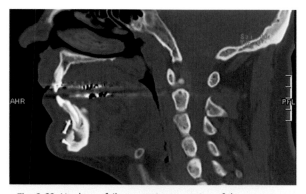

Fig. 8.69 Hardware failure, causing nonunion of the geniotubercle advancement.

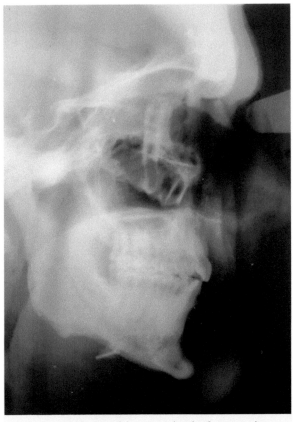

Fig. 8.70 Detachment of the geniotubercle after genioglossus advancement.

GA is a procedure performed as a solitary hypopharyngeal procedure or in combination with MMA.[285] The technique places the genioglossus under tension and this tension may be sufficient to keep the base of tongue region open during sleep (▶Fig. 8.71). This procedure does not gain more room for the tongue and thus must be considered a limited procedure that is dependent on the thickness of the individual's anterior mandible (mean thickness 12–18 mm). In addition, the existing laxity to the tongue during sleep is a factor on how much tension is gained when the genial tubercle is moved. In a flaccid tongue, the movement may all or partially be taken up by the advancement and little or no improvement may be attained. Paucity exists in determining the amount of tension needed or the critical distance the genial tubercle needs to move for effective PAS improvement. A recent study has determined that the tension to width ratio associated with GA surgery may be an indicator for surgical response in OSA patients.[286] These two factors limit our preoperative ability to accurately or consistently predict clinical outcomes. A meta-analysis evaluated success rates of GA to be between 39 to 78%.[219] Results of GA as a sole procedure for treatment of hypopharyngeal obstruction has been published in severe OSA patients with success over 60% in three studies and oxyhemoglobin saturation results in two studies showing improvement in low oxyhemoglobin saturation in both studies. Only one study controlled for BMI and all four studies were level 4 EBM (see ▶Table 8.17). The overall success rate was 62%. Our recent published article demonstrates clinical outcomes for success for GA with UPPP to be 61%.[284,286,287]

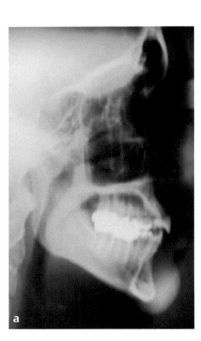 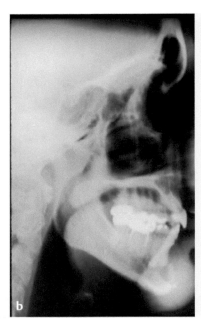

Fig. 8.71 Lateral X-ray. (a) A patient's preoperative posterior airway space. (b) A patient's postoperative posterior airway space after genioglossus advancement.

▶ Table 8.17 Genioglossal advancement evidence base review

Study	BMI (mean)	AHI (pre)	AHI (post)	Success rate, No./ total no. of cases (%)	LSAT	EBM
Riley et al[260]	NR	NR	NR	9/23[51]		4
Johnson and Chinn[410]	NR	59	14§	7/9[102]	Yes	4
Lee et al[414]	NR	53	19§	24/35[80]		4
Miller et al[422]	30	53	19§	16/24[78]	Yes	4

Abbreviations: AHI, apnea–hypopnea index; BMI, body mass index; LSAT, lowest oxygen saturation; NR, not reported.
Note: EBM = level of evidence-based medicine.

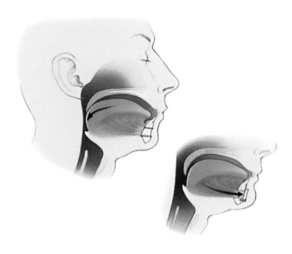

Fig. 8.72 Tension to width ratio as a predictive measure in genioglossus advancement surgery.

Key Points

We have noted that decreased tension and increased mandibular width are positive predictive factors for postoperative success.[287] Conversely, increased tension and narrow mandibular width are negative predictive factors for postoperative success. Thus, the tension to bicortical width ratio may be an independent predictor of postoperative success following GA, which trends toward significance. A significant difference in the tension to bicortical width ratio between responders and nonresponders, $p = 0.07$, exists. Responders show a significant reduction in the average AHI (25.1 event per hour) compared to nonresponders (0.3 events per hour), $p = 0.005$, as delineated by the tension to width ratio. This novel approach to determine the force applied to the genioglossus muscle during advancement and its correlation to postoperative outcomes may be an indicator for surgical success.

Other centers have reported similar results with this procedure.

Our center has previously published clinical outcomes for success rates for GA with UPPP as 62.5% and our responder rate was 87.5%.[283] GA with UPPP surgery was clinically effective in reducing the mean AHI from 48.3 ± 48.45 events per hour with a median of 48.5 (range: 12.4–76) in this study evaluating swallow function after GA and UPPP. Postoperatively the mean AHI was 11.6 ± 10.7 events per hour with a median of 10.75 (range: 3.8–29; $p = 0.003$). The procedure did not significantly affect the hyolaryngeal function of patients. There was no reported pre- or postoperative dysphagia or aspiration. Radiographic evidence of silent aspiration was not seen.[283] The ability to determine how tension of the genioglossus muscle and genial width contribute to surgical response is essential in understanding why patients respond or fail in surgery (▶Fig. 8.72).[287] More so, ESS scores decreased from 13.2 ± 4.5 to 7.6 ± 3.4 ($p = 0.002$).

Hypoglossal Nerve Stimulation

Joachim T. Maurer, Nico de Vries, and Clemens Heiser

Definition

The impact of tongue muscle relaxation during sleep on upper airway collapse has been discussed since OSA has been first described. During the late 1970s, Remmers et al already hypothesized that disturbed neuromuscular control would lead to impaired airway stability.[288] They considered an insufficient genioglossus muscle tone during sleep as a major contributor to upper airway obstructions. During the last two decades, impaired neuromuscular responses to airflow obstructions could be attributed in part to alterations of afferent and efferent pharyngeal nerve fibers.[289] Consequently, the idea of increasing the genioglossus muscle tone by electric stimulation became obvious.

Stimulation of the genioglossus muscle leads not only to an opening of the tongue base but the upper portion of the pharynx (soft palate) can also be opened due to the so-called "palatoglossus coupling." The palatoglossus muscle forms the anterior pillar from the uvula and extends into the sides of the tongue.[290,291] A protrusion

213

of the stiffened tongue by stimulation anchors the palatoglossus muscle to open the soft palate. This prevents airflow obstruction during sleep over all pharyngeal levels. Oliven and Schwartz could demonstrate in early animal studies that exogenous electrical stimulation of the genioglossus muscle augmented its activity and improved airway patency.[292,293] This was reproduced in humans by activating the genioglossus muscle using direct stimulation of the hypoglossal nerve with fine needle electrodes placed sublingually.[294] Then hypoglossal nerve stimulation therapy was designed to recruit genioglossus activity and relieve airflow obstruction in sleeping patients with OSA. In this chapter, we present different implantable devices and surgical techniques for hypoglossal nerve stimulation that are commercially available so far.

Closed-Loop Technique

This technique was developed in the 1990s by initially Medtronic (Minneapolis, Minnesota, USA), and since 2007 Inspire Medical Systems (Maple Grove, MN, USA). Today the therapy is often called Upper Airway Stimulation ("UAS"). It tries to mimic neuromuscular upper airway control during wakefulness as much as possible. Respiration is measured using an intercostal pressure sensor. If the implantable pulse generator (IPG) detects the onset of inspiration through the pressure sensor between the ribs, a stimulation cuff electrode placed around the protruding fibers of the hypoglossal nerve will stimulate selectively those distal branches that protrude and stiffen the tongue to keep the airway open. At the end of inspiration, the stimulation stops. This feedback mechanism shall avoid stimulation during the wrong phase of the respiratory cycle as well as muscle fatigue. (See also Video 8.4 for a presentation of this technique.)

Open-Loop Technique

This technique was developed in the beginning of 2000 by ImThera Medical, San Diego, CA, USA and it is called Targeted Hypoglossal Neurostimulation ("THN"). The nerve is stimulated via an electrode containing six circumferential contacts, which can be separately and alternatingly addressed. It intends to continuously increase the tone of several muscles innervated by the hypoglossal nerve in order to stabilize the upper airway throughout the entire respiratory cycle. This means that while one contact is stimulating certain muscle fiber groups other muscle fibers remain relaxed. When changing to another selected contact different muscle fibers will be relaxed and activated. This mode of action shall not only get rid of the necessity to synchronize with respiration but also avoid fatigue.

Indications, Contraindications, and Patient Selection

Both existing techniques are only indicated in adult patients with moderate to severe OSA who fail or reject

positive pressure therapy. If other SRBDs are present to a clinically relevant degree, the patient should only be implanted if there is an appropriate treatment available addressing the coexisting SRBD or if a relevant improvement of OSA is considered to benefit the patient's overall health status.

Patients with contralateral preexisting hypoglossal nerve palsy are considered to be at specific risk if the remaining functioning hypoglossal nerve were harmed during the implantation.

Upper Airway Stimulation (Closed-Loop Technique)

There are different additional inclusion criteria according to the country practicing medicine. In the United States, current FDA approval is granted for patients with a BMI ≤ 32 kg/m², an AHI between 15 and 65/h, and the exclusion of a complete circumferential palatal collapse during DISE. In Europe (CE label), there is no regulatory limit for the BMI; only the AHI is limited to 15 to 65/h. Even though this is allowed, implanting patients without a circumferential palatal collapse during DISE is not recommended in Europe either.

In 2017, approval for reimbursement was obtained in the Netherlands, the second country after Germany in Europe. For 2018, limits are set for AHI to be from 20 to 50, but it is expected that these inclusion criteria will be widened soon.

Targeted Hypoglossal Neurostimulation (Open-Loop Technique)

There are no additional and specific regulatory exclusion criteria in Europe. According to the feasibility trial (THN 2), an AHI < 65, an AI ≤ 30, a desaturation index (>10% desaturation) < 15, and a BMI < 35 kg/m² seem to be predictors of success[295] and are used as relevant PSG selection criteria in the multicenter pivotal trial (THN 3). In the United States, the technique cannot be used outside of the aforementioned premarketing study.

Diagnostic Workup

PSG or related measures are used to assess the severity of OSA and other respiratory variables, thorough upper airway ENT examination including endoscopy to rule out a relevant anatomical reason for airway obstruction and hypoglossal function during wakefulness, followed by DISE to gather information of the level, pattern, and degree of obstruction. The latter is mandatory for Inspire UAS. BMI and comorbidities have to be noted.

System Components Inspire UAS for the Closed-Loop Technique

The implantable parts (▶Fig. 8.73) are comprised of a stimulation lead, a sensing lead, and an IPG, which

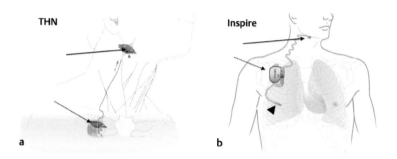

THN   Inspire

a   b

Fig. 8.73 The two different systems and components. **(a)** This image shows the open-loop technique (THN system from ImThera). **(b)** This image shows the closed-loop technique (Inspire 2 from Inspire Medical Systems). The *black arrow* in both images indicates the stimulation lead; meanwhile the *dashed arrow* indicates the implantable pulse generator. The *black arrowhead* shows the sensing lead in the closed-loop system. **(a)** Courtesy of ImThera. **(b)** Courtesy of Inspire.

together sense respiration patterns and deliver stimulation to the hypoglossal nerve synchronously with inspiration. The external parts are comprised of a physician programmer and a patient programmer.

Sensing Lead

The sensing lead incorporates a differential pressure sensor and two tissue anchors. The respiratory cycles are detected by their pressure variations, which are monitored by the IPG (see ▸Fig. 8.73, *black arrowhead*).

Stimulation Lead

The stimulation lead incorporates a cuff section with a shorter inner and a longer outer flap including three electrodes parallel to the cuff, which can be configured in a variety of unipolar or bipolar settings for stimulation. One tissue anchor is attached to the lead acting as a strain relief for the cuff portion around the nerve (see ▸Fig. 8.73, *black arrow*).

Implantable Pulse Generator

The IPG is connected to both leads and contains an algorithm that synchronizes hypoglossal nerve stimulation with respiration signals. The IPG's electronics and non-rechargeable battery are sealed inside a titanium case (see ▸Fig. 8.73, *dashed arrow*).

Physician Programmer

The physician programmer communicates via short-range radiofrequency telemetry unit with the IPG. Telemetry communication allows the physician to interrogate IPG status (e.g., battery status, system patient usage, respiratory waveforms, and programming log) and adjust settings (e.g., stimulation, sensing, refractory periods, and patient programmable settings such as start delay).

Patient Programmer

The patient programmer is used by the patient to activate nerve stimulation before sleep or temporarily pause it, if desired. The patient can also make adjustments to the stimulation amplitude within the physician's preselected limits.

System Components ImThera THN for the Open-Loop Technique

The implantable parts (▸Fig. 8.73) are comprised of a stimulation lead and an IPG. They deliver cyclical stimulation to sectorial parts of the hypoglossal nerve. The external parts are comprised of physician programming software, a charging antenna, and a remote control.

Stimulation Lead

The stimulation lead incorporates a cuff section with a shorter inner and a longer outer flap including six electrodes located in a circular pattern inside the cuff, which can be separately configured in unipolar settings for alternating stimulation. One movable tissue anchor is to be attached to the lead acting as a strain relief for the cuff portion around the nerve.

Implantable Pulse Generator

The IPG Aura6000 is connected to the lead and contains an algorithm that delivers hypoglossal nerve stimulation. The IPG's electronics and rechargeable battery are sealed inside a titanium case. The battery needs a recharge of approximately 20 minutes for every night in use; recharging should ideally be done daily, at least every third day. If the battery is completely depleted recharging will take 2 to 3 hours.

Physician Programming Software

The physician programming software should be installed on a portable laptop. It communicates via short-range telemetry unit with the IPG. Telemetry communication allows the physician to remotely check IPG status (e.g., battery status, system patient usage, and programming log) and adjust settings (e.g., activation of each electrode, stimulation parameters, pauses, and patient programmable settings such as start delay) via the remote control that needs to be connected to the laptop.

Remote Control

The patient can activate and terminate the therapy or temporarily pause it, if desired, by using the remote control. The patient can also make adjustments to the stimulation amplitude within the physician's preselected upper limit. In addition, the remote control contains a rechargeable battery, which itself is used to recharge the battery of the IPG via a charging antenna. The physician uses the remote control for advanced interrogation and titration purposes.

Specific Risks, Patient Information, and Consent

Patients have to be informed about procedure- and treatment-related adverse events (see ▶ Table 8.18 and ▶ Table 8.19).

A possible pneumothorax while placing the intercostal pressure sensor should be mentioned even though this has never been reported thus far. For the first 2 to 4 weeks some pain may occur while moving the right shoulder.

IPG migration requiring refixation may occur in rare cases if the IPG sutures get loose. Using the Inspire UAS device diving depth may be limited to 10 m (old device) or 30 m (new device), respectively. MRI conditionality is granted for the new Inspire UAS device but not for the old one (until 2017 or 2018, there may be different release

▶ Table 8.18 Nonserious adverse events in the STAR trial during 4 years after implantation

Adverse events (126 participants)	No. of events (0–12 mo)	No. of events (12–36 mo)	No. of events (36–48 mo)
Procedure-related nonserious adverse events			
Postoperative discomfort related to incisions	47	3	1
Postoperative discomfort independent of incisions	41	1	0
Temporary tongue weakness	34	0	0
Intubation effects	18	0	0
Headache	8	0	0
Other postoperative symptoms	22	0	0
Mild infection	1	0	0
Treatment-related nonserious adverse events			
Discomfort due to electrical stimulation	81	48	7
Tongue abrasion	28	16	3
Dry mouth	10	7	0
Mechanical pain associated with presence of the device	7	6	0
Temporary internal device usability or functionality complaint	12	9	3
Temporary external device usability or functionality complaint	11	19	9
Other acute symptoms	21	15	2
Mild infection	1	0	0

Abbreviation: STAR, stimulation treatment for apnea reduction.
Modified from Gillespie et al.[455]

▶ Table 8.19 Serious and nonserious adverse events during the first month (short term) and 6 months (long term) after THN implantation

Description of event	Nonserious		Serious	
	Short term	Long term	Short term	Long term
Anesthesia complication	1	—	—	—
Hematoma	1	2	1	—
Infection	4	—	—	—
Pain	7	12	1	2
Paresis	5	—	—	—
Paresthesia	5	1	—	—
Bleeding	—	—	1	—
No stimulation	—	—	1	—
Device migration	—	—	—	1
Other	1	16	2	3
Total	24 (17 pts./37.0%)	31 (20 pts/43.5%)	6 (6 pts./13.0%)	6 (5 pts./10.9%)

Modified from Friedman et al.[295]

months according to country and center) or the ImThera THN system. The patients have to understand that they have an active implant being recognized by security scanning systems (e.g., at airports).

The implant is not very thick. However, the bulk may be visible in skinny patients. Both IPGs will need to be exchanged if the battery reaches its end of life. Inspire calculates the expiry of the nonrechargeable battery after 8 to 12 years. ImThera calculates a life span of the rechargeable battery of 11 to 15 years. The life span might be even longer in real life when looking at battery power levels after regular use for 6 to 7 years.

Anesthesia and Positioning

Both techniques are performed under general anesthesia. Nasal intubation is recommended, especially in UAS in order to better visualize tongue motions.[296,297,298] The patient's neck is extended with a shoulder roll and turned to the left as for submandibulectomy. For UAS, an additional positioning cushion is placed under the patient's right chest to facilitate insertion of the sensing lead. Prophylactic antibiotics (e.g., 2 mg cephazoline or other drugs, if an allergy to cephalosporins is present) are given intravenously at the onset of anaesthesia. Long-acting muscle relaxants have to be avoided. Furthermore, a cylindrical gauze packing is again placed between the molar teeth of the left side to enable visualization of tongue movement during surgery.

Two paired intraoral neuromonitoring electrodes (18 mm long) are then placed.[299] The tongue and the mouth should be disinfected prior to placing the EMG electrodes. The first is placed in the right anterior floor of mouth, directed in a vertical direction just posterior to the mandible to monitor the genioglossus muscle. The second is placed along the ventrolateral aspect of the right tongue directed posteriorly, just underneaththe mucosa, to monitor the hyoglossus and styloglossus muscle. The electrodes are finally connected to a nerve integrity monitoring system. Instead of a nerve integrity monitoring, some surgeons use a simple nerve locator when implanting the ImThera device.

The surgical field is prepared with a sterile wash and eventually covered with an Ioban drape. The mouth is always covered with a transparent drape of sufficient size to allow for visualization of the tongue and its movement during the procedure.

Equipment

Standard oncology net, with nerve dissection instruments, is required. Magnification via loupes or microscope is mandatory. Nerve integrity monitoring is done with two channels. For Inspire UAS, longer retractors are necessary to sufficiently expose the ribs and a 0.6 cm malleable retractor for the intercostal space when placing the sensing lead.

Procedural Steps

The implantation can be divided into different steps. Steps 3 and 6 involving the pressure sensing lead are only required for the UAS device and not for the THN system.

1. Placement of stimulation lead
2. Pocket preparation for IPG
3. *Placement of sensing lead*
4. Tunneling and connecting lead(s) to IPG
5. Verification of tongue response to stimulation and impedance testing
6. *Verification of sensing*
7. Securing of IPG in pocket
8. Closure of incisions without drain

The entire surgery lasts between 90 and 150 minutes in most cases of UAS implantation. As there is no sensing lead required, THN implantation is typically finished within 60 to 120 minutes.

▶ Fig. 8.74 gives an overview of the nerve anatomy and stimulation lead positioning on the hypoglossal nerve.

Placement of the Stimulation Lead

The implantation always starts with the placement of the stimulation lead. It is the most important and technically demanding part of the procedure. If a tongue response cannot be obtained, then the surgeon should consider discontinuing the implantation and perform a troubleshooting surgery.[299]

The 2- to 5-cm incision for the stimulation lead placement is in the right submental neck, one fingers' breadth below the mandible and more anterior than a submandibulectomy approach. It starts 1 cm right to the midline for the UAS and 2 cm for the THN.

When dissecting through the platysma down toward the hyoid tendon, the anterior edge of the submandibular gland and anterior and posterior belly of the digastric muscle become visible.

Gently retracting the gland superoposteriorly and the anterior belly of the digastric muscle inferoanteriorly will present the posterior margin of the mylohyoid muscle, which then can be lifted to see the hyoglossus muscle underneath.

Placement of the Cuff Electrode for THN

The trunk of the hypoglossal nerve can be identified on the hyoglossus muscle indicating the *proximal placement* between the branch to the ansa cervicalis and the styloglossus for THN. The nerve is dissected off the muscle creating a pocket of 1 cm length with an angled blunt dissector and the red silicone thread attached to the longer sleeve of the electrode is pulled around the nerve from medial to lateral. Grasping the blue silicone thread attached to the shorter inner sleeve with another forceps and thus opening the cuff can facilitate this. The longer outer sleeve is put around the shorter inner sleeve so that the six electrodes will get in close contact to the nerve surface. At the end the silicone threads can be cut off and disposed. The cuff is rotated clockwise to have the lead exit the cuff on the superficial side. A fillet type movable anchor is placed around the lead 4 to 5 cm from the cuff creating a gentle loop and secured on the deep fascia. The cuff electrode is irrigated with physiological sodium chloride for elimination of air bubbles and improvement if electrical conductivity.

Placement of the Cuff Electrode for UAS

When separating the anterior belly from the gland and the subcutaneous tissue further anteriorly one will reach the anterior margin of the hyoglossus muscle for the *distal placement* of the cuff electrode. The surgeon will now isolate all retracting branches (hyoglossus and styloglossus) to be excluded from all protruding branches (genioglossus and geniohyoideus, the latter a branch of the root C1 travelling with the hypoglossal nerve) to be included (see ►Fig. 8.74, ►Fig. 8.75).

This area of interest is often accompanied or even crossed by a ranine vein (vena comitans nervi hypoglossi) making the placement of the cuff electrode difficult or impossible.

C1 is often attached to the perivascular tissue under the ranine vein. Therefore, careful separation from the nerve or even ligation is regularly required. Nerve integrity monitoring is mandatory to clearly select between the different sometimes closely coupled branches. A bipolar probe is recommended for this purpose, providing a narrower field of stimulation. In addition to the NIM-signals, watching tongue motion through the transparent drape covering the mouth is helpful—right sided or bilateral protrusion of the tongue for inclusion branches as a positive predictor versus contralateral protrusion or tongue retraction for exclusion branches as a negative predictor of therapy success. Once the inclusion fibers are clearly identified, isolated, and prepared the cuff electrode is placed around the nerve. It might be considered to use vessel loops to lift the nerve gently to facilitate cuff placement.

An angled blunt dissector is passed under the nerve from medial to lateral through the 1 cm pocket; the thin and long, outer sleeve is presented with a forceps, grasped, and pulled through the pocket. The inner shorter sleeve is furled around all the selected branches and covered with the long outer sleeve. One has to be careful not

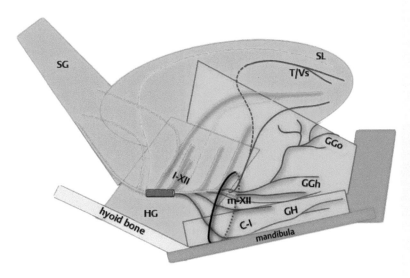

Fig. 8.74 A schematic sagittal section through the tongue, presenting the terminating distal branches of the hypoglossal nerve (XII). The black circle shows the selective cuff placement of the closed-loop technique (Inspire) and the blue tube the placement of the open-loop technique (THN). The green muscles (GGo, GGh, GH) are the main protrusors of the tongue and tongue base to open the upper airway. The orange marked muscles are mainly the upper airway stiffeners and tongue retractors to close the upper airway or stabilizing the upper airway. C-1, first cervical nerve; GGh and GGo, genioglossus muscle horizontal and oblique; GH, geniohyoid muscle; HG, fibers to hyoglossus muscle; l-XII, lateral branches of the hypoglossal nerve; m-XII, medial branches of the hypoglossal nerve; SG, styloglossus muscle; T/V, transverse and vertical intrinsic muscles.

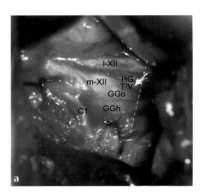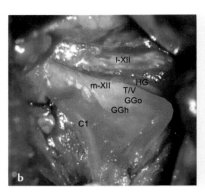

Fig. 8.75 (a, b) An intraoperative view of the terminating branches of the hypoglossal nerve. In (b), the green field shows the nerve fibers which need to be included in the stimulation lead, and the red field shows the fibers which need to be excluded. l-XII, lateral branches of the hypoglossal nerve; m-XII, medial branches of the hypoglossal nerve; C-1, first cervical nerve; GGh and GGo, fibers to genioglossus muscle horizontal and oblique; T/V, fibers to transverse and vertical intrinsic muscles.

to let nerve branches slip between both sleeves impairing electric conductivity between electrode and nerve. The lead is passed under the digastric muscle and, in a gentle loop, guided to the tendon or anterior belly of the digastric muscle whereto the fixed anchor is sutured with a 3–0 or 4–0 nonresorbable, braided suture. Sodium chloride irrigation around the cuff reduces trapped air inside the cuff and improves conductivity.

Pocket Preparation for the IPG

The 5-cm long incision is at the right anterior chest wall, as medial as esthetically possible, about 2 to 4 cm inferior and parallel to the clavicle along relaxed skin tension lines. The pocket is created on the fascia of the pectoralis major muscle and should be small enough to avoid too much movement of the IPG. On the other hand, the pocket should be large enough to avoid direct contact of the IPG to the incision.

Placement of the Sensing Lead (Inspire UAS Only)

The third incision, 5-cm long, is positioned horizontally along the relaxed skin tension lines at about the fourth to sixth intercostal space. The mid-axillary line marks its lateral extent. The inferolateral border of the pectoralis major should not be passed medially. When dissecting down to the ribs the anterior serratus and the external oblique muscle may be mistaken for the external intercostal muscle. They need to be separated from the ribs to find the external and internal intercostal muscle. At the upper edge of the fifth rib a channel of 6 cm length is created between both muscle layers using a malleable retractor or a curved clamp. One should prevent the pressure sensor from sliding over the rib because this would disturb the pressure signal and impair respiratory sensing. With the same intention, the pressure sensor has to face toward the pleura, which can be verified when the small humps on the first fixed anchor are visible facing superficially. This fixed anchor is sutured to the periosteum or intercostal fascia just outside the intercostal channel with a nonresorbable braided suture 3–0 or 4–0. The lead is then guided cranially in a gentle loop. The second anchor is fixed at the entrance of the subcutaneous tunnel toward the IPG pocket with the same suture.

Tunneling and Connecting Lead(s) to IPG

The leads are blindly tunneled with blunt tunneling tools for both techniques. This is easier done if the tunnel is initially dissected with a Kelly clamp or alike. In UAS, the surgical kit contains a disposable tunneling device with a blunt tip and a connector for the lead plugs. In THN, a commercially available shunt passer (e.g., Codman Disposable Catheter Passer) is used. The internal obturator with the blunt tip needs to be withdrawn leaving behind the metal tube, which acts as a safe guide for the lead.

The sensing lead (UAS only) is tunneled first, coming from the lateral chest wall incision toward the IPG pocket in the subcutaneous plane. In women, care should be taken not to penetrate through the breast.

The stimulation lead may be tunneled from the IPG pocket to the submandibular incision or vice versa. The devices are bent to match the individual anatomy and to stay above the clavicle in the subcutaneous or, in skinny patients, the subplatysmal plane. The external jugular vein should be identified to avoid hemorrhage. (Alternatively, a tunnel can be created in the plane above the platysm. The advantage is that the risk for vessel injury is lower; the down side is, in particular patients with a thin skin, that the wire might be visible.) The tunnel as well as the lead should be brought out at the superomedial corner of the IPG pocket in order to minimize stretching of the lead while extending and turning the head.

The leads are finally connected to the IPG so that the plugs are fully inserted dry and clean. The torque for correct fixing of the screws is respected.

Verification of Tongue Response to Stimulation, Impedance Testing, and Sensing

Now impedances of the stimulation lead, thresholds for EMG signal, and motor responses are obtained using the specific hardware and software of the manufacturers. For THN, each contact needs to be checked separately. In UAS, a bipolar configuration (+ − +) is used as a standard. A bilateral or right-sided tongue protrusion and flattening is considered to be a positive predictor.[300] Furthermore, in UAS respiratory sensing is verified in order to allow good synchronization between respiration and stimulation.

If the surgeon has any suspicion of stimulation lead misplacement or dislocation during the other steps of the implantation or weak or nonphysiologic pressure signals, revision of the leads is still possible at this stage.

Securing of IPG in Pocket and Closure of Incisions without Drain

Now the IPG is sutured into the pocket with two nonabsorbable, braided 2–0 sutures. In UAS, both are secured at the single existing hole; for THN there are two holes for one suture each. A loose sling is created on the deep fascia of the pectoralis major muscle first and the suture is tied to the device hole next. The manufacturer logo faces superficially for proper connection between the device and programmer. The lead in THN is shorter and exits toward the cranial side; it is longer in UAS and must be stored under the IPG. We advise to extend and turn the patient's neck to the left as much as possible. This allows us to understand whether there is any strain on the stimulation lead, so we can correct it before closing. Finally, a two-layer incision closure is performed, taking care not to suture and damage the leads. Drains are not recommended, as microbial colonization of the implanted parts might occur along the drains. Instead, pressure dressings are applied.

Complications

In general, the morbidity associated with hypoglossal nerve stimulation is minor and low. The most relevant procedure-related adverse events are bleeding, infection, and temporary tongue weakness. More severe (venous) bleeding may take place when tunneling the stimulation lead too superficially and hitting the external jugular vein. Temporary tongue weakness resolved in all cases spontaneously during the first weeks after the procedure. Permanent tongue weakness and pneumothorax have never been reported so far. Tension on the cervical lead or scar rarely happens; however, it can be difficult to treat if it arises eventually requiring surgical revision and repositioning of the lead at the IPG pocket or even the submandibular region. We had a single patient with UAS recently where pain along the stimulation lead made us reposition the stimulation lead. Finally, the cuff electrode had to be replaced as well. Postoperative hypoglossal nerve function remained completely normal after this revision surgery. In the stimulation treatment for apnea reduction (STAR) trial there have been a total of five serious adverse events (5 patients of 126, 4.0%) during the 48-month follow-up. Three patients underwent elective explantation due to untreatable insomnia, suspicion of causing a septic sternoclavicular joint (finally unrelated to the sterile IPG), and nonresponse, respectively. Two needed a replacement of malfunctioning device components (one sensing lead and one stimulation lead with IPG to reposition the electrode's location and improve therapy response) during the fourth year. The revision operations were without complications or significant sequelae.

Treatment-related morbidity is mainly due to the stiffening or movement of the tongue during stimulation. This may lead to tongue soreness, pain, or abrasions, which can be resolved by reprogramming, wearing a dental guard, or smoothening sharp tooth edges. As with every device, malfunction may occur. In THN, some patients had trouble with the charging antenna risking device depletion. This was resolved by exchanging the antenna. Treatment-related adverse events are typically bothering the patient only during the night when the therapy is active. After switching off the therapy in the morning, the patient does not suffer from altered anatomy or pharyngeal malfunction (e.g., scarring, numbness, and dry throat) as is known in palatal or tongue base surgeries.

Adverse events as reported over 4 years with UAS in the STAR trial (see ▶ Table 8.18) and over 6 months with THN in the THN 2 trial (see ▶ Table 8.19) show that there are no surgical long-term sequelae and that the treatment-related morbidity continuously decreases over the years with UAS.

The low morbidity is supported for UAS in a German postmarket study in 60 patients with 1-year follow-up.[298,301] During two surgeries (3.3%) cervical venous bleeding occurred while tunneling. Postoperative pain in five (8%), tongue numbness in one (1.6%), and dysarthria in one patient (1.6%) resolved spontaneously within 2 months. Another patient (1.6%) requested device removal due to personal nonacceptance of wearing an implant and for cosmetic reasons toward the end of the first year. Three patients (5%) reported painful stimulation and one (1.6%) reported speech difficulties during stimulation, which was resolved by acclimatizing to the therapy or reprogramming.

Postoperative Care

According to the local standards of care, antibiotic prophylaxis may be extended. The day of or after surgery a lateral neck X-ray is made to document lead and cuff position. For UAS, an additional AP chest X-ray will not only document the sensor lead position but also the absence of a pneumothorax. The pressure dressings are removed after 48 hours and the sutures after 7 to 10 days. Patients are discharged with clear instructions regarding postoperative behavior. They should limit right arm movements and heavy lifting for 2 weeks starting at the end of surgery. An arm sling attaching the right arm to the chest wall can facilitate this but is not mandatory. Patients incompliant to this instruction may risk seroma evolution and delayed fibrotic pocket formation around the implant.

There are no requirements regarding diet. Simple painkillers (e.g., paracetamol 3 × 500 to 3 × 1,000 mg or ibuprofen 3 × 600 mg) for a few days typically are sufficient.

Therapy Initiation

The IPG will be activated for the first time 1 month after surgery, allowing sufficient time for healing. This is done in an outpatient setting during wakefulness. The activation is done in a sitting position with the telemetry taped or held onto the skin over the IPG. Impedances are checked. The activation and titration during sleep are different in UAS and THN. Even though this is a surgical handbook, the surgeon has to know the major aspects. More advanced titration settings than explained here are needed in a smaller portion of the patient population. Successful titration may need more than one night. Therefore, early follow-up sleep studies may be necessary. Effect on AHI and therapy comfort have to be balanced for individual therapy success.

Activation and Titration in UAS

The physician programmer is used in the standard settings (bipolar + − +) to define the amplitudes of three thresholds (voltage): first sensation by the patient, clear tongue protrusion over the incisors (functional), and subdiscomfort.[300] The tongue motion (right-sided or bilateral) and any change due to varying amplitudes are documented. One can select other bipolar settings or switch to monopolar stimulation, changing the electrical field produced at the cuff electrode and thus affecting outcome.[302] Typical functional stimulation amplitudes in the standard setting range between 1.3 and 2.5 V. Start delay (e.g., 20 minutes), pause time when waking up during the night (e.g., 10 minutes), and lower and upper limit for home use are set. The lower limit typically is set to 0.2 V below the functional threshold and the upper limit to 0.2 V below the subdiscomfort threshold. Furthermore, the respiratory signal is checked and with that the stimulation is started. Now, synchronization between respiration and stimulation is verified and, if needed, thresholds and sensitivity for the detection of inhalation and exhalation are adjusted in arbitrary units. When synchronized stimulation is achieved the final settings are saved and the IPG is configured for home use. The patient is advised to slowly increase the amplitude in the preset range and adapt to the therapy at home. After 4 weeks of adaptation, the therapy is fine-tuned during the first titration sleep study.

Activation and Titration in THN

The software is used to program each of the six electrode contacts separately in a monopolar setting. Sensory threshold and therapeutic level (in µA) are defined for each contact. Therapeutic level while awake in THN is comparable to subdiscomfort in UAS. The positive or negative effect of stimulation of a specific contact on breathing while awake can be assessed by subjective patient feedback or by flexible pharyngoscopy. The same night, the necessary amplitudes, duration of activation, and ramp-up and ramp-down time for each contact will be defined. Typically, two to four contacts will provide airway stabilization and improve or normalize airflow while asleep. The activation sequence of the selected contacts is defined. Start delay (e.g., 20 minutes), pause time when waking up during the night (e.g., 10 minutes), and lower and upper limit for home use are set. The upper limit is equivalent to the therapeutic level. The different therapeutic levels of all activated contacts are defined as 100%. The lower limit typically is set at 80% of the therapeutic level. The patient is instructed on how to increase this master amplitude for all activated contacts.

Outcomes

Upper Airway Stimulation

In 2001, a first-in-man study was published presenting eight patients who were implanted with the first generation of the Inspire device.[303] All but one patient showed an improvement of their respiratory indices without disturbing sleep, proving the concept. Technical failures such as lead breakage and poor synchronization with respiration due to cardiovascular pressure artifacts caused by the transsternal positioning of the pressure sensor led to therapy termination in five patients. Designing a new device as described in the paragraphs above solved those technical and conceptual problems. A feasibility trial with 20 patients in its first phase had only six responders but revealed first predictors of treatment response. Another eight selected patients with an AHI from 20 to 50/h, a BMI ≤32 kg/m^2, and the absence of a complete concentric collapse at the soft palate during DISE[304] served as a small validation cohort with only one nonresponder.[305] Applying these main selection criteria, a multicenter phase III pivotal trial (e.g., STAR) demonstrated a significant reduction of median AHI from 29.3 to 9.0 and ODI from 25.4 to 7.4 as primary endpoints after 12 months. About 66% of the 126 patients enrolled fulfilled the Sher's criteria of therapy success. A significant and clinically meaningful improvement of sleep-related quality of life (median FOSQ [functional outcomes of sleep questionnaire] from 14.6 to 18.2) and daytime sleepiness (median ESS from 11.0 to 6.0) could be presented.[306] At 12 months ($n = 124$), a randomized therapy withdrawal study over 7 days in the first 46 therapy responders made OSA relapse in the withdrawal group, proving that the treatment response was related to the stimulation treatment.[307] Subjective and objective outcome remained stable after 18 ($n = 123$), 24 ($n = 123$), 36 ($n = 116$), 48 ($n = 109$), and 60 ($n = 97$) months without any increase in stimulation amplitudes.[301,308,309,310] Overall, there was an acceptably low number of patient drop-outs during the follow-up. This study demonstrated sustainable and favorable long-term results of upper airway stimulation.

Three German centers could confirm the subjective and objective outcome of the pivotal trial in a postmarketing study in 60 patients averaging 2 nights of seven-channel home sleep test at baseline and 6 and 12 months after implantation.[311,312] The study population was defined using extended selection criteria close to the CE approval (AHI 15–65, BMI ≤35 kg/m^2) and using less titration nights than in the STAR trial. The AHI dropped from a median of 28.6 to 8.3 after 6 and 9.5 after 12 months. About 68% reached AHI response status after 6 months and 73% after 12 months, respectively. No patient worsened the respiratory parameters during the follow-up. Median ESS and FOSQ improved from 13 to 6.0 and finally to 6.5 and from 13.7 to 18.6 and finally to 18.6, respectively. The average use per week was 39.16 ± 14.9 hours during the first year, which is more than 5.5 hours per night.

Currently, 12 centers in the United States, in Germany, and the Netherlands are recruiting 2,500 patients in a registry during the first year of treatment.

In this registry, no specific study visits were scheduled. Treatment and follow-up were conducted in each center according to their local standards of care. So far, the first 301 patients (248 m, 53 f; 59.2 ± 11.2 years; BMI 29.2 ± 3.8 kg/m²) have been evaluated.[313] Comparably to the pivotal trial and the postmarketing study, the AHI dropped from 35.6 ± 15.3 at baseline to 10.2 ± 12.9 at posttitration ($p < 0.0001$) with median AHI decreasing from 32.5 to 5.5, achieving a posttitration AHI < 15 in 81% of the patients. Daytime sleepiness improved from 11.9 ± 5.5 to 7.5 ± 4.7 ($p < 0.0001$) with median ESS reduced from 12 to 7. Average home device use was 6.5 ± 2.3 hours per night. In this study, physicians were asked about the overall clinical impression with the therapy. About 94% rated the patient's condition as improved compared to before. Around 92% of the patients were satisfied with the treatment.

There are other single- or multicenter publications showing comparable subjective and objective results.

UAS shows consistent subjective and objective short- and long-term success with high therapy adherence in association with high patient satisfaction.

Targeted Hypoglossal Neurostimulation

There are only three publications available regarding the open-loop technique so far. The first-in-man study published in 2013 by Mwenge et al presented 13 implanted patients (12 m, 1 f; AHI > 20; BMI 25–40 kg/m²) during a 12 month follow-up. Stimulation could reduce average AHI from 45.2 ± 17.8 at baseline to 21.7 ± 19.9 after 3 months and 21.0 ± 16.5 after 12 months. According to Sher's criteria, 10 of the 13 patients responded to the therapy. ODI was reduced similarly from 29.2 ± 19.6 to 14.2 ± 16.7 and 15.3 ± 16.2 as well as arousal index from 36.8 ± 12.5 to 24.9 ± 14.4 and 24.9 ± 13.7, respectively. Sleep stages and ESS did not change significantly.[314] The 10 responders were asked to stop stimulation for one night. Average AHI, ODI, and arousal index did not relapse indicating a certain residual and ongoing effect.[315]

A feasibility trial in 46 patients (43 m, 3f; 54.9 ± 11.1 years; BMI 30.8 ± 3.7 kg/m²) evaluated the safety and efficacy over 6 months in order to define predictors of success. Whereas the changes in AHI (from 34.9 ± 22.5 to 25.4 ± 23.1) were not satisfatory for the whole group, patients with a BMI < 35 kg/m², an AHI < 65, an apnea index (AI) ≤ 30, and an ODI (10% desaturations) < 15 responded best to the therapy. Daytime sleepiness (ESS) improved significantly; quality of life measures did not change.[296] The response predictors found here became selection criteria for the RCT THN 3. Recruitment has been finished by the end of 2017.

THN has shown promising results in the first two trials. Therefore, the RCT outcome is eagerly awaited at the beginning of 2019.

Key Points

Hypoglossal nerve stimulation offers a completely novel treatment concept by directly addressing the impaired airway patency in contrast to surgeries modifying upper airway anatomy. There are two types of hypoglossal nerve stimulation: closed-loop synchronized to respiration (Inspire, "UAS") and open-loop (ImThera, "THN"). Both devices are marketed in the European Union and some other countries worldwide. So far the US FDA has approved Inspire UAS only. A randomized, controlled pivotal trial for ImThera (THN 3) is still running. The number of publications, scientific basis, and level of evidence achieved regarding all aspects of the therapy are more advanced for the closed-loop technique UAS.

Both therapies are indicated in adult OSA as an alternative treatment if positive pressure ventilation therapy fails or is not tolerated or refused. Further, inclusion and exclusion criteria as well as required BMI and PSG findings differ slightly according to country and device. Overall, a BMI above 35 kg/m² seems less favorable. For the closed-loop technique a complete concentric palatal collapse has to be ruled out during DISE, which has not been evaluated for the open-loop technique so far. Both techniques are considered as stand-alone procedures, yet can be used in a staged surgical concept as well.

Surgery of UAS requires a nerve-monitoring guided placement of the cuff electrode around selected distal hypoglossal nerve branches and the placement of an intercostal respiratory sensor, whereas the cuff is placed at the proximal nerve when using THN without any respiratory sensing. The morbidity of the procedures seems comparable.

First activation is done 1 month after surgery; first titration is performed during PSG shortly after requiring specific training and expertise for each of the devices. Titration may be adjusted over the years.

Adherence to the therapy is important; average daily use lies above 6 hours per night in UAS in clinical routine. Long-term therapy success with UAS over a period of 5 years is achieved in approximately 75% of properly selected patients. For THN, there are only feasibility trials with 6 or 12 months follow-up available.

The open-loop technique "THN" is available for specific patients. The results of the pivotal RCT are eagerly awaited. The closed-loop technique "UAS" has entered clinical routine with clearly defined selection criteria, surgical technique, and predictable as well as favorable long-term outcome.

8.2.3 Larynx and Trachea

Partial Epiglottidectomy

Thomas Verse and Filippo Montevecchi

Definition

Since the introduction of DISE as a routine procedure prior to sleep apnea surgery, laryngeal infections in adult OSA are diagnosed much more frequently than before the DISE era.[221] Supraglottic collapse also has been identified as a potential cause of sleep surgery failure.[193]

In Forli, Italy, we started DISE in November 2005 for selected patients, using Propofol (initially by bolus technique and later by infusion pump) with an anaesthesiologist in the operating room. In 2010, a retrospective study of 250 consecutive patients was investigated, making a comparison between awake and DISE findings.[246] In this study, we found significant differences between the degree and pattern of hypopharyngeal obstruction (59 and 49%, respectively) and we discovered up to 30% of cases with laryngeal obstruction by DISE. In Hamburg, we analyzed 100 consecutive cases.[316] As in Forli, 30% of our Hamburg patients showed laryngeal obstructions at the level of the epiglottis. In 28% of the patients, the epiglottis was sucked to the posterior pharyngeal wall obstructing the upper airway without changing its shape. In the other 2% of our patients, the epiglottis was instable and fell into the larynx. Again, Kezirian and colleagues described an involvement of the epiglottis in airway collapse during DISE of 29 to 30% in a cohort of 108 sleep apnea patients.[317] A recent review about epiglottic collapse in adult OSA reports about a prevalence between 9.7 and 73.5% in sleep apnea patients during DISE.[318]

There are some early case reports about the so-called floppy epiglottis. A laxity of the epiglottis was described as cause for CPAP failure in these cases.[319,320,321] A floppy epiglottis can be defined as an instable epiglottis that collapses during inspiration independently from the tongue. Obviously this finding occurs most frequently in elderly men. However, a floppy epiglottis has also been described secondary after epiglottic cancer,[322] trauma, or oropharyngeal surgery.[323]

In conclusion, we think it is crucial to classify epiglottis involvement into two categories: *primary* and *secondary* epiglottis collapse. In the first pattern (primary), the epiglottis collapses itself causes obstruction over the larynx. As described earlier, this is possible in two ways: (1) the epiglottis falls back and obstructs the upper airway by touching the posterior pharyngeal wall (▶ Fig. 8.76; Video 8.5) or (2) the epiglottis collapses into the larynx,

obstructing it. In contrast to children, the latter type of primary collapse of the epiglottis is a rare condition in adults, and of which little is known regarding its role in OSA. This chapter will focus on the former collapse type. Treatment of choice is partial epiglottidectomy (PE). In children, especially in premature children, other findings are much more frequent. For pediatric laryngeal OSA and its treatment, please refer to Chapter 6.

In the second pattern (secondary), the epiglottic collapse is secondary to tongue base collapse. The latter condition requires tongue base treatments. Please refer to Chapter 8.2.2.

Indications, Contraindications, and Patient Selection

All patients that show primary epiglottis collapse during DISE are potential candidates for PE.

As PE is performed transorally, patients need to be able to open their mouths wide enough in order to insert the surgical instruments. To a certain extend, a limited mouth opening can be managed by the use of the CO_2-laser and a distending operating laryngoscope.

Dental pathologies might interfere with insertion of the laryngoscope and need to be taken into account. Please check preoperatively and address this issue in the informed consent.

As in any sleep apnea case, severe comorbidities need to be excluded. The patient must be suitable for surgery under general anaesthesia.

PE might affect swallowing within the first couple of days, rarely even longer. This potential complication needs to be mentioned in the informed consent.

In addition, neuromuscular diseases, neurological or psychiatric illnesses in need of treatment, cleft palate, chronic alcoholism, soporific drug abuse, severe bite misalignments, preexisting swallowing disturbances, and severe craniofacial deformities are regarded as contraindications.

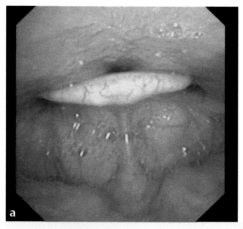 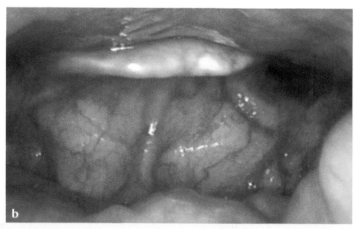

Fig. 8.76 (a, b) Two cases of primary collapse of the epiglottis in adult males.

Diagnostic Workup

Any kind of sleep apnea surgery requires objective preoperative sleep studies. Without a preoperative sleep study, the effect of the surgery on the AHI and other objective parameters cannot be determined after surgery. Apart from this, subjective complaints need to be recorded pre- and postoperatively. Please refer to Chapter 5 to find the instruments that are available for this purpose.

Please screen for dysphagia prior to surgery.

Specific Risks, Patient Information, and Consent

The general risks of surgery (i.e., pain, scarring, infection, wound healing problems, and postoperative hemorrhage) need to be addressed preoperatively.

Patients usually develop swallowing problems only for a few days. Usually, patients can return to normal diet immediately after surgery. Corticosteroids can help improve swallowing. Since we usually perform PE in combination with other soft palate and/or tongue base surgery complications of these other surgeries need to be explained prior to surgery.

Painkillers will be necessary for up to 1 week after surgery. Postoperative pain distinctively varies interindividually. Please check for intolerances prior to surgery. However, patients usually report low pain after PE.

Please verify the patient's ability to open his/her mouth and inspect the dental status. Address damages of the teeth and hematoma within the tongue as potential complications induced by the laryngoscope.

Anesthesia and Positioning

We only perform PE under general anesthesia with the patient being orally intubated and lying in supine position with the head slightly extended. Some authors use a special laser intubation tube for safety reasons. It is sufficient to protect the conventional intubation tube with armed, damp swabs.

We always prefer CO_2-laser surgery via a distending operating laryngoscope. Please mind the usual laser surgery safety arrangements (protection of the eyes, sufficient covering of the patient with damp cloth, etc.).

For PE, the patient is required to be relaxed.

Some authors prefer nasal intubation. Oral intubation works fine and saves nasal trauma.

Equipment

For laser surgery, we use a distending operating laryngoscope (see ▶ Fig. 8.51). We prefer the CO_2-laser (AcuPulse, Lumenis) with a power setting of 8 W (continuous mode). For blood control, a monopolar electrocautery system is strongly recommended. A surgical suction system is necessary as well.

A toothed rack helps to avoid damage of the teeth.

Operative Technique/Steps

We prefer the CO_2-laser for surgery (AcuPulse, Lumenis) with a power setting of 8 W (continuous mode). The epiglottis will be exposed using the distending operating laryngoscope (▶ Fig. 8.77). Needless to say that you need to include laser precaution measures, as mentioned earlier.

We usually resect two-thirds of the free epiglottis (▶ Fig. 8.78). The cutting of the mucosa is easy to perform. For the cartilage we sometimes use microscissors. Electrocautery might be needed for blood control.

▶ Fig. 8.79 shows completion of surgery. The situation 3 months after surgery is shown in ▶ Fig. 8.80.

Risks, Tips, and Tricks

- Use the CO_2-laser and microscissors in addition.
- Mind the upper teeth and lower lip while inserting the distending laryngoscope.
- You might need electrocautery for blood control.

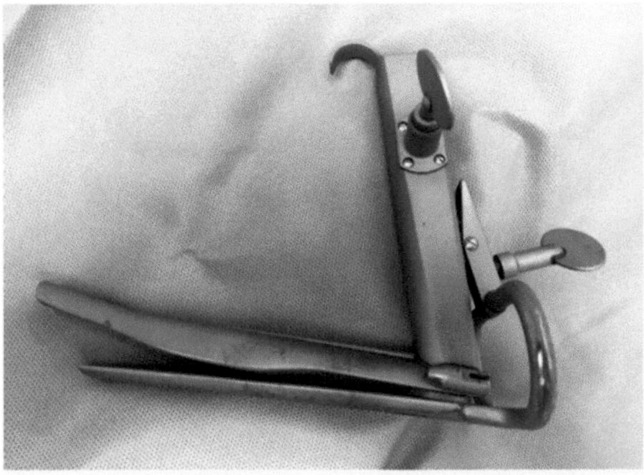

Fig. 8.77 Distending operating laryngoscope used for exposure of epiglottis.

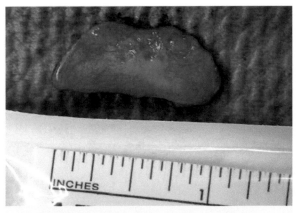
Fig. 8.78 Resection of two-thirds of the free epiglottis.

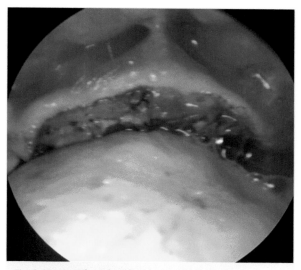

Fig. 8.79 Partial epiglottidectomy: end of surgery.

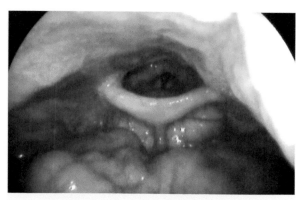

Fig. 8.80 Three months after epiglottidectomy.

Complications

Postoperative Pain

In contrast to other OSA surgeries, PE induces less postoperative pain. However, there is a need for postoperative analgetic drug treatment for a couple of days. Intensity and duration of pain show a high interindividual variability. Under medication, patients should be free of pain unless during swallowing. Use VASs separately for swallowing and not swallowing in order to record treatment success.

Hot, spicy, and sour foods and drinks are not recommended during the first 1 to 2 weeks after surgery.

Hemorrhage

So far, we did not have one single case with a relevant postoperative bleeding.

Dysphagia

Almost every patient can return to a normal diet on the first evening after surgery. If not, please make sure that the patient gets sufficient fluid intravenously until he/she returns to normal fluid intake.

Wound Infection

To avoid wound infection, we only apply one single-shot of cefuroxime (1.5 or 3.0 g depending on the body weight) intraoperatively. In addition, we provide a local antiseptic mouth solution (e.g., chlorhexidine solution, 0.2%) to improve the patient's mouth hygiene.

Postoperative Care

As in any other sleep apnea surgery, the severity of OSA has a significant impact on postoperative care and monitoring. This is why sleep apnea patients undergoing surgery under general anaesthesia or under sedation are at an increased risk for perioperative complications.[105,106,107]

This perioperative risk is particularly increased if OSA is treated surgically, as postoperative bleeding and swellings within the pharynx need to be taken into account. According to a review, postoperative complications are rare and occur within the first 4 hours after extubation. This result is in accordance with our own experience.[108] As a result, we keep our sleep apnea patients in the recovery room for 4 hours after extubation. If there are no complications during that time, the patients are regarded to be safe and will be discharged to the regular ward. In case of complications, the patient is monitored overnight.[109]

Management of postoperative pain is always crucial in sleep apnea surgery. A basic treatment with ibuprofen (four times 400–600 mg) in addition with metamizole (four times 0.5–1 g) works fine in adults. However, there are huge interindividual differences that require individual adaptations. If the basic treatment is not sufficient in time opioids might be added (e.g., three times 10 mg oxycodone). Please refer to Section 10.2 for further information about the postoperative care and medication.

As stated earlier, a postoperative antibiotic prophylaxis is not regarded necessary after PE.

Outcomes

Unfortunately, information about the outcome of isolated PE for OSA is very limited, as currently PE is usually combined with lingual surgery and/or palatal surgery.

There is one case series about 12 adult patients after unsuccessful UPPP.[324] In all these patients, a DISE showed a lax epiglottis that was sucked backward during inspiration against the posterior wall of the hypopharynx as origin of the persisting airway obstruction. All patients underwent a laser PE. There were no serious complications. Immediately after surgery, mean oxygen saturation increased from an average of 82% to an average of 93%. Subjectively, seven patients (58.3%) regarded the surgery as successful, another two patients (16.6%) as partially successful, and the other three patients (25%) as not successful. Nine out of 12 patients showed up for postoperative PSG 1 year after surgery. The AI decreased significantly from a mean of 42 ± 16.4 (± SD) at baseline to a mean of 8 ± 3.2 after surgery.

A second case series included 27 patients.[325] PE was performed in a similar fashion as described earlier. The mean RDI at baseline was 45 ± 14.6 and decreased to 14 ± 5.1 after surgery.

Apart from case reports, there is no information about the isolated use of PE in sleep apnea patients. ▶ Table 8.20 summarizes the present data.

In addition, PE has been described as part of various successful multilevel-surgery concepts.[238,326,327,328]

Key Points

Since the introduction of DISE into the presurgical workup in patients, sleep apnea laryngeal OSA is diagnosed much more frequently. In adults, a laxity of the epiglottis is the most frequent origin of laryngeal OSA. PE is an easy to perform, safe, and effective treatment to solve this problem.

In our centers, we perform PE under general anaesthesia using the CO_2-laser. Dysphagia and postoperative pain are usually not extensive, but may require medical treatment. PE can easily be combined with other sleep apnea surgeries within the same surgery.

Nasal intubation is a good option but not a necessary one. In order to avoid nasal trauma, we usually have our patients orally intubated.

Skin-Lined Tracheostomy

Filippo Montevecchi, Claudio Vicini, and Khai Beng Chong

Definition

In the 1950s, the OSAS had not yet been identified from a pathogenic and physiopathological point of view and the clinical pattern, characterized by pathological daytime sleepiness and its cardiac and cerebrovascular complications, was erroneously correlated with a status of chronic alveolar hypoventilation related to the grade of obesity of the patients studied (the so-called Pickwickian syndrome).[329] Later in the 1960s, the first PSG recordings demonstrating the pathogenesis of the daytime sleepiness

typical of Pickwickian syndrome was due to repeated episodes of prolonged obstruction at upper airways and not because of status of chronic carbonarcosis.[329] Kulho et al, in 1968,[184] who was among the first to perform PSG recordings in patients with Pickwickian syndrome, proposed that the "shunt" of upper airways should be carried out by means of permanent tracheostomy in order to exclude the anatomic parts in which the obstructive events occur. This is a surgical proposal that appears extremely "radical" and certainly not completely satisfying to the patient, but that was a pioneering age in which subjects with morbid obesity and severe grade of OSAS (RDI > 60, SaO_2 < 60%) were studied and there were no other instrumental or surgical alternatives such as CPAP. The surgical procedure proposed by Kulho was a classical tracheostomy with the positioning of a fenestrated cannula, which was maintained closed during the day time to allow phonation.[184] The permanent tracheotomy has unequivocally demonstrated the obstructive cause of clinical patterns previously interpreted differently and it was the first surgical procedure proposed to solve these apneas and is still the only surgical option which ensures, even in very severe cases, complete disappearance of apneas and thus remission of the clinical symptoms. When a permanent tracheostomy is necessary, the most interesting surgical technique is the so-called Skin-Lined procedure, described by Mayer and Penta in the 1960s and proposed in conditions of chronic severe respiratory failure with indications for tracheostomy (myasthenia gravis, lateral amyotrophic sclerosis [LAS], severe emphysema, etc.).[330,331] In 1977, Fee and Ward were the first to use Skin-Lined Tracheostomy (SLT) in patients with OSAS in order to reduce the risk of development of granulation tissue at tracheal stoma level and improve management of the cannula by the patient himself/herself.[332] Despite the current availability of numerous and heterogeneous therapeutic options, both surgical and nonsurgical, for the treatment of OSAS, permanent tracheostomy still has some specific indications even if limited to selected cases of severe obstructive apneas.

Indication

Permanent tracheotomy (tracheostomy) is used in extreme conditions, as far as concerns the range of options for snoring surgery, and is indicated only in rare

▶ Table 8.20 Objective results of isolated PE in adults

Author	N	Add. proc.	Follow-up (months)	AHI (pre)	AHI (post)	Success (%)	ESS (pre)	ESS (post)	EBM
Catalfumo et al[324]	9	None	12	42	8	No data	No data	No data	4
Golz et al[325]	27	None	12	45	14	85.2	No data	No data	4
All	36		12	44.25	12.5	85.2	No data	No data	C

Abbreviations: Add. proc, additional procedure; AHI, apnea–hypopnoea index; ESS, Epworth sleepiness scale.
Notes: N = number of patients enrolled; EBM =level of evidence-based medicine.

conditions of life-threatening OSAS in which n-CPAP is ineffective or not tolerated,[333] for example:

- Severe hypoxiemia (<60%)
- Severe hypercapnia
- Severe RDI (>50)
- Severe OSAS-correlated arrhythmias (bradycardia, asystolia, ventricular tachycardia, etc.)
- Severe EDS
- Severe overweight (BMI > 40 kg/m^2)
- Ischemic cardiopathy exacerbated by OSAS
- Ischemic encephalopathy exacerbated by OSAS
- Obstructive pneumopathy exacerbated by OSAS
- Severe OSAS with little possibility of solution with other surgical procedures, or failure of the latter

Of the indications, apart from OSAS (besides severe laryngeal or tracheal stenosis, laryngeal nerve palsy, myasthenia gravis, LAS, intractable aspiration, severe emphysema), in our experience, multisystemic atrophy has become increasingly indicated, due to severe nocturnal laryngospasm with risk of sudden death during sleep. Therapeutic tracheotomy has to be permanent and therefore it is preferable to use a specific technique (SLT) that will be able to guarantee the following:

- *Greater stability*—the presence of an epithelialized bridge between the anterior cervical skin and the tracheal mucosa prevents retracting and scarring, which can lead to spontaneous closure without a cannula, as seen in many nonskin-lined tracheostomies.
- *Less risk of granulation tissue*—the seal provided by the skin-mucosa continuity is the best guarantee of a slight, but not absent, tendency of the peristomal connective tissue to penetrate into the lumen in the form of granulation tissue, with all the practical consequences, as well as difficulties in management of the case.
- *Larger opening of tracheostomy* for easier and safer management of the cannula in the home setting (removal, cleaning, reinsertion) (1) to allow the stoma to be maintained without a cannula, particularly in the daytime hours, without the risk of untoward stenosis during the day and (2) to allow safe use of personalized obturator, "custom made," to be used, instead of the cannula, and exclusively during the hours the patient is awake, for better phonation (an improved solution compared to simple closure of the cannula, which often gives rise to a consistent leakage of peristomal air).
- Sufficient *reversibility*, if necessary, due to perfect preservation of the structures of the trachea.

Anesthesia and Positioning

General anesthesia was used in every procedure on account of the complex technique, the long and delicate manipulation of the tracheal structures, the dissection of long cutaneous flaps, and the not infrequent severe obesity with a consequently more difficult approach to the tracheal wall for which a similar procedure is not feasible under local anesthesia.

Positioning of the patient is the same as in standard tracheotomy, with a pillow under the shoulders and neck hyperextended and not turned. To reduce the venous congestion of the neck, it is advisable to position the operating table with the headend of the table raised by at least 20 degrees. In some cases, it is necessary to tape the chin of the patient to the table in order to guarantee hyperextension of the head, especially in obese patients. Furthermore, it could be necessary to use the same method in cases of severe obesity and extremely voluminous breasts, which would otherwise have obstructed the operating field.

Surgical Technique

A surgical marking pen is used to mark the incisions in the anterior cervical region. The first step is to decide the area from where the skin flaps should be harvested, bearing in mind the distance between the suprasternal notch and the cricoid cartilage. The positioning of the flaps should take into consideration the following needs, at times contrasting:

- Convenience for the patient to have a stoma as low and less visible as possible.
- Need for the surgeon to work in the subisthmic site.
- Need for the surgeon to work on a trachea that is not yet fully positioned in the mediastinum.
- Need to accommodate the drawing of the flaps in a sometimes minimal cricoid-suprasternal notch space.
- Care to bear in mind that when the neck returns from the extended to the normal position, the incision line tends to slip below.
- The final choice is a compromise since the surgeon will have to reflect upon all these aspects also bearing in mind personal experience.
- Drawing of the incisions will include the following:
  - Identify the landmarks like the thyroid notch, cricoid cartilage, suprasternal notch.
  - Draw two parallel transverse lines which are slightly concave (2 or 3 cm in length; 1 to 1.5 cm apart).
  - A median vertical line that joins the two transverse lines (1 to 1.5 cm in length).

The design is virtually a capital "H" rotated 90 degrees with respect to the vertical position (▶ Fig. 8.81). The length of the incisions is empirically calculated in proportion to the adipose tissue in the neck. In the case of a particularly voluminous neck, a longer flap is necessary to reach the trachea that is relatively further away from the skin layer.

Infiltration of the incision lines is then carried out with anesthetic and vasoconstrictor. The operative field is disinfected and delimited.

A 15 number scalpel is used for the incisions in order to lift, from the superficial cervical bundle, two skin flaps together with the subcutaneous tissue. The flaps are then positioned laterally with two sutures on each side.

Fatty tissue is then removed from the flaps, ensuring to remove all the adipose tissue from the distal tips, progressively leaving a larger amount of fat, as the root of the flap is approached. This should ensure the maximum afferent and efferent vascularization possible. Dissection along the linea alba as far as the pretracheal fascia is then carried out.

Management of the thyroid isthmus is, in effect, related to the opening in the anterior tracheal wall. If sufficient space is present, the isthmus is pulled upward. Rarely, it may be necessary to perform thyroid isthmectomy, which allows ample exposure of the tracheal axis. At this stage, use of strong, flat, and sufficiently long retractors offers optimal exposure placing, two on each side and, possibly, a third in correspondence to the suprasternal notch.

Incision of the two tracheal flaps, superior and inferior, is then performed. To this end, in the midpoint of the open tracheal area, three "H-shaped" incisions are made, respectively, two paramedian vertical parallel incisions, 2.5 cm in height, symmetrical, 1.5 cm one from the other (▶Fig. 8.82). The final result is of two upper and lower adjacent tracheal flaps; the superior flap involving one tracheal ring and the inferior flap involving two tracheal rings. These two flaps will be ready to be sutured to the skin superiorly and inferiorly (▶Fig. 8.83). The cutaneous lateral flaps previously prepared are sutured with the lateral walls of the trachea (▶Fig. 8.84), completely isolating the subcutaneous and connective tissue of the neck from the skin surface.

At this stage, the endotracheal tube is removed and the trachea cannula is introduced.

A cuffed tracheal cannula is then introduced, as big as possible, for the first 3 to 4 days, after which an uncuffed

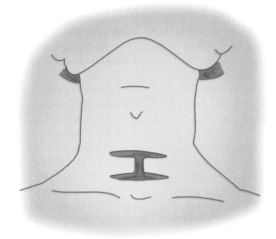

Fig. 8.81 Skin incision forms an "H" 90 degree rotated from the vertical position.

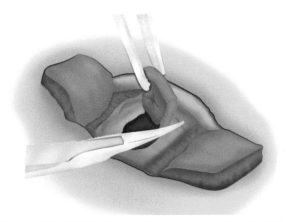

Fig. 8.82 Tracheal flaps incision, "H" shaped.

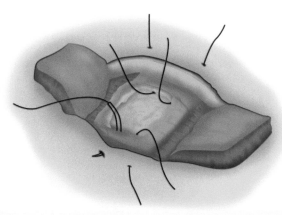

Fig. 8.83 Tracheal ring flaps sutured to the skin superiorly and inferiorly.

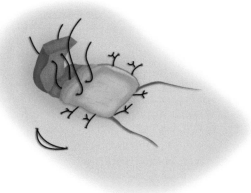

Fig. 8.84 Cutaneous lateral flaps previously prepared are sutured with the lateral walls of the trachea.

fenestrated cannula of the same diameter is used (unlike in standard tracheotomies, the well-known effect promoting granulation due to fenestration is improbable due to epithelialization of the stoma).

Within approximately 1 month, the stabilization of the tracheostomy is achieved, which is concentrically narrowed (about one-third of the original diameter). At this stage, if the local stoma condition and the social-educational level of the patient and his family allow, it is possible to leave the stoma uncovered and functioning, with or without the cannula during the night. During the day, it is possible to cover the stoma with a waterproof patch, or to close the stoma with a cannula and its button or close the stoma with a silicone "custom-made" obturator made of dental impression material.

> ### Risks, Tips, and Tricks
>
> - Use a pen to mark the landmarks and to draw the cutaneous flaps.
> - Perform cutaneous flaps as big as possible to have a big stoma.
> - If necessary, perform a thyroid isthmectomy.
> - Remove sutures after 12 to 15 days.
> - The excessive overweight could lead to an unexpected event such as partial obstruction of the external orifice of the cannula.

Complications

Usually no intra- or postoperative complications were observed. The formation of granulation tissue is almost negligible. The excessive overweight could lead to an unexpected event such as partial obstruction of the external orifice of the cannula on account of bulky cervical skin folds due to the abnormal fat tissue. The physiological circular narrowing of the stoma usually does not give rise to significant stenosis.

Postoperative Care

The tracheal cannula is almost always necessary to guarantee adequate opening of the tracheostomy in any sleeping position, particularly in those patients with presenting OSAS due to a cervical conformation (short and wide circumference) and the large skin plications due to abnormal fat tissue. Management of the cannula in the home setting did not present any difficulty, similar to a case of total laryngectomy.

For better phonation, and only while awake, it is advised to remove the cannula and to apply the personalized obturator, which is obtained by shaping the material for dental impression material on the tracheostomy tract, thus obtaining a cone-shaped obturator. This solution was found to be better than simple closure of the cannula (which often gives rise to consistent output of peristomal air leak), which is fairly well accepted and used in various ways.

Outcomes

The efficacy of permanent tracheotomy is demonstrated by reports in the literature. Motta et al, comparing PSG parameters in six patients (cardiac frequency, systemic and pulmonary blood pressure, SaO_2), before and after tracheostomy, observed a significant improvement in all hemodynamic parameters.[334] Partinen et al studied a population of 198 patients with severe OSAS, for 8 years, of whom 71 underwent tracheostomy and 127 were treated for weight loss. After 5 years, the death rate was 11% in the 127 patients who had opted for conservative therapy versus no deaths in patients submitted to tracheostomy.[335] Haapaniemi et al, in a longitudinal study on seven obese patients with severe OSAS submitted to tracheostomy, observed an improvement in the clinical pattern as well as in the postoperative PSG findings, which remained stable after 5 years.[336] Campanini et al described a total of 10 cases, seven patients presented with nocturnal laryngeal stridor, a form of laryngospasm with severe respiratory insufficiency due to a very rare neurological disease, multisystemic atrophy (MSA), and the other three patients had severe OSAS. In OSAS patients (patients with massive obesity and a variable degree of hypoventilation of the restrictive type), it was found to have a complete disappearance of apnea (RDI < 10) and related symptoms (immediate and astonishing effects on sleep and daily symptoms).[333]

▶ Table 8.21 highlights the available PSG data. In addition, there are two recent reviews about the objective success of tracheostomy in OSA patients.[337,338] The first review includes PSG data about 161 OSA patients before and after surgery (see ▶ Table 8.22).[337] The more recent one provides somehow inhomogenous data about another 14 morbidly obese patients.

Conclusions

By a better understanding of OSAS and a significant improvement in the treatment options available (instrumental, medical and surgical) it is, nowadays, extremely rare to encounter cases in which tracheotomy is the only feasible treatment. These conditions occur only in severe OSAS, at high risk (even life threatening) and in which n-CPAP is not tolerated or ineffective. In these selected cases, tracheostomy is carried out by using the skin-lined technique, which offers several advantages, such as a greater opening of the stoma, higher stability over time, less risk of granulation tissue, and reversibility. The procedure did not appear to give rise to any serious complications. The expected functional results are achieved with immediate disappearance of daytime symptoms and satisfactory recovery as far as nocturnal apneas are concerned. This technique would be suitable for use in patients with sleep disordered breathing of neurological origin (laryngeal stridor due to multisystemic atrophy). Besides sleep-related disorders, various clinical

▶ Table 8.21 Polysomnographic data before and after tracheostomy

Author	N	Follow-up (months)	Success (%)	Definition of success	EBM grade
Guilleminault et al[339]	50	9–72 (mean 32)	100.0	AI < 5	4
Haapaniemi et al[336]	7	30–108	100.0	No data	4
Kim et al[340]	23	no data	73.9	AHI < 20	3b
Thatcher and Maisel[341]	79	3–240	100.0	No data	4
All	159	3–240	96.2	No data	C

Abbreviations: AI, apnea index; AHI, apnea–hypopnea index.
Note: EBM = level of evidence-based medicine.

▶ Table 8.22 Polysomnographic data before and after tracheostomy

Author	N	Follow-up (months)	Age	BMI	AI (pre)	AI (post)
Camacho et al[337]	120	9.1 ± 12.4	49.4 ± 10.1	34.0 ± 7.8	73.0 ± 27.1	0.2 ± 1.2
					AHI pre	AHI post
	41	0.4 ± 0.5	48.2 ± 10.9	no data	92.0 ± 34.8	17.3 ± 20.5

Abbreviations: AI: apnea index; AHI: apnea–hypopnea index.

conditions, for which permanent tracheotomy is indicated, may benefit from the skin-lined technique, such as severe laryngeal or tracheal stenoses, laryngeal diplegia, myasthenia gravis, LAS, intractable aspiration, and severe emphysema.[342]

8.3 Maxillofacial Surgeries

Aarnoud Hoekema and Jan de Lange

8.3.1 Introduction

In 1979, Kuo et al were the first to describe the effects of orthognathic surgery for the treatment of OSA.[343] They described a case in which mandibular advancement surgery was reported to reverse the symptoms of sleep apnea. In 1986, Riley et al were the first to describe the combination of advancement of both maxilla and mandible in order to improve airway patency in OSA patients.[344] Although trial-based evidence is still scarce, MMA surgery is currently regarded as a highly effective and safe surgical treatment modality for OSA.[345,346] MMA surgery in OSA patients generally consists of a bilateral sagittal split osteotomy (BSSO) of the mandible and a Le Fort 1 osteotomy of the maxilla (▶ Fig. 8.85). In OSA patients, MMA surgery generally requires a minimum advancement of the mandible of 10 mm.[347,348] Consequently, several upper airway muscles and ligaments are repositioned anteriorly including the anterior belly of the digastric, mylohyoid, genioglossus, and geniohyoid muscles. The advancement of the maxilla pulls the soft tissue of the palate forward, tightens the palatoglossal and palatopharyngeal muscles, and increases tongue support. Moreover, "adding" the maxillary advancement also increases the amount of mandibular advancement that can be accomplished with surgery. In order to achieve additional improvements in oro- and hypopharyngeal airway patency, MMA surgery may be combined with a GA or a modified genioplasty[349,350] (▶ Fig. 8.86, ▶ Fig. 8.89). In order to decrease the patient's cervical fat mass and to further improve airway patency, cervicomental liposuction may be added to the surgical plan in selected cases.[350] The resultant of this maxillary, mandibular, and chin advancement is a structural enlargement of the naso/oro/hypopharyngeal airway and enhanced tension and decreased collapsibility of the pharyngeal dilator musculature. Because this is not aimed at correcting dentofacial abnormalities, MMA surgery in OSA patients is sometimes also referred to as "telegnathic surgery."

Indications, Contraindications, and Patient Selection

In general, prerequisites for MMA surgery include clinically "significant" OSA that is not susceptible to conservative management (e.g., CPAP), a medically and psychologically stable condition and the patient's informed consent prior to surgery.[351] MMA surgery is successful in a high proportion of patients and comparable to CPAP therapy in terms of effectiveness.[345,346] One of the possible advantages of surgical management is that treatment efficacy is not dependent on adherence like CPAP therapy. It should however be noted that studies evaluating surgical interventions in OSA generally incorporate methodological deficits. Further bias is introduced with the use of divergent criteria

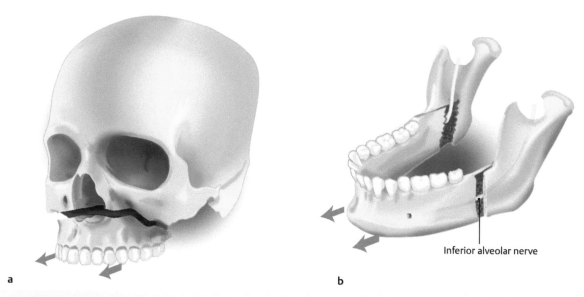

a   b

Fig. 8.85 Maxillomandibular advancement surgery. Maxillomandibular advancement surgery for obstructive sleep apnea syndrome provides enlargement of the upper airway by means of a Le Fort I advancement osteotomy of the maxilla (**a**) and a bilateral sagittal split advancement osteotomy of the mandible (**b**). (Used with permission from Rosenberg AJ, Damen GW, Schreuder KE, et al. Ned Tijdschr Geneeskd. 2005; 149:1223–1226.)

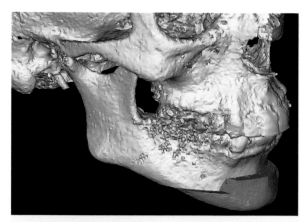

Fig. 8.86 Modified genioplasty. In a modified genioplasty, the tongue is put under anterior traction by performing a trapezoid-shaped osteotomy with advancement of the chin and the genial tubercle/genioglossus muscle complex.

for surgical success. Therefore, in clinical practice surgical interventions for OSA are usually reserved for patients who are "nonresponsive" or "nonadherent" to noninvasive therapies such as CPAP or oral appliances. Exceptions to this "rule" are patients characterized by a severe malocclusion, retrognathia, or a bimaxillary retrusion. In these patients, MMA surgery will not only be likely to correct their OSA, it will also result in a more harmonic dentofacial composition. This subgroup of patients may therefore be offered MMA surgery as a primary treatment. In addition, young patients that

wish for a more "permanent" solution for their OSA instead of a lifelong treatment with noninvasive therapies like CPAP or an oral appliance are generally also good candidates for MMA surgery.

Several different treatment algorithms have been adopted for the selection of surgical candidates for MMA surgery in OSA. Riley et al employ a phased protocol based on the specific site of upper airway obstruction.[352] Depending on the level of airway obstruction (soft palate and/or base of tongue), patients are treated with a UPPP and/or a GA with hyoid myotomy and suspension in the first phase of this protocol. The second phase consists of MMA surgery and is generally reserved for phase I failures. Because the majority of patients failing the first surgical phase tend to have more severe OSA, obesity, and mandibular deficiency,[348] others (patients with severe OSA and/or craniofacial dysmorphy) directly proceed with MMA surgery.[353,354] Prinsell et al adopt a "site-specific" approach in which OSA patients with "orohypypharyngeal narrowing caused by macroglossia with a retropositioned tongue base" are considered eligible for MMA surgery.[355] Both Waite et al and Hochban et al adopt a protocol in which MMA surgery is considered the first surgical option in patients with specific "craniofacial deformities" (e.g., abnormal PAS).[356,357] Finally, the response to an oral appliance may also be used to select suitable candidates for MMA surgery. Patients demonstrating a substantial reduction in baseline AHI (i.e., >50%) with oral appliance therapy appear good candidates for MMA surgery.[358]

Several studies including two systematic reviews have evaluated the most relevant patient characteristics and clinical factors predictive of a surgical success or cure following MMA surgery in OSA patients. Holty et al found in a univariate analyses that patients who are younger and have a lower preoperative AHI are more likely to achieve a surgical success with surgery (i.e., AHI reduction >50% to a value <20).[345] Also, the amount of advancement of the maxilla appears to correlate with the degree of reduction in AHI.[345,359] Patients with a surgical success are more likely to have their maxilla advanced to 10 mm or more.[345] Conversely, the amount of mandibular advancement does not appear to correlate with a successful outcome following surgery.[345] A surgical cure (i.e., AHI <5) was seen more often in patients with lower baseline AHI values[345,346] and in patients in whom no preceding upper airway surgeries have been performed.[3] However, patients with higher baseline AHI values generally display a more pronounced reduction in AHI following surgery.[346] Zaghi et al found in their systematic review that female gender, higher preoperative BMI and ESS values, and lower preoperative SpO$_2$ nadir were associated with a favorable outcome of surgery in a univariate analyses.[346] With respect to possible cephalometric predictors, an increased postoperative PAS, determined from lateral cephalometric radiographs, appears to be the only relevant variable of predictive value for a successful outcome of MMA surgery.[345] In multivariate analysis by Holty et al, independent predictors of surgical success or cure included a lower pre-MMA BMI and a greater degree of maxillary advancement.[345] In the multivariate analyses by Zaghi et al, the only predictor of a surgical success was a lower preoperative AHI, whereas a surgical cure was associated with younger age, lower preoperative AHI, and lower preoperative SpO$_2$ nadir.[346] Despite the variety of treatment protocols and predictors of favorable surgical outcomes, a precise treatment algorithm for MMA surgery in OSA management is currently indefinite.

Diagnostic Workup

Before proceeding with the MMA surgery, a general workup and thorough sleep history of each patient should be documented. Former OSA treatments and their clinical and PSG result should also be evaluated in this workup. The PSG recording should not be older than 12 months and not concern a split-night study. Before proceeding with the surgery, a comprehensive medical workup of every patient should be performed. This should identify confounding factors that can increase the medical, anaesthetic, and surgical risk of the procedure. The preoperative evaluation should also include a clinical examination of the head and neck region including nasal airway obstruction, the palatal region, the LPWs, and the size and character of the tonsils. An intraoral examination is performed to assess dental status, soft tissues including tongue and tongue base, malocclusions, and skeletal abnormalities. A lateral cephalometric head film and a preoperative PSG recording are mandatory to plan an MMA surgery. Surgery may also be planned using 3D imaging techniques like (cone beam) CT (see Video 8.6). Subsequently, virtual surgical planning can be conducted, which offers the surgeon valuable information on the anticipated skeletal, airway, and facial aesthetic changes (▶ Fig. 8.87).[360] Finally, fiberoptic nasopharyngoscopy awake or during drug-induced sleep is also recommended before surgery. This can further help to identify nasal, RP, or tongue base pathology that may affect the outcome of the MMA surgery.

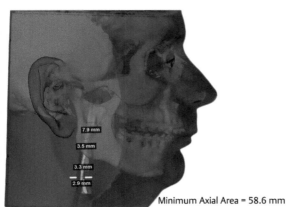
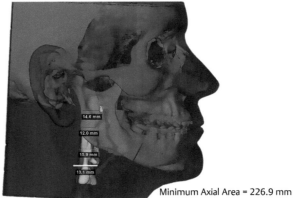

a

b

Fig. 8.87 Three-dimensional planning of maxillomandibular advancement surgery. A preoperative (a) and postoperative (b) morph illustrating the anticipated skeletal, airway and facial aesthetic changes following maxillomandibular advancement surgery with a genioplasty in a patient with sleep disordered breathing. (Courtesy Mr. D. Brock; 3D Systems, Inc.)

Specific Risks, Patient Information, and Consent

Simultaneous advancement of the maxilla and mandible changes the skeletal framework of the face, thereby resulting in a possible rejuvenation of the middle and lower third of the face. This concept of a "reverse face lift" with positive effects on facial aesthetics following MMA surgery in OSA patients is observed in the majority of patients (▶Fig. 8.88). Li et al found that 6 months after surgery, 50% of patients reported a younger and 36% reported a more attractive facial appearance.[349,361] It should be noted that 9% of the patients in this study reported a less attractive facial appearance following surgery. Conversely, in two other studies OSA patients indicated not to be bothered by their appearance following MMA surgery.[362,363] Although patients seeking treatment for their OSA generally do not desire a facial aesthetic improvement, it is important to communicate the anticipated facial changes before surgery. The magnitude of facial soft-tissue changes of the lips and chin has been shown to correlate with 90% of the underlying dental and skeletal movement.[364] Because the majority of OSA patients exhibit normal craniofacial skeletal morphology, profound advancements should not result in an unacceptable deformity of a patient's facial aesthetics. A surgical technique involving a so called "counterclockwise" rotation of the occlusal plane, which has previously been used in correcting severe "bird-face" deformity, may be used to achieve both aesthetic goals and to fulfill the main objective in the treatment of OSA patients, an optimal increase in airway patency.[365]

Anesthesia and Positioning

MMA surgery is performed under general anesthesia. The patient's head should be positioned in slight hyperextension resting in a head positioning cushing or a maxillofacial headrest. Body position should be in a slight reverse Trendelenburg position for head and neck procedures. Most patients will have less blood loss during the procedure if the mean arterial pressure is decreased to 65 mm Hg, provided there are no contraindications for this deliberate hypotensive anesthesia (e.g., underlying organ dysfunction).[366] The use of tranexamic acid following intubation may further reduce blood loss during surgery.[366] A bolus of 20 mg/kg or 1,000 mg of tranexamic acid intravenously following intubation are commonly used dosages. Furthermore, the use of cocaine hydrochloride topically applied via gauze nasal packing may also further reduce the blood loss from the Le Fort 1 osteotomy.

Equipment

Orthognathic surgery equipment net is used for the procedure. Orthognathic miniplates and miniscrews are used for rigid fixation of the mandible and maxilla, following the osteotomy. For fixation of the chin after a genioplasty, either straight miniplates or prebent chin plates can be used. The surgical set is complemented with a straight dental surgical bur and reciprocating saw. The use of a piezoelectric surgical device is encouraged as this may minimize soft-tissue trauma during surgery.

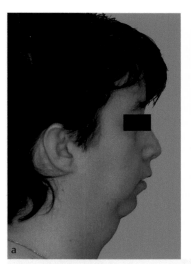 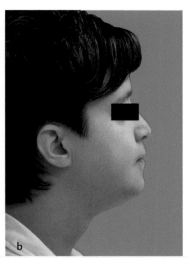 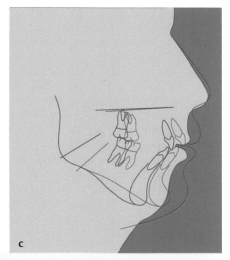

Fig. 8.88 Effects of maxillomandibular advancement surgery on facial aesthetics. A preoperative (**a**) and postoperative (**b**) photograph illustrating the rejuvenation of the middle and lower third of the face following maxillomandibular advancement surgery combined with a modified genioplasty and cervicomental liposuction in a severe obstructive sleep apnea patient. The profound advancement of the lower third of the patients profile can be appreciated when the pre- and postsurgical cephalometric radiographs are superimposed (**c**). (Used with permission from Doff MH, Jansma J, Schepers RH, Hoekema A. Maxillomandibular advancement surgery as alternative to continuous positive airway pressure in morbidly severe obstructive sleep apnea: a case report. Cranio 2013;31:246–251.)

Operative Technique

MMA surgery combined with a modified genioplasty requires a nasoendotracheal tube exiting superiorly over the forehead as the preferred position (see Video 8.7). When performing a "clockwise" rotation of the occlusal plane with MMA surgery, the cortical bone cuts for the BSSO are performed first with subsequent completion of the Le Fort 1 osteotomy. However, since "counterclockwise" rotation of the occlusal plane results in a more optimal increase in airway patency, surgery will usually start with completion of the BSSO. Following intubation, a local anaesthetic is applied from the ascending ramus area up to the second premolar region of the mandible on each side. A local anaesthetic with vasoconstrictor should be used, as this will reduce blood loss during surgery. During the procedure, application of the local anaesthetic is repeated 20 minutes before starting the Le Fort 1 osteotomy or genioplasty. For this reason, the buccal sulcus from the third molar up to the third molar in the maxilla and the buccal sulcus from canine to canine in the mandible are infiltrated, respectively. Following the administration of the local anaesthetic, the operating area is washed with chlorhexidine 0.5% in alcohol 70%. This includes the anterior facial skin from the forehead area to the level of the thyroid cartilage posteriorly limited by the ears. Care should be taken not to apply the solution to the eyes. To minimize this risk, an ophthalmic ointment should be applied beneath the eyelids and the eyes should be taped closed preceding the skin disinfection. Draping should provide for adequate exposure of the glabella area, the eyes, the preauricular area, the face, and the neck. Subsequently, the forehead area up to the nose is draped with a transparent foil. A 20-mm long, 1.4-mm-diameter Kirschner wire is placed in the glabella area. The distance between the Kirschner wire and the mid-maxillary incisor crown is recorded with a calliper and used for controlling vertical maxillary height when performing the Le Fort 1 osteotomy.

Starting with the right-side BSSO, an incision is performed in the vestibular sulcus from the ascending ramus up to the second premolar down to the bone.[367] Subsequently, subperiostal dissection is performed in order to expose the anterior aspect of the ramus and the posterior body of the mandible down to the inferior border. After adequate exposure has been accomplished, three bone cuts are performed by using the surgical bur, reciprocating saw, and/or piezosurgery. The first cut is made horizontally through the medial cortex of the ramus just above the level of the mandibular occlusal plane and does not exceed 2 cm in length (i.e., a Hunsuck modification). The second cut runs up laterally from the inferior border of the mandible between the first and second molar (i.e., the Dal Point modification). On the inferior border of the mandible this bone cut should extend 2 to 3 mm into the lingual cortex. This will facilitate a so-called "short lingual split," which will be beneficial when a counterclockwise rotation of the mandible is performed. The third bone cut is made in such a way that it connects the first two cuts, running just laterally to the molars. Once the same procedure is completed on the left side, the osteotomy can be completed on both sides. By using a sagittal splitter and separator, the split is initiated. Periosteal elevators or fine osteotomes can be used to complete the split. Care is taken to avoid injury to the inferior alveolar nerve during this procedure. After the split is completed, further freeing of the neurovascular bundle from the proximal segment is sometimes desirable. Pressing down on the molar-baring fragment while simultaneously pulling the incisor-baring fragment upward may be performed to stretch the periosteal tissue attached to the distal mandible. This will further facilitate the counterclockwise rotation of the mandible ultimately minimizing the risk of surgical relapse. The distal mandible is placed into occlusion through a prefabricated intermediate splint and the jaws are wired together by means of 0.4 or 0.5 mm surgical steel wire loops. After removal of possible bony interferences between the proximal and distal mandibular fragments, the proximal segment of the mandible is fixated to the distal mandible by means of straight miniplates. Some surgeons prefer fixation with bicortical minscrews. However, this may result in a less optimal surgical stability. When counterclockwise rotations or large advancements of the mandible (i.e., >10 mm) are planned, preferably two miniplates are used on each side. Instead of two miniplates, some surgeons prefer to use one miniplate combined with two or three bicortical screws, which may also be sufficient to prevent surgical relapse or a nonunion. First, the miniplates are bent to accustom the proximal and distal segment of the mandible with the condyle seated in the terminal hinge position. Subsequently, the miniplates are first fixated to the proximal segment of the mandible. Second, the proximal segment of the mandible is seated in the terminal hinge position with the application of a posterior–superior vector force (i.e., bivector seating of the condyles) whereupon the miniplates are fixed to the distal segment of the mandible. The same procedure is completed on the contralateral side whereafter the jaws are unwired. It is examined if the occlusion is even and passive into the dental splint. If not, the screw fixation is removed from the distal segment of the mandible and the process of fixation is repeated. When the proper repositioning of the mandible has been obtained, the procedure is continued with the Le Fort 1 osteotomy.

The le Fort 1 osteotomy is initiated with a circumvestibular incision from the first premolar region toward the maxillary midline.[367] Once the mucosa is incised the scaple is directed toward the dentoalveolar region down to the bone. Subsequently, a subperiosteal dissection is performed with elevators exposing the anterior maxilla on both sides up to the level of the infraorbital nerve. The dissection is then extended anteriorly just to expose the inferior aspect of the anterior nasal spine and posteriorly up to the pterygomaxillary junction. An elevator and a flat Ash are used to free the anterior nasal mucosa from the lateral nasal walls and the nasal floor. The anterior nasal spine is then released from the anterior aspect of the nasal floor by means of a fine osteotome (i.e., a subspinal approach). Using a curved freer elevator, the nasal mucosa on the lateral, medial, and inferior aspect is further freed from the underlying bone. Care is taken not to create any perforations in the nasal mucosa. With a reciprocating saw the le Fort 1 horizontal osteotomy is completed through the anterior, medial, and lateral maxillary walls on each side. When doing so the nasal mucosa and the buccal periosteal tissue should be protected with retractors. If segmentation of the maxilla is planned, interdental osteotomies should be initiated in this phase of the surgery. With a curved le Fort 1 chisel and mallet, the pterygomaxillary suture is separated on each side. Then the septum of the nose (i.e., cartilage and bone) is separated from the maxilla with a guarded chisel and mallet. With a Tessier zygomatic hook placed on the ledge of the nasal sill, force is applied to down-fracture the le Fort 1 osteotomy unit. The down-fracture may be facilitated by placing a separator at the osteotomy at the anterior maxilla near the lateral nasal wall. While down-fracturing a suction tip, periosteal elevator are used (by the assistant) to further separate and limit tearing of the nasal mucosa. Now the down-fracture is complete, further mobilization of the Le Fort 1 osteotomy unit is realized by performing a disimpaction. For this purpose Rowe nasomaxillary disimpaction forceps and Tessier hooks behind the maxillary tuberosity are used. Following the desimpaction of the maxilla, a septoplasty and reduction of the inferior turbinates may be performed when indicated. If segmentation of the maxilla is planed the interdental cuts will be completed at this stage as well as parasagittal osteotomies through the hard palate. Next the maxilla is placed into final occlusion by means of a prefabricated final splint and the jaws are wired together with 0.4 or 0.5 mm surgical steel wire-loops. With the condyles seated in the terminal hinge position, the maxillomandibular complex is rotated to achieve the vertical dimension that was planned preoperatively. For this purpose the distance between the Kirschner wire in the glabella area and the mid-maxillary incisor crown is checked by means of a calliper set in the planned vertical movement of the mid-maxillary incisor tip. If vertical shortening (impaction) of the maxilla is planned, this will require removal of bony interferences with a straight dental surgical bur and a piezoelectric surgical device. Attention should also be paid to the possible indication for bone removal at the region of the anterior nasal spine, the nasal aperture and the floor of the nose. With the condyles remaining in the terminal hinge position and with the maxilla in the preferred vertical position, appropriately sized and individually contoured L-shaped titanium miniplates are placed at the lateral nasal rim and zygomatic buttress on

each side. When the extent of horizontal advancement and vertical lengthening are judged to be significant, interpositioning a single or combination of autogenous bone grafts and alloplastic or heterogenous bone substitutes should be performed. Autogenous bone may be harvested locally (i.e., during the le Fort 1 or BSSO) or if required in significant quantities from the anterior iliac crest. Grafting should be performed at the anterior, lateral, and posterior maxillary walls. Subsequently, maxillary wound closure is initiated. This should include an alar cinch suture passing through a predrilled hole in the anterior nasal spine. This will prevent widening of the nasal base following the le Fort 1 osteotomy. Two to three additional V-Y plasty sutures in the midline are subsequently performed to enhance upper lip projection. Finally the wound is closed in a one or two layer fashion with interrupted and running sutures.

As a final procedure the (modified) genioplasty may be performed.[349,350,367] The incision is through the mucosa in the depth of the facial vestibule area of the chin. It extends from cuspid to cuspid region with the center two-thirds of the incision extending through the mentalis muscles down to the bone. Dissection with an elevator now exposes the anterior surface of the chin. The dissection should extend laterally inferiorly and remain inferior and end just posterior to the mental foramen. The midline on the chin should be marked for orientation with a straight line by means of a dental surgical bur or piezoelectric surgical device. Subsequently, a curved elevator is placed on one side just anterior to the mental foramen and the oblique osteotomy is initiated in the central portion using a reciprocating saw. The osteotomy should be continued and extend through the inferior border and the lingual cortex. The design of the osteotomy depends on the presenting chin morphology and the planned displacement of the chin but should always respect the position of the dental roots and the mental foramen on each side. In addition, when performing a modified genioplasty the design of the osteotomy should be at least 10 mm below the roots of the central incisors. This will leave enough space to perform an additional trapezoid-shaped osteotomy in the mid-symphyseal area required for advancement of the genial tubercle/genioglossus muscle complex. However, many different modifications of this so-called modified genioplasty have been described including a design where the trapezoid-shaped tubercle-baring fragment is included in the genioplasty. An osteotome is now inserted in the horizontal osteotomy line with a twisting motion in order to complete the osteotomy separation. Now the procedure is modified from a conventional genioplasty by performing the trapezoid-shaped osteotomy in the mid-symphyseal area. For this purpose two drill holes are placed with a round surgical bur approximately 5 mm bellow the dental roots about 5 mm out of the midline of the chin. These drill holes should be continued so to extend through the lingual cortex in a diverting direction. Subsequently, the drill holes on the buccal and lingual aspect of the anterior mandible are connected with a reciprocating saw with a horizontally placed osteotomy line. Now a vertical osteotomy line is placed on each side from inferior aspect of the mandible extending into the drill holes following the diverting direction of the drill hole. With an osteotome inserted with a twisting motion a trapezoid shaped bone block is now mobilized. After mobilization the lingual cortex is fixated with a toothed clamp and the medullary bone and buccal cortex are removed using a reciprocating saw. The lingual cortex of the trapezoid bone block is now advanced pulling the genial tubercle and genioglossal muscle forward and fixated on the outer symphyseal cortex. Because the lingual cortex is a bit wider than the buccal defect, it will usually lock itself on the buccal cortex. The position of the displaced lingual cortex can be further secured by means of one bicortical screw. Should there be any instability the fragment may also be fixated by means of two laterally placed miniplates with screws. Subsequently, the chin-bearing fragment of the mandible is now displaced in the planned position and fixated by means of miniplate fixation or a chin plate. Significant bony defects may now be grafted with bone grafts and/or bone substitutes whereupon the wound is closed in a two-layer fashion. The mentalis muscle on each side is generally closed with one or two interrupted sutures whereupon the mucosa is closed with a running suture.

Following completion of the modified genioplasty, attention is directed toward closure of the BSSO on each side. Before doing so the intermaxillary fixation is released and the final occlusion is checked. It is highly unlikely that repositioning of the maxilla has been inappropriate and that refixation of the maxilla is required. The gap between the proximal and distal fragment of the BSSO is now grafted on each side. For this purpose any remaining bone is grinded in a bone mill. If the amount of bone is not sufficient for grafting a demineralized bone matrix of alloplastic origin may be added including 1 to 2 cc of the patient's venous blood. After grafting the inferior border of the gap with an alloplastic bone substitute the space in between the proximal and distal segment of the mandible is grafted with the autogenous bone mix. Then the wound is closed in a two layer fashion with running sutures that should yield a watertight closure. Before removal of the nasoendotracheal tube the nasal packing and Kirschner wire in the glabella area should be removed. If a throat was inserted this should now be removed and any gastric accumulation of fluid and blood should be removed via a gastric tube. The patient is now placed in light intermaxillary fixation or class 2 traction by means of orthodontic elastics. Since most postoperative swelling will be located peripherally a postoperative tracheostomy is not required in most cases.

Complications

Major complications following MMA surgery in OSA patients are rare.[345] Individual and nonfatal cases of cardiac arrest or dysrhythmia have been described following surgery.[368] One study described a case of a life-threatening airway obstruction after extubation that required reintubation.[369] However, no cases of immediate postoperative death have been reported following this type of surgery in OSA patients.[345] One study reported a case of transient central sleep apnea following MMA surgery that resolved spontaneously 6 months postoperatively.[370] Minor complication rate has been reported to be approximately 3%.[345] Minor complications include haemorrhage or local infections that are generally cured with either antibiotics or surgical drainage. The presence of postoperative malocclusions or facial paraesthesia is not included in this minor complication rate. Facial paraesthesia is present in almost all patients following surgery but resolves in approximately 85% of patients at the 1-year follow-up.[345] Conversely, some studies indicate that half of the patients treated report a persistence of facial paraesthesia.[371] Although malocclusions may be seen in up to 44% of patients, they can generally be resolved with (prosthetic) dental treatment or equilibration of the dental occlusion.[368] However, when patients have been orthodontically prepared for MMA surgery, malocclusions are generally no long-term problem. Some studies report a trend for poor bone healing and increased foreign body reactions after MMA surgery in OSA patients.[372] Since increased age has been associated with an increased complication rate, older OSA patients appear more at risk of surgical complications.[353] In addition, subtle subjective changes in speech and swallowing have been reported following surgery in 24 and 12% of patients, respectively.[361] All of the patients in this study had undergone previous upper airway surgery (e.g., UPPP), which probably contributes to these changes. Nasal regurgitation has been reported in 10% of patients following MMA surgery that completely resolved at the 1-year follow-up.[349] All patients developing nasal regurgitation in the latter study have had a previous UPPP. Patient perceived pain following MMA surgery is generally not profound and usually less when compared with the complaints from other upper airway surgeries.[353] With 3.5 days, average hospital stay is slightly longer following MMA surgery in OSA patients when compared with "conventional" orthognathic patients.[345] Most OSA patients are able to return to full-work within 2 to 10 weeks following surgery.[353,355]

Postoperative Care

Medical surgical management of the postsurgical patient with OSA is more complicated than with conventional orthognathic patients, despite the profound postsurgical improvement in upper airway patency. Although the majority of OSA patients are stable when awake postoperatively, this may change dramatically with postoperative sedative medication or when the patient is asleep. ICU placement and the logical use of analgesic and hypertensive medication are therefore mandatory. Furthermore, the use of nasal CPAP in the postoperative period may be helpful to maintain the airway and control postoperative oedema, if tolerated by the patient. If recovery is sufficient discharge is up to the surgeon and patient but requires proper pain control and oral intake. Because younger patients tend to recover quicker, discharge is usually earlier in this group of patients.

Follow-up of patients depends on the surgeon's individual protocol and specific patient characteristics. It should be noted that postoperative oedema will usually be maximum 72 hours after surgery. The effect of swelling following MMA surgery rarely compromises the upper airway since it is located more peripherally. However, swelling can sometimes be significant which could worry patients. Frequent postoperative follow-up visits are recommended until patients are fully recovered. Since in sporadic cases patients may develop transient central sleep apnea following MMA surgery, PSG follow-up studies before a 6-month follow-up are not recommended.[370] Furthermore, it should be stressed to all overweight patients that weight loss is an important part of their pre- and posttreatment OSA management, since even modest weight change will affect the outcome.

Outcomes

OSA management following MMA surgery is generally successful in a high proportion of patients. A meta-analyses from Holty in 2010 studying 627 patients from 22 studies demonstrated that the median surgical success, defined by a postoperative AHI < 20 with a > 50% reduction in the AH, is 86%.[345] Surgical cure, defined more stringent by a postoperative AHI < 5, was observed in 43% of patients in this meta-analyses. After a mean follow-up of 5 months a statistically and clinically significant reduction in the mean AHI from 63.9 to 9.5 and improvement in the lowest nocturnal oxyhemoglobin saturation from 71.9 to 87.7% is observed.[345] Similar improvements in most other PSG outcomes like sleep efficiency and sleep stages are observed following MMA surgery. It should be noted that in about two thirds of the studies in this meta-analyses previous or concurrent upper airway surgeries like UPPP, GA and/or hyoid myotomy and suspension have been performed. Interestingly patients that have had these previous upper airway surgeries performed were less likely to achieve a surgical cure with MMA surgery.[345] Another and more recent meta-analysis by Zaghi et al only included studies evaluating the outcomes of MMA surgery excluding studies in patients who underwent adjunctive surgical

procedures at the time of surgery (e.g., tonsillectomy, UPPP or partial glossectomy).[346] They included 45 observational studies evaluating the outcomes of MMA surgery in 518 OSAS patients. Surgical success and surgical cure was observed in 85 and 39% of patients respectively. After a median follow-up of 6 months a statistically and clinically significant reduction in the mean AHI from 57.2 to 9.5 and improvement in the lowest nocturnal oxyhemoglobin saturation from 70.1 to 87.0% was observed.[346]

Although the number of studies evaluating long-term outcomes of MMA surgery is still limited, long-term results appear relatively stable over follow-up periods exceeding 2 to 5 years.[347,348,361,373,374] In addition, several studies found statistically and clinically significant improvements in blood pressure following MMA surgery in OSA patients.[355,375] Finally, evidence for the medium to long-term stability of the skeletal advancements with MMA surgery in OSAS patients has been corroborated by several cephalometric studies.[348,376,377,378]

When evaluating subjective outcomes following MMA surgery for OSA, most patients report improvements in snoring, witnessed apneas and EDS, morning headaches, memory loss, and impaired concentration.[345] The percentage of patients with elevated ESS values (i.e., >10) has been reported to decrease from 72 to 10%.[379] Also the meta-analyses by Holty and Zaghi showed significant reductions in ESS values from 13.2 to 5.1 and from 13.5 to 3.2, respectively.[345,346] Significant improvements in all domains of the FOSQ have also been reported (summary score presurgically 14.4 vs. postsurgically 18.9).[361] Another study reported a 72% absolute reduction in subjective symptoms of depression or irritability following MMA surgery.[355] Most patients will be able to discontinue their CPAP following MMA surgery with patients overall reporting that treatment was worthwhile and recommendable to others.[379]

As with many surgical interventions for OSA, randomized trials comparing MMA surgery with other interventions are scarce. There are however several cohort studies comparing the outcomes of MMA surgery with UPPP and CPAP, respectively.[352,355,380,381,382] When MMA surgery (n = 37) is compared with the results of a UPPP (n = 34), the mean change in AHI is significantly larger with MMA surgery (mean AHI reduction 40.5 vs. 19.4).[380] This study could also not demonstrate a favorable effect of a UPPP preceding MMA surgery on the final outcome.[380] When the AHI with CPAP therapy is compared with the AHI following MMA surgery, five cohort studies do not demonstrate significant differences between these two interventions.[345] To date, only one study performed a prospective RCT that compared the therapeutic efficacy of MMA surgery with CPAP in 50 patients with severe OSAS (mean AHI: 56.8).[383] Although both CPAP and MMA surgery showed profound and significant improvements in AHI and ESS values after a 1-year treatment period, the degree of improvement was not clinical or statistical significantly different between these interventions. The AHI reduced with CPAP from 50.3 to 6.3 whereas with MMA surgery from 56.8 to 8.1, thereby suggesting equivalence of these treatments.

The effects of MMA surgery on the upper airway and surrounding structures have been extensively studied.[384] Two-dimensional cephalometric studies generally show a significant increase in velo-, oro-, and hypopharyngeal airway space following MMA surgery[359] (▶ Fig. 8.89). Furthermore, surgery may result in an increase in intermaxillary space, a decreased tongue proportion and a more superior and anterior position of the hyoid bone.[359,384] These improvements in upper airway dimensions are confirmed by three-dimensional CT studies showing enlargement of the entire upper airway calibre following MMA surgery[384,385] (▶ Fig. 8.90). The increase in airway volume appears to be most pronounced in the velopharynx followed by the oropharynx.[385] In addition, CT studies of the upper airway have also observed profound improvements in the lateral dimension and a considerable reduction of the upper airway length following surgery.[384,385] The latter phenomenon is suggested to

contribute structurally to a decreased airway collapsibility following MMA surgery.[386] Many of the above mentioned changes in upper airway dimensions and skeletal structures have been correlated with OSA improvements. However, at present there is unfortunately insufficient data to support a relation between OSA improvements like AHI values and changes in the upper airway and its surrounding bony structures.[384]

Key Points

MMA surgery plays an important role in the correction of OSA that is refractive to noninvasive therapies. Since large advancements of the maxillomandibular complex are required in medically compromised patients, MMA surgery in OSA patients is generally more complex than "conventional" orthognathic surgery. With proper precautions it is however a safe and highly effective treatment modality for OSA. MMA surgery is probably the most effective surgical intervention in patients who are skeletally compromised (e.g., severe malocclusions, retrognathia, or bimaxillary retrusion). These patients, especially when they are relatively young, should therefore be informed of MMA surgery as primary surgical treatment modality.

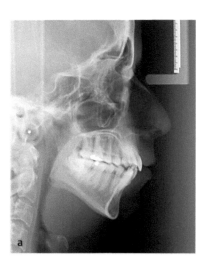
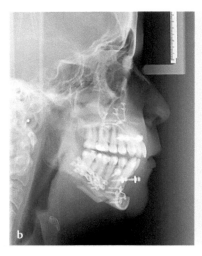

Fig. 8.89 Two-dimensional airway changes following maxillomandibular advancement surgery. A preoperative (**a**) and postoperative (**b**) lateral cephalometric radiograph indicating the sagittal changes in upper airway space following maxillomandibular advancement surgery combined with a modified genioplasty and cervicomental liposuction in a severe obstructive sleep apnea patient. (Used with permission from Doff MH, Jansma J, Schepers RH, Hoekema A. Maxillomandibular advancement surgery as alternative to continuous positive airway pressure in morbidly severe obstructive sleep apnea: a case report. Cranio 2013;31:246–251.)

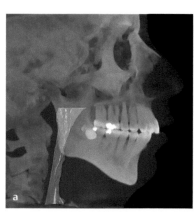
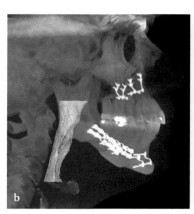

Fig. 8.90 Three-dimensional airway changes following maxillomandibular advancement surgery. A preoperative (**a**) and postoperative (**b**) conebeam computed tomography reconstruction of the upper airway indicating the three-dimensional changes in upper airway space, following maxillomandibular advancement surgery combined with a modified genioplasty and cervicomental liposuction in a severe obstructive sleep apnea patient.

8.3.2 Distraction Osteogenesis Maxillary Expansion

Stanley Yung-Chuan Liu, Christian Guilleminault, and Audrey Jung-Sun Yoon

Definition

The concept of distraction osteogenesis maxillary expansion (DOME) originated from the need to expand high-arched and narrow maxilla in adult patients with OSA.[387] There is strong evidence from pediatric studies that show resolution of OSA with maxillary expansion using orthodontic expanders, especially for treating persistent disease after tonsillectomy and adenoidectomy.[388,377,390] While there were no reliable maxillary skeletal expansion procedures for adults, the narrow maxilla is also an anatomic risk factor for adult OSA. A likely mechanism for improved sleep-disordered breathing from maxillary expansion includes an increase of the nasal floor, decrease in nasal resistance, and promotion of an anterior and superior tongue position.[391,392,393,394]

Christian Guilleminault of Stanford University had observed for years that adult OSA patients with the same phenotype (high-arch, narrow palate) also needed maxillary expansion. In these patients with skeletal hypoplasia, advancements are commonly performed, and while that increases intraoral volume for the soft tissue, there is persistent high nasal resistance and flow limitation.

Craniomaxillofacial surgeons conventionally perform surgically assisted rapid palatal expansion (SARPE) for adult skeletal transverse hypoplasia, which combines Lefort I level osteotomies, pterygoid disjunction, and orthodontic tooth-anchored expander.[395] Limitations of the SARPE procedure include: (1) conventional tooth-anchored expanders exert lateralizing forces on the dentition and expansion forces concentrate more on the dentoalveolar segments, but not on the nasal floor or the roof of palate,[396] and (2) the jaw movement with the highest relapse rate. Alternatively, the upper jaw can be split into multiple segments to gain width. Yet, multipiece LeFort osteotomies move the dentoalveolar segments, but frequently leaves behind a separate bone segment that is free floating and attached to the palatal soft tissue. These movements focus on moving teeth for correction of malocclusion, but do not address key areas for sleep-disordered breathing in adults.

The need was clear. A method was needed to expand the upper jaw in adults the same way that pediatric OSA patients are expanded, that is (1) predictable, (2) fast, (3) stable, and (4) addresses the nasal cavity and intraoral volume specifically for sleep-disordered breathing. Anecdotally, the lead surgeon describes the process to patients that the goal is to change a high-arch palate to a *dome*-shaped palate. Hence, DOME was coined in

2014 by Christian Guilleminault (sleep medicine), Audrey Yoon (orthodontics), and Stanley Liu (sleep surgery) at Stanford University. Since then, DOME has become an integral part of the revised Stanford sleep surgery protocol.

Indications, Contraindications, and Patient Selection

DOME is generally recommended for three phenotypes of adult with OSA:

1. OSA patient who presents with absolute skeletal transverse hypoplasia presenting with crossbite.
2. Mild OSA or upper airway resistance syndrome (UARS) patients who do not have malocclusion, but complain of persistent nasal obstruction in the setting of narrow, high-arch palate, and who either have underwent previous nasal surgery, or do not present with significant septal deviation or inferior turbinate hypertrophy.
3. Moderate to severe OSA patients as phase I, preceding other operations including palatal surgery (e.g., UPPP, MMA, or upper airway stimulation).

Relative contraindications include patients with:

1. Periodontal disease.
2. Inability or unwillingness to undergo perioperative orthodontic care.
3. Difficulty turning the expander device once daily for approximately 1 month.

Diagnostic Workup

We strongly encourage the patient to have undergone an attended PSG, particularly to assess for flow limitation in the setting of UARS. Maxillofacial CT is necessary for visualization of relevant surgical landmarks (thickness of premaxilla, position of nasopalatine nerve, and distance between central incisors roots). For the orthodontist, the thickness of the maxilla may dictate the lengths of implants used on the expander. Pre- and posttreatment photos are routine in orthodontic offices. It is important to note that DOME does not change one's facial appearance significantly upon completion of treatment. Minor changes may be seen with improved support of the premaxilla.

Specific Risks, Patient Information, and Consent

Patients must be informed about the goals of treatment. From our clinical outcomes data, the most significant and reproducible outcome is decrease in subjective nasal obstruction, measured by the nasal obstruction symptom evaluation (NOSE) scale.[397] For patients with severe OSA, surgical success is approximately 70%, and these patients will continue to receive further interventions including palatopharyngoplasty, upper airway stimulation, and MMA. For UARS, the decrease in AHI is significant, but surgical success cannot be defined by the Sher's criteria because pretreatment AHI is usually less than 10 events per hour.

Surgical risks include loss of vitality to a central incisor, asymmetric maxillary expansion, inadequate expansion, periodontal recession, palatal fistula, and persistent paresthesia of the vestibular incision.

Pain is minimal after DOME. Most patients are managed with over-the-counter NSAIDs. Some require narcotic medication for the first few days postoperatively.

Anesthesia and Positioning

The procedure usually takes less than 45 minutes from skin to skin. Oral intubation with total intravenous anesthesia is preferred to decrease postoperative nausea and vomiting. An oral flexible and reinforced tube taped to one side of the commissure is the least intrusive position. The patient is turned 180 degrees away from the anesthesia cart. Hypotensive anesthesia is not required as only Lefort 1 level osteotomies are made without pterygoid disjunction. Preemptive analgesia is performed with bilateral V2 level blocks at the infraorbital nerve region.

Equipment

A standard head and neck or maxillofacial set including bovie electrocautery, nine periosteal elevator, toe-out retractor, curved freer elevator, reciprocating saw, Piezo-electric saw (optional), several straight osteotomes, and 3–0 chromic sutures.

Procedural Steps

Prior to surgery, the collaborating orthodontist has designed and sometimes placed the expander with the transpalatal implants. It is crucial that the implants are placed as medially as possible, straddling the mid-palatal suture. Additional implants can be placed against the sides of the alveolus bilaterally near the molar region.

Vestibular approach to the maxilla is performed with bovie electrocautery set to 32. A curvilinear incision 1 cm above the mucogingival junction is made with broader posterior pedicles. Attention is taken not to violate the Stenson's ducts bilaterally. Subperiosteal dissection is made toward the piriform rim medially, and maxillary buttress laterally. The infraorbital nerve foramen is the superior extent of dissection. Le Fort level 1 osteotomies are created with the reciprocating saw, medially to the piriform rim and laterally to the maxillary buttress.

The primordial groove of the mid-palatal suture is seen inferior to the anterior nasal spine, and between the apices of the maxillary central incisors. Piezoelectric saw, which does not cut the mucosa of the palate across the maxillary alveolus, is used to deepen the groove. Osteotomes are used in sequential fashion to wedge open the mid-palatal suture from the groove. A diastema between the central incisors is seen immediately as the suture opens. The expander is then turned to ensure symmetric and easy separation of the maxilla bilaterally, until a 2 mm separation is created (see Video 8.8).

Closure of the vestibular wound is performed by 3–0 chromic sutures.

Complications

Major complications such as nonunion, malunion, oronasal fistula, and skeletal, nasal, sinus, or odontogenic infections have not been reported with DOME. Minor asymmetric maxillary expansion has occurred, but within range of orthodontic correction. Resolution of V_2 paresthesia in the anterior maxilla takes place ranging from 1 to 6 months. Maxillary central incisors occasionally show signs of decreased perfusion. Loss of central incisor vitality requiring root canal treatment (but no loss of dentition) is less than 5%. Palatal fistula has been seen in 2% of the patients. Most have self-resolved with completion of distraction and healing by secondary intention. Rare is the occasion that a bone graft and repair of the fistula is required.

Postoperative Care

Depending on the severity of OSA, patients can either be discharged on the day of surgery, or monitored overnight. Pain control with a combination of oral NSAID and narcotic medication is adequate. Regular diet is resumed within a week. Limited epistaxis and nasal congestion are expected from the Le Fort I osteotomies in the early postoperative period.

Patients turn the expander daily, resulting in an expansion of 0.25 mm per day. For most patients, 7 to 12 mm of expansion at the nasal floor is achieved within 4 to 6 weeks. Orthodontic brackets are then placed to close the diastema, while the skeletal expander is left in place to prevent relapse during the bony consolidation period. The consolidation period is between cessation of traction forces and removal of distractor. Typically, the consolidation phase is 3 months[398,399,400] for pediatric craniofacial distraction, but we recommend a consolidation period of 6 to 8 months stability in adults. The distractor does not interfere with tooth movement and allows the expander to remain in place while the orthodontist restores proper occlusion. Average orthodontic treatment required is 12 to 18 months. Following the active orthodontic treatment, the expansion needs to be maintained passively by a removable retainer. ▸Fig. 8.91 illustrates pre-DOME, post-DOME and final postorthodontic treatment progress.

Outcomes

At Stanford, 72 patients (25 women) underwent DOME since January of 2015. The mean age is 28.5 ± 9. Perioperative change in BMI is not significant. Mean preoperative ESS score was 11.6 ± 5. The mean postoperative ESS was 8 ± 4. The preoperative NOSE score was 11.6 ± 5.3,

and postoperative NOSE score was 4.4 ± 4.3. Mean AHI decreased from 22.4 ± 22 to 11.3 ± 8. This decrease achieves greater surgical success if the patients with UARS are excluded (as they start with low AHI and creates a bimodal distribution in the outcomes data). For moderate to severe patients, the mean decrease in AHI is from 60 ± 20 to 19 ± 7. The mean decrease in the oxygen desaturation index (ODI) is from 14 ± 2 to 6.1 ± 6.2. For the moderate to severe group, the decrease is from 48 ± 14 to 10 ± 3. The mean expansion of the nasal floor at the internal nasal valve is from 22.7 ± 4 to 28.2 ± 5 mm.

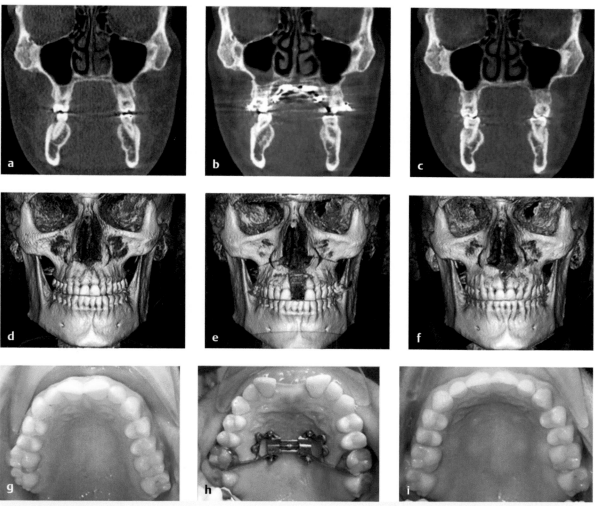

Fig. 8.91 A 31-year-old male with upper airway resistant syndrome who presents with normal occlusion, narrow nasal floor, and high arched palate. Coronal view at palatal cusps of the first molar level: pre-DOME (distraction osteogenesis maxillary expansion) (**a**), post-DOME (**b**) and postorthodontic treatment (**c**) shows that the nasal floor was expanded and nasal cavity become more patent after expansion. Three-dimensional surface rendering from CBCT: pre-DOME (**d**), post-DOME (**e**) and final postorthodontic treatment (**f**) show DOME does not change mid-facial profile with 10 mm nasal floor expansion. Occlusal view: pre-DOME (**g**), post-DOME (**h**) and final postorthodontic treatment (**i**) show that 14 mm of diastema expanded (**h**) and spaces closed with orthodontic treatment with palatal roof expansion maintained.

8.4 Multilevel Surgery

Nico de Vries, Peter van Maanen, and Thomas Verse

8.4.1 Definition

Multilevel surgery is defined as any combination of invasive surgical procedures of different collapsible segments of the upper airway. These procedures are restricted to the same four levels: Velum (soft palate and uvula), Oropharynx (including tonsils), base of Tongue and Epiglottis, as designated in DISE VOTE classification. In this perspective, multilevel surgery is a logical and consequent extension and translation of the sites, severity and direction of the obstruction(s) as assessed by DISE, while the disease severity of the patient is taken into account at the same time. While in multilevel surgery almost always at least one palatal and one base of tongue procedure are included, the rare combination of a tonsillar and epiglottis procedure would fall within the definition as well.

This definition excludes however any combination of *nasal surgery* with only palatal or only base of tongue interventions, and such combinations will not be discussed in this chapter. Simultaneous *intralaryngeal surgery* as part of "multilevel surgery" is excluded as well. In our institutions, both such combinations are hardly ever indicated and are performed only in extremely rare occasions.

We regard a combination of minimally invasive procedures (e.g., simultaneous radiofrequency of the palate and base of tongue) or any kind of invasive palatal surgery (e.g., UPPP/ZPP, ESP) combined with only radiofrequency of the base of tongue not as a "multilevel surgery" because minimally invasive surgeries are designed to treat simple snoring and mild OSA only. We propose to use the term minimally invasive multilevel surgery for these surgeries, as there are some articles about minimally invasive multilevel surgeries (refer to ▶Table 8.23 for details).

MMA and hypoglossal nerve stimulation, in our definition, are also not regarded as multilevel surgeries. In contrast, we regard TORS (transoral robotic resection of the base of tongue) as a tongue base procedure. Thus, combinations of TORS with invasive palatal surgery will be regarded as multilevel surgeries.

We are aware that different levels of airway obstruction could be treated step-wise as well. Our philosophy of multilevel surgery relies on three aspects: (1) if the patient shows moderate to severe complaints, (2) if the patient's disease severity is confirmed by PSG, and (3) if the patient's subsequent DISE assesses multilevel obstruction, a logical approach dictates simultaneous intervention of the levels of obstruction as assessed by DISE. We are convinced that our philosophy helps to avoid repeated surgery and related side effects and morbidity.

We would like to stress that PSG and DISE findings should be in agreement and make sense—in case of only mild disease, one should expect only limited obstruction during DISE (e.g., more often multilevel than unilevel obstruction, more often partial than total obstruction, more often anteroposterior [AP] than concentric collapse, no complete concentric collapse on palatal level). In case of moderate and in particular severe OSA, more serious forms of obstruction should be expected—more often multilevel than one level only, more often total than partial, more often concentric than AP, etc.

In case of unexplained discrepancies between mild OSA complaints and subsequent PSG recording and significant DISE findings, one should be alert, and oversedation during DISE should be ruled out. We do not advocate the use of multilevel surgery in mild OSA in combination with unexpected and unexplained quite severe DISE findings.

Evolutionary speaking, multilevel surgery in one tempo is one step further than "staged surgery." We do not see any point in performing surgery at only one level at a time, in case DISE shows obstruction at more levels. Multilevel surgery has proven to be safe, if the patients are selected carefully and monitored thoroughly in the perioperative period. For perioperative monitoring please refer to Chapter 10.

As outlined in previous chapters, many invasive palatal and base of tongue procedures are being explored and can be combined during multilevel surgery. When VOTE findings are consequently being followed, any combination of the procedures mentioned below might fit in a surgical treatment planning in the framework of invasive multilevel surgery:

VOTE (V): Palatal interventions include UPPP, ZPP, UPF techniques, ESP, barbed wire sphincter pharyngoplasty (BSP), palatal advancement, and other modifications of UPPP.

VOTE (O): In case of obstruction of the tonsils only, tonsillectomy or tonsillotomy can be indicated. In most palatal procedures the tonsils are removed as well. In the rare case of tonsil size 3 of 4 (kissing tonsils) without collapse at palatal level, isolated total removal or partial removal of the tonsils can be indicated.

VOTE (T): In case of base of tongue obstruction, interventions include RFTs (usually reserved for partial obstruction at base of tongue level), hyoidthyroidpexia (we almost always then perform radiofrequency of the base of tongue at the same time), hyoid suspension (surgical or with wires), GA, tongue stiffening procedures, LT, midline glossectomy (independent of the technique and surgical instruments used), tongue implants and others.

VOTE (E): In case of epiglottis collapse partial removal of the epiglottis or epiglottopexia can be considered.

This approach has other consequences as well—in case of severe OSA DISE shows only one level of total obstruction (e.g., complete concentric palatal collapse), we would *not* embark on multilevel surgery, but address the palate only first.

In multilevel surgery any combination, that combines at least one velum or oropharynx surgery with at least one tongue base or epiglottis surgery, is possible (see ▶ Table 8.24). This great variety of combinations explains to a large extent the wide variation of success rates of multilevel surgery as reported in the literature. Other reasons for the large variation in success rates reported so far are differences in patient selection. In many earlier studies, DISE was not used as a selection tool. Apart from this, in some studies patients with high BMIs were included while not in others, and some of the older surgical techniques have now been replaced by more modern modifications.

▶ Table 8.23 Results of minimally invasive multilevel surgery

Author	N	Surgeries	Device	Follow-up (mos)	AHI (pre)	AHI (post)	Success	ESS (pre)	ESS (post)	EBM
Fischer et al[401]	15	RFT SP, TB, Tons	Somnus	4.8	32.6	22.0	20.0	11.1	8.2	4
Woodson et al[402]	26	RFT SP, TB	Somnus	1.0	21.3	16.8	no data	11.9	9.8	2b
Stuck et al[403]	18	RFT SP, TB	Somnus	2	25.3	16.7	33.3	9.3	6.1	4
Steward[404]	22	RFT SP, TB	Somnus	2.5	31.0	18.8	59.0	11.4	7.0	3b
Friedman et al[405]	122	Pillars, RFT TB	Somnus	12.2	23.2	14.5	47.5	9.7	6.9	4
Ceylan et al[406]	26	RFT Nose, SP, TB	Somnus	12.0	29.6	16.1	53.8	10.8	8.2	3b
Bäck et al[407]	13	RFT SP, TB	Celon	4.0	31.0	33.0	23.1	7.0	4.0	4
Neruntarat[265]	72	RFT SP, TB	Sutter	3.0	35.6	12.5	66.7	14.2	7.9	4
		RFT SP, TB	Sutter	14.2	35.6	16.8	55.6	14.2	8.2	4
All	314			6.5	19.8	13.1	33.8	7.8	5.6	B

Abbreviations: ESS, Epworth sleepiness scale; RFT, (interstitial) radiofrequency treatment; SP: soft palate; TB: tongue base.
Notes: EBM = level of evidence-based medicine; mos = months; Pillars = soft palate implants; Tons = tonsils.

▶ Table 8.24 Four levels of the collapsible segment of the upper airway

VOTE	Velum	Oropharynx	Tongue base	Epiglottis
	UPPP	Tonsillectomy	Radiofrequency	Partial epiglottectomy
	modifications of UPPP	Tonsillotomy	Hyoid suspension type 1 (to the mandible)	Epiglottopexy
	Palatal advancement		Hyoid suspension type 2 (to the thyroid cartilage)	
			Genioglossal advancement	
			Lingual tonsillectomy	
			Midline glossectomy	
			Tongue implants	

Abbreviation: UPPP, uvulopalatopharyngoplasty.
Note: In multilevel surgery, any combination of the procedures of the four levels of the collapsible segment of the upper airway (Velum, Oropharynx, base of Tongue and Epiglottis) is possible.

8.4.2 Indications, Contraindications, and Patient Selection

For the indications, techniques, success rates, and complications of the various individual procedures the reader is referred to the chapters where these procedures are described. Multilevel surgery is a combined procedure that is usually applied in moderate to severe OSA, with CPAP failure or upfront refusal to even trying it.

In severe OSAS, the likelihood that obstruction is present on both the palatine-oropharyngeal level as well as on the retrolingual level is high. In fact, obstruction at both levels is usually responsible for the high AHI. This is confirmed by DISE in large series of patients with OSAS, where retropalatinal/oropharyngeal and retrolingual obstructions are found in a large percentage of cases. For more information refer to Section 3.4.2.

An older therapeutic dilemma is whether patients should undergo intervention (and what form of surgery) at both levels staged (and in which sequence) or simultaneously. To our opinion, multilevel surgery in the case of multilevel obstruction performed in a staged sequence will lead to an unnecessary prolonged path to success. Eliminating obstruction at one level while leaving the other obstruction untreated makes no sense, especially in patients suffering from moderate to severe OSA. We have since long abandoned this kind of staged surgery and embarked on multilevel surgery in case DISE reveals multilevel collapse directly. Contrariwise, if DISE only shows one level of obstruction, we prefer to address this first even in severe OSA.

In case of mild OSA, it depends on the DISE findings. We often perform an invasive technique on the main obstruction level and add a minimally invasive procedure to the minor obstruction level (maybe UPPP plus tonsillectomy combined with an RFT of the base of tongue in patients with mainly oropharyngeal collapse during DISE).

Another grey area is the upper limit of the AHI. In our experience, the results of multilevel surgery are often not good in patients with AHIs above 55 to 60, and as a rule we often do not embark on multilevel surgery in such cases, but rather advise more aggressive surgeries such as MMA or TORS upfront. Again, there may be exceptions. The real difficulty lies where to try multilevel surgery first, and keep MMA or TORS in reserve, or do not try multilevel surgery first and opt for MMA directly.

Since nobody knows where the AHI cut-off point should be put, and since the consequences are so substantial, shared decision-making, with the patient and his/her relatives, is crucial. These are individual choices. Patients should be informed how the change of success of multilevel surgery in his/her specific circumstances is estimated (e.g., in the given situation at around 60%) and this should be weighted to the in general higher success rate of MMA (85%), in combination with its often significantly higher morbidity. Some patients will opt for multilevel surgery first with MMA in reserve, while others prefer to go for the higher success rates of MMA directly and accept its often more serious consequences. Here, more research is needed. In sum, multilevel surgery can be considered in patients with an AHI[32] of 15 to 60 and BMI of less than 32.

A relative contraindication is professional speakers and singers.

8.4.3 Diagnostic Workup

PSG or related measures to assess the severity of OSA is necessary, followed by DISE to gather information of the level(s) of obstruction. Multilevel surgery is mostly considered in patients with a BMI <32 kg/m², but there might be exceptions where even in case of higher BMIs multilevel surgery might be indicated.

For any further information, refer to the specific chapters describing the isolated procedures.

8.4.4 Specific Risks, Patient Information, and Consent

In our experience, when discussing consent, before even starting to discuss the potential complications individually, the best beginning is to give an honest and reasonable estimation of the chance of success in the patient's unique individual situation, based on the surgeons experience with the selected techniques, and taking factors such as disease severity, AHI, BMI, and DISE findings into account. If the chance of success is regarded too low to even consider the procedure, it is not useful to discuss any potential complications in the first place.

The expected treatment outcome is much more relevant (e.g., "scenario 1 estimates a 65% of success rate") to start with, than detailed information of the chance of a bleeding ("2–4% chance").

Only after the patient and relatives have been informed about the success rates and when they are willing to take the risk in their specific situation, the next step is to discuss the expected and potential side effects and complications. The best way is to systemically address the different components of the procedures and discuss the respective complications per procedure individually.

For the indications, techniques, success rates, and complications of the various procedures the reader is referred to the chapters where these procedures are individually described. This great variety of possible combinations explains to a large extent the wide variation of success rates and complications of multilevel surgery as reported in the literature. Patients should be informed accordingly.

Definitely, all potential candidates for surgical treatments need to be informed about all the conservative alternatives. In doubt, appliances can be given a try, while surgery is not reversible. We mostly perform multilevel surgery in moderate to severe disease, and CPAP failure. In well-selected patients who refuse CPAP upfront, multilevel surgery might be applied as a first-line treatment.

8.4.5 Anesthesia and Positioning

The different components of the specific form of multilevel surgery dictate the anesthesia, tube placement, and positioning. It might be needed to reposition the tube one or two times.

As an example, a common combination is RFT of the tongue, followed by a palatal procedure and hyoidthyroidpexia. In this situation, we start with the RFT of the tongue base, and the tube is first placed in the corner of the mouth. For the subsequent palatal procedure the tube is repositioned to the midline, still in a downward direction. After the palatal procedure, a second repositioning of the tube is needed in an upward direction for the hyoidthyroidpexia. To perform the neck procedure, the head ideally should be in slight hyperextension (pillow under shoulders) with an armed tube diverted upward.

8.4.6 Equipment

The different components of the multilevel surgery dictate which equipment is needed. The reader is referred to the individual chapters.

8.4.7 Operative Technique/Steps

Please refer to the individual chapters that describe the single surgical techniques.

Risks, Tips, and Tricks

- Change positioning of the patient for each surgical step.
- Change tube placement for each surgical step.
- As combined surgeries may predispose for airway obstruction after extubation, monitor the patients carefully in the perioperative period (refer to Chapter 10).
- Antibiotic prophylaxis seems helpful to avoid complications.
- Discuss the case carefully with your anesthesiologist.
- Corticosteroids may be useful.

8.4.8 Complications

For the complications of the various procedures the reader is referred to the chapters where these procedures are individually described. In multilevel surgery all complications are possible that may occur in the isolated procedures of which the multilevel procedure is composed.

It is even likely that the combination of procedures might induce complications that rarely occur in isolated procedures. As an example, after multilevel surgery—composed of UPPP, radiofrequency of the tongue and hyoidthyroidpexia—we have encountered a few cases of long-term swallowing disturbances that we have not seen with the isolated procedures.

The most feared direct postoperative complication is a bleeding either in the mouth, pharynx, or neck. This should be considered an absolute emergency. Reintubation might be extremely difficult, or impossible. Reopening of the neck to evacuate the blood and/or hematoma, before starting new general anesthesia, or even tracheostomy, should be considered.

8.4.9 Postoperative Care

As in any other sleep apnea surgery the severity of OSA has a significant impact on postoperative care and monitoring. This is why sleep apnea patients undergoing surgery under general anaesthesia or under sedation are at an increased risk for perioperative complications.[106,107,108]

This perioperative risk is particularly increased if OSA is treated surgically, as postoperative bleeding and swellings within the pharynx need to be taken into account. According to a recent review, postoperative complications are rare and occur within the first 4 hours after extubation.[109] This result is in accordance with our own experience. As a result, in Hamburg, we keep our sleep apnea patients in the recovery room for 4 hours after extubation. If there are no complications, the patients are regarded to be safe and will be discharged to the regular ward. In case of complications, the patients are monitored overnight.[324] We always act in agreement with the executive anesthesiologist, who is responsible for the recovery room.

As stated earlier, management of postoperative pain is crucial after soft palate surgery. A basic treatment with ibuprofen (four times 400–600 mg) in addition with metamizole (four times 0.5–1 g) works fine in adults. However, there are huge interindividual differences that require individual adaptations. If the basic treatment is not sufficient in time add opioids might be added (e.g., three times 10 mg oxycodone). Please refer to Section 10.2 for further information about the postoperative care and medication.

Antibiotics for the perioperative period and perioperative antibiotic prophylaxis are routinely necessary in multilevel surgery patients. The use of corticosteroids depends on the individual case.

Patients are discharged as soon as pain treatment is sufficient and patients returned to normal diet (approximately 48–96 hours postoperatively).

8.4.10 Outcomes

As stated earlier, data about multilevel surgery are very difficult to compare due to different patient selection criteria and different surgical components. However, ▶Table 8.25 presents all the pre- and postoperative PSG data on AHI. So far, it is not possible to detect the best combination of surgical techniques. Every surgeon needs to decide for himself or herself which combination works best in their hands.

▶ **Table 8.25** Results of multilevel surgery

Author	N	Soft palate	Hypopharynx	Follow-up (mos)	AHI (pre)	AHI (post)	Success (%)	ESS (pre)	ESS (post)	EBM
Riley et al[408]	55	UPPP	GA, HS	3.0	58	23.2	67.3	no data	no data	4
Djupesland et al[409]	19	UPPP	GP	8.7	54.0	31.0	31.6	no data	no data	4
Riley et al[272]	223	UPPP	GA, HS	9.0	48.3	9.5	60.1	no data	no data	4
Riley et al[260]	12	UPPP	GA	3.0	71.2	46.7	0.0	no data	no data	4
Johnson and Chinn[410]	9	UPPP	GA	39.0	58.7	14.5	77.8	no data	no data	4
Ramirez and Loube[411]	12	UPPP	GA, HS	6.0	49.0	23.0	41.7	no data	no data	4
Utley et al[412]	14	UPPP	GA, HS	4.0	46.6	23.3	57.0	no data	no data	4
Elasfour et al[413]	18	UPPP	MLG	3–21	65.0	29.2	44.4	no data	no data	3b
Lee et al[414]	35	UPPP	GA	4–6	55.2	21.7	66.7	no data	no data	4
Bettega et al[353]	44	UPPP	GA, HS	6.0	45.2	42.8	22.7	no data	no data	4
Hsu and Brett[415]	13	UPPP	GA, HS	12.6	52.8	15.6	76.9	18.2	6.4	4
Hendler et al[354]	33	UPPP	GA	6.0	60.2	28.8	45.5	no data	no data	4
Terris et al[416]	19	UPPP	TBS	3	33.2	17.9	67	no data	no data	4
Vilaseca et al[274]	20	UPPP	GA, HS	6.0	60.5	44.6	35.0	12.0	7.9	4
Miller et al[417]	15	UPPP	TBS	3.8	38.7	21.0	20.0	no data	no data	4
Neruntarat[418]	31	Flap	GA, HS	8.0	48.2	14.5	71.0	14.9	8.2	4
Neruntarat[265]	32	Flap	HS	8.1	44.5	15.2	78.0	14.1	8.2	4
Neruntarat[419]	46	Flap	GA, HS	6.0	47.9	14.2	78.0	no data	no data	4
		Flap	GA, HS	39.4	47.9	18.6	65.2	no data	no data	4
Sorrenti et al[420]	15	UPPP	TBS	4.0	44.5	24.2	40.0	11.2	6.6	4
Sorrenti et al[421]	8	UPPP	oTBR	3.0	55.1	9.7	87.5	14.3	5.3	4
Miller et al[422]	24	UPPP	GA	4.7	52.9	15.9	66.7	no data	no data	4
Dattilo and Drooger[423]	37	UPPP	GA, HS	1.5	38.7	16.2	70.3	10.0	7.5	4
Hörmann et al[424]	66	UPPP/Flap	RFT, HS	no data	38.9	19.3	57.6	9.6	6.4	4
Li et al[425]	6	EUPF	MLG	6.0	50.7	14.3	83.3	no data	no data	4
	6	EUPF	LLT	6.0	56.2	62.8	0.0	no data	no data	4
Verse et al[426]	45	Flap	RFT, HS	4.7	38.3	20.6	51.1	10.4	7.1	4
Omur et al[427]	22	UPPP	TBS	6.0	47.5	17.3	81.8	13.9	5.4	4
Hsieh et al[428]	6	EUPF	MLG	6.0	50.7	11.6	no data	no data	no data	4
Bowden et al[266]	29	UPPP	HS	12.0	36.5	37.6	17.2	13.8	10.9	4
Liu et al[429]	44	UPPP	GA	3.0	62.0	29.6	52.3	14.3	6.3	4
Baisch et al[273]	67	Flap	RFT, HS	1.0	38.3	18.9	59.7	9.7	6.6	3b
Verse et al[262]	45	Flap	RFT, HS	4.3	38.9	20.7	51.1	9.4	7.2	3b
Jakobowitz[430]	37	UPPP	RFT, HS, GA	3.0	46.5	14.9	70.3	12.1	6.7	4
Vicente et al[431]	55	UPPP	TBS	36.0	52.8	14.1	78.0	12.2	8.2	4
Sorrenti et al[238]	10	UPPP	oTBR +	14.6	54.7	9.4	100.0	14.3	5.3	4
Yin et al[432]	18	UPPP	GA, HS	6.0	63.8	21.4	67.0	no data	no data	4
Richard et al[269]	22	UPPP	RFT, HS, GA	no data	48.7	28.8	45.5	8.6	3.6	4

▶ Table 8.25 (*Continued*)

Author	N	Soft palate	Hypopharynx	Follow-up (mos)	AHI (pre)	AHI (post)	Success (%)	ESS (pre)	ESS (post)	EBM
Sun et al[433]	31	UPPP	GA, HS	6	65.9	28.6	no data	17.1	8.9	4
Benazzo et al[268]	109	UPPP	HS	6	37.0	18.7	61.5	10.5	7.2	4
Fernández-Julián et al[434]	28	UPPP	TBS	3	33.1	15.1	57.1	13.5	9.1	2b
Kezirian et al[435]	30	UPPP	GA, HS	3	44.9	27.8	43.0	no data	no data	2b
Babademez et al[436]	15	EUPF	TBR (Coblation)	3	22.7	10.4	no data	7.6	3.2	2b
	15	EUPF	harmonic scalpel	3	29.9	11.0	no data	8.4	4.8	2b
Yi et al[166]	26	UPPP	GA, HS	6	65.6	30.1	46.0	13.5	6.9	4
Sezen et al[437]	12	Flap	TBS	12	28.8	15.3	50.0	14.8	7.6	4
Emara et al[277]	23	UPPP	GA	6	40.7	15.4	86.9	14.2	8.3	4
van Maanen et al[438]	94	UPPP/ZPP	HS	no data	38.4	26.5	no data	no data	no data	4
Hou et al[439]	34	UPPP	MLG	60	56	17.0	70.6	no data	no data	4
Tunçel et al[440]	35	lat PP/ZPP	TBS	6	14.6	6.2	no data	no data	no data	3b
Friedman et al[441]	27	ZPP	TORS MLG	6	54.6	18.6	66.7	14.4	5.4	3b
Lee et al[226]	20	UPPP	TORS	8	55.6	24.1	45	13.4	5.9	4
Berg et al[442]	30	UPPP	TBS, HS	4	43.4	23.9	63.3	no data	no data	4
Li et al[443]	45	UPPP	TBS	6	39.4	8.9	51.1	12.9	3.4	3b
Cillo et al[444]	13	UPPP	GA, HS	18	28.3	12.1	no data	15.2	6.3	4
Gunawardena et al[445]	27	UPPP, PA	MLG	3	44.0	12.5	74.1	8.3	5.8	4
Suh[446]	50	UPPP	MLG+LT	3–6	55.3	26.9	56.0	no data	no data	4
Lin et al[169]	35	ZPPP	midline glossectomy	3	50.6	26.5	62.9	11.0	8.7	4
Vicini et al[196]	12	ESP	TORS	6	38.5	9.9	83.3	12	4.4	3b
	12	UPPP	TORS	6	38.4	19.8	33.3	13.8	7.6	3b
Vicini et al[240]	243	div.	TORS	3	43	17.9	66.9	12.3	5.7	4
Li et al[447]	34	Han-UPPP	div.	12	41.5	12	no data	11.1	4.4	3b
Chen et al[144]	24	UPPP	GA	12	46.1	26.2	no data	10	no data	2b
	26	UPPP	TBS	12	51.8	25.2	no data	9.5	no data	2b
Hoff et al[448]	121	div.	TORS LT	3	42.7	22.2	51.2	no data	no data	4
Toh et al[328]	20	UPPP	TORS TBR	6	41.3	13.5	55	13	5.6	4
Lin et al[449]	39	UPPP	TORS	4–6	43.9	21.9	53.8	15.6	5.7	4
Roher et al[284]	8	Flap	GA	4	48.3	11.6	62.5	no data	no data	4
Vicini et al[185]	10	barbed rPP	div.	6	43.7	13.6	90	11.6	4.3	4
Turhan et al[450]	90	UPPP	TBS	6	51.8	20.5	74.4	no data	no data	4
Verse et al[227]	58	UPPP	LT	2	34.5	17.4	58.6	10.4	6.3	3b
	50	UPPP	HS + RFT ZG	2	32.9	17	54	11.8	7.6	3b
Chiffer et al[451]	18	UPPP	TORS	6	53.9	19.8	61.1	no data	no data	4
Yüksel et al[452]	14	mod. UPPP	TBS	24	33.2	18	57.1	11.9	5	3b
Thaler et al[453]	75	UPPP	TORS	3	57.5	31.4	45	12.8	5.8	3b

▶ Table 8.25 (Continued)

Author	N	Soft palate	Hypopharynx	Follow-up (mos)	AHI (pre)	AHI (post)	Success (%)	ESS (pre)	ESS (post)	EBM
Barrera et al[287]	18	Flap	GA	6	41.1	22.9	61.1	13.2	6.7	4
Li et al[454]	25	mod. UPPP	CELL	6	45.7	12.8	80.0	9.6	7.5	4
All	2,808			1–39.4	44.74	19.99	58.08	12.03	6.55	B

Abbreviations: barbed rPP, barbed suture relocation pharyngoplasty; CELL, Coblation endoscopic lingual lightening; ESS, Epworth sleepiness scale; ESP, expansion sphincter palatoplasty; EUPF, extended uvulopalatal flap; GA, genioglossal advancement; HS, hyoid suspension; lat PP, lateral palatoplasty; LLT, laser lingual tonsillectomy; LT, lingual tonsillectomy; MLG, midline glossectomy; mod. UPPP, modification of uvulopalatopharyngoplasty; oTBR, open transcollar tongue base resection; PA, palatal advancement; RFT, radiofrequency treatment; TBS, tongue base suspension; TBR, tongue base resection; TORS, transoral robotic resection of the base of tongue; UPPP, uvulopalatopharyngoplasty; ZPP, z-palatoplasty; ZPPP, z-palatopharyngoplasty.
Notes: div. = diverse; EBM: level of evidence-based medicine; flap: uvulopalatal flap; mos = months.

References

[1] Powell NB, Riley RW, Troell RJ, Blumen MB, Guilleminault C. Radiofrequency volumetric reduction of the tongue. A porcine pilot study for the treatment of obstructive sleep apnea syndrome. Chest. 1997; 111(5):1348–1355

[2] Stuck BA, Maurer JT, Hörmann K. Tongue base reduction with radiofrequency tissue ablation: preliminary results after two treatment sessions. Sleep Breath. 2000; 4(4):155–162

[3] Blumen MB, Coquille F, Rocchicioli C, Mellot F, Chabolle F. Radiofrequency tongue reduction through a cervical approach: a pilot study. Laryngoscope. 2006; 116(10):1887–1893

[4] Powell NB, Riley RW, Troell RJ, Li K, Blumen MB, Guilleminault C. Effects of new technology on subjects with sleep disordered breathing—radiofrequency volumetric tissue réduction of the palate. Chest. 1998; 113(5):1163–1174

[5] Troell RJ, Powell NB, Riley RW, Li KK, Guilleminault C. Comparison of postoperative pain between laser-assisted uvulopalatoplasty, uvulopalatopharyngoplasty, and radiofrequency volumetric tissue reduction of the palate. Otolaryngol Head Neck Surg. 2000; 122(3):402–409

[6] Blumen MB, Chalumeau F, Gauthier A, Bobin S, Coste A, Chabolle F. Comparative study of four radiofrequency generators for the treatment of snoring. Otolaryngol Head Neck Surg. 2008; 138(3):294–299

[7] Balsevičius T, Uloza V, Vaitkus S, Sakalauskas R, Miliauskas S. Controlled trial of combined radiofrequency-assisted uvulopalatoplasty in the treatment of snoring and mild to moderate OSAS (pilot study). Sleep Breath. 2013; 17(2):695–703

[8] Atef A, Mosleh M, Hesham M, Fathi A, Hassan M, Fawzy M. Radiofrequency vs laser in the management of mild to moderate obstructive sleep apnoea: does the number of treatment sessions matter? J Laryngol Otol. 2005; 119(11):888–893

[9] Blumen MB, Vezina JP, Bequignon E, Chabolle F. Snoring intensity after a first session of soft palate radiofrequency: predictive value of the final result. Laryngoscope. 2013; 123(6):1556–1559

[10] Terris DJ, Chen V. Occult mucosal injuries with radiofrequency ablation of the palate. Otolaryngol Head Neck Surg. 2001; 125(5):468–472

[11] Farrar J, Ryan J, Oliver E, Gillespie MB. Radiofrequency ablation for the treatment of obstructive sleep apnea: a meta-analysis. Laryngoscope. 2008; 118(10):1878–1883

[12] Birkent H, Soken H, Akcam T, Karahatay S, Gerek M. The effect of radiofrequency volumetric tissue reduction of soft palate on voice. Eur Arch Otorhinolaryngol. 2008; 265(2):195–198

[13] Franklin KA, Anttila H, Axelsson S, et al. Effects and side-effects of surgery for snoring and obstructive sleep apnea—a systematic review. Sleep. 2009; 32(1):27–36

[14] Stuck BA, Sauter A, Hormann K, Verse T, Maurer JT. Radiofrequency surgery of the soft palate in the treatment of snoring: a placebo-controlled trial. Sleep. 2005; 28:847–850

[15] Stuck BA, Maurer JT, Hein G, Hörmann K, Verse T. Radiofrequency surgery of the soft palate in the treatment of snoring: a review of the literature. Sleep. 2004; 27(3):551–555

[16] Bäck LJ, Hytönen ML, Roine RP, Malmivaara AO. Radiofrequency ablation treatment of soft palate for patients with snoring: a systematic review of effectiveness and adverse effects. Laryngoscope. 2009; 119(6):1241–1250

[17] Balsevičius T, Uloza V, Vaitkus S, Sakalauskas R, Miliauskas S. Controlled trial of combined radiofrequency-assisted uvulopalatoplasty in the treatment of snoring and mild to moderate OSAS (pilot study). Sleep Breath. 2013; 17(2):695–703

[18] Stuck BA. Radiofrequency-assisted uvulopalatoplasty for snoring: long-term follow-up. Laryngoscope. 2009; 119(8):1617–1620

[19] De Kermadec H, Blumen MB, Engalenc D, Vezina JP, Chabolle F. Radiofrequency of the soft palate for sleep-disordered breathing: a 6-year follow-up study. Eur Ann Otorhinolaryngol Head Neck Dis. 2014; 131(1):27–31

[20] Blumen MB, Dahan S, Fleury B, Hausser-Hauw C, Chabolle F. Radiofrequency ablation for the treatment of mild to moderate obstructive sleep apnea. Laryngoscope. 2002; 112(11):2086–2092

[21] Baba RY, Mohan A, Metta VV, Mador MJ. Temperature controlled radiofrequency ablation at different sites for treatment of obstructive sleep apnea syndrome: a systematic review and meta-analysis. Sleep Breath. 2015; 19(3):891–910

[22] D'Souza A, Hassan S, Morgan D. Recent advances in surgery for snoring—somnoplasty (radiofrequency palatoplasty) a pilot study: effectiveness and acceptability [in French]. Rev Laryngol Otol Rhinol. 2000; 12:111–115

[23] Pessey JJ, Rose X, Michenet F, Calmels MN, Lagleyre S. Treatment of simple snoring by radiofrequency velar coblation [in French]. Ann Otolaryngol Chir Cervicofac. 2005; 122:21–26

[24] Bäck LJ, Koivunen P, Pyykkö I, Stene BK, Mäkitie AA. The impact of pretreatment assessment of oropharynx on interstitial soft palate radiofrequency surgery outcome: a multi-center study in patients with habitual snoring. Sleep Breath. 2012; 16(1):199–204

[25] Sonsuwan N, Rujimethabhas K, Sawanyawisuth K. Factors associated with successful treatment by radiofrequency treatment of the soft palate in obstructive sleep apnea as the first-line treatment. Sleep Disord. 2015; 2015:690425

[26] Kotecha B, Kumar G, Sands R, Walden A, Gowers B. Evaluation of upper airway obstruction in snoring patients using digital video stroboscopy. Eur Arch Otorhinolaryngol. 2013; 270(7):2141–2147

[27] Wassmuth Z, Mair E, Loube D, Leonard D. Cautery-assisted palatal stiffening operation for the treatment of obstructive sleep apnea syndrome. Otolaryngol Head Neck Surg. 2000; 123 (1 Pt 1):55–60

[28] Brietzke SE, Mair EA. Injection snoreplasty: how to treat snoring without all the pain and expense. Otolaryngol Head Neck Surg. 2001; 124(5):503–510

[29] Brietzke SE, Mair EA. Injection snoreplasty: investigation of alternative sclerotherapy agents. Otolaryngol Head Neck Surg. 2004; 130(1):47–57

[30] Poyrazoglu E, Dogru S, Saat B, Güngör A, Çekin E, Cincik H. Histologic effects of injection snoreplasty and radiofrequency in the rat soft palate. Otolaryngol Head Neck Surg. 2006; 135(4):561–564

[31] Lafrentz JR, Brietzke SE, Mair EA. Evaluation of palatal snoring surgery in an animal model. Otolaryngol Head Neck Surg. 2003; 129(4):343–352

[32] Al-Jassim AH, Lesser THJ. Single dose injection snoreplasty: investigation or treatment? J Laryngol Otol. 2008; 122(11):1190–1193

[33] Brietzke SE, Mair EA. Injection snoreplasty: extended follow-up and new objective data. Otolaryngol Head Neck Surg. 2003; 128(5):605–615

[34] Iseri M, Balcioglu O. Radiofrequency versus injection snoreplasty in simple snoring. Otolaryngol Head Neck Surg. 2005; 133(2):224–228

[35] Olszewska E, Panek J, O, ', Day J, Rogowski M. Usefulness of snoreplasty in the treatment of simple snoring and mild obstructive sleep apnea/hypopnea syndrome—preliminary report. Otolaryngol Pol. 2014; 68(4):184–188

[36] Labra A, Haro-Valencia R, Huerta-Delgado A-D, Jimenez-Correa U, Sanchez-Narvaez F. Efficacy of submucosal sodium tetradecyl sulfate in the soft palate as a treatment of the mild obstructive sleep apnea syndrome: a pilot study. Sleep Disord. 2012; 2012:597684

[37] Nordgård S, Wormdal K, Bugten V, Stene BK, Skjøstad KW. Palatal implants: a new method for the treatment of snoring. Acta Otolaryngol. 2004; 124(8):970–975

[38] Friedman M, Schalch P, Joseph NJ. Palatal stiffening after failed uvulopalatopharyngoplasty with the Pillar Implant System. Laryngoscope. 2006; 116(11):1956–1961

[39] Akpinar ME, Yigit O, Kocak I, Altundag A. Does the length of uvula affect the palatal implant outcome in the management of habitual snoring? Laryngoscope. 2011; 121(5):1112–1116

[40] Rotenberg BW, Luu K. Four-year outcomes of palatal implants for primary snoring treatment: a prospective longitudinal study. Laryngoscope. 2012; 122(3):696–699

[41] Akpinar ME, Kocak I, Gurpinar B, Esen HE. Effects of soft palate implants on acoustic characteristics of voice and articulation. J Voice. 2011; 25(3):381–386

[42] Gillespie MB, Wylie PE, Lee-Chiong T, Rapoport DM. Effect of palatal implants on continuous positive airway pressure and compliance. Otolaryngol Head Neck Surg. 2011; 144(2):230–236

[43] Choi JH, Kim SN, Cho JH. Efficacy of the Pillar implant in the treatment of snoring and mild-to-moderate obstructive sleep apnea: a meta-analysis. Laryngoscope. 2013; 123(1):269–276

[44] Lin H-C, Friedman M, Chang H-W, et al. Effects of Pillar implants for sleep-related breathing disorders on middle ear function. Eur Arch Otorhinolaryngol. 2013; 270(8):2339–2343

[45] Fujita S, Conway W, Zorick F, Roth T. Surgical correction of anatomic azbnormalities in obstructive sleep apnea syndrome: uvulopalatopharyngoplasty. Otolaryngol Head Neck Surg. 1981; 89(6):923–934

[46] Carenfelt C. Laser uvulopalatoplasty in treatment of habitual snoring. Ann Otol Rhinol Laryngol. 1991; 100(6):451–454

[47] Littner M, Kushida CA, Hartse K, et al. Practice parameters for the use of laser-assisted uvulopalatoplasty: an update for 2000. Sleep. 2001; 24(5):603–619

[48] Kamami YV. Laser CO_2 for snoring. Preliminary results. Acta Otorhinolaryngol Belg. 1990; 44(4):451–456

[49] Coleman JA Jr. Laser-assisted uvulopalatoplasty: long-term results with a treatment for snoring. Ear Nose Throat J. 1998; 77(1):22–24, 26–29, 32–34

[50] Bassiouny A, El Salamawy A, Abd El-Tawab M, Atef A. Bipolar radiofrequency treatment for snoring with mild to moderate sleep apnea: a comparative study between the radiofrequency assisted uvulopalatoplasty technique and the channeling technique. Eur Arch Otorhinolaryngol. 2007; 264(6):659–667

[51] Wedman J, Miljeteig H. Treatment of simple snoring using radio waves for ablation of uvula and soft palate: a day-case surgery procedure. Laryngoscope. 2002; 112(7 Pt 1):1256–1259

[52] Baisch A, Maurer JT, Hörmann K, Stuck BA. Combined radiofrequency assisted uvulopalatoplasty in the treatment of snoring. Eur Arch Otorhinolaryngol. 2009; 266(1):125–130

[53] Camacho M, Nesbitt NB, Lambert E, et al. Laser-assisted uvulopalatoplasty for obstructive sleep apnea: a systematic review and meta-analysis. Sleep. 2017; 40(3)

[54] Fabiani M. Surgery for Snoring and Obstructive Sleep Apnea Syndrome. Amsterdam: Kugler Publications; 2003: 463–474

[55] Krespi Y, et al. The ef cacy of laser-assisted uvulopalatoplasty in the management of obstructive sleep apnea syndrome and upper airway resistance syndrome. Oper Tech Otolaryngol–Head Neck Surg. 1994; 5:235–243

[56] Friedman M, Wilson MN, Pulver T, et al. Screening for obstructive sleep apnea/hypopnea syndrome: subjective and objective factors. Otolaryngol Head Neck Surg. 2010; 142(4):531–535

[57] Finkelstein Y, Stein G, Ophir D, Berger R, Berger G. Laser-assisted uvulopalatoplasty for the management of obstructive sleep apnea: myths and facts. Arch Otolaryngol Head Neck Surg. 2002; 128(4):429–434

[58] Göktas Ö, Solmaz M, Göktas G, Olze H. Long-term results in obstructive sleep apnea syndrome (OSAS) after laser-assisted uvulopalatoplasty (LAUP). PLoS One. 2014; 9(6):e100211

[59] Iyngkaran T, Kanagalingam J, Rajeswaran R, Georgalas C, Kotecha B. Long-term outcomes of laser-assisted uvulopalatoplasty in 168 patients with snoring. J Laryngol Otol. 2006; 120(11):932–938

[60] Rombaux P, Hamoir M, Bertrand B, Aubert G, Liistro G, Rodenstein D. Postoperative pain and side effects after uvulopalatopharyngoplasty, laser-assisted uvulopalatoplasty, and radiofrequency tissue volume reduction in primary snoring. Laryngoscope. 2003; 113(12):2169–2173

[61] Kaluskar SK, Kaul GH. Long-term results of KTP/532 laser uvulopalatopharyngoplasty. Rev Laryngol Otol Rhinol (Bord). 2000; 121(1):59–62

[62] Wang Z, Rebeiz EE, Shapshay SM. Laser soft palate "stiffening": an alternative to uvulopalatopharyngoplasty. Lasers Surg Med. 2002; 30(1):40–43

[63] Hörmann K, Verse T. Surgery for Sleep Disordered Breathing. 2 ed. Heidelberg: Springer Verlag, 2010

[64] Thorn C, Faber A, Schultz JD, Hörmann K, Stuck BA. Prophylactic antibiotic use in ENT surgery HNO. 2015; 63(2):118–124

[65] Ferguson KA, Heighway K, Ruby RR. A randomized trial of laser-assisted uvulopalatoplasty in the treatment of mild obstructive sleep apnea. Am J Respir Crit Care Med. 2003; 167(1):15–19

[66] Larrosa F, Hernandez L, Morello A, Ballester E, Quinto L, Montserrat JM. Laser-assisted uvulopalatoplasty for snoring: does it meet the expectations? Eur Respir J. 2004; 24(1):66–70

[67] Verse T, Dreher A, Heiser C, et al. S2e-guideline: "ENT-specific therapy of obstructive sleep apnea in adults" short version : sleep medicine task force of the german society for otorhinolaryngology, head and neck surgery HNO. 2016; 64(5):310–319

[68] Stuck BA. Radiofrequency-assisted uvulopalatoplasty for snoring: long-term follow-up. Laryngoscope. 2009; 119(8):1617–1620

[69] Lee KD, Lee HS, Hong JC, et al. Diameter of vessels across the tonsillar capsule as an anatomical consideration for tonsillectomy. Clin Anat. 2008; 21(1):33–37

[70] Lourijsen ES, Wong Chung JE, Koopman JP, Blom HM. Postoperative morbidity and 1-year outcomes in CO_2-laser tonsillotomy versus dissection tonsillectomy. Acta Otolaryngol. 2016; 136(10):983–990

[71] Deak L, Saxton D, Johnston K, Benedek P, Katona G. Comparison of postoperative pain in children with two intracapsular tonsillotomy techniques and a standard tonsillectomy: microdebrider and radiofrequency tonsillotomies versus standard tonsillectomies. Sultan Qaboos Univ Med J. 2014; 14(4):e500–e505

[72] Acevedo JL, Shah RK, Brietzke SE. Systematic review of complications of tonsillotomy versus tonsillectomy. Otolaryngol Head Neck Surg. 2012; 146(6):871–879

[73] Walton J, Ebner Y, Stewart MG, April MM. Systematic review of randomized controlled trials comparing intracapsular tonsillectomy with total tonsillectomy in a pediatric population. Arch Otolaryngol Head Neck Surg. 2012; 138(3):243–249

[74] Windfuhr JP, Savva K, Dahm JD, Werner JA. Tonsillotomy: facts and fiction. Eur Arch Otorhinolaryngol. 2015; 272(4):949–969

[75] Stuck BA, Starzak K, Verse T, Hörmann K, Maurer JT. Complications of temperature-controlled radiofrequency volumetric tissue reduction for sleep-disordered breathing. Acta Otolaryngol. 2003; 123(4):532–535

[76] Barone DA, Krieger AC. Stroke and obstructive sleep apnea: a review. Curr Atheroscler Rep. 2013; 15(7):334

[77] Drager LF, Togeiro SM, Polotsky VY, Lorenzi-Filho G. Obstructive sleep apnea: a cardiometabolic risk in obesity and the metabolic syndrome. J Am Coll Cardiol. 2013; 62(7):569–576

[78] Stiefel P, Sánchez-Armengol MA, Villar J, Vallejo-Vaz A, Moreno-Luna R, Capote F. Obstructive sleep apnea syndrome, vascular pathology, endothelial function and endothelial cells and circulating microparticles. Arch Med Res. 2013; 44(6):409–414

[79] Konecny T, Kara T, Somers VK. Obstructive sleep apnea and hypertension: an update. Hypertension. 2014; 63(2):203–209

[80] Maurer JT. Update on surgical treatments for sleep apnea. Swiss Med Wkly. 2009; 139(43–44):624–629

[81] Orr WC, Martin RJ. Obstructive sleep apnea associated with tonsillar hypertrophy in adults. Arch Intern Med. 1981; 141(8):990–992

[82] Rubin AH, Eliaschar I, Joachim Z, Alroy G, Lavie P. Effects of nasal surgery and tonsillectomy on sleep apnea. Bull Eur Physiopathol Respir. 1983; 19(6):612–615

[83] Moser RJ III, Rajagopal KR. Obstructive sleep apnea in adults with tonsillar hypertrophy. Arch Intern Med. 1987; 147(7):1265–1267

[84] Aubert-Tulkens G, Hamoir M, Van den Eeckhaut J, Rodenstein DO. Failure of tonsil and nose surgery in adults with long-standing severe sleep apnea syndrome. Arch Intern Med. 1989; 149(9):2118–2121

[85] Houghton DJ, Camilleri AE, Stone P. Adult obstructive sleep apnoea syndrome and tonsillectomy. J Laryngol Otol. 1997; 111(9):829–832

[86] Miyazaki S, Itasaka Y, Tada H, Ishikawa K, Togawa K. Effectiveness of tonsillectomy in adult sleep apnea syndrome. Psychiatry Clin Neurosci. 1998; 52(2):222–223

[87] Verse T, Kroker BA, Pirsig W, Brosch S. Tonsillectomy as a treatment of obstructive sleep apnea in adults with tonsillar hypertrophy. Laryngoscope. 2000; 110(9):1556–1559

[88] Martinho FL, Zonato AI, Bittencourt LR, et al. Obese obstructive sleep apnea patients with tonsil hypertrophy submitted to tonsillectomy. Braz J Med Biol Res. 2006; 39(8):1137–1142

[89] Nakata S, Noda A, Yanagi E, Suzuki K, Yamamoto H, Nakashima T. Tonsil size and body mass index are important factors for efficacy of simple tonsillectomy in obstructive sleep apnoea syndrome. Clin Otolaryngol. 2006; 31(1):41–45

[90] Nakata S, Miyazaki S, Ohki M, et al. Reduced nasal resistance after simple tonsillectomy in patients with obstructive sleep apnea. Am J Rhinol. 2007; 21(2):192–195

[91] Stow NW, Sale PJ, Lee D, Joffe D, Gallagher RM. Simultaneous tonsillectomy and nasal surgery in adult obstructive sleep apnea: a pilot study. Otolaryngol Head Neck Surg. 2012; 147(2):387–391

[92] Tan LT, Tan AK, Hsu PP, et al. Effects of tonsillectomy on sleep study parameters in adult patients with obstructive sleep apnea—a prospective study. Sleep Breath. 2014; 18(2):265–268

[93] Senchak AJ, McKinlay AJ, Acevedo J, et al. The effect of tonsillectomy alone in adult obstructive sleep apnea. Otolaryngol Head Neck Surg. 2015; 152(5):969–973

[94] Verse T, Brus J, Wenzel S. Effect of tonsil size on AHI in sleep surgery patients. Own unpublished data

[95] Fukuda N, Abe T, Katagiri M, Yokoba M, Okamoto M, Tomita T. Effects of uvulopalatopharyngoplasty on patients with obstructive sleep apnea—the severity of preoperative tonsillar hypertrophy Nihon Kokyuki Gakkai Zasshi. 1998; 36(1):34–40

[96] Friedman M, Ibrahim H, Bass L. Clinical staging for sleep-disordered breathing. Otolaryngol Head Neck Surg. 2002; 127(1):13–21

[97] Windfuhr JP. Serious complications following tonsillectomy: how frequent are they really? ORL J Otorhinolaryngol Relat Spec. 2013; 75(3):166–173

[98] Brosch S, Matthes C, Pirsig W, Verse T. Uvulopalatopharyngoplasty changes fundamental frequency of the voice—a prospective study. J Laryngol Otol. 2000; 114(2):113–118

[99] Friedman M, Tanyeri H, La Rosa M, et al. Clinical predictors of obstructive sleep apnea. Laryngoscope. 1999; 109(12):1901–1907

[100] Cardozo AA, Hallikeri C, Lawrence H, Sankar V, Hargreaves S. Teenage and adult tonsillectomy: dose-response relationship between diathermy energy used and morbidity. Clin Otolaryngol. 2007; 32(5):366–371

[101] Habermann W, Müller W. Tissue penetration of bipolar electrosurgical currents: Joule overheating beyond the surface layer. Head Neck. 2013; 35(4):535–540

[102] Windfuhr JP, Verspohl BC, Chen YS, Dahm JD, Werner JA. Post-tonsillectomy hemorrhage—some facts will never change. Eur Arch Otorhinolaryngol. 2015; 272(5):1211–1218

[103] Gysin C, Dulguerov P. Hemorrhage after tonsillectomy: does the surgical technique really matter? ORL J Otorhinolaryngol Relat Spec. 2013; 75(3):123–132

[104] Numanoğlu KV, Ayoğlu H, Er DT. Efficacy of tramadol as a pre-incisional infiltration anesthetic in children undergoing inguinal hernia repair: a prospective randomized study. Ther Clin Risk Manag. 2014; 10:753–758

[105] Vasu TS, Grewal R, Doghramji K. Obstructive sleep apnea syndrome and perioperative complications: a systematic review of the literature. J Clin Sleep Med. 2012; 8(2):199–207

[106] Bahammam A, Delaive K, Ronald J, Manfreda J, Roos L, Kryger MH. Health care utilization in males with obstructive sleep apnea syndrome two years after diagnosis and treatment. Sleep. 1999; 22(6):740–747

[107] McNicholas WT, Ryan S. Obstructive sleep apnoea syndrome: translating science to clinical practice. Respirology. 2006; 11(2):136–144

[108] Rotenberg B, Theriault J, Pang K. Is overnight monitoring required for adult patients undergoing surgery for obstructive sleep apnea? Laryngoscope. 2011; 121(4):692–693

[109] Rösslein M, Bürkle H, Walther A, Stuck BA, Verse T. Position paper: perioperative management of adult patients with obstructive sleep apnea in ENT surgery Laryngorhinootologie. 2015; 94(8):516–523

[110] Rotenberg BW, Wickens B, Parnes J. Intraoperative ice pack application for uvulopalatoplasty pain reduction: a randomized controlled trial. Laryngoscope. 2013; 123(2):533–536

[111] Bellis JR, Pirmohamed M, Nunn AJ, et al. Dexamethasone and haemorrhage risk in paediatric tonsillectomy: a systematic review and meta-analysis. Br J Anaesth. 2014; 113(1):23–42

[112] Stevenson EW, Turner GT, Sutton FD, Doekel RC, Pegram V, Hernandez J. Prognostic significance of age and tonsillectomy in uvulopalatopharyngoplasty. Laryngoscope. 1990; 100(8):820–823

[113] Schwartz AR, Schubert N, Rothman W, et al. Effect of uvulopalatopharyngoplasty on upper airway collapsibility in obstructive sleep apnea. Am Rev Respir Dis. 1992; 145(3):527–532

[114] McGuirt WF Jr, Johnson JT, Sanders MH. Previous tonsillectomy as prognostic indicator for success of uvulopalatopharyngoplasty. Laryngoscope. 1995; 105(11):1253–1255

[115] Boot H, van Wegen R, Poublon RM, Bogaard JM, Schmitz PI, van der Meché FG. Long-term results of uvulopalatopharyngoplasty for obstructive sleep apnea syndrome. Laryngoscope. 2000; 110(3 Pt 1):469–475

[116] Hessel NS, de Vries N. Results of uvulopalatopharyngoplasty after diagnostic workup with polysomnography and sleep endoscopy: a report of 136 snoring patients. Eur Arch Otorhinolaryngol. 2003; 260(2):91–95

[117] Fujita S, Conway WA, Zorick FJ, et al. Evaluation of the effectiveness of uvulopalatopharyngoplasty. Laryngoscope. 1985; 95(1):70–74

[118] Kezirian EJ, Maselli J, Vittinghoff E, Goldberg AN, Auerbach AD. Obstructive sleep apnea surgery practice patterns in the United States: 2000 to 2006. Otolaryngol Head Neck Surg. 2010; 143(3):441–447

[119] Kezirian EJ, Weaver EM, Yueh B, et al. Incidence of serious complications after uvulopalatopharyngoplasty. Laryngoscope. 2004; 114(3):450–453

[120] American Sleep Disorders Association. Practice parameters for the treatment of obstruc-tive sleep apnea in adults: the efficacy of surgical modifications of the upper airway. Re-port of the American Sleep Disorders Association. Sleep. 1996; 19(2):152–155

[121] Sundaram S, Bridgman SA, Lim J, Lasserson TJ. Surgery for obstructive sleep apnoea. Cochrane Database Syst Rev. 2005(4):CD001004

[122] Ishman SL, Wakefiel TL, Collop NA. Sleep apnea and sleep disprders. I Flint PW, Haughey BH, Lund VJ, et al, eds. Cummings

Otolaryngology-Head and Neck Surgery. 5th ed. Philadelphia, PA: Mosby; 2010

[123] Li HY, Wang PC, Lee LA, Chen NH, Fang TJ; Li HY1. Prediction of uvulopalatopharyngoplasty outcome: anatomy-based staging system versus severity-based staging system. Sleep. 2006; 29(12):1537–1541

[124] Friedman M, Vidyasagar R, Bliznikas D, Joseph N. Does severity of obstructive sleep apnea/hypopnea syndrome predict uvulopalatopharyngoplasty outcome? Laryngoscope. 2005; 115(12):2109–2113

[125] Friedman M, Ibrahim H, Joseph NJ. Staging of obstructive sleep apnea/hypopnea syndrome: a guide to appropriate treatment. Laryngoscope. 2004; 114(3):454–459

[126] Laffont F, Lecendreux B, Minz M, et al. Efficacy of uvulopalatopharyngoplasty (UPPP) and modifications in sleep structure in the sleep apnea syndrome (SAS) Neurophysiol Clin. 1989; 19(6):477–488

[127] Gislason T, Lindholm CE, Almqvist M, et al. Uvulopalatopharyngoplasty in the sleep apnea syndrome. Predictors of results. Arch Otolaryngol Head Neck Surg. 1988; 114(1):45–51

[128] Shie DY, Tsou YA, Tai CJ, Tsai MH. Impact of obesity on uvulopalatopharyngoplasty success in patients with severe obstructive sleep apnea: a retrospective single-center study in Taiwan. Acta Otolaryngol. 2013; 133(3):261–269

[129] Heiser C, Landis BN, Giger R, et al. Taste disorders after tonsillectomy: a long-term follow-up. Laryngoscope. 2012; 122(6):1265–1266

[130] Hessel NS, Vries N. Increase of the apnoea-hypopnoea index after uvulopalatopharyngoplasty: analysis of failure. Clin Otolaryngol Allied Sci. 2004; 29(6):682–685

[131] Aktas O, Erdur O, Cirik AA, Kayhan FT. The role of drug-induced sleep endoscopy in surgical planning for obstructive sleep apnea syndrome. Eur Arch Otorhinolaryngol. 2015; 272(8):2039–2043

[132] Ikeda K, Oshima T, Shimomura A, Takasaka T. Surgical criteria for obstructive sleep apnea syndrome based on localization of upper airway collapse during sleep: a preliminary study. Tohoku J Exp Med. 1998; 185(1):1–8

[133] Osnes T, Rollheim J, Hartmann E. Effect of UPPP with respect to site of pharyngeal obstruction in sleep apnoea: follow-up at 18 months by overnight recording of airway pressure and flow. Clin Otolaryngol Allied Sci. 2002; 27(1):38–43

[134] Stuck BA, Ravesloot MJL, Eschenhagen T, de Vet HCW, Sommer JU. Uvulopalatopharyngoplasty with or without tonsillectomy in the treatment of adult obstructive sleep apnea: a systematic review. Sleep Med 2018;50:152–165

[135] Kim JA, Lee JJ, Jung HH. Predictive factors of immediate postoperative complications after uvulopalatopharyngoplasty. Laryngoscope. 2005; 115(10):1837–1840

[136] Lundkvist K, Januszkiewicz A, Friberg D. Uvulopalatopharyngoplasty in 158 OSAS patients failing non-surgical treatment. Acta Otolaryngol. 2009; 129(11):1280–1286

[137] Kezirian EJ, Weaver EM, Yueh B, Khuri SF, Daley J, Henderson WG. Risk factors for serious complication after uvulopalatopharyngoplasty. Arch Otolaryngol Head Neck Surg. 2006; 132(10):1091–1098

[138] Browaldh N, Nerfeldt P, Lysdahl M, Bring J, Friberg D. SKUP3 randomised controlled trial: polysomnographic results after uvulopalatopharyngoplasty in selected patients with obstructive sleep apnoea. Thorax. 2013; 68(9):846–853

[139] Browaldh N, Bring J, Friberg D. SKUP(3) RCT; continuous study: changes in sleepiness and quality of life after modified UPPP. Laryngoscope. 2016; 126(6):1484–1491

[140] Sommer UJ, Heiser C, Gahleitner C, et al. Tonsillectomy with uvulopalatopharyngoplasty in obstructive sleep apnea. Dtsch Arztebl Int. 2016; 113(1–02):1–8

[141] Wilhelmsson B, Tegelberg A, Walker-Engström ML, et al. A prospective randomized study of a dental appliance compared with uvulopalatopharyngoplasty in the treatment of obstructive sleep apnoea. Acta Otolaryngol. 1999; 119(4):503–509

[142] Santamaria JD, Prior JC, Fleetham JA. Reversible reproductive dysfunction in men with obstructive sleep apnoea. Clin Endocrinol (Oxf). 1988; 28(5):461–470

[143] Shin HW, Park JH, Park JW, et al. Effects of surgical vs. non-surgical therapy on erectile dysfunction and quality of life in obstructive sleep apnea syndrome: a pilot study. J Sex Med. 2013; 10(8):2053–2059

[144] Chen S, Shi S, Xia Y, et al. Changes in sleep characteristics and airway obstruction in OSAHS patients with multi-level obstruction following simple UPPP, UPPP-GA, or UPPP-TBA: a prospective, single-center, parallel group study. ORL J Otorhinolaryngol Relat Spec. 2014; 76(4):179–188

[145] Keenan SP, Burt H, Ryan CF, Fleetham JA. Long-term survival of patients with obstructive sleep apnea treated by uvulopalatopharyngoplasty or nasal CPAP. Chest. 1994; 105(1):155–159

[146] Browaldh N, Friberg D, Svanborg E, Nerfeldt P. 15-year efficacy of uvulopalatopharyngoplasty based on objective and subjective data. Acta Otolaryngol. 2011; 131(12):1303–1310

[147] Powell N, Riley R, Guilleminault C, Troell R. A reversible uvulopalatal flap for snoring and sleep apnea syndrome. Sleep. 1996; 19(7):593–599

[148] Li HY, Li KK, Chen NH, Wang PC. Modified uvulopalatopharyngoplasty: the extended uvulopalatal flap. Am J Otolaryngol. 2003; 24(5):311–316

[149] Neruntarat C. Uvulopalatal flap for snoring on an outpatient basis. Otolaryngol Head Neck Surg. 2003; 129(4):353–359

[150] Hörmann K, Erhardt T, Hirth K, Maurer JT. Modified uvula flap in therapy of sleep-related breathing disorders HNO. 2001; 49(5):361–366

[151] Neruntarat C. Uvulopalatal flap for obstructive sleep apnea: short-term and long-term results. Laryngoscope. 2011; 121(3):683–687

[152] Verse T, Stuck BA. Modern modifications of uvulopalatopharyngoplasty HNO. 2017; 65(2):90–98

[153] Elbassiouny AM. Soft palatal webbing flap palatopharyngoplasty for both soft palatal and oropharyngeal lateral wall collapse in the treatment of snoring and obstructive sleep apnea: a new innovative technique without tonsillectomy. Sleep Breath. 2015; 19(2):481–487

[154] Li HY, Chen NH, Lee LA, Shu YH, Fang TJ, Wang PC. Use of morphological indicators to predict outcomes of palatopharyngeal surgery in patients with obstructive sleep apnea. ORL J Otorhinolaryngol Relat Spec. 2004; 66(3):119–123

[155] Li HY, Chen NH, Shu YH, Wang PC. Changes in quality of life and respiratory disturbance after extended uvulopalatal flap surgery in patients with obstructive sleep apnea. Arch Otolaryngol Head Neck Surg. 2004; 130(2):195–200

[156] Li HY, Huang YS, Chen NH, Fang TJ, Liu CY, Wang PC. Mood improvement after surgery for obstructive sleep apnea. Laryngoscope. 2004; 114(6):1098–1102

[157] Li HY, Li KK, Chen NH, Wang CJ, Liao YF, Wang PC. Three-dimensional computed tomography and polysomnography findings after extended uvulopalatal flap surgery for obstructive sleep apnea. Am J Otolaryngol. 2005; 26(1):7–11

[158] Lin SW, Chen NH, Li HY, et al. A comparison of the long-term outcome and effects of surgery or continuous positive airway pressure on patients with obstructive sleep apnea syndrome. Laryngoscope. 2006; 116(6):1012–1016

[159] Lin HC, Friedman M, Chang HW, Gurpinar B. The efficacy of multilevel surgery of the upper airway in adults with obstructive sleep apnea/hypopnea syndrome. Laryngoscope. 2008; 118(5):902–908

[160] Sher AE, Schechtman KB, Piccirillo JF. The efficacy of surgical modifications of the upper airway in adults with obstructive sleep apnea syndrome. Sleep. 1996; 19(2):156–177

[161] Friedman M, Ibrahim HZ, Vidyasagar R, Pomeranz J, Joseph NJ. Z-palatoplasty (ZPP): a technique for patients without tonsils. Otolaryngol Head Neck Surg. 2004; 131(1):89–100

[162] Cahali MB. Lateral pharyngoplasty: a new treatment for obstructive sleep apnea hypopnea syndrome. Laryngoscope. 2003; 113(11):1961–1968

[163] Pang KP, Woodson BT. Expansion sphincter pharyngoplasty: a new technique for the treatment of obstructive sleep apnea. Otolaryngol Head Neck Surg. 2007; 137(1):110–114

[164] Friedman M, Duggal P, Joseph NJ. Revision uvulopalatoplasty by Z-palatoplasty. Otolaryngol Head Neck Surg. 2007; 136(4):638–643

[165] Lin HC, Friedman M, Chang HW, Su MC, Wilson M. Z-palato-pharyngoplasty plus radiofrequency tongue base reduction for moderate/severe obstructive sleep apnea/hypopnea syndrome. Acta Otolaryngol. 2010; 130(9):1070–1076

[166] Yi HL, Sun XQ, Chen B, et al. Z-palatopharyngoplasty plus genio-glossus advancement and hyoid suspension for obstructive sleep apnea hypopnea syndrome. Otolaryngol Head Neck Surg. 2011; 144(3):469–473

[167] Xiong YP, Yi HL, Yin SK, et al. Predictors of surgical outcomes of uvulopalatopharyngoplasty for obstructive sleep apnea hypopnea syndrome. Otolaryngol Head Neck Surg. 2011; 145(6):1049–1054

[168] Liu SR, Yi HL, Yin SK, et al. Associated predictors of therapeutic response to uvulopharyngopalatoplasty for severe obstructive sleep apnea hypopnea syndrome. Eur Arch Otorhinolaryngol. 2013; 270(4):1411–1417

[169] Lin HC, Friedman M, Chang HW, Yalamanchali S. Z-palato-pharyngoplasty combined with endoscopic coblator open tongue base resection for severe obstructive sleep apnea/hypopnea syndrome. Otolaryngol Head Neck Surg. 2014; 150(6):1078–1085

[170] Lin HC, Friedman M, Chang HW, Shao CH, Pulver TM, Chen YC. Effects of obstructive sleep apnea surgery on middle ear func-tion. Arch Otolaryngol Head Neck Surg. 2011; 137(4):373–376

[171] Friedman M, Hwang MS. Z-palatopharyngoplasty. Oper Tech Otolaryngol–Head Neck Surg. 2015; 26:90–94

[172] van Maanen JP, Witte BI, de Vries N. Theoretical approach to-wards increasing effectiveness of palatal surgery in obstructive sleep apnea: role for concomitant positional therapy? Sleep Breath. 2014; 18(2):341–349

[173] Li HY, Lee LA. Relocation pharyngoplasty for obstructive sleep apnea. Laryngoscope. 2009; 119(12):2472–2477

[174] Li HY, Cheng WN, Chuang LP, et al. Positional dependency and surgical success of relocation pharyngoplasty among patients with severe obstructive sleep apnea. Otolaryngol Head Neck Surg. 2013; 149(3):506–512

[175] Verse T, Stuck BA. Modern modifications of uvulopaltopharyn-goplasty. HNO. 2016

[176] Hsu PP, Tan AK, Gan EC, et al. Computer-assisted quantitative upper airway analysis following modified uvulopalatal flap and lateral pharyngoplasty for obstructive sleep apnoea: a prospective case-controlled study. Clin Otolaryngol. 2012; 37(3):188–196

[177] Cahali MB, Formigoni GG, Gebrim EM, Miziara ID. Lateral pharyngoplasty versus uvulopalatopharyngoplasty: a clinical, polysomnographic and computed tomography measurement comparison. Sleep. 2004; 27(5):942–950

[178] de Paula Soares CF, Cavichio L, Cahali MB. Lateral pharyngoplas-ty reduces nocturnal blood pressure in patients with obstructive sleep apnea. Laryngoscope. 2014; 124(1):311–316

[179] Sorrenti G, Piccin O. Functional expansion pharyngoplasty in the treatment of obstructive sleep apnea. Laryngoscope. 2013; 123(11):2905–2908

[180] Chi JCY, Chiang RPY, Chou TY, Shu CH, Shiao AS, Lin CM. The role of lateral pharyngoplasty in obstructive sleep apnea syndrome. Eur Arch Otorhinolaryngol. 2015; 272(2):489–496

[181] Han D, Ye J, Lin Z, Wang J, Wang J, Zhang Y. Revised uvulopala-topharyngoplasty with uvula preservation and its clinical study. ORL J Otorhinolaryngol Relat Spec. 2005; 67(4):213–219

[182] Huang TW, Cheng PW. Microdebrider-assisted extended uvu-lopalatopharyngoplasty. Arch Otolaryngol Head Neck Surg. 2008; 134:141–145

[183] Ikematsu T. Study of snoring, 4th report: therapy. Journal of Japanese Otorhinolaryngology. 1964; 64:434–435

[184] Kuhlo W, Doll E, Franck MC. Successful management of Pickwickian syndrome using long-term tracheostomy Dtsch Med Wochenschr. 1969; 94(24):1286–1290

[185] Vicini C, Hendawy E, Campanini A, et al. Barbed reposition pha-ryngoplasty (BRP) for OSAHS: a feasibility, safety, efficacy and teachability pilot study. "We are on the giant's shoulders". Eur Arch Otorhinolaryngol. 2015; 272(10):3065–3070

[186] Mesti JJ, Cahali MB. Evolution of swallowing in lateral pharyn-goplasty with stylopharyngeal muscle preservation. Rev Bras Otorrinolaringol (Engl Ed). 2012; 78(6):51–55

[187] Sforza E, Bacon W, Weiss T, Thibault A, Petiau C, Krieger J. Upper airway collapsibility and cephalometric variables in pa-tients with obstructive sleep apnea. Am J Respir Crit Care Med. 2000; 161(2 Pt 1):347–352

[188] Hoffstein V, Mateika S. Differences in abdominal and neck circumferences in patients with and without obstructive sleep apnoea. Eur Respir J. 1992; 5(4):377–381

[189] Welch KC, Foster GD, Ritter CT, et al. A novel volumetric magnet-ic resonance imaging paradigm to study upper airway anatomy. Sleep. 2002; 25(5):532–542

[190] Schwab RJ, Pasirstein M, Pierson R, et al. Identification of upper airway anatomic risk factors for obstructive sleep apnea with volumetric magnetic resonance imaging. Am J Respir Crit Care Med. 2003; 168(5):522–530

[191] Huon LK, Liu SY, Shih TT, Chen YJ, Lo MT, Wang PC. Dynamic upper airway collapse observed from sleep MRI: BMI-matched severe and mild OSA patients. Eur Arch Otorhinolaryngol. 2016; 273(11):4021–4026

[192] Lan MC, Liu SY, Lan MY, Modi R, Capasso R. Lateral pharyngeal wall collapse associated with hypoxemia in obstructive sleep ap-nea. Laryngoscope. 2015; 125(10):2408–2412

[193] Soares D, Sinawe H, Folbe AJ, et al. Lateral oropharyngeal wall and supraglottic airway collapse associated with failure in sleep apnea surgery. Laryngoscope. 2012; 122(2):473–479

[194] Liu SY, Huon LK, Lo MT, et al. Static craniofacial measurements and dynamic airway collapse patterns associated with severe obstructive sleep apnoea: a sleep MRI study. Clin Otolaryngol. 2016; 41(6):700–706

[195] Liu SY, Huon LK, Iwasaki T, et al. Efficacy of maxillomandibu-lar advancement examined with drug-induced sleep endoscopy and computational fluid dynamics airflow modeling. Otolaryn-gol Head Neck Surg. 2016; 154(1):189–195

[196] Vicini C, Montevecchi F, Pang K, et al. Combined transoral robotic tongue base surgery and palate surgery in obstructive sleep apnea-hypopnea syndrome: expansion sphincter pharyngoplasty versus uvulopalatopharyngoplasty. Head Neck. 2014; 36(1):77–83

[197] Ulualp SO. Modified expansion sphincter pharyngoplasty for treatment of children with obstructive sleep apnea. JAMA Oto-laryngol Head Neck Surg. 2014; 140(9):817–822

[198] Carrasco-Llatas M, Marcano-Acuña M, Zerpa-Zerpa V, Dalmau-Galofre J. Surgical results of different palate techniques to treat oropharyngeal collapse. Eur Arch Otorhinolaryngol. 2015; 272(9):2535–2540

[199] Pang KP, Siow JK, Tseng P. Safety of multilevel surgery in obstruc-tive sleep apnea: a review of 487 cases. Arch Otolaryngol Head Neck Surg. 2012; 138(4):353–357

[200] Young T, Palta M, Dempsey J, et al. The occurrence of SDB among middle-aged adults. N Engl J Med. 1993; 328:1230–1235

[201] Young T, Evans L, Finn L, Palta M. Estimation of the clinically diagnosed proportion of sleep apnea syndrome in middle-aged men and women. Sleep. 1997; 20(9):705–706

[202] Ellis PD. Laser palatoplasty for snoring due to palatal flutter: a further report. Clin Otolaryngol Allied Sci. 1994; 19(4):350–351

[203] Mair EA, Day RH. Cautery-assisted palatal stiffening operation. Otolaryngol Head Neck Surg. 2000; 122(4):547–556

[204] Pang KP, Terris DJ. Modified cautery-assisted palatal stiffening operation: new method for treating snoring and mild obstructive sleep apnea. Otolaryngol Head Neck Surg. 2007; 136(5):823–826

[205] Pang KP, Tan R, Puraviappan P, Terris DJ. Anterior palatoplasty for the treatment of OSA: three-year results. Otolaryngol Head Neck Surg. 2009; 141(2):253–256

[206] Salamanca F, Costantini F, Mantovani M, et al. Barbed anterior pharyngoplasty: an evolution of anterior palatoplasty. Acta Oto-rhinolaryngol Ital. 2014; 34(6):434–438

[207] Mantovani M, Minetti A, Torretta S, Pincherle A, Tassone G, Pignataro L. The "Barbed Roman Blinds" technique: a step forward. Acta Otorhinolaryngol Ital. 2013; 33(2):128

[208] Mantovani M, Minetti A, Torretta S, Pincherle A, Tassone G, Pignataro L. The velo-uvulo-pharyngeal lift or "roman blinds" technique for treatment of snoring: a preliminary report. Acta Otorhinolaryngol Ital. 2012; 32(1):48–53

[209] Marzetti A, Tedaldi M, Passali FM. Preliminary findings from our experience in anterior palatoplasty for the treatment of

obstructive sleep apnea. Clin Exp Otorhinolaryngol. 2013; 6(1):18–22

[210] Ugur KS, Kurtaran H, Ark N, Kizilbulut G, Yuksel A, Gunduz M. Comparing anterior palatoplasty and modified uvulopalatopharyngoplasty for primary snoring patients: preliminary results. B-ENT. 2013; 9(4):285–291

[211] Ugur KS, Ark N, Kurtaran H, Kizilbulut G, Yuksel A, Gunduz M. Anterior palatoplasty for selected mild and moderate obstructive sleep apnea: preliminary results. Eur Arch Otorhinolaryngol. 2014; 271(6):1777–1783

[212] Beyers J, Vanderveken O, Van de Heyning P, Hamans E. The role of soft-tissue surgery of the tongue in obstructive sleep apnea. Current otorhinolaryngology reports. Curr Otorhinolaryngol Rep. 2016; 4:13–25

[213] Vroegop AV, Vanderveken OM, Boudewyns AN, et al. Drug-induced sleep endoscopy in sleep-disordered breathing: report on 1,249 cases. Laryngoscope. 2014; 124(3):797–802

[214] Hamans E, Boudewyns A, Stuck BA, et al. Adjustable tongue advancement for obstructive sleep apnea: a pilot study. Ann Otol Rhinol Laryngol. 2008; 117(11):815–823

[215] Handler E, Hamans E, Goldberg AN, Mickelson S. Tongue suspension: an evidence-based review and comparison to hypopharyngeal surgery for OSA. Laryngoscope. 2014; 124(1):329–336

[216] Pavelec V, Rotenberg BW, Maurer JT, Gillis E, Verse T. A novel implantable device for the treatment of obstructive sleep apnea: clinical safety and feasibility. Nat Sci Sleep. 2016; 8:137–144

[217] Kühnel TS, Schurr C, Wagner B, Geisler P. Morphological changes of the posterior airway space after tongue base suspension. Laryngoscope. 2005; 115(3):475–480

[218] Senders CW, Strong EB. The surgical treatment of obstructive sleep apnea. Clin Rev Allergy Immunol. 2003; 25(3):213–220

[219] Kezirian EJ, Goldberg AN. Hypopharyngeal surgery in obstructive sleep apnea: an evidence-based medicine review. Arch Otolaryngol Head Neck Surg. 2006; 132(2):206–213

[220] Zerpa Zerpa V, Carrasco Llatas M, Agostini Porras G, Dalmau Galofre J. Drug-induced sedation endoscopy versus clinical exploration for the diagnosis of severe upper airway obstruction in OSAHS patients. Sleep Breath. 2015; 19(4):1367–1372

[221] Eichler C, Sommer JU, Stuck BA, Hörmann K, Maurer JT. Does drug-induced sleep endoscopy change the treatment concept of patients with snoring and obstructive sleep apnea? Sleep Breath. 2013; 17(1):63–68

[222] Hewitt RJB, Dasgupta A, Singh A, Dutta C, Kotecha BT. Is sleep nasendoscopy a valuable adjunct to clinical examination in the evaluation of upper airway obstruction? Eur Arch Otorhinolaryngol. 2009; 266(5):691–697

[223] Son EL, Underbrink MP, Qiu S, Resto VA. The surgical plane for lingual tonsillectomy: an anatomic study. J Otolaryngol Head Neck Surg. 2016; 45:22

[224] Leitzbach SU, Bodlaj R, Maurer JT, Hörmann K, Stuck BA. Safety of cold ablation (coblation) in the treatment of tonsillar hypertrophy of the tongue base. Eur Arch Otorhinolaryngol. 2014; 271(6):1635–1639

[225] Wee JH, Tan K, Lee WH, Rhee CS, Kim JW. Evaluation of coblation lingual tonsil removal technique for obstructive sleep apnea in Asians: preliminary results of surgical morbidity and prognosticators. Eur Arch Otorhinolaryngol. 2015; 272(9):2327–2333

[226] Lee JM, Weinstein GS, O'Malley BW Jr, Thaler ER. Transoral robot-assisted lingual tonsillectomy and uvulopalatopharyngoplasty for obstructive sleep apnea. Ann Otol Rhinol Laryngol. 2012; 121(10):635–639

[227] Verse T, Wenzel S, Brus J. Multi-level surgery for obstructive sleep apnea. Lingual tonsillectomy vs. hyoid suspension in combination with radiofrequency of the tongue base. Sleep Breath. 2015; 19(4):1361–1366

[228] Kang KT, Koltai PJ, Lee CH, Lin MT, Hsu WC. Lingual tonsillectomy for treatment of pediatric obstructive sleep apnea: a meta-analysis. JAMA Otolaryngol Head Neck Surg. 2017; 143(6):561–568

[229] DeMarcantonio MA, Senser E, Meinzen-Derr J, Roetting N, Shott S, Ishman SL. The safety and efficacy of pediatric lingual tonsillectomy. Int J Pediatr Otorhinolaryngol. 2016; 91:6–10

[230] O'Malley BW Jr, Weinstein GS, Snyder W, Hockstein NG. Transoral robotic surgery (TORS) for base of tongue neoplasms. Laryngoscope. 2006; 116(8):1465–1472

[231] Weinstein GS, O'Malley BW Jr, Magnuson JS, et al. Transoral robotic surgery: a multicenter study to assess feasibility, safety, and surgical margins. Laryngoscope. 2012; 122(8):1701–1707

[232] Friedman M, Soans R, Gurpinar B, Lin HC, Joseph N. Evaluation of submucosal minimally invasive lingual excision technique for treatment of obstructive sleep apnea/hypopnea syndrome. Otolaryngol Head Neck Surg. 2008; 139(3):378–384, discussion 385

[233] Fujita S, Woodson BT, Clark JL, Wittig R. Laser midline glossectomy as a treatment for obstructive sleep apnea. Laryngoscope. 1991; 101(8):805–809

[234] Maturo SC, Mair EA. Coblation lingual tonsillectomy. Otolaryngol Head Neck Surg. 2006; 135(3):487–488

[235] Michelson SA. Radiofrequency tissue volume reduction of the tongue. In: Terris DJ, Goode RL. Surgical Management of Sleep Apnoea and Snoring. Boca Raton, FL: Taylor & Francis; 2005

[236] Woodson BT. Innovative technique for lingual tonsillectomy and midline posterior glossectomy for obstructive sleep apnea. Oper Tech Otolaryngol–Head Neck Surg. 2007; 18:20–28

[237] Chabolle F, Wagner I, Blumen MB, Séquert C, Fleury B, De Dieuleveult T. Tongue base reduction with hyoepiglottoplasty: a treatment for severe obstructive sleep apnea. Laryngoscope. 1999; 109(8):1273–1280

[238] Sorrenti G, Piccin O, Mondini S, Ceroni AR. One-phase management of severe obstructive sleep apnea: tongue base reduction with hyoepiglottoplasty plus uvulopalatopharyngoplasty. Otolaryngol Head Neck Surg. 2006; 135(6):906–910

[239] Vicini C, ed. Tongue-base reduction with hyoepiglottoplasty [TBRHE di Chabolle]. In: Chirurgia della RoncopatiaA. 1st ed. Lucca: Eureka; 2007: 253–259

[240] Vicini C, Montevecchi F, Campanini A, et al. Clinical outcomes and complications associated with TORS for OSAHS: a benchmark for evaluating an emerging surgical technology in a targeted application for benign disease. ORL J Otorhinolaryngol Relat Spec. 2014; 76(2):63–69

[241] Vicini C, Hoff P, Montevecchi F, eds. TransOral Robotic Surgery for Obstructive Sleep Apnea. Springer, New York: NY; 2016.

[242] Young T, Peppard PE, Gottlieb DJ. Epidemiology of obstructive sleep apnea: a population health perspective. Am J Respir Crit Care Med. 2002; 165(9):1217–1239

[243] Giles TL, Lasserson TJ, Smith BH, White J, Wright J, Cates CJ. Continuous positive airways pressure for obstructive sleep apnoea in adults. Cochrane Database Syst Rev. 2006; 3(3):CD001106

[244] Barkdull GC, Kohl CA, Patel M, Davidson TM. Computed tomography imaging of patients with obstructive sleep apnea. Laryngoscope. 2008; 118(8):1486–1492

[245] Abdullah VJ, Van Hasselt CA. Video sleep nasendoscopy. In: Terris DJ, Goode RL, eds. Surgical Management of Sleep Apnoea and Snoring. 1st ed. Taylor & Francis, Boca Raton: FL; 2005

[246] Campanini A, Canzi P, De Vito A, Dallan I, Montevecchi F, Vicini C. Awake versus sleep endoscopy: personal experience in 250 OSAHS patients. Acta Otorhinolaryngol Ital. 2010; 30(2):73–77

[247] Pringle MB, Croft CB. A comparison of sleep nasendoscopy and the Muller manoeuvre. Clin Otolaryngol Allied Sci. 1991; 16(6):559–562

[248] Kezirian EJ. Nonresponders to pharyngeal surgery for obstructive sleep apnea: insights from drug-induced sleep endoscopy. Laryngoscope. 2011; 121(6):1320–1326

[249] Hillman DR, Loadsman JA, Platt PR, Eastwood PR. Obstructive sleep apnoea and anaesthesia. Sleep Med Rev. 2004; 8(6):459–471

[250] Campanini A, De Vito A, Frassineti S, Vicini C. Temporary tracheotomy in the surgical treatment of obstructive sleep apnea syndrome: personal experience. Acta Otorhinolaryngol Ital. 2003; 23(6):474–478

[251] Sun H, Lou W, Wang L, Wu Y. Clinical significance of preoperative tracheotomy in preventing perioperative OSAHS severe complications Lin Chuang Er Bi Yan Hou Ke Za Zhi. 2005; 19(9):394–395

[252] Cormack RS, Lehane J. Difficult tracheal intubation in obstetrics. Anaesthesia. 1984; 39(11):1105–1111

[253] Vicini C, Montevecchi F, Tenti G, Canzi P, Dallan I, Tod H. Huntley. Transoral robotic surgery: tongue base reduction and supraglottoplasty for obstructive sleep apnea. Operative Technique in Otolaryngology. 2012; 23(1):45–47

[254] Vicini C, Dallan I, Canzi P, Frassineti S, La Pietra MG, Montevecchi F. Transoral robotic tongue base resection in obstructive sleep apnoea-hypopnoea syndrome: a preliminary report. ORL J Otorhinolaryngol Relat Spec. 2010; 72(1):22–27

[255] Vicini C, Dallan I, Canzi P, et al. Transoral robotic surgery of the tongue base in obstructive sleep Apnea-Hypopnea syndrome: anatomic considerations and clinical experience. Head Neck. 2012; 34(1):15–22

[256] Sequert C, Lestang P, Baglin AC, Wagner I, Ferron JM, Chabolle F. Hypoglossal nerve in its intralingual trajectory: anatomy and clinical implications Ann Otolaryngol Chir Cervicofac. 1999; 116(4):207–217

[257] Lauretano AM, Li KK, Caradonna DS, Khosta RK, Fried MP. Anatomic location of the tongue base neurovascular bundle. Laryngoscope. 1997; 107(8):1057–1059

[258] Riley R, Guilleminault C, Powell N, Derman S. Mandibular osteotomy and hyoid bone advancement for obstructive sleep apnea: a case report. Sleep. 1984; 7(1):79–82

[259] Riley RW, Powell NB, Guilleminault C. Inferior sagittal osteotomy of the mandible with hyoid myotomy-suspension: a new procedure for obstructive sleep apnea. Otolaryngol Head Neck Surg. 1986; 94(5):589–593

[260] Riley RW, Powell NB, Guilleminault C. Obstructive sleep apnea and the hyoid: a revised surgical procedure. Otolaryngol Head Neck Surg. 1994; 111(6):717–721

[261] Hörmann K, Baisch A. The hyoid suspension. Laryngoscope. 2004; 114(9):1677–1679

[262] Verse T, Baisch A, Maurer JT, Stuck BA, Hörmann K. Multilevel surgery for obstructive sleep apnea: short-term results. Otolaryngol Head Neck Surg. 2006; 134(4):571–577

[263] Tschopp KP. Modification of the Hörmann technique of hyoid suspension in obstructive sleep apnoea. J Laryngol Otol. 2007; 121(5):491–493

[264] Piccin O, Scaramuzzino G, Martone C, Marra F, Gobbi R, Sorrenti G. Modified hyoid suspension technique in the treatment of multilevel related obstructive sleep apnea. Otolaryngol Head Neck Surg. 2014; 150(2):321–324

[265] Neruntarat C. Hyoid myotomy with suspension under local anesthesia for obstructive sleep apnea syndrome. Eur Arch Otorhinolaryngol. 2003; 260(5):286–290

[266] Bowden MT, Kezirian EJ, Utley D, Goode RL. Outcomes of hyoid suspension for the treatment of obstructive sleep apnea. Arch Otolaryngol Head Neck Surg. 2005; 131(5):440–445

[267] den Herder C, van Tinteren H, de Vries N. Hyoidthyroidpexia: a surgical treatment for sleep apnea syndrome. Laryngoscope. 2005; 115(4):740–745

[268] Benazzo M, Pagella F, Matti E, et al. Hyoidthyroidpexia as a treatment in multilevel surgery for obstructive sleep apnea. Acta Otolaryngol. 2008; 128(6):680–684

[269] Richard W, Kox D, den Herder C, van Tinteren H, de Vries N. One stage multilevel surgery (uvulopalatopharyngoplasty, hyoid suspension, radiofrequent ablation of the tongue base with/without genioglossus advancement), in obstructive sleep apnea syndrome. Eur Arch Otorhinolaryngol. 2007; 264(4):439–444

[270] Stuck BA, Neff W, Hörmann K, et al. Anatomic changes after hyoid suspension for obstructive sleep apnea: an MRI study. Otolaryngol Head Neck Surg. 2005; 133(3):397–402

[271] Safiruddin F, Mourits DL, de Vries N. Thyroglossal duct cysts and obstructive sleep apnoea: three case reports and review of the literature. J Laryngol Otol. 2014; 128(8):738–741

[272] Riley RW, Powell NB, Guilleminault C. Obstructive sleep apnea syndrome: a review of 306 consecutively treated surgical patients. Otolaryngol Head Neck Surg. 1993; 108(2):117–125

[273] Baisch A, Maurer JT, Hörmann K. The effect of hyoid suspension in a multilevel surgery concept for obstructive sleep apnea. Otolaryngol Head Neck Surg. 2006; 134(5):856–861

[274] Vilaseca I, Morelló A, Montserrat JM, Santamaría J, Iranzo A. Usefulness of uvulopalatopharyngoplasty with genioglossus and hyoid advancement in the treatment of obstructive sleep apnea. Arch Otolaryngol Head Neck Surg. 2002; 128(4):435–440

[275] Richard W, Timmer F, van Tinteren H, de Vries N. Complications of hyoid suspension in the treatment of obstructive sleep apnea syndrome. Eur Arch Otorhinolaryngol. 2011; 268(4):631–635

[276] Lewis MR, Ducic Y. Genioglossus muscle advancement with the genioglossus bone advancement technique for base of tongue obstruction. J Otolaryngol. 2003; 32(3):168–173

[277] Emara TA, Omara TA, Shouman WM. Modified genioglossus advancement and uvulopalatopharyngoplasty in patients with obstructive sleep apnea. Otolaryngol Head Neck Surg. 2011; 145(5):865–871

[278] den Herder C, van Tinteren H. de Vries, Nico. Sleep endoscopy versus Mallampati score in sleep apnea and scoring. Laryngoscope. 2005; 115:735–739

[279] Rodriguez-Bruno K, Goldberg AN, McCulloch CE, Kezirian EJ. Test-retest reliability of drug-induced sleep endoscopy. Otolaryngol Head Neck Surg. 2009; 140(5):646–651

[280] Barrera JE, Holbrook AB, Santos J, Popelka GR. Sleep MRI: novel technique to identify airway obstruction in obstructive sleep apnea. Otolaryngol Head Neck Surg. 2009; 140(3):423–425

[281] Barrera JE. Sleep magnetic resonance imaging: dynamic characteristics of the airway during sleep in obstructive sleep apnea syndrome. Laryngoscope. 2011; 121(6):1327–1335

[282] Partinen M, Guilleminault C, Quera-Salva MA, Jamieson A. Obstructive sleep apnea and cephalometric roentgenograms. The role of anatomic upper airway abnormalities in the definition of abnormal breathing during sleep. Chest. 1988; 93(6):1199–1205

[283] Riley RW, Powell NB, Guilleminault C. Maxillary, mandibular, and hyoid advancement for treatment of obstructive sleep apnea: a review of 40 patients. J Oral Maxillofac Surg. 1990; 48(1):20–26

[284] Rohrer JW, Eller R, Santillan PG, Barrera JE. Geniotubercle advancement with a uvulopalatal flap and its effect on swallow function in obstructive sleep apnea. Laryngoscope. 2015; 125(3):758–761

[285] Barrera JE, Powell NB, Riley RW. Facial skeletal surgery in the management of adult obstructive sleep apnea syndrome. Clin Plast Surg. 2007; 34(3):565–573

[286] Andrews J, Barrera JE. Does tension matter? A study of tension in geniotubercle advancement surgery. Otolaryngol Head Neck Surg. 2012; 145(2, suppl):270

[287] Barrera JE, Dion GR. Predicting surgical response using tensiometry in osa patients after genioglossus advancement with uvulopalatopharyngoplasty. Otolaryngol Head Neck Surg. 2016; 154(3):558–563

[288] Remmers JE, deGroot WJ, Sauerland EK, Anch AM. Pathogenesis of upper airway occlusion during sleep. J Appl Physiol. 1978; 44(6):931–938

[289] Schwartz AR, Smith PL, Oliven A. Electrical stimulation of the hypoglossal nerve: a potential therapy. J Appl Physiol (1985). 2014; 116(3):337–344

[290] Safiruddin F, Vanderveken OM, de Vries N, et al. Effect of upper-airway stimulation for obstructive sleep apnoea on airway dimensions. Eur Respir J. 2015; 45(1):129–138

[291] Heiser C, Edenharter G, Bas M, Wirth M, Hofauer B. Palatoglossus coupling in selective upper airway stimulation. Laryngoscope. 2017; 127(10):E378–E383

[292] Oliven A, Odeh M, Schnall RP. Improved upper airway patency elicited by electrical stimulation of the hypoglossus nerves. Respiration. 1996; 63(4):213–216

[293] Schwartz AR, Thut DC, Russ B, et al. Effect of electrical stimulation of the hypoglossal nerve on airflow mechanics in the isolated upper airway. Am Rev Respir Dis. 1993; 147(5):1144–1150

[294] Schwartz AR, Eisele DW, Hari A, Testerman R, Erickson D, Smith PL. Electrical stimulation of the lingual musculature in obstructive sleep apnea. J Appl Physiol (1985). 1996; 81(2):643–652

[295] Friedman M, Jacobowitz O, Hwang MS, et al. Targeted hypoglossal nerve stimulation for the treatment of obstructive sleep apnea: Six-month results. Laryngoscope. 2016; 126(11):2618–2623

[296] Maurer JT, Van de Heyning P, Lin HS, et al. Operative technique of upper airway stimulation—an implantable treatment of obstructive sleep apnea. Oper Tech Otolaryngol—Head Neck Surg. 2012; 23:227–233

[297] Heiser C, Thaler E, Boon M, Soose RJ, Woodson BT. Updates of operative techniques for upper airway stimulation. Laryngoscope. 2016; 126(Suppl 7):S12–S16

[298] Heiser C, Thaler E, Soose RJ, Woodson BT, Boon M. Technical tips during implantation of selective upper airway stimulation. Laryngoscope. 2018; 128(3):756–762

[299] Heiser C, Hofauer B, Lozier L, Woodson BT, Stark T. Nerve monitoring-guided selective hypoglossal nerve stimulation in obstructive sleep apnea patients. Laryngoscope. 2016; 126(12):2852–2858

[300] Heiser C, Maurer JT, Steffen A. Functional outcome of tongue motions with selective hypoglossal nerve stimulation in patients with obstructive sleep apnea. Sleep Breath. 2016; 20(2):553–560

[301] Strollo PJ, Soose R, Badr M, Strohl KP. Upper airway stimulation for obstructive sleep apnea: objective and patient reported outcomes after five years of follow-up. Sleep. 2017; 40:A209

[302] Heiser C. Advanced titration to treat a floppy epiglottis in selective upper airway stimulation. Laryngoscope. 2016; 126(Suppl 7):S22–S24

[303] Schwartz AR, Bennett ML, Smith PL, et al. Therapeutic electrical stimulation of the hypoglossal nerve in obstructive sleep apnea. Arch Otolaryngol Head Neck Surg. 2001; 127(10):1216–1223

[304] Vanderveken OM, Maurer JT, Hohenhorst W, et al. Evaluation of drug-induced sleep endoscopy as a patient selection tool for implanted upper airway stimulation for obstructive sleep apnea. J Clin Sleep Med. 2013; 9(5):433–438

[305] Van de Heyning PH, Badr MS, Baskin JZ, et al. Implanted upper airway stimulation device for obstructive sleep apnea. Laryngoscope. 2012; 122(7):1626–1633

[306] Strollo PJ Jr, Soose RJ, Maurer JT, et al. STAR Trial Group. Upper-airway stimulation for obstructive sleep apnea. N Engl J Med. 2014; 370(2):139–149

[307] Woodson BT, Gillespie MB, Soose RJ, et al. STAR Trial Investigators. STAR Trial Investigators. Randomized controlled withdrawal study of upper airway stimulation on OSA: short- and long-term effect. Otolaryngol Head Neck Surg. 2014; 151(5):880–887

[308] Strollo PJ Jr, Gillespie MB, Soose RJ, et al. Stimulation Therapy for Apnea Reduction (STAR) Trial Group. Upper airway stimulation for obstructive sleep apnea: durability of the treatment effect at 18 months. Sleep. 2015; 38(10):1593–1598

[309] Soose RJ, Woodson BT, Gillespie MB, et al. STAR Trial Investigators. Upper airway stimulation for obstructive sleep apnea: self-reported outcomes at 24 months. J Clin Sleep Med. 2016; 12(1):43–48

[310] Woodson BT, Soose RJ, Gillespie MB, et al. STAR Trial Investigators. Three-year outcomes of cranial nerve stimulation for obstructive sleep apnea: the STAR trial. Otolaryngol Head Neck Surg. 2016; 154(1):181–188

[311] Steffen A, Sommer JU, Hofauer B, Maurer JT, Hasselbacher K, Heiser C. Outcome after one year of upper airway stimulation for obstructive sleep apnea in a multicenter German post-market study. Laryngoscope. 2018; 128(2):509–515

[312] Heiser C, Maurer JT, Hofauer B, Sommer JU, Seitz A, Steffen A. Outcomes of upper airway stimulation for obstructive sleep apnea in a multicenter german postmarket study. Otolaryngol Head Neck Surg. 2017; 156(2):378–384

[313] Boon M, Huntley C, Steffen A, et al. Upper airway stimulation for obstructive sleep apnea—results from the adhere registry. Otolaryngol Head Neck Surg. 2017

[314] Mwenge GB, Rombaux P, Dury M, Lengelé B, Rodenstein D. Targeted hypoglossal neurostimulation for obstructive sleep apnoea: a 1-year pilot study. Eur Respir J. 2013; 41(2):360–367

[315] Rodenstein D, Rombaux P, Lengele B, Dury M, Mwenge GB. Residual effect of THN hypoglossal stimulation in obstructive sleep apnea: a disease-modifying therapy. Am J Respir Crit Care Med. 2013; 187(11):1276–1278

[316] Meyer zu Natrup C, Verse T. The VOTE-classification to describe findings during drug-induced sleep endoscopy in patients with sleep related breathing disorders. Results of the first 100 patients. [In German] Abstract. German ENT congress Berlin, 13–16.5. Abstract Book. 2015; 2015:260–261

[317] Kezirian EJ, White DP, Malhotra A, Ma W, McCulloch CE, Goldberg AN. Interrater reliability of drug-induced sleep endoscopy. Arch Otolaryngol Head Neck Surg. 2010; 136(4):393–397

[318] Torre C, Camacho M, Liu SY, Huon LK, Capasso R. Epiglottis collapse in adult obstructive sleep apnea: A systematic review. Laryngoscope. 2016; 126(2):515–523

[319] Andersen AP, Alving J, Lildholdt T, Wulff CH. Obstructive sleep apnea initiated by a lax epiglottis. A contraindication for continuous positive airway pressure. Chest. 1987; 91(4):621–623

[320] Verse T, Pirsig W. Age-related changes in the epiglottis causing failure of nasal continuous positive airway pressure therapy. J Laryngol Otol. 1999; 113(11):1022–1025

[321] Chetty KG, Kadifa F, Berry RB, Mahutte CK. Acquired laryngomalacia as a cause of obstructive sleep apnea. Chest. 1994; 106(6):1898–1899

[322] Golz A, Goldenberg D, Netzer A, Westerman ST, Joachims HZ. Epiglottic carcinoma presenting as obstructive sleep apnea. J Otolaryngol. 2001; 30(1):58–59

[323] Woo P. Acquired laryngomalacia: epiglottis prolapse as a cause of airway obstruction. Ann Otol Rhinol Laryngol. 1992; 101(4):314–320

[324] Catalfumo FJ, Golz A, Westerman ST, Gilbert LM, Joachims HZ, Goldenberg D. The epiglottis and obstructive sleep apnoea syndrome. J Laryngol Otol. 1998; 112(10):940–943

[325] Golz A, Goldenberg D, Westerman ST, et al. Laser partial epiglottidectomy as a treatment for obstructive sleep apnea and laryngomalacia. Ann Otol Rhinol Laryngol. 2000; 109(12 Pt 1):1140–1145

[326] Mickelson SA, Rosenthal L. Midline glossectomy and epiglottidectomy for obstructive sleep apnea syndrome. Laryngoscope. 1997; 107(5):614–619

[327] Lin HS, Rowley JA, Badr MS, et al. Transoral robotic surgery for treatment of obstructive sleep apnea-hypopnea syndrome. Laryngoscope. 2013; 123(7):1811–1816

[328] Toh ST, Han HJ, Tay HN, Kiong KL. Transoral robotic surgery for obstructive sleep apnea in Asian patients: a Singapore sleep centre experience. JAMA Otolaryngol Head Neck Surg. 2014; 140(7):624–629

[329] Coccagna G. Il Sonno e i suoi disturbi. 2nd ed. Padova: Piccin Editore; 2000

[330] Mayer E. Permanent tracheostomy for pulmonary cripples. Dis Chest. 1961; 39:581–584

[331] Penta AQ, Mayer E. Permanent tracheostomy in the treatment of pulmonary insufficiency. Ann Otol Rhinol Laryngol. 1960; 69:1157–1169

[332] Fee WE Jr, Ward PH. Permanent tracheostomy: a new surgical technique. Ann Otol Rhinol Laryngol. 1977; 86(5 Pt 1):635–638

[333] Campanini A, De Vito A, Frassineti S, Vicini C. Role of skin-lined tracheotomy in obstructive sleep apnoea syndrome: personal experience. Acta Otorhinolaryngol Ital. 2004; 24(2):68–74

[334] Motta J, Guilleminault C, Schroeder JS, Dement WC. Tracheostomy and hemodynamic changes in sleep-inducing apnea. Ann Intern Med. 1978; 89(4):454–458

[335] Partinen M, Jamieson A, Guilleminault C. Long-term outcome for obstructive sleep apnea syndrome patients. Mortality. Chest. 1988; 94(6):1200–1204

[336] Haapaniemi JJ, Laurikainen EA, Halme P, Antila J. Long-term results of tracheostomy for severe obstructive sleep apnea syndrome. ORL J Otorhinolaryngol Relat Spec. 2001; 63(3):131–136

[337] Camacho M, Certal V, Brietzke SE, Holty JE, Guilleminault C, Capasso R. Tracheostomy as treatment for adult obstructive sleep apnea: a systematic review and meta-analysis. Laryngoscope. 2014; 124(3):803–811

[338] Camacho M, Teixeira J, Abdullatif J, et al. Maxillomandibular advancement and tracheostomy for morbidly obese obstructive sleep apnea: a systematic review and meta-analysis. Otolaryngol Head Neck Surg. 2015; 152(4):619–630

[339] Guilleminault C, Simmons FB, Motta J. Obstructive sleep apnea syndrome and tracheostomy. Long-term follow-up experience. Arch Intern Med. 1981; 141(8):985–988

[340] Kim SH, Eisele DW, Smith PL, Schneider H, Schwartz AR. Evaluation of patients with sleep apnea after tracheotomy. Arch Otolaryngol Head Neck Surg. 1998; 124(9):996–1000

[341] Thatcher GW, Maisel RH. The long-term evaluation of tracheostomy in the management of severe obstructive sleep apnea. Laryngoscope. 2003; 113(2):201–204

[342] Mickelson SA. Upper airway bypass surgery for obstructive sleep apnea syndrome. Otolaryngol Clin North Am. 1998; 31(6):1013–1023

[343] Kuo PC, West RA, Bloomquist DS, McNeil RW. The effect of mandibular osteotomy in three patients with hypersomnia sleep apnea. Oral Surg Oral Med Oral Pathol. 1979; 48(5):385–392

[344] Riley RW, Powell NB, Guilleminault C, Nino-Murcia G. Maxillary, mandibular, and hyoid advancement: an alternative to tracheostomy in obstructive sleep apnea syndrome. Otolaryngol Head Neck Surg. 1986; 94(5):584–588

[345] Holty JE, Guilleminault C. Maxillomandibular advancement for the treatment of obstructive sleep apnea: a systematic review and meta-analysis. Sleep Med Rev. 2010; 14(5):287–297

[346] Zaghi S, Holty JE, Certal V, et al. Maxillomandibular advancement for treatment of obstructive sleep apnea: a meta-analysis. JAMA Otolaryngol Head Neck Surg. 2016; 142(1):58–66

[347] Conradt R, Hochban W, Brandenburg U, Heitmann J, Peter JH. Long-term follow-up after surgical treatment of obstructive sleep apnoea by maxillomandibular advancement. Eur Respir J. 1997; 10(1):123–128

[348] Riley RW, Powell NB, Li KK, Troell RJ, Guilleminault C. Surgery and obstructive sleep apnea: long-term clinical outcomes. Otolaryngol Head Neck Surg. 2000; 122(3):415–421

[349] Li KK, Riley RW, Powell NB, Guilleminault C. Patient's perception of the facial appearance after maxillomandibular advancement for obstructive sleep apnea syndrome. J Oral Maxillofac Surg. 2001; 59(4):377–380, discussion 380–381

[350] Doff MH, Jansma J, Schepers RH, Hoekema A. Maxillomandibular advancement surgery as alternative to continuous positive airway pressure in morbidly severe obstructive sleep apnea: a case report. Cranio. 2013; 31(4):246–251

[351] Prinsell JR. Primary and secondary telegnathic maxillomandibular advancement, with or without adjunctive procedures, for obstructive sleep apnea in adults: a literature review and treatment recommendations. J Oral Maxillofac Surg. 2012; 70(7):1659–1677

[352] Riley RW, Powell NB, Guilleminault C. Obstructive sleep apnea syndrome: a surgical protocol for dynamic upper airway reconstruction. J Oral Maxillofac Surg. 1993; 51(7):742–747, discussion 748–749

[353] Bettega G, Pépin JL, Veale D, Deschaux C, Raphaël B, Lévy P. Obstructive sleep apnea syndrome. Fifty-one consecutive patients treated by maxillofacial surgery. Am J Respir Crit Care Med. 2000; 162(2 Pt 1):641–649

[354] Hendler BH, Costello BJ, Silverstein K, Yen D, Goldberg A. A protocol for uvulopalatopharyngoplasty, mortised genioplasty, and maxillomandibular advancement in patients with obstructive sleep apnea: an analysis of 40 cases. J Oral Maxillofac Surg. 2001; 59(8):892–897, discussion 898–899

[355] Prinsell JR. Maxillomandibular advancement surgery in a site-specific treatment approach for obstructive sleep apnea in 50 consecutive patients. Chest. 1999; 116(6):1519–1529

[356] Waite PD, Wooten V, Lachner J, Guyette RF. Maxillomandibular advancement surgery in 23 patients with obstructive sleep apnea syndrome. J Oral Maxillofac Surg. 1989; 47(12):1256–1261, discussion 1262

[357] Hochban W, Conradt R, Brandenburg U, Heitmann J, Peter JH. Surgical maxillofacial treatment of obstructive sleep apnea. Plast Reconstr Surg. 1997; 99(3):619–626, discussion 627–628

[358] Hoekema A, de Lange J, Stegenga B, de Bont LG. Oral appliances and maxillomandibular advancement surgery: an alternative treatment protocol for the obstructive sleep apnea-hypopnea syndrome. J Oral Maxillofac Surg. 2006; 64(6):886–891

[359] Lye KW, Waite PD, Meara D, Wang D. Quality of life evaluation of maxillomandibular advancement surgery for treatment of obstructive sleep apnea. J Oral Maxillofac Surg. 2008; 66(5):968–972

[360] Barrera JE. Virtual surgical planning improves surgical outcome measures in obstructive sleep apnea surgery. Laryngoscope. 2014; 124(5):1259–1266

[361] Li KK, Riley RW, Powell NB, Gervacio L, Troell RJ, Guilleminault C. Obstructive sleep apnea surgery: patient perspective and polysomnographic results. Otolaryngol Head Neck Surg. 2000; 123(5):572–575

[362] Smatt Y, Ferri J. Retrospective study of 18 patients treated by maxillomandibular advancement with adjunctive procedures for obstructive sleep apnea syndrome. J Craniofac Surg. 2005; 16(5):770–777

[363] De Dieuleveult T, Wagner I, Meulien P, Fleury B, Hausser-Hawn C, Chabolle F. Retrospective cephalometric analysis for surgically treated obstructive sleep apnea: therapeutic deductions Ann Otolaryngol Chir Cervicofac. 2000; 117(6): 339–348

[364] Conley RS, Boyd SB. Facial soft tissue changes following maxillomandibular advancement for treatment of obstructive sleep apnea. J Oral Maxillofac Surg. 2007; 65(7):1332–1340

[365] Brevi BC, Toma L, Pau M, Sesenna E. Counterclockwise rotation of the occlusal plane in the treatment of obstructive sleep apnea syndrome. J Oral Maxillofac Surg. 2011; 69(3):917–923

[366] Posnick JC. Anesthesie techniques, blood loss/fluid replacement, airway management and convalescence in the treatment of dentofacial deformities. In: Posnick, JC, ed. Orthognathic Surgery Principles and Practice. St Louis, MO: Elsevier Saunders; 2014:308–336, chapter 11

[367] Posnick JC. A sequencing of orthognathic procedures: step-by-step approach. In: Posnick, JC, ed. Orthognathic Surgery Principles and Practice. St Louis, MO: Elsevier Saunders; 2014:441–476, chapter 15

[368] Waite PD, Wooten V. Maxillomandibular advancement: a surgical treatment of obstructive sleep apnea. In: Bell WH, ed. Modern Practice in Orthognathic and Reconstructive Surgery. Philadelphia, PA: W.B. Saunders; 1992; 2042–2059

[369] Hogan PW, Argalious M. Total airway obstruction after maxillomandibular advancement surgery for obstructive sleep apnea. Anesth Analg. 2006; 103(5):1267–1269

[370] Corcoran S, Mysliwiec V, Niven AS, Fallah D. Development of central sleep apnea after maxillofacial surgery for obstructive sleep apnea. J Clin Sleep Med. 2009; 5(2):151–153

[371] Blumen MB, Buchet I, Meulien P, Hausser Hauw C, Neveu H, Chabolle F. Complications/adverse effects of maxillomandibular advancement for the treatment of OSA in regard to outcome. Otolaryngol Head Neck Surg. 2009; 141(5):591–597

[372] Gregg JM, Zedalis D, Howard CW, Boyle RP, Prussin AJ. Surgical alternatives for treatment of obstructive sleep apnoea: review and case series. Ann R Australas Coll Dent Surg. 2000; 15:181–184

[373] Dekeister C, Lacassagne L, Tiberge M, Montemayor T, Migueres M, Paoli JR. Mandibular advancement surgery in patients with severe obstructive sleep apnea uncontrolled by continuous positive airway pressure. A retrospective review of 25 patients between 1998 and 2004 Rev Mal Respir. 2006; 23(5 Pt 1):430–437

[374] Raunio A, Rauhala E, Kiviharju M, Lehmijoki O, Sándor GK, Oikarinen K. Bimaxillary advancement as the initial treatment of obstructive sleep apnea: five years follow-up of the pori experience. J Oral Maxillofac Res. 2012; 3(1):e5

[375] Goh YH, Lim KA. Modified maxillomandibular advancement for the treatment of obstructive sleep apnea: a preliminary report. Laryngoscope. 2003; 113(9):1577–1582

[376] Louis PJ, Waite PD, Austin RB. Long-term skeletal stability after rigid fixation of Le Fort I osteotomies with advancements. Int J Oral Maxillofac Surg. 1993; 22(2):82–86

[377] Miles PG, Nimkarn Y. Maxillomandibular advancement surgery in patients with obstructive sleep apnea: mandibular morphology and stability. Int J Adult Orthodon Orthognath Surg. 1995; 10(3):193–200

[378] Nimkarn Y, Miles PG, Waite PD. Maxillomandibular advancement surgery in obstructive sleep apnea syndrome patients: long-term surgical stability. J Oral Maxillofac Surg. 1995; 53(12):1414–1418, discussion 1418–1419

[379] Goodday R, Bourque S. Subjective outcomes of maxillomandibular advancement surgery for treatment of obstructive sleep apnea syndrome. J Oral Maxillofac Surg. 2012; 70(2): 417–420

[380] Boyd SB, Walters AS, Song Y, Wang L. Comparative effectiveness of maxillomandibular advancement and uvulopalatopharyngoplasty for the treatment of moderate to severe obstructive sleep apnea. J Oral Maxillofac Surg. 2013; 71(4):743–751

[381] Conradt R, Hochban W, Heitmann J, et al. Sleep fragmentation and daytime vigilance in patients with OSA treated by surgical maxillomandibular advancement compared to CPAP therapy. J Sleep Res. 1998; 7(3):217–223

[382] Riley RW, Powell NB, Guilleminault C. Maxillofacial surgery and obstructive sleep apnea: a review of 80 patients. Otolaryngol Head Neck Surg. 1989; 101(3):353–361

[383] Vicini C, Dallan I, Campanini A, et al. Surgery vs ventilation in adult severe obstructive sleep apnea syndrome. Am J Otolaryngol. 2010; 31(1):14–20

[384] Hsieh YJ, Liao YF. Effects of maxillomandibular advancement on the upper airway and surrounding structures in patients with obstructive sleep apnoea: a systematic review. Br J Oral Maxillofac Surg. 2013; 51(8):834–840

[385] Hsieh YJ, Liao YF, Chen NH, Chen YR. Changes in the calibre of the upper airway and the surrounding structures after maxillomandibular advancement for obstructive sleep apnoea. Br J Oral Maxillofac Surg. 2014; 52(5):445–451

[386] Susarla SM, Abramson ZR, Dodson TB, Kaban LB. Upper airway length decreases after maxillomandibular advancement in patients with obstructive sleep apnea. J Oral Maxillofac Surg. 2011; 69(11):2872–2878

[387] Liu SY, Guilleminault C, Huon LK, Yoon A. Distraction osteogenesis maxillary expansion (DOME) for adult obstructive sleep apnea patients with high arched palate. Otolaryngol Head Neck Surg. 2017; 157(2):345–348

[388] Pirelli P, Saponara M, Guilleminault C. Rapid maxillary expansion in children with obstructive sleep apnea syndrome. Sleep. 2004; 27(4):761–766

[389] Pirelli P, Saponara M, Guilleminault C. Rapid maxillary expansion (RME) for pediatric obstructive sleep apnea: a 12-year follow-up. Sleep Med. 2015; 16(8):933–935

[390] Cistulli PA, Palmisano RG, Poole MD. Treatment of obstructive sleep apnea syndrome by rapid maxillary expansion. Sleep. 1998; 21(8):831–835

[391] Iwasaki T, Takemoto Y, Inada E, et al. The effect of rapid maxillary expansion on pharyngeal airway pressure during inspiration evaluated using computational fluid dynamics. Int J Pediatr Otorhinolaryngol. 2014; 78(8):1258–1264

[392] Iwasaki T, Saitoh I, Takemoto Y, et al. Tongue posture improvement and pharyngeal airway enlargement as secondary effects of rapid maxillary expansion: a cone-beam computed tomography study. Am J Orthod Dentofacial Orthop. 2013; 143(2):235–245

[393] Zambon CE, Ceccheti MM, Utumi ER, et al. Orthodontic measurements and nasal respiratory function after surgically assisted rapid maxillary expansion: an acoustic rhinometry and rhinomanometry study. Int J Oral Maxillofac Surg. 2012; 41(9):1120–1126

[394] Cistulli PA, Richards GN, Palmisano RG, Unger G, Berthon-Jones M, Sullivan CE. Influence of maxillary constriction on nasal resistance and sleep apnea severity in patients with Marfan's syndrome. Chest. 1996; 110(5):1184–1188

[395] Pogrel MA, Kaban LB, Vargervik K, Baumrind S. Surgically assisted rapid maxillary expansion in adults. Int J Adult Orthodon Orthognath Surg. 1992; 7(1):37–41

[396] Krebs A. Midpalatal suture expansion studies by the implant method over a seven-year period. Rep Congr Eur Orthod Soc. 1964; 40:131–142

[397] Stewart MG, Witsell DL, Smith TL, Weaver EM, Yueh B, Hannley MT. Development and validation of the nasal obstruction symptom evaluation (NOSE) scale. Otolaryngol Head Neck Surg. 2004; 130(2):157–163

[398] Yu JC, Fearon J, Havlik RJ, Buchman SR, Polley JW. Distraction Osteogenesis of the Craniofacial Skeleton. Plast Reconstr Surg. 2004; 114(1):1E–20E

[399] Swennen G, Schliephake H, Dempf R, Schierle H, Malevez C. Craniofacial distraction osteogenesis: a review of the literature: Part 1: clinical studies. Int J Oral Maxillofac Surg. 2001; 30(2):89–103

[400] Günbay T, Akay MC, Günbay S, Aras A, Koyuncu BO, Sezer B. Transpalatal distraction using bone-borne distractor: clinical observations and dental and skeletal changes. J Oral Maxillofac Surg. 2008; 66(12):2503–2514

[401] Fischer Y, Khan M, Mann WJ. Multilevel temperature-controlled radiofrequency therapy of soft palate, base of tongue, and tonsils in adults with obstructive sleep apnea. Laryngoscope. 2003; 113(10):1786–1791

[402] Woodson BT, Steward DL, Weaver EM, Javaheri S. A randomized trial of temperature-controlled radiofrequency, continuous positive airway pressure, and placebo for obstructive sleep apnea syndrome. Otolaryngol Head Neck Surg. 2003; 128(6):848–861

[403] Stuck BA, Starzak K, Hein G, Verse T, Hörmann K, Maurer JT. Combined radiofrequency surgery of the tongue base and soft palate in obstructive sleep apnoea. Acta Otolaryngol. 2004; 124(7):827–832

[404] Steward DL. Effectiveness of multilevel (tongue and palate) radiofrequency tissue ablation for patients with obstructive sleep apnea syndrome. Laryngoscope. 2004; 114(12):2073–2084

[405] Friedman M, Lin HC, Gurpinar B, Joseph NJ. Minimally invasive single-stage multilevel treatment for obstructive sleep apnea/hypopnea syndrome. Laryngoscope. 2007; 117(10):1859–1863

[406] Ceylan K, Emir H, Kizilkaya Z, et al. First-choice treatment in mild to moderate obstructive sleep apnea: single-stage, multilevel, temperature-controlled radiofrequency tissue volume reduction or nasal continuous positive airway pressure. Arch Otolaryngol Head Neck Surg. 2009; 135(9):915–919

[407] Bäck LJ, Liukko T, Rantanen I, et al. Hypertonic saline injections to enhance the radiofrequency thermal ablation effect in the treatment of base of tongue in obstructive sleep apnoea patients: a pilot study. Acta Otolaryngol. 2009; 129(3):302–310

[408] Riley RW, Powell NB, Guilleminault C. Inferior mandibular osteotomy and hyoid myotomy suspension for obstructive sleep apnea: a review of 55 patients. J Oral Maxillofac Surg. 1989; 47(2):159–164

[409] Djupesland G, Schrader H, Lyberg T, Refsum H, Lilleås F, Godtlibsen OB. Palatopharyngoglossoplasty in the treatment of patients with obstructive sleep apnea syndrome. Acta Otolaryngol Suppl. 1992; 492:50–54

[410] Johnson NT, Chinn J. Uvulopalatopharyngoplasty and inferior sagittal mandibular osteotomy with genioglossus advancement for treatment of obstructive sleep apnea. Chest. 1994; 105(1):278–283

[411] Ramirez SG, Loube DI. Inferior sagittal osteotomy with hyoid bone suspension for obese patients with sleep apnea. Arch Otolaryngol Head Neck Surg. 1996; 122(9):953–957

[412] Utley DS, Shin EJ, Clerk AA, Terris DJ. A cost-effective and rational surgical approach to patients with snoring, upper airway resistance syndrome, or obstructive sleep apnea syndrome. Laryngoscope. 1997; 107(6):726–734

[413] Elasfour A, Miyazaki S, Itasaka Y, Yamakawa K, Ishikawa K, Togawa K. Evaluation of uvulopalatopharyngoplasty in treatment of obstructive sleep apnea syndrome. Acta Otolaryngol Suppl. 1998; 537:52–56

[414] Lee NR, Givens CD Jr, Wilson J, Robins RB. Staged surgical treatment of obstructive sleep apnea syndrome: a review of 35 patients. J Oral Maxillofac Surg. 1999; 57(4):382–385

[415] Hsu PP, Brett RH. Multiple level pharyngeal surgery for obstructive sleep apnoea. Singapore Med J. 2001; 42(4):160–164

[416] Terris DJ, Kunda LD, Gonella MC. Minimally invasive tongue base surgery for obstructive sleep apnoea. J Laryngol Otol. 2002; 116(9):716–721

[417] Miller FR, Watson D, Malis D. Role of the tongue base suspension suture with The Repose System bone screw in the multilevel surgical management of obstructive sleep apnea. Otolaryngol Head Neck Surg. 2002; 126(4):392–398

[418] Neruntarat C. Genioglossus advancement and hyoid myotomy under local anesthesia. Otolaryngol Head Neck Surg. 2003; 129(1):85–91

[419] Neruntarat C. Genioglossus advancement and hyoid myotomy: short-term and long-term results. J Laryngol Otol. 2003; 117(6):482–486

[420] Sorrenti G, Piccin O, Latini G, Scaramuzzino G, Mondini S, Rinaldi Ceroni A. Tongue base suspension technique in obstructive sleep apnea: personal experience. Acta Otorhinolaryngol Ital. 2003; 23(4):274–280

[421] Sorrenti G, Piccin O, Scaramuzzino G, Mondini S, Cirignotta F, Ceroni AR. Tongue base reduction with hyoepiglottoplasty for the treatment of severe OSA. Acta Otorhinolaryngol Ital. 2004; 24(4):204–210

[422] Miller FR, Watson D, Boseley M. The role of the Genial Bone Advancement Trephine system in conjunction with

uvulopalatopharyngoplasty in the multilevel management of obstructive sleep apnea. Otolaryngol Head Neck Surg. 2004; 130(1):73–79

[423] Dattilo DJ, Drooger SA. Outcome assessment of patients undergoing maxillofacial procedures for the treatment of sleep apnea: comparison of subjective and objective results. J Oral Maxillofac Surg. 2004; 62(2):164–168

[424] Hörmann K, Maurer JT, Baisch A. [Snoring/sleep apnea—surgically curable] HNO. 2004; 52(9):807–813

[425] Li HY, Wang PC, Hsu CY, Chen NH, Lee LA, Fang TJ. Same-stage palatopharyngeal and hypopharyngeal surgery for severe obstructive sleep apnea. Acta Otolaryngol. 2004; 124(7):820–826

[426] Verse T, Baisch A, Hörmann K. [Multi-level surgery for obstructive sleep apnea. Preliminary objective results] Laryngorhinootologie. 2004; 83(8):516–522

[427] Omur M, Ozturan D, Elez F, Unver C, Derman S. Tongue base suspension combined with UPPP in severe OSA patients. Otolaryngol Head Neck Surg. 2005; 133(2):218–223

[428] Hsieh TH, Fang TJ, Li HY, Lee SW. Simultaneous midline laser glossectomy with palatopharyngeal surgery for obstructive sleep apnoea syndrome. Int J Clin Pract. 2005; 59(4):501–503

[429] Liu SA, Li HY, Tsai WC, Chang KM. Associated factors to predict outcomes of uvulopharyngopalatoplasty plus genioglossal advancement for obstructive sleep apnea. Laryngoscope. 2005; 115(11):2046–2050

[430] Jacobowitz O. Palatal and tongue base surgery for surgical treatment of obstructive sleep apnea: a prospective study. Otolaryngol Head Neck Surg. 2006; 135(2):258–264

[431] Vicente E, Marín JM, Carrizo S, Naya MJ. Tongue-base suspension in conjunction with uvulopalatopharyngoplasty for treatment of severe obstructive sleep apnea: long-term follow-up results. Laryngoscope. 2006; 116(7):1223–1227

[432] Yin SK, Yi HL, Lu WY, Guan J, Wu HM, Cao ZY. Genioglossus advancement and hyoid suspension plus uvulopalatopharyngoplasty for severe OSAHS. Otolaryngol Head Neck Surg. 2007; 136(4):626–631

[433] Sun X, Yi H, Cao Z, Yin S. Reorganization of sleep architecture after surgery for OSAHS. Acta Otolaryngol. 2008; 128(11):1242–1247

[434] Fernández-Julián E, Muñoz N, Achiques MT, García-Pérez MA, Orts M, Marco J. Randomized study comparing two tongue base surgeries for moderate to severe obstructive sleep apnea syndrome. Otolaryngol Head Neck Surg. 2009; 140(6):917–923

[435] Kezirian EJ, Malhotra A, Goldberg AN, White DP. Changes in obstructive sleep apnea severity, biomarkers, and quality of life after multilevel surgery. Laryngoscope. 2010; 120(7):1481–1488

[436] Babademez MA, Yorubulut M, Yurekli MF, et al. Comparison of minimally invasive techniques in tongue base surgery in patients with obstructive sleep apnea. Otolaryngol Head Neck Surg. 2011; 145(5):858–864

[437] Sezen OS, Aydin E, Eraslan G, Haytoglu S, Coskuner T, Unver S. Modified tongue base suspension for multilevel or single tract obstructions in sleep apnea: clinical and radiologic results. Auris Nasus Larynx. 2011; 38(4):487–494

[438] van Maanen JP, Ravesloot MJ, Witte BI, Grijseels M, de Vries N. Exploration of the relationship between sleep position and isolated tongue base or multilevel surgery in obstructive sleep apnea. Eur Arch Otorhinolaryngol. 2012; 269(9):2129–2136

[439] Hou J, Yan J, Wang B, et al. Treatment of obstructive sleep apnea-hypopnea syndrome with combined uvulopalatopharyngoplasty and midline glossectomy: outcomes from a 5-year study. Respir Care. 2012; 57(12):2104–2110

[440] Tunçel U, Inançlı HM, Kürkçüoğlu SS, Enoz M. A comparison of unilevel and multilevel surgery in obstructive sleep apnea syndrome. Ear Nose Throat J. 2012; 91(8):E13–E18

[441] Friedman M, Hamilton C, Samuelson CG, et al. Transoral robotic glossectomy for the treatment of obstructive sleep apnea-hypopnea syndrome. Otolaryngol Head Neck Surg. 2012; 146(5):854–862

[442] Berg EE, Bunge F, Delgaudio JM. Multilevel treatment of moderate and severe obstructive sleep apnea with bone-anchored pharyngeal suspension sutures. Ear Nose Throat J. 2013; 92(8):E1

[443] Li S, Wu D, Shi H. Treatment of obstructive sleep apnea hypopnea syndrome caused by glossoptosis with tongue-base suspension. Eur Arch Otorhinolaryngol. 2013; 270(11):2915–2920

[444] Cillo JE Jr, Dalton PS, Dattilo DJ. Combined elliptical window genioglossus advancement, hyoid bone suspension, and uvulopalatopharyngoplasty decrease apnea hypopnea index and subjective daytime sleepiness in obstructive sleep apnea. J Oral Maxillofac Surg. 2013; 71(10):1729–1732

[445] Gunawardena I, Robinson S, MacKay S, et al. Submucosal lingualplasty for adult obstructive sleep apnea. Otolaryngol Head Neck Surg. 2013; 148(1):157–165

[446] Suh GD. Evaluation of open midline glossectomy in the multilevel surgical management of obstructive sleep apnea syndrome. Otolaryngol Head Neck Surg. 2013; 148(1):166–171

[447] Li S, Wu D, Bao J, Qin J. Nasopharyngeal tube: a simple and effective tool to screen patients indicated for glossopharyngeal surgery. J Clin Sleep Med. 2014; 10(4):385–389

[448] Hoff PT, Glazer TA, Spector ME. Body mass index predicts success in patients undergoing transoral robotic surgery for obstructive sleep apnea. ORL J Otorhinolaryngol Relat Spec. 2014; 76(5):266–272

[449] Lin HS, Rowley JA, Folbe AJ, Yoo GH, Badr MS, Chen W. Transoral robotic surgery for treatment of obstructive sleep apnea: factors predicting surgical response. Laryngoscope. 2015; 125(4):1013–1020

[450] Turhan M, Bostanci A, Bozkurt S. Predicting the outcome of modified tongue base suspension combined with uvulopalatopharyngoplasty. Eur Arch Otorhinolaryngol. 2015; 272(11):3411–3416

[451] Chiffer RC, Schwab RJ, Keenan BT, Borek RC, Thaler ER. Volumetric MRI analysis pre- and post-Transoral robotic surgery for obstructive sleep apnea. Laryngoscope. 2015; 125(8):1988–1995

[452] Yüksel A, Ugur KS, Kizilbulut G, et al. Long-term results of one staged multilevel surgery with tongue suspension surgery or one level palatal surgery for treatment of moderate and severe obstructive sleep apnea. Eur Arch Otorhinolaryngol. 2016; 273(5):1227–1234

[453] Thaler ER, Rassekh CH, Lee JM, Weinstein GS, O'Malley BW Jr. Outcomes for multilevel surgery for sleep apnea: Obstructive sleep apnea, transoral robotic surgery, and uvulopalatopharyngoplasty. Laryngoscope. 2016; 126(1):266–269

[454] Li HY, Lee LA, Kezirian EJ. Coblation endoscopic lingual lightening (CELL) for obstructive sleep apnea. Eur Arch Otorhinolaryngol. 2016; 273(1):231–236

[455] Gillespie MB, Soose RJ, Woodson BT, et al. STAR Trial Investigators. Upper airway stimulation for obstructive sleep apnea: patient-reported outcomes after 48 months of follow-up. Otolaryngol Head Neck Surg. 2017; 156(4):765–771

[456] Campanini A, Canzi P, De Vito A, Dallan I, Montevecchi F, Vicini C. Awake versus sleep endoscopy: personal experience in 250 OSAHS patients. Acta Otorhinolaryngol Ital. 2010; 30(2):73–77

Recommended Readings

den Herder C, Kox D, van Tinteren H, de Vries N. Bipolar radiofrequency induced thermotherapy of the tongue base: its complications, acceptance and effectiveness under local anesthesia. Eur Arch Otorhinolaryngol. 2006; 263(11):1031–1040

Li KK, Powell NB, Riley RW, Troell R, Guilleminault C. Overview of phase I surgery for obstructive sleep apnea syndrome. Ear Nose Throat J. 1999; 78(11):836–837, 841–845

Oksenberg A, Silverberg DS, Arons E, Radwan H. Positional vs. nonpositional obstructive sleep apnea patients: anthropomorphic, nocturnal polysomnographic, and multiple sleep latency test data. Chest. 1997; 112(3):629–639

Peppard PE, Young T, Palta M, Dempsey J, Skatrud J. Longitudinal study of moderate weight change and sleep-disordered breathing. JAMA. 2000; 284(23):3015–3021

Richard W, Kox D, den Herder C, Laman M, van Tinteren H, de Vries N. The role of sleep position in obstructive sleep apnea syndrome. Eur Arch Otorhinolaryngol. 2006; 263(10):946–950

Stuck BA, Köpke J, Maurer JT, et al. Lesion formation in radiofrequency surgery of the tongue base. Laryngoscope. 2003; 113(9):1572–1576

9 Bariatric Surgery

Christel de Raaff, Bart van Wagensveld, and Nico de Vries

Abstract

Obesity is a problem worldwide. Bariatric surgery has shown to be the only effective treatment for morbid obesity in the long term. The two most performed procedures are the laparoscopic Roux-en-Y gastric bypass and laparoscopic sleeve gastrectomy. Overall, around 10% of patients experience a postoperative complication varying in severity. The incidence of anastomotic leakage is 1% and mortality rate is 0.25%. One of the most common comorbidities in morbidly obese patients is obstructive sleep apnea (OSA). Since two-third of bariatric surgery patients have OSA and one-third have moderately severe disease, all bariatric patients should be screened for OSA prior to surgery. The gold standard for diagnosing OSA is polysomnography. After surgery, mean excess weight loss is around 70% (target body mass index 25 kg/m²). The apnea-hypopnea-index (AHI) decreases from 66 to 25/hour in the severe OSA group, from 21 to 9/hour in the moderate OSA group, and from 10 to 5/hour in the mild OSA group. OSA is cured in 54, 25, and 18% of the preoperatively diagnosed severe, moderate, and mild OSA patients, respectively. At least 75% of the moderately severe OSA patients achieve AHI levels below 15/hour and could, therefore, become independent of continuous positive airway pressure therapy.

Keywords: morbid obesity, bariatric surgery, metabolic surgery; weight loss surgery; laparoscopic Roux-en-Y gastric bypass, laparoscopic sleeve gastrectomy

9.1 Definition

Obesity is defined as body mass index (BMI) greater than or equal to 30 kg/m² (▶Table 9.1). This disease is affecting more than 600 million adults worldwide.[1] In 2014, the World Health Organization stated that 13% of adults aged 18 years and over were obese.[1] Obesity predisposes to comorbidities affecting every organ system. Examples are obstructive sleep apnea (OSA), type II diabetes, dyslipidemia, hypertension, several types of cancer, depression, urinary incontinence, and infertility. Moreover, BMI is positively correlated with mortality rate.[2]

Bariatric surgery, also known as metabolic surgery or weight loss surgery, includes a variety of surgical procedures as treatment for morbid obesity. These procedures result in significant weight loss by restricting the amount of food by reducing the stomach and/or causing malabsorption of nutrients by bypassing the small intestines. Additionally, this weight loss improves or even cures obesity-related comorbidities. At present, all procedures include minimal invasive techniques, that is, laparoscopic surgery.

9.2 Indications, Contraindications, and Patient Selection

According to the National Institutes of Health consensus conference in 1991, patients are candidates for bariatric surgery if they are morbidly obese, had failed conservative therapies including diets and exercise programs, are motivated to change their lifestyle, and have no significant psychological diseases.[3] Additional criteria of the International Federation for the Surgery of Obesity (IFSO) and metabolic disorders are age between 18 and 65 years, no drug dependency problems, and no pregnancy anticipation in the first 2 years following surgery.[4]

Surgery is contraindicated when there is no last resort, meaning that weight loss could still be achieved by other conservative therapies than surgery. Relative contraindications may include severe cardiac diseases, end-stage pulmonary diseases, malignant diseases, cirrhosis with portal hypertension, uncontrolled alcohol or drug dependency, and severely impaired intellectual capacity.

In most hospitals, patients are invited for a preoperative screening by a multidisciplinary team of dieticians, psychologists, physicians (i.e., surgeons), and if necessary internal medicine specialists. This team evaluates whether a patient is suitable for surgery and whether the benefits of operation outweigh the risks.

In consultation with a surgeon, a patient can select a specific bariatric surgical procedure. Nowadays, all procedures are performed laparoscopically. The gold standard is the Roux-en-Y gastric bypass (RYGB). Other procedures are the sleeve gastrectomy (SG), adjustable gastric banding (AGB), biliopancreatic diversion (BD), and one anastomosis gastric bypass (OAGB), also known as Mini or Omega loop gastric bypass.

9.3 Diagnostic Workup

Candidates for bariatric surgery should undergo a diagnostic workup:
- Screening for OSA. The gold standard is polysomnography. Alternatives are a portable type 3 polygraphy or in case of financial, capacity, or time limitations, the

▶ Table 9.1 Body mass index and weight categories

Body mass index (kg/m²)	Weight category
<18	Underweight
18–24.9	Normal weight
25–29.9	Overweight
30–34.9	Obesity
35–49.9	Morbid obesity
≥50	Super obesity

STOP-Bang questionnaire. When moderate or severe OSA is detected, patients should be referred to a pulmonologist for continuous positive airway pressure (CPAP).

- Screening for *Helicobacter pylori* in the stomach, for example, with a feces test.
- Preoperative laboratory tests such as lipid status, vitamins, electrolytes, and minerals.
- Preoperative consultation by an anesthesiologist.
- When necessary, preoperative consultation by a subspecialist (endocrinologist, gastroenterologist).
- Esophagogastroduodenoscopy in patients with previous gastric banding.

9.4 Specific Risks, Patient Information, Consent

Before bariatric surgery, patients receive extensive information regarding the scheduled surgical procedure and its results and complication risks. Patients' medical history and medication use are evaluated in order to assess additional operative risks.

9.5 Anesthesia and Positioning

The most common type of anesthesia used in bariatric surgery is general anesthesia. The ramped position, referred to as the ear-to-sternum position, is the preferred position for intubation and induction. In addition, best laparoscopic view is achieved when the patient is in reversed Trendelenburg position (▶Fig. 9.1).

9.6 Equipment

All bariatric surgeries are performed laparoscopically. Stapler devices and suturing material are required to create staple lines and anastomoses.

9.7 Operative Technique/ Operative Steps

In this section, the two most performed procedures will be described. The RYGB procedure starts with the creation of a 30-mL gastric pouch by using a stapler device. This pouch is connected to the small intestine with staplers and suturing material, generating the first anastomosis, namely the gastrojejunostomy. Additionally, a second anastomosis, the jejunojejunostomy is made after bypassing 150 cm of the small intestines (▶Fig. 9.2).

For an SG, around 85% of the stomach is removed. This is performed with a stapler device alongside the smaller curvature using a gastric tube (▶Fig. 9.3).

Risks, Tips, and Tricks

The benefits of bariatric surgery, namely weight loss and improvement of comorbidities, must outweigh the risks of surgery such as anastomotic leakage and respiratory distress. Following are the tips and tricks to consider bariatric surgery and reduce perioperative risks:

- Patients opting for bariatric surgery should be screened preoperatively by a multidisciplinary team of dieticians, psychologists, and physicians.
- Bariatric surgery should always be considered "last resort."
- Indications for bariatric surgery are according to IFSO criteria.
- Anesthesiologists should provide a perioperative plan adjusted to morbidly obese patients with accompanying comorbidities such as OSA.
- Monitoring of vital parameters, especially heart rate, is important in the first 24 to 48 hours.
- Perioperative management of OSA in bariatric patients is according to a recently published consensus guideline.[5]

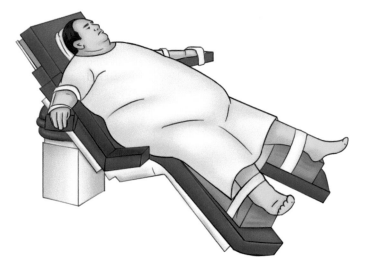

Fig. 9.1 Positioning of bariatric patient. OR, operating room.

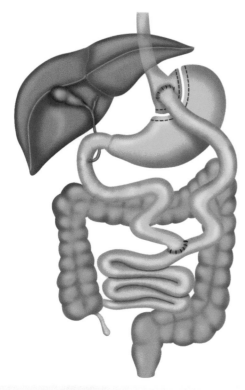

Fig. 9.2 Roux-en-Y gastric bypass.

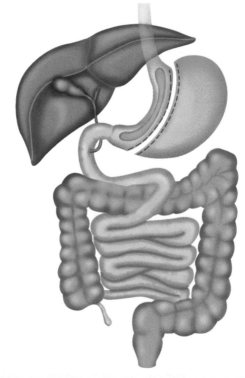

Fig. 9.3 Sleeve gastrectomy.

9.8 Complications (Including Measures for Specific Complications)

The overall complication rate is 10% for RYGB, 6.3% for SG, and 2.4% for AGB.[6] These complications vary in severity and include both surgical and nonsurgical complications. General complications in laparoscopic abdominal surgery are infection, bleeding, conversion to laparotomy, venous thromboembolic events, and iatrogenic injury. The overall mortality rate is 0.25%.[7] Insufficient weight loss or weight regain is a risk after all surgical procedures.

RYGB-specific complications include anastomotic leakage, stenosis, marginal ulcer, internal herniation, dumping syndrome, intra-abdominal abscess, and nutritional deficiencies.

SG-specific complications include staple line leak, stenosis, stricture, increased reflux, intra-abdominal abscess, and nutritional deficiencies.

9.9 Postoperative Care (Including Medications and Drainage)

After surgery, patients are admitted to the surgical ward, postanesthesia care unit, or intensive care unit. This depends on patient characteristics, postoperative complication risks, and hospital capabilities. In general, all patients are discharged 24 to 48 hours postoperatively. In order to decrease the risk of respiratory depression in the direct postoperative period, anesthesiologists are advised to avoid use of opioids. Direct postoperative usage of CPAP is recommended for all moderate to severe OSA patients.

With the exception of AGB, all bariatric surgery patients require life-long multivitamins and calcium supplements. Patients with gastric sutures should receive prophylactic proton pump inhibitors for 6 months postoperatively to decrease the risk of developing marginal ulcers.

Approximately 2 weeks after surgery, patients are reevaluated at the outpatient clinic. Weight loss and metabolic effects should be carefully monitored during the first 2 years in order to adjust medication use.

9.10 Outcomes (Including Data for Apnea–Hypopnea Index and Epworth Sleepiness Scale)

Weight loss and improvement of comorbidities are important outcomes of bariatric surgery.

The amount of excess weight loss is similar between RYGB (76.6%) and SG (72.3%) groups, 1 year postoperative. This effect was still found 5 years after surgery (69.8% for RYGB and 67.3% for SG).[8,9]

Bariatric surgery has shown to be superior in OSA improvement compared to nonsurgical weight loss.[10] In 2014, Ravesloot et al investigated the effect of bariatric surgery on OSA. After 7.7 months, the mean BMI decreased from 45 to 36 kg/m² and the mean apnea–hypopnea index (AHI) from 40 to 16/h. In the severe OSA group, the mean AHI decreased from 66 to 25/h, in the moderate group from 21 to 9/h, and in the mild group from 10 to 5/h (▶Fig. 9.4). Furthermore, postoperative AHI levels below 5/h (i.e., "curated OSA") were seen in 54% of the mild OSA patients, 25% of the moderate OSA patients, and 18% of the severe OSA patients.[11]

An important clinical outcome for both patients and surgeons is the risk of persistent moderately severe disease and consequently CPAP dependency after surgery. A recent study has shown that one-third of all bariatric patients have moderately severe OSA and in most cases patients would benefit from CPAP therapy (▶Table 9.2).[12] In at least 75% of these patients, the AHI decreases below 15/h representing curated of mild residual disease after surgery.

Additionally, the majority (90.4%) of patients with moderate OSA (AHI 15–30/h) achieved a postoperative AHI below 15/h after surgery. In the groups with a preoperative AHI of 30 to 60/h, 60 to 90/h, and more than 90/h, this was achieved in 70.3, 56.8, and 10%, respectively (▶Fig. 9.5).[13]

The Epworth Sleepiness Scale (ESS) is considered a useful screening tool in the adult population. However, studies have shown that ESS is not significantly related to the presence of OSA patients scheduled for bariatric surgery, and hence is not a reliable predictor for OSA in this specific surgical population.[14]

▶ Table 9.2 Number of patients with preoperative AHI more than or equal to 5, 15, 30, 60, and 90 per hour

Variable	Bariatric surgery patients	Number needed to screen[a]
AHI ≥ 5/h	61.6%	2
AHI ≥ 15/h	31.6%	4
AHI ≥ 30/h	16.7%	6
AHI ≥ 60/h	6.2%	17
AHI ≥ 90/h	1.3%	77

Abbreviation: AHI, apnea–hypopnea index.
[a]Number of bariatric patients who should undergo sleep registration to detect AHI more than or equal to 5, 15, 30, 60, and 90 per hour.

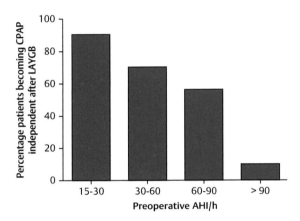

Fig. 9.5 Percentage of patients with preoperative moderately severe OSA achieving postoperative AHI less than 15/h, that is, curated or mild OSA. AHI, apnea–hypopnea index; CPAP, continuous positive airway pressure; LRYGB, laparoscopic Roux-en-Y gastric bypass; OSA, obstructive sleep apnea.

Key Points

- Bariatric surgery is considered a successful treatment for morbid obesity in the long-term.
- All procedures are minimally invasive/laparoscopically performed.
- The two most performed procedures are the RYGB and SG.
- All patients should be screened for OSA before surgery.
- Around 10% of patients experience a complication (varying in severity).
- Mean excess weight loss is around 70%.
- Bariatric surgery is superior in OSA improvement compared to nonsurgical weight loss treatments.
- At least 75% of moderately severe OSA patients achieve AHI levels below 15/h after surgery.

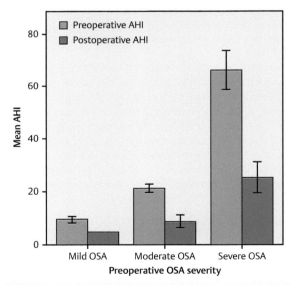

Fig. 9.4 OSA improvement after bariatric surgery. AHI, apnea–hypopnea index; OSA, obstructive sleep apnea.

References

[1] World Health Organization. Fact Sheet. Obesity and overweight. Available at: http://www.who.int/mediacentre/factsheets/fs311/en/Updated June 2016

[2] Whitlock G, Lewington S, Sherliker P, et al. Prospective Studies Collaboration. Body-mass index and cause-specific mortality in 900 000 adults: collaborative analyses of 57 prospective studies. Lancet. 2009; 373(9669):1083–1096

[3] Guidelines for Clinical Application of Laparoscopic Bariatric Surgery. Available at: http://www.sages.org/publications/guidelines/guidelines-for-clinical-application-of-laparoscopic-bariatric-surgery/Accepted: 25 March 2008 ©SAGES 2008

[4] International Federation for the Surgery of Obesity and Metabolic Disorders. Are you a candidate. Selection criteria. Available at: http://www.ifso.com/are-you-a-candidate/ ©2014

[5] de Raaff CAL, Gorter-Stam MAW, de Vries N, et al. Perioperative management of obstructive sleep apnea in bariatric surgery: a consensus guideline. Surg Obes Relat Dis. 2017; 13(7):1095–1109

[6] Carlin AM, Zeni TM, English WJ, et al. Michigan Bariatric Surgery Collaborative. The comparative effectiveness of sleeve gastrectomy, gastric bypass, and adjustable gastric banding procedures for the treatment of morbid obesity. Ann Surg. 2013; 257(5):791–797

[7] Morino M, Toppino M, Forestieri P, Angrisani L, Allaix ME, Scopinaro N. Mortality after bariatric surgery: analysis of 13,871 morbidly obese patients from a national registry. Ann Surg. 2007; 246(6):1002–1007, discussion –1007–1009

[8] Peterli R, Borbély Y, Kern B, et al. Early results of the Swiss Multicentre Bypass or Sleeve Study (SM-BOSS): a prospective randomized trial comparing laparoscopic sleeve gastrectomy and Roux-en-Y gastric bypass. Ann Surg. 2013; 258(5):690–694, discussion 695

[9] Leyba JL, Llopis SN, Aulestia SN. Laparoscopic Roux-en-Y gastric bypass versus laparoscopic sleeve gastrectomy for the treatment of morbid obesity. a prospective study with 5 years of follow-up. Obes Surg. 2014; 24(12):2094–2098

[10] Ashrafian H, Toma T, Rowland SP, et al. Bariatric surgery or non-surgical weight loss for obstructive sleep apnoea? A systematic review and comparison of meta-analyses. Obes Surg. 2015; 25(7):1239–1250

[11] Ravesloot MJ, Hilgevoord AA, van Wagensveld BA, de Vries N. Assessment of the effect of bariatric surgery on obstructive sleep apnea at two postoperative intervals. Obes Surg. 2014; 24(1):22–31

[12] de Raaff CA, Pierik AS, Coblijn UK, de Vries N, Bonjer HJ, van Wagensveld BA. Value of routine polysomnography in bariatric surgery. Surg Endosc. 2016

[13] de Raaff CA, Coblijn UK, Ravesloot MJ, de Vries N, de Lange-de Klerk ES, van Wagensveld BA. Persistent moderate or severe obstructive sleep apnea after laparoscopic Roux-en-Y gastric bypass: which patients? Surg Obes Relat Dis. 2016; 12(10):1866–1872

[14] Ravesloot MJ, van Maanen JP, Hilgevoord AA, van Wagensveld BA, de Vries N. Obstructive sleep apnea is underrecognized and underdiagnosed in patients undergoing bariatric surgery. Eur Arch Otorhinolaryngol. 2012; 269(7):1865–1871

10 Postoperative Care and Follow-Up

Abstract

This chapter deals with perioperative care and follow-up, both from the perspective of the anesthesiologist and surgeon. Perioperative complications of OSA, preoperative management, intraoperative management, and postoperative management are discussed in detail.

Keywords: preoperative management, perioperative management, postoperative management

10.1 Perioperative Care and Follow-Up: Anesthesiologist's Aspects

Martin Roesslein

10.1.1 Introduction

The impact of adequate treatment in patients with obstructive sleep apnea (OSA) and other sleep-related breathing disorders has been progressively recognized.

Depending on the pathophysiology and severity of OSA along with patient's anatomy, risk factors, and preferences, surgical therapy may serve as primary therapy, adjunctive therapy in order to increase patient compliance with other therapeutic options, or second-line therapy when adherence to conservative treatment is inadequate.[1]

A wide array of surgical procedures and approaches are available that principally aim at enlarging or stabilizing the upper airway. These procedures can be categorized as nasal, upper pharyngeal, lower pharyngeal, and global upper airway procedures.[2,3,4]

The surgical evaluation of patients with OSA depends on careful patient and procedure selection, especially related to the anatomy, physiology, and function of the upper aerodigestive tract.

Emphasis should also be placed on adequate perioperative management including preoperative evaluation, intraoperative anesthesia technique, and postoperative care because OSA patients undergoing surgery are at an increased risk for perioperative complications.[5,6,7,8,9,10,11,12,13]

10.1.2 Perioperative Complications of OSA

Surgical treatment of OSA may place patients at risk to suffer perioperative complications for two reasons.

First, OSA patients undergoing any procedure requiring the use of opioids, sedation, or general anaesthesia have an increased risk of developing a variety of pulmonary, cardiovascular, and other complications throughout the perioperative period (▶Table 10.1).[6,7,8,9,10,11,12,13] The fact that OSA patients may be afflicted with

▶ **Table 10.1** Postoperative complications in patients with OSA[5,6,13,144,145]

Organ system	Postoperative complication
Respiratory	• Hypoxia • Hypercapnia • Pneumonia • Atelectasis • Bronchospasm • ARDS • Pulmonary edema • Need for noninvasive ventilation and/or reintubation
Cardiovascular	• Arrhythmia • Myocardial ischemia • Pulmonary embolism
Central nervous system	• Delirium • Encephalopathy • Apoplexy
Other organ systems	• Acute renal failure • Gastrointestinal bleeding • Wound hematoma
Other complications	• Unscheduled transfer to a higher care level • Increased duration or hospital stay

Abbreviations: ARDS, acute respiratory distress syndrome; OSA, obstructive sleep apnea.

comorbidities (systemic and/or pulmonary hypertension, coronary artery disease, atrial fibrillation, cerebral vascular accidents, and type 2 diabetes mellitus) may contribute to their perioperative risk.[14,15,16,17]

Secondly, individual techniques of OSA surgery may be associated with specific complications and the risk of airway obstruction leading to respiratory failure.[18] For example, postobstructive pulmonary edema in the early postoperative period has been associated with laryngospasm after uvulopalatopharyngoplasty (UPPP).[19]

Several factors related to anesthesia, positioning of the patient, or the procedure may contribute to a perioperative aggravation of OSA:

- Negative influence of hypnotics, opioids, and muscle relaxants on the tone of the upper airway dilating muscles, protective airway reflexes, central respiratory drive, and arousal response.[20,21,22,23,24,25,26]
- Narrowing of upper airway caused by surgery and/or intubation-related pharyngeal edema, bleeding, hematoma, or protracted prone positioning of the patient.[27,28]
- Increased collapsibility of the airway caused by protracted postoperative supine positioning of the patient[29] and/or perioperative discontinuation of positive airway pressure (PAP) therapy.[30]
- Disruption of sleep architecture with increased occurrence of rapid eye movement (REM); phases favoring apneas between postoperative nights 3 and 5.[31]

▶ Table 10.2 Elements of preoperative evaluation for OSA

Preoperative evaluation for OSA	
Past medical history	• Severity of OSA (results of PSG and information about treatment and compliance if available) • Information about past perioperative difficulties or complications related to sedation or general anaesthesia • Existence of (OSA-related) comorbidities (systemic and/or pulmonary hypertension, coronary artery disease, atrial fibrillation, cerebral vascular accidents, and type 2 diabetes mellitus)
Physical examination	• Information about the existence of an expected difficult airway
OSA diagnosis	• Oximetry, PG, or PSG

Abbreviations: OSA, obstructive sleep apnea; PG, polygraphy; PSG, polysomnography.

10.1.3 Preoperative Management of Patients with OSA

As preoperative recognition of OSA may lead to less perioperative complications,[32,33,34] OSA patients undergoing sleep surgery should be presented to the anesthetist after sleep medical and surgical evaluation to facilitate the best possible perioperative management.[35]

OSA severity, anatomical deviations predisposing for an airway that may be difficult to manage, and other known risks of the projected surgery should be communicated preoperatively between surgeon and anesthetist. Clinical guidelines also suggest considering additional evaluation to allow preoperative cardiopulmonary optimization in patients with signs of uncontrolled systemic disease or additional problems with ventilation or gas exchange such as hypoventilation syndromes, severe pulmonary hypertension, or resting hypoxemia.[36]

▶Table 10.2 presents preoperative anesthesiological elements to be taken into consideration when evaluating an OSA patient for surgery.

Preoperative Positive Airway Pressure Therapy

While PAP is considered first-line therapy in the treatment for OSA,[37,38,39,40,41,42,43,44,45] the impact of its use before hospitalization in preventing postoperative complications is less clear.[5,7,46,47,48,49] In addition, long-time compliance to this treatment is limited, partly for reasons manageable by sleep surgery.[3,50] However, continued preoperative application of PAP therapy is recommended and its initiation should be considered in severe cases according to current clinical guidelines.[32,36]

Preoperative Premedication

Anxiolytic and/or sedating drugs such as benzodiazepines should only be given preoperatively with clear indication and adequate means of respiratory monitoring as these substances may predispose OSA patients to airway collapse and/or respiratory depression.[51] Alpha 2 agonists may be preferable, as their use has not been shown to increase the incidence of respiratory complications in this context.[52]

10.1.4 Intraoperative Management of Patients with OSA

Anesthesia Regimen

Intravenous (IV) and volatile anesthetics as well as opioids have been shown to negatively affect the tone of the pharyngeal muscles,[20,21,22,23,26] ventilatory drive in response to hypercapnia,[24,25] and arousal in response to airway obstruction.[53]

In order to minimize these effects in the postoperative period, it may be advantageous to use anesthetics and opioids with a favorable pharmacokinetic profile, that is, short context-sensitive half-time.[51]

Depending on the specific surgical procedure for the treatment of OSA, supplementary application of local anesthetics may be advisable.[54]

Usage of Muscle Relaxants

The fact that the overall risk for postoperative pulmonary complications due to incomplete reversal of muscle relaxants is generally increased in surgical patients may relate to OSA patients in particular.[55] In consequence, patients undergoing OSA surgery under general anesthesia should be extubated only after full recovery of muscle tone as proven by neuromuscular monitoring.[32] Short-acting muscle relaxants and/or antagonizing drugs with a low profile of adverse side effects should be used under these circumstances. In this context, Sugammadex, a modified gamma-cyclodextrin, which selectively reverses aminosteroid-induced neuromuscular blockade, may be advantageous as it may decrease the incidence of postoperative respiratory complications and related costs in OSA.[56]

Airway Management

OSA patients are known to have an increased risk for presenting a difficult airway including difficult or impossible mask ventilation, intubation, or both, which seems to be independent of body mass index (BMI) or Mallampati status.[57,58,59,60,61,62,63,64] This underlines the essential requirement to be prepared with equipment for difficult airway management and to provide adequate preoxygenation and patient positioning before induction of anesthesia.[65]

In this context, general anesthesia with a secured airway is favored over deep sedation without airway securement in OSA patients.[32] If sedation is performed, the use of an oro- or nasopharyngeal airway or continuous positive airway pressure (CPAP) should be considered.[32]

10.1.5 Postoperative Management of Patients with OSA

Oxygenation

As OSA patients are at an increased risk of hypoxemia in the early postoperative period, continuous application of supplemental oxygen should be sustained until basal levels of oxygen saturation haven been reached under room air.[31,66,67]

In order to minimize the associated risk of hypoventilation, adequate ventilation should be monitored, for example, by capnography, and supplemental oxygen should be reduced as circumstances permit.[68]

Postoperative Positive Airway Pressure Therapy

Use of immediate postoperative PAP has been shown to attenuate OSA severity and may be associated with less postoperative complications.[30,33,69] Therefore, clinical guidelines generally recommend resumption or even commencement of PAP therapy in the postoperative period.[32,36] Of note, isolated nasal surgery in patients with OSA and nasal obstruction has been shown to reduce therapeutic PAPs and to increase long-term PAP adherence.[70]

However, nasal packing or swelling in the upper airway may aggravate measures of OSA in the immediate postoperative period while making PAP therapy using conventional facemasks impossible.[71]

Postoperative Analgesia

While it is not clear whether withholding or minimizing the usage of opioids leads to less postoperative complications in patients with (or without) OSA,[72] the 72-hour postoperative opioid dose has been identified to be one of the factors associated with worsening sleep-disordered breathing in OSA patients as measured by apnea–hypopnea index (AHI).[66] Of note, intermittent hypoxia and sleep disruption—both commonly seen in postoperative OSA patients—have been demonstrated to enhance pain, while intermittent hypoxia itself may aggravate opioid-mediated analgesic effects.[73,74] This underlines the complex pathophysiology of individual OSA phenotypes.[75,76]

Nonopioid analgesics and local anesthetics as well as coanalgesics, especially when combined, have been shown to reduce the demand for systemically applied opioids in the postoperative period and should be considered the first-line therapy in this situation.[32,77] It is noteworthy in this context that nonsteroidal anti-inflammatory drugs (NSAIDs) have not been associated with increased bleeding in cases of tonsillectomy.[78] In cases where opioids are indispensable for achieving adequate analgesia, their application should be individually titrated.[32]

Patient Positioning

Avoiding the supine position has been shown to increase oxygenation while decreasing AHI in nonsurgical OSA patients and may therefore be advantageous in the postoperative period.[29,79]

Postoperative Monitoring of Patients with OSA

Despite the increased risk of OSA patients for postoperative complications, it is unclear from the literature, to what extent and duration postoperative monitoring should be sustained.[32] This is of interest considering the growing disparity of high demand for postoperative monitoring in these patients and limited health care resources.[9] In this context, neither using a telemetry systems nor transfer to a monitored setting has been able to show a clear benefit in OSA patients.[32]

Several retrospective studies investigated rate and onset of postoperative complications after surgical OSA treatment.[35] Complication rates were between 1.1 and 7.1%. Except for bleeding, onset of all complications was within the first 4 hours after extubation.

Therefore, respiratory monitoring should be rigorous, especially in the immediate postoperative period. Some patients may experience an extended recurrence of respiratory events in the postoperative period such as apnea, bradypnea, hypoxemia, or pain combined with reduced wakefulness.[80] In these cases, PAP therapy, if feasible, should be resumed or started as soon as possible using appropriate masks, and/or transfer to the intensive care unit (ICU) should be considered in order to prevent the occurrence of further respiratory complications.[80,81]

Until high-level evidence and respective recommendations become available, duration and extent of postoperative monitoring remains to be determined using clinical judgment based on the individual clinical scenario.

10.1.6 Outpatient Surgery for Patients with OSA

An increasing number of OSA patients consider surgery in an outpatient setting. Existing guidelines recommend evaluating the adequacy of a surgical procedure to be performed under these circumstances based on factors related to the patient, the type of surgery/anesthesia, and the outpatient facility (▶Table 10.3).[32]

Relevant comorbidities should be optimized and use of PAP and requirement of minimal doses of postoperative opioids be considered for OSA patients to be eligible for ambulatory anesthesia.[82,83]

Patients with high AHI and BMI or uncontrolled medical comorbidities undergoing OSA surgery who require postoperative nasal packing are at increased risk of postoperative complications in an outpatient setting.[84,85] These cases should be referred to an inpatient facility.

▶ **Table 10.3** Factors to be considered in determining the adequacy of performing surgical procedures in OSA patients in an outpatient setting according to the American Society of Anesthesiologists Task Force on Perioperative Management of Patients with Obstructive Sleep Apnea[32]

Scope	Factor
Patient	Age
	Sleep apnea status
	Anatomical and physiologic abnormalities
	Status of coexisting diseases
Surgery/ anaesthesia	Need for postoperative opioids
	Adequacy of postdischarge observation
Outpatient facility	Availability of: • Emergency difficult airway equipment • Respiratory care equipment • Radiology facilities • Clinical laboratory facilities
	Transfer agreement with an inpatient facility

10.1.7 Conclusion

Patients suffering from OSA are at an increased risk for various perioperative complications.

A diligent perioperative management of OSA patients should focus on the individual patient's OSA status and existing comorbidities, type and invasiveness of surgery, and required anesthesia as well as appropriate postoperative monitoring, including resumption or commencement of PAP therapy.

10.2 Perioperative Management: Surgeon's Perspective

Christel de Raaff, Bart van Wagensveld, and Nico de Vries

10.2.1 Introduction to OSA

OSA is a disease that is characterized by repetitive complete or partial obstruction of the upper airway during sleep (Chapter 2). Resultant sleep disruption following these events results in severe clinical symptoms such as excessive daytime sleepiness, cognitive disorders, or even depression. Furthermore, pathophysiologic changes such as hypoxemia, hypercapnia, and metabolic disturbances lead to cardiovascular, neurovascular, pulmonary, and metabolic disorders in the long term.[86] OSA treatment aims to reduce these symptoms, long-term risks, and the preventable risk of traffic, domestic, or workplace accidents caused by excessive daytime sleepiness (mean crash-rate ratio between 1.21 and 4.89).[36]

Additionally, it is important to reduce the risk of perioperative complications in patients undergoing surgery requiring general anesthesia (▶ Table 10.4). A recent

▶ **Table 10.4** Reasons for diagnosing and treating OSA in surgical patients

Reason	Examples
Reduce clinical symptoms	Excessive daytime sleepiness and cognitive disorders, depression
Reduce long-term complication risks	Hypertension, myocardial infarction, arrhythmias, pulmonary hypertension, congestive heart failure, metabolic syndrome
Reduce risk of accidents	Traffic, domestic, workplace
Reduce perioperative risks	Postoperative desaturations, cardiac events, and respiratory failure

meta-analysis including 17 studies with a total of 7,162 patients showed that OSA patients are at increased risk of postoperative desaturations, cardiac events, and respiratory failure.[87] The increased risks of these complications are partly caused by coexistence of comorbidities such as obesity, diabetes, hypoventilation syndrome, hypertension, and cardiac diseases. Hypoventilation and breathing obstruction following unrecognized OSA result in hypoxemia in the immediate postoperative period. Furthermore, specific anesthetic problems can occur during induction of anesthesia such as difficulties with ventilation and intubation, and the OSA severity may worsen during thepostoperative period.[31]

Therefore, physicians and hospitals facing surgical patients should be aware of the risk factors for OSA and its perioperative management to reduce the risk of perioperative complications.

10.2.2 Definition of OSA

An apnea is defined as a cessation of airflow for at least 10 seconds. A hypopnea is defined as a reduction of airflow. The number of apneas and hypopneas per hour during sleep represent the AHI. OSA is present when the AHI is more than or equal to 5/hour. The generally accepted definitions of OSA severity levels are:
• No OSA: AHI 0 to 4.9/hour.
• Mild OSA: AHI 5 to 14.9/hour.
• Moderate OSA: AHI 15 to 29.9/hour.
• Severe OSA: AHI more than or equal to 30/hour.[36]

10.2.3 Prevalence of OSA

The prevalence of OSA varies depending on the definitions used and specific populations. Due to its strong association with gender and age, literature mostly describes the prevalence of subgroups rather than estimating the overall prevalence. A recent guideline of Chung and colleagues reported that 9% of women and 26% of men aged between 30 and 49 years suffers from OSA. This percentage has increased to 27 and 43%, respectively, in the age group of 50 to 70 years.[36] The prevalence of OSA is even higher in specific groups with risk factors for OSA such as morbid obesity. In the bariatric population, around two-thirds have OSA and one-third have moderately to severe disease, suggesting need for therapy.[88,89]

10.2.4 Clinical Symptoms Suggesting Presence of OSA

- Snoring.
- Witnessed apneas.
- Excessive daytime sleepiness.
- Dry mouth.
- Less intellectual performance.
- Sexual dysfunction.
- Depression or burn-out.

10.2.5 General Clinical Signs Suggesting Presence of OSA

- Male sex.
- (Morbid) obesity.
- Advanced age.
- High blood pressure.

10.2.6 Head- and Neck-Specific Clinical Signs Suggesting Presence of OSA

- Increased neck circumference (men >42 cm; women >37).
- Craniofacial abnormalities, for example, mandibular retrognathia, affecting the airway.
- Large tonsil size.
- Large tongue size.
- Long soft palate and uvula.
- Nasopharyngeal stenosis as a result of previous palatal surgery for OSA, cleft palate, and as side effect of ritual uvulectomy.

Less strong predictive factors are excessive use of alcohol, menopause, ethnicity, and smoking. Although decreased nasal obstruction is often thought to cause OSA, this is not an important risk factor for OSA. Literature has shown that improving decreased nasal obstruction, either medically or surgically, gives no improvement of the AHI. Yet, temporarily complete nasal obstruction as a result of nasal surgery with nasal packing can give temporary increase of the AHI and should be recognized (Chapter 7). While the pathophysiology of OSA is multifactorial and complex, it should be suspected when above-mentioned signs are present. Nevertheless, absence of these signs does not rule out OSA, which also has shown to be present in nonobese subjects and children. To diagnose OSA, objective measurements remain essential.

10.2.7 Surgical Groups

Head and Neck Surgery for OSA

In patients undergoing palatal surgery, base of tongue surgery, or multilevel surgery for OSA, all relevant information (history, clinical features, Mallampati stage, sleep study results) concerning OSA severity and anatomy of the upper airway should be obtained. The very fact that the same clinical features that might lead to difficult intubation (Mallampati stage) also lead to OSA, makes the combination of OSA and head and neck surgery risky. After head and neck surgery for OSA, there is risk for both postoperative edema of the upper airway and postoperative bleedings. Some procedures are riskier than others; for example, for the palate, procedures in which the tonsils are removed, (UPPP, expansion sphincter pharyngoplasty [ESP]) have more risk of bleeding than procedures in which no tonsillectomy is performed (Z-palatoplasty [ZPP]).

Bleedings are extremely rare after radiofrequency ablation for base of tongue surgery, however, the risk of bleeding is increased after midline glossectomy and transoral robotic setting (TORS). After hyoidthyroidpexia, a bleeding in the neck might occur, making reintubation extremely difficult.

Severe OSA due to kissing tonsils is a special situation. In such cases, in spite of a preoperatively high AHI, one can reason that after tonsillectomy the upper airway should be open.

Nasal surgery in a patient with OSA is another special situation, necessitating surgeons to use nasal packs. Nasal surgery can be indicated in order to improve CPAP compliance. In such cases, nasal packing should be avoided; however, if not possible, it should be kept in mind that complete nasal obstruction might increase the AHI during the period when the packs are in situ. In patients on CPAP, temporarily switching to a full face mask is recommended.

Bariatric Surgery

According to several guidelines, patients who are scheduled for bariatric surgery are at high risk of OSA and should routinely be evaluated for this comorbidity preoperatively.[90,91] Perioperative tasks such as induction and intubation for patients with OSA as well as morbid obesity are challenging for anesthesiologists.

General Surgery

A more challenging group is the general surgery population. As these patients do not undergo routine OSA screening, risk stratification is an important task in this group. Many surgeons lack knowledge about OSA and its perioperative management, increasing the importance of adequate risk stratification by anesthesiologists. Signs and symptoms mentioned earlier in this chapter could provide guidance in the preoperative phase. Surgeons should describe the position of the patient during surgery and in the immediate postoperative period. Extra precautions should be taken in patients who have a high AHI in supine position and undergo surgery requiring supine position or should be in supine position in the immediate postoperative period.

10.2.8 Methods of OSA Screening

Although the signs and symptoms discussed earlier in this chapter could indicate the risk of OSA, there is no clinical model that accurately predicts the presence of OSA. Therefore, diagnosing definitive OSA requires objective testing. This section describes the gold standard for diagnosing OSA, that is, polysomnography (PSG), alternatives including objective and subjective testing, and future perspectives such as biomarkers. These alternatives can be considered when PSG is not applicable in a clinical setting due to time, cost, or capacity reasons.

There are four types of sleep studies to diagnose OSA:

Type 1: PSG with observation.
Type 2: PSG without observation.
Type 3: Polygraphy (PG).
Type 4: Other objective sleep measurements such as pulse oximetry and heart rate.

Type 1 and 2: PSG

The gold standard for diagnosing definitive OSA is an overnight laboratory PSG.[36,90,91] This sleep study determines the frequency and duration of apneas and hypopneas during a full night of documented sleep. Subsequently, it generates the AHI, indicating OSA severity.

Moreover, a PSG generates the total time of sleep in different sleeping positions as well as the AHI in a specific position. As the AHI might be increased in supine position, this information is valuable to provide adequate treatment and to predict perioperative risks.

Over the past years, there has been an increasing interest in other PSG-generated severity metrics besides AHI. The oxygen desaturation index (ODI) or cumulated duration of oxygen desaturation below 90% have shown to be useful parameters in detecting OSA and predicting perioperative risks.[92,93] One study showed that patients with mean preoperative overnight SpO_2 below 92.7%, ODI above 28.5 events/hour, or cumulative time percentage with SpO_2 below 90% and ODI above 7.2% are at higher risk for postoperative events.[94] These studies show that PSG is not only successful in diagnosing OSA, but also in specifying OSA severity and additional parameters that are needed to provide optimal treatment and foresee perioperative risks.

Unfortunately, most hospitals and clinics performing surgeries on patients at high risk of OSA have not accepted mandatory preoperative PSG as standard of care due to capacity, costs, and time management. Furthermore, patients undergoing PSG are attached to many electrodes and wires, resulting in patient burden (▶Fig. 10.1).

Type 3: PG

Type 3 PG is a less time-consuming and patient-friendly sleep study (▶Fig. 10.2). While this test records less physiological signs and lacks sleep information, it has been shown to be a reliable OSA screening tool. In a recent meta-analysis of 19 studies, the area under the curve varied between 0.85 and 0.99 across different levels of disease severity. Sensitivity ranged between 0.79 and 0.97 and specificity between 0.60 and 0.93 across different AHI cutoffs.[95]

Its use is also reliable in bariatric surgery population. For an AHI cutoff of 5/hour, PG has a sensitivity of 93% and specificity of 71%. This increases to a sensitivity and specificity of 94% and 94% for an AHI cutoff of 15/hour.[96]

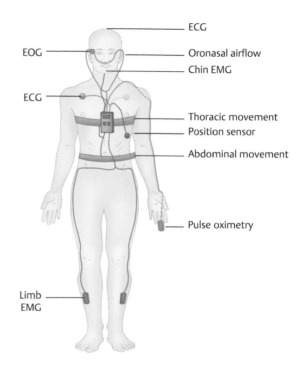

Fig. 10.1 Type 1 and 2 sleep studies—polysomnography.

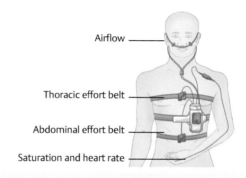

Fig. 10.2 Type 3 sleep study—polygraphy.

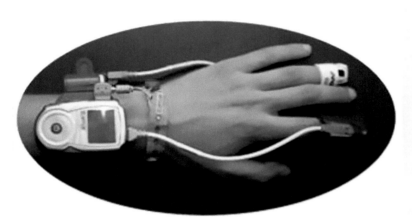

Fig. 10.3 Type 4 sleep study—WatchPAT.

For the severe class, one study found a sensitivity of 89% and 67% in laboratory and home, respectively, with a specificity of 100%.[97]

Type 4: Other Sleep Studies

All other sleep studies are defined as Type 4 studies. These include objective measurements such as oxygen saturation and heart rate. An example is WatchPAT, Itamar Medical Ltd., Israel (▶Fig. 10.3).[98]

Subjective Testing

The overall evaluation of patients suspected of having OSA begins with a sleep history of snoring, daytime sleepiness, and evaluation of presence of obesity or hypertension.[90] If these tests are positive, additional symptoms are evaluated during a comprehensive sleep evaluation.[90] Questionnaires are often used to stratify patients at risk of OSA and hence indicates the need for objective testing.

A frequently used and validated questionnaire is the STOP-Bang (▶Table 10.5). This questionnaire includes eight questions all covering one point. A recently published meta-analysis calculated the predictive parameters of STOP-Bang more than or equal to 3 as cutoff in the surgical population. The prevalence of AHI more than or equal to 5/hour, more than or equal to 15/hour, and more than or equal to 30/hour was 68.4%, 39.2%, and 18.7%, respectively. Corresponding sensitivity scores were 90%, 94%, and 96% and specificity scores were 43%, 32%, and 29%, respectively.[99]

Other questionnaires are the Berlin questionnaire, American Society of Anesthesiologists (ASA) checklist, and Epworth Sleepiness Scale (ESS). In the surgical population, the Berlin questionnaire has a sensitivity of 68.9% and specificity of 56.4%. The ASA checklist has a higher sensitivity (72.1%) and lower specificity (38.2%).[36] The lowest sensitivity scores were found for the ESS. At a cutoff of 8, 10, and 12, sensitivity scores were 76%, 66%, and 53%, respectively. Respective specificities scores were 31%, 48%, and 62%.[100] These questionnaires are inferior to the STOP-Bang questionnaire.

▶ **Table 10.5** The STOP-Bang questionnaire[101]

STOP-Bang questions	
Snoring	Yes/No
Tiredness	Yes/No
Observed apnea	Yes/No
Blood Pressure	Yes/No
BMI >35 kg/m²	Yes/No
Age >50 years	Yes/No
Neck circumference >40 cm	Yes/No
Gender male	Yes/No

Predicting OSA in the morbidly obese population is an even more challenging task. Characteristics such as obesity and neck circumference are not reliable in this specific population, as all bariatric patients suffer from severe obesity and have an increased neck circumference. Additionally, OSA and obesity are both related to type II diabetes, hypertension, tiredness, and snoring, decreasing the ability to differentiate participants on their OSA status. This results in different sensitivities and specificities. For stratifying an AHI more than 15/hour in the morbidly obese population, a score above or equal to 5 points has a sensitivity of 65.2% and specificity of 64.9%.[101] Although a high sensitivity is found for a score above or equal to 3 (97%), this goes along with a low specificity (6.8%). Due to its high sensitivity, the STOP-Bang questionnaire is considered useful in stratifying OSA in the morbidly obese population.[91]

Future Developments: Biomarkers

A biomarker is a characteristic that can be objectively measured in blood and indicates a condition. Several studies have tried to find potential biomarkers for OSA providing information concerning diagnosis and (response to) treatment. Although potential biomarkers including inflammatory (tumor necrosis factor [TNF]-α, interleukin [IL]-6), metabolic (HbA1C), and oxidative markers

(8-isoprostane, nitric oxide) were previously investigated, no ideal biomarker currently exists.[102,103] Discovery of an accurate OSA biomarker would provide an opportunity for all clinics to perform routine OSA screening before performing surgery and during follow-up.

10.2.9 Treatment of OSA

OSA has multiple treatment options. In more severe OSA, treatment with CPAP is the gold standard. It is also the most prescribed therapy for OSA in patients scheduled for surgery. Perioperative CPAP usage reduces the postoperative AHI compared with the preoperative AHI, may reduce cardiorespiratory complications, and shows a trend toward a shorter length of hospital stay.[36]

Advantages of CPAP compared to other OSA treatments are a short acclimatization period in the preoperative period and ability to evaluate compliance. Furthermore, in the bariatric population, CPAP goes along with low costs due to the ability to return the device after OSA improvement following weight loss postoperatively.

Next to CPAP, positional therapy (PT) is considered a successful treatment for patients with positional OSA (POSA). POSA is defined as an AHI twice as high in supine position than in other positions. PT can be considered in patients with POSA when CPAP is not tolerated (▶Fig. 10.4). In the bariatric population more than 50% of the mild OSA patients have POSA. As POSA is not considered a predictive value for 30-day complications, perioperative treatment is not required for such patients.[104] More detailed information regarding treatment of OSA is given in previous chapters of this book.

10.2.10 Intraoperative Management

Although OSA is an important risk factor for difficult intubation when not managed appropriately, literature has shown that neither obesity nor OSA nor neck circumference predicts difficult intubation, when applying the ramped position.[105,106] Mallampati 3 or 4 (see ▶Fig. 3.4) and male gender are significant risk factors. Additional instruments, such as videolaryngoscopy, should be available in every operating room if there is a concern for a difficult intubation in patients.[91] Another excellent tool when faced with a difficult airway is the Eschmann tracheal tube introducer, also known as the gum elastic bougie (▶Fig. 10.5). This tool allows blind passage when the

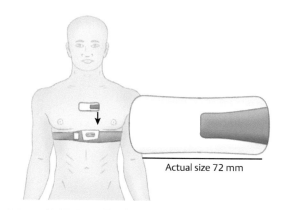

Actual size 72 mm

Fig. 10.4 Positional therapy.

Fig. 10.5 Gum elastic bougie.

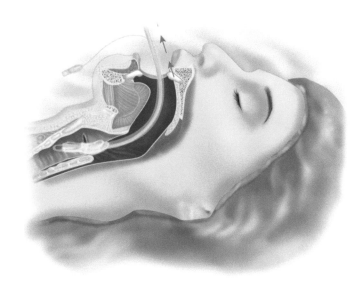

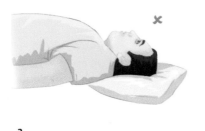
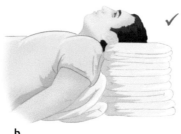

Fig. 10.6 Supine position (**a**; wrong) versus ramped position (**b**; right).

a   b

vocal cords are not visualized. The anterior positioned angled tip provides "clicks" when touching the cartilaginous rings of the trachea.

Other positions, such as the supine position, should be avoided in patients who may rapidly desaturate to difficult mask fit and/or reduced functional residual capacity (▶Fig. 10.6).[91] Nevertheless, several surgical procedures such as head and neck surgeries and orthopedic surgeries are only feasible in the supine position. For orthopedic procedures, supine position is advised in the immediate postoperative period as well. Extra precautions must be taken in patients who underwent orthopedic procedures and when the AHI in supine position is of clinical significance.

CPAP usage at induction is highly recommended in moderately severe OSA patients to maintain lung capacity and reduce time to oxygen desaturation.[91]

Extubation should only be performed in those who are fully awake, have no sedative and opioid effects, and have full reversal of neuromuscular function.[91]

Sedatives and Opioids

OSA patients have an abnormal sensitivity to sedatives that can lead to hypoventilation, apneas, and cardiopulmonary adverse events.[107] Therefore, careful perioperative management includes avoidance of routine use of sedatives as premedication and analgesia. If used, recommendations include slow titration and continuous monitoring.[91,107]

In addition to sedatives, OSA patients have a significant degree of opioid sensitivity because of its respiratory-depressant effects. Acute tolerance to its analgesic effect can occur after the first opioid dose, whereas tolerance to its side effects develops more slowly. This results in increased obstructive breathing postoperatively.[66]

Depending on the type of surgery, a subgroup of patients are discharged 24 to 48 hours after surgery. Delayed occurrence of respiratory depression would occur at home without adequate monitoring. As total IV opioid-free strategies are available, avoidance of opioid usage is recommended.[91,108]

However, pain management is different among surgical patient groups. The majority of bariatric patients become free of pain with paracetamol and NSAIDs, whereas patients who underwent palatal surgery experience more pain resulting in taking stronger analgesics.

▶ Table 10.6 Opioid-free analgesia

Effective analgesics	Promising analgesics
Paracetamol	Ketamine
Nonsteroidal anti-inflammatory drugs	Alpha 2 agonists (clonidine; dexmedetomidine)
Incisional infiltration	Magnesium
Epidural analgesia	Intravenous lidocaine
Peripheral nerve blocks	-

Multimodal Analgesic Model

The use of short-acting opioids such as remifentanil appeared promising; however, they increased postoperative pain due to central sensitization, resulting in additional opioid requirements.[108]

Other methods have been identified as multimodal analgesic model minimizing the need for opioid administration (▶Table 10.6). Multiple studies showed that paracetamol and NSAIDs decrease opioid requirements in the postoperative period. NSAIDs are superior to paracetamol, regarding opioid requirements and additionally might have advantages reducing inflammation. Best results are seen when paracetamol and NSAIDs are combined.[108,109,110] Nevertheless, NSAID usage should be restricted to several days to avoid the risk of gastric perforation after bariatric surgery. Other opioid-free successful methods are local anesthetics for incisional infiltration, epidural analgesia, and peripheral nerve blocks.

Additional analgesics including ketamine and alpha 2 agonists such as clonidine and dexmedetomidine are increasingly being administered. Yet, high quality evidence regarding their use in this setting is missing.[91,110]

10.2.11 Postoperative Management

Important aspects of the immediate postoperative period are adequate monitoring of vital parameters and pain management. Recommendations for postoperative care depend on the type of surgery (length of operation, OSA-specific surgery in the head and neck area, general surgery—laparoscopic or open approach, level of expertise of the center, etc.) and type of anesthesia (use of sedatives/opioids).

Recovery Room

Patients are transferred from operating room to the recovery room or postanesthesia care unit (PACU) after surgery. This department is located in the operation complex and provides continuous monitoring and expertise of anesthesiologists when necessary. In the PACU, patients are prepared to be transferred to another department with less or more monitoring capabilities, that is, surgical ward or ICU. As OSA patients are at increased risk of hypoxemia in the early postoperative period, continuous application of supplemental oxygen should be sustained until basal levels of oxygen saturation haven been reached under room air.[31,66,67] In order to minimize the associated risk of hypoventilation, adequate ventilation should be monitored, for example by capnography, and supplemental oxygen should be reduced as circumstances permit.[68] There may be a role for prolonged stay in the PACU to identify high-risk patients and to determine subsequent appropriate management.[91]

General Ward versus Medium/Intensive Care Unit

Admission of a postsurgical patient to a general ward, medium care unit (MCU), or ICU depends on the type of surgery and following risk stratification. In 2013, the ASA published a scoring system for the perioperative risk from OSA (▶Table 10.7). This system indicates whether there is an increased perioperative risk from OSA (4 or more points) and hence a need for ICU admission. Topics include severity of OSA, invasiveness of surgery and anesthesia, and requirements of postoperative opioids. This system is considered a useful and applicable tool for anesthesiologists in the clinical setting. However, still some improvements are required in this system. A more common definition of moderate and severe OSA is an AHI of more than or equal to 15/hour (instead of 20/hour) and more than or equal to 30/hour (instead of 40/hour), respectively.[32] Additionally, monitoring recommendations are different between surgical groups for example head and neck, bariatric, and general surgical groups, and should be further specified.[32] OSA position dependency is not mentioned as well, while in surgeries after which patients are forced to be positioned on their back, the AHI in supine position might be more relevant than the overall AHI.

Head and Neck Surgery for OSA

These surgical procedures are not necessarily always an indication for ICU admission postsurgery. Moderately severe OSA patients are often admitted to the ICU, depending on the type of surgery. Palatal surgery is mostly not an indication for ICU admission, whereas invasive tongue base surgery (midline glossectomy) is. Noninvasive tongue procedures (radiofrequency of the base of tongue) are not an indication for ICU admission. Hyoid suspension with or without radiofrequency ablation of the base of tongue is regarded as indication for ICU admission, particularly

▶ **Table 10.7** Scoring system perioperative risk from obstructive sleep apnea of American Society of Anesthesiologists Task Force[36]

a) Severity of sleep apnea based on sleep study

Severity of OSA[a]	Points
• None	0
• Mild	1
• Moderate	2
• Severe	3

b) Invasiveness of surgery and anesthesia

Type of surgery and anesthesia	Points
• Superficial surgery under local or peripheral nerve block anesthesia without sedation	0
• Superficial surgery with moderate sedation or general anesthesia	1
• Peripheral surgery with spinal or epidural anesthesia	1
• Peripheral surgery with general anesthesia	2
• Airway surgery with moderate sedation	2
• Major surgery, general anesthesia	3
• Airway surgery, general anesthesia	3

c) Requirements for postoperative opioids

Opioid requirement	Points
• None	0
• Low-dose oral opioids	1
• High-dose oral opioids, parental, or neuraxial opioids	3

d) Estimation of perioperative risk

• Overall point score: the score for A plus the greater score for either B or C[b]

[a]One point may be subtracted if a patient has been on therapy before surgery and is compliant during the postoperative period; One point should be added if a patient with mild of moderate OSA also has a resting $PaCO_2 > 50$ mm Hg.
[b]Patients with a score of 4 may be at increased perioperative risk from OSA; patients with a score of 5 or 6 may be at significantly increased perioperative risk from OSA.

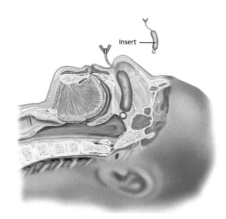

Fig. 10.7 Nasal pack causing complete nasal obstruction.

because these procedures are usually reserved for more serious diseases. Nasal surgery requires ICU admission only when nasal packs result in complete nasal blockage (▶Fig. 10.7). Therefore, it is preferable to avoid the use of nasal packs in rhinoplasty and septoplasty if possible.

If not, temporarily application of a full face CPAP interface should be considered to avoid ICU admittance. In functional endoscopic sinus surgery, specific nasal packs placed in the middle meatus allow patients to still breathe through their nose. Regarding turbinate surgery, it is preferred to use techniques that do not necessitate nasal packs (radiofrequency instead of cold steel surgery; Chapter 7). Patients who undergo multilevel head and neck surgery should be admitted to the ICU for the first postoperative night; however, exceptions can be made on individual basis.

Bariatric Surgery

In similarity with the head and neck surgery group, routine ICU admission is not required for bariatric surgery patients with OSA.[91,111] However, as these patients are at increased risk of perioperative complications due to both their obesity and OSA, an important aspect of the postoperative care of these patients is continuous monitoring in which the minimum required monitoring is by pulse oximeter (▶ Fig. 10.8). Early recognition of desaturations could prevent the occurrence of cardiorespiratory complications in moderately severe OSA patients after bariatric surgery. In a recent study, all severe OSA patients were admitted to the ICU for continuous oxygen saturation monitoring after bariatric surgery. Desaturations occurred in 17.4%, whereas no cardiopulmonary complications, reintubations, or deaths occurred.[112] The additive value of other vital parameters such as blood pressure needs to be further evaluated. To avoid the need for ICU admission, designated surgical wards are becoming more popular in high-volume bariatric centers. These wards include rooms with equipment, that is, pulse oximeter, monitors, and alarm systems, to provide continuous monitoring for OSA patients after bariatric surgery.

Other Surgical Groups

For other nonspecified surgical groups, the following factors could result in an increased postoperative complication risk and should be included in an anesthetists' consideration for ICU admission:
- Difficult intubation.
- Large tongue, upper airway edema.
- Use of sedatives and/or opioids.
- Male gender.
- Age above 50 years.
- BMI above 60 kg/m².

OSA Treatment

Chung et al published an overview of the effectiveness of CPAP in the perioperative setting.[69] Moreover, a recent meta-analysis including 6 studies resulting in 904 patients showed that patients with CPAP had a risk ratio of 0.88 (95% CI, 0.73–1.06) and a 12% risk reduction of postoperative complications with a corresponding number to treat of 45.[30] According to the authors, the nonsignificant benefit of CPAP could have been a result of the suboptimal compliance of CPAP and the relative small sample size and low incidence of complications in the meta-analysis. As many more studies support the evidence of CPAP benefits, preoperatively prescribed CPAP therapy (or other therapies such as PT or mandibular advancement device) should be continued in the direct postoperative period.[30]

It is important to realize that previously mentioned monitoring recommendations are independent from CPAP usage, as CPAP compliance is not guaranteed. This applies to all types of surgical patients.

The use of CPAP is not associated with an increased complication risk after head and neck surgery. Patients who underwent nasal surgery should receive full face CPAP instead of nasal CPAP (▶ Fig. 10.9).

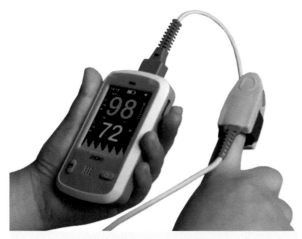

Fig. 10.8 Example of pulse oximeter generating heart rate and oxygen saturation.

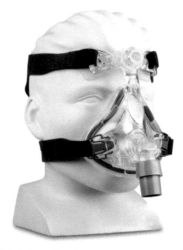

Fig. 10.9 Full face continuous positive airway pressure (CPAP).

In bariatric surgery, the pressure given by CPAP is often thought to increase the risk of leakage of the gastrointestinal anastomosis or staple line in the upper abdomen. However, several studies have shown that there is no increased risk, and consequently the use of CPAP is safe in the postoperative period.[113,114,115]

Admission Time/Discharge

Most patients undergoing head and neck surgery for OSA, that is, palatinal surgery are discharged after the first night. Patients who underwent multilevel surgery and include a drain might be discharged after 2 nights when the drain has been removed. Same-day surgery is rare in head and neck surgery for OSA. An exception could be radiofrequency of the base of tongue in a patient with a low AHI, for example, 7/hour. The most feared complication in the direct postoperative period is a bleeding after tonsillectomy, in the neck after hyoid suspension, or in the tongue (midline glossectomy, TORS, lingual tonsillectomy) (▶Fig. 10.10) (see Hyoid Bone Surgeries in Chapter 8).[116] Edema is a less common complication.

According to enhanced recovery after bariatric surgery (ERABS) principles the admission time of bariatric surgery patients is 1 (same-day surgery) to 2 days.[117] There is no AHI cutoff for same-day surgery.[111] The most feared complications in the first week after surgery are anastomotic leakage, stenosis, intra-abdominal abscesses and pulmonary embolism (Chapter 9) (▶Fig. 10.11). As bariatric surgery is mostly performed in certified centers, patients are advised to return to their bariatric center in case of adverse events.

As most surgical patients are discharged after 12 to 48 hours, long-term effects of anesthesia, such as apneas, could develop at home when patients are not monitored. Several anesthetics and the use of opioids could result in respiratory depression in the first few days after surgery. Therefore, adequate treatment with CPAP and optimized anesthesia without sedatives and opioids is preferable in these patients.

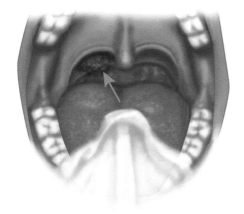

Fig. 10.10 Bleeding after tonsillectomy.

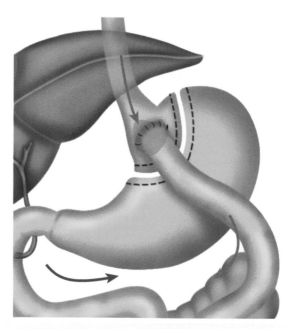

Fig. 10.11 Leakage of the gastrojejunostomy in gastric bypass surgery.

Factors to be considered in determining the adequacy of performing surgical procedures in OSA patients in an outpatient setting have been described by the ASA Task Force[32] (see ▶Table 10.3).

10.2.12 Postoperative Follow-Up

After discharge, follow-up of surgical patients is arranged through the outpatient clinic. This department enables evaluation of clinical status and arrangements of both diagnostics and treatment without requiring hospital admission or overnight care. First medical follow-up after surgery is mostly after 1 to 2 weeks, dependent on the type of surgery. During this visit, surgical outcome and complications are evaluated and sutures/agraves are removed when necessary. This section describes the outpatient care of OSA patients who underwent surgery.

OSA Follow-Up: When and How?

Patients who underwent surgery visit the outpatient clinic to evaluate surgical outcome and adverse events. However, one must not forget that those with OSA should receive adequate postoperative follow-up for their OSA as well. Timing for OSA follow-up depends on the type and expected outcome of surgery and is further discussed. As no reliable screening tools have been identified to assess residual disease in the postoperative setting, PSG is the recommended test in the postoperative phase (▶Table 10.8). In the Netherlands, according to the Dutch guideline for "diagnosis and treatment of OSA in adults," it is customary to repeat a sleep study in patients

▶ Table 10.8 OSA follow-up for different surgical groups

Type of surgery	Follow-up requirements
Head and neck surgery for OSA	PSG CPAP compliance report
Bariatric surgery	PSG CPAP compliance report
General (non-OSA) surgery	Annual clinical appointment CPAP compliance report

Abbreviations: CPAP, continuous positive airway pressure; OSA, obstructive sleep apnea; PSG, polysomnography.

▶ Table 10.9 Timing of postoperative PSG in moderately severe OSA patients

Type of surgery	Time of postoperative PSG
Head and neck surgery for OSA	3–6 mo 12 mo When considered necessary
Bariatric surgery	6–12 mo When considered necessary
General (non-OSA) surgery	Only indicated when changes in AHI are expected, (e.g., due to weight loss)

Abbreviations: AHI, apnea–hypopnea index; CPAP, continuous positive airway pressure; OSA, obstructive sleep apnea; PSG, polysomnography.

who had an AHI above 15 before treatment or in patients with mild disease (AHI < 15), whenever there is doubt about clinical improvement.

As a PSG has several cost-efficient disadvantages, future perspectives are to develop a less time-consuming, less expensive, and more patient-friendly test that is applicable in all clinics, such as high-volume bariatric centers.

The most commonly used therapy for OSA is CPAP.[69] This device is mostly prescribed for patients diagnosed with an AHI more than 15/hour, indicating moderately severe disease. Well-selected patients who undergo site-specific surgical interventions achieve AHI levels below 15/hour. Criteria for surgical success are discussed in Chapters 5.2 and 5.3. Prior to reevaluation PSG, one must consider the presence of CPAP washout. This effect has been previously described (Chapter 5.1).

Patients with moderately severe and severe OSA are usually nonpositional; their AHI is high in all positions. However, when the postoperative AHI is reduced, patients with residual mild disease (AHI 5–15/hour) could develop POSA, in which the AHI is at least twice as high in supine position than in other positions; their AHI dropped more in lateral as compared with supine sleeping position. When patients become positional (i.e., mean AHI 15/hour, but AHI in supine position 60/hour) after OSA-specific head and neck or bariatric surgery, and a significant percentage of their total sleeping time is in supine position, they might experience clinical symptoms and be at risk of cardiovascular complications. For this subgroup, additional PT might be indicated (Chapter 4).

Head and Neck Surgery for OSA

For patients with a preoperative AHI greater than 15/hour (moderately severe disease), a follow-up PSG is recommended at 3 to 6 months and, on indication, 12 months after surgery (▶Table 10.9).[118] At least 3 months are required for a patient to reduce the postoperative swelling in the pharyngeal area and to adapt to a new situation, whereas a preliminary effect should be seen 6 months after surgery. Ideally one should not wait much longer, since in case of a negative treatment outcome, additional measures are indicated. Additional follow-up moments should be planned when further success is expected. This might be the case after bariatric surgery,

when additional weight loss between 6 and 12 months postoperative is accomplished. Additional PT is prescribed when after partial effective surgery severe nonpositional OSA reverses to less severe POSA, requiring the effect of this combined treatment modality (surgery and PT) to be evaluated. A temporary rise in the proportion central and mixed sleep apneic events is another reason to repeat sleep studies after head and neck surgery in the long term. This is a reversal phenomenon, with or without (medical) intervention. Repeated PSG might show reduction in the central and mixed component after another 6 months. Patients with a preoperative AHI 5 to 15/hour (mild disease) with subjective clinical improvement are thought to be curated after surgery, and postoperative PSG is only indicated when there are doubts about surgical success.

Bariatric Surgery

Since bariatric patients experience major changes such as weight loss and improved physical and mental status after surgery, differentiating OSA improvements such as less tiredness and lower BMI from these changes remains a difficult task. For this reason, PSG is superior to screening questionnaires in the postbariatric setting. There is an ongoing debate regarding timing of postoperative PSG. Several studies performing PSG before and after bariatric surgery have been reported. Greenburg and colleagues published a systematic review of 12 studies representing 342 patients. While the included studies had varying follow-up criteria, the effect of timing was not analyzed by the authors.[119] A recent study used follow-up data of more than 12 months, another study of 7 and 12 months, while another group reported at 6 and 9 months.[120,121,122,123] One study evaluated the AHI improvement at two postoperative intervals. A total of 50 patients underwent a PSG at 7.1 and 16.9 months, respectively, after bariatric surgery. The mean AHI decreased from 49.1 to 22.7 to 17.4/hour.[121] The largest study including 205 patients showed that nearly three-quarter of the moderately severe OSA (AHI ≥15/hour) patients were curated (AHI < 5/hour) or had residual mild OSA (AHI

5–14.9/hour). This result was seen after a mean follow-up of 8.6 months (standard deviation 4.8). While this and previous studies have not succeeded in finding a correlation between weight loss and AHI reduction, the most recent study has found excess weight loss below 60% to be a significant predictive factor for persistent moderately severe OSA after bariatric surgery.[122] Hence, timing of postoperative PSG should be dependent on excess weight loss and patients' symptoms, though this is not 100% accurate. A reasonable time for follow-up PSG seems between 6 and 12 months postoperatively.

General Surgery

There are many patients who undergo surgery for other reasons than OSA, most common being orthopedic surgery. Although no improvement is expected post-surgery, OSA patients should receive adequate follow-up for their OSA. This includes a clinical appointment at the outpatient clinic and a compliance report of CPAP annually.[118]

CPAP and Compliance

One of the most challenging parts of follow-up is maintaining CPAP compliance. Multiple definitions of compliance exist. A frequently used definition of compliance is more than 4 hours of CPAP use per night for at least 5 days a week.[118] Another definition of compliance is more than 4 hours of CPAP use for 7 nights a week. Maintaining CPAP compliance is highly important in all OSA patients after surgery. Patients who underwent surgery for reducing OSA severity, for example head and neck surgery for OSA or bariatric surgery, often assume CPAP compliance is of little importance after surgery. However, previous sections have shown that significant reduction of the AHI may require several months, while clinical improvement first needs to be confirmed by a sleep study. During these months, adequate follow-up is essential to monitor any reduction in OSA-related clinical symptoms and risks. As CPAP pressures might change due to surgical success, frequent pressure evaluations are necessary to avoid mask complaints and to improve effectiveness and compliance.[123] In case of persistent OSA, patients should be managed as any other OSA patient. One small study showed that patients with persistent OSA after bariatric surgery experienced increase of the BMI when not using CPAP at long-term follow-up compared to those with continued CPAP usage (6.8% vs. −1.8%, p = 0.05).[124]

Patients who underwent surgery without effect on OSA severity require long-term OSA treatment. Maintaining long-term compliance is essential for this group. Predictive factors for long-term (5 year) compliance are:
- AHI above 15/hour.
- ESS score > 10.
- CPAP usage > 4 hours/night at 3 months of follow-up.[86]

Key components to increasing compliance are:
- Education regarding CPAP usage.
- Motivation.
- Insight of the consequences of untreated OSA.
- Mask interface/mask fit.
- CPAP pressure.
- (Warm) humidifier.
- Regular follow-up with PSG and compliance reports.

Risks and Tips and Tricks

Recognition and anticipation of OSA is highly important in patients undergoing surgery. Surgeons and anesthesiologists need to be aware of different patient groups such as patients undergoing head and neck surgery for OSA, bariatric patients, and patients undergoing general surgery. Perioperative management should be arranged based on patient characteristics, type of surgery, and hospital arrangements. OSA can be diagnosed with a formal sleep study (Type I–IV); screening questionnaires may be used with precaution to screen patients for OSA when sleep studies are not available/applicable. Several intraoperative tools exist to optimize OSA patients and minimize the risk of perioperative complications. Examples are usage of CPAP, preoxygenation, and avoidance of sedatives and opioids. Postoperative monitoring is essential in the early postoperative period to monitor vital parameters, early complaints, and to prevent further complications.

10.3 Follow-Up

Armin Steffen

10.3.1 Definition

This section focusses on follow-up in a more long-term definition with regard to outcome measurements and the identification of adverse events. So, postoperative care for the first 24 to 48 hours is addressed extensively in previous chapters for the particular surgical technique.

The protocol about the extent of the follow-up is highly influenced by the severity of the underlying OSA, the invasiveness and technical approach of the intervention, and the comorbidities of the patient. The time range is mostly regarded as the end of wound healing, which is strongly dependent on OSA treatment and the question whether any implants are used, especially active tools. Therefore, the following can offer some general thinking and experiences, but will never fully meet the individual case.

10.3.2 Follow-Up for Outcome Measurements

The time for performing the reevaluation needs to consider that (1) wound healing has finished and (2) the result of the surgery on the upper airway could affect the health state, especially the daytime sleepiness. In most cases, there is a difference between both points in time.

For the most interventions with resections at the soft palate and minimal invasive techniques at the tongue base, wound healing is finished within 8 to 10 weeks. At this time, early changes can be detected for daytime sleepiness and snoring reduction. Having time with a now more stable effect on the operated airway, most short-term evaluation for reduction of daytime sleepiness are done after 3 months.[125] In more invasive procedures with longer wound healing such as tongue base reduction and interruption of bone continuity such as in maxillomandibular advancement,[126,127] 6 months and more are appropriate. Depending on the early short-term results and the comorbidities in the particular patient, repeated evaluation should be scheduled in a 12-month period. Especially in unfavorable results, this approach of fix revisits supports the relation between patient and surgeon and avoids unwanted changes of treatment centers. For long-term follow-up, it is important to know and instruct the patient for decreasing effects with restarting daytime sleepiness and snoring.[125] A regular long-term follow-up in classic surgical approaches outside of clinical studies depends on the individual situation.

A follow-up should concentrate on the major complaints of the patient which led to the surgery of OSA. An answer should be possible to the procedure's success in patient's perspective. A minimum standard is to document the condition during daytime and whether sleep is regarded as restorative in patient's words, for better comparability additionally assessed in ESS. The effect of snoring in patient's and in bed partner's point of view cannot be overestimated. A strong indicator in reduction of OSA severity is when bed partners can sleep in the same room with the patient having OSA. Adverse events of surgical therapy should be documented with focus on swallowing or speech problems or globus sensation.[128]

Especially in surgical centers, where the OSA diagnostic is done outside, special care is recommended with regard to the type of diagnostic—screening, PG, PSG—and the visual validation of the tests. In the analysis of the OSA tests, there are typical pitfalls, for example the washout effect after CPAP usage[129] or the assessment of POSA.[130,131] So it is not only important to compare the AHI of the total night recording and the AHI in supine position, but also to consider the time spent in supine position as this influences the total night AHI in cases with strong positional dependency. Special attention should be paid to patients with clear benefit with regard to OSA reduction but persisting daytime sleepiness.[1,32] Therefore, a broader evaluation before surgery is helpful if the patient who reports nonrestorative sleep with well-adjusted PAP therapy. Especially a potential depression should be addressed.[133]

In cases with no or insufficient reduction of OSA in the follow-up, a whole workup of sleep diagnostic and the detecting of persisting obstruction sites in the upper airway is recommended. Here, a newly developed sleep endoscopy is of great help.[1,34] Especially considering an escalation of surgical ladder might draw attention to other aspects of sleep endoscopy than before initial surgery.[1,35] Nevertheless, it is important to understand the upper airway not as a rigid pipe what may explain the persistence or newly appeared obstructions after intervention.[1,36] In general, a CT scan or MRI of the neck after insufficient sleep surgery should be reserved for clinical studies or in cases, where a maxillomandibular advancement is taken into account.[126,134] Before starting revision cases, patient should be updated that PAP might be a proper solution without surgical and failure risks, especially as there are reports about restored PAP adherence after failed multilevel surgery.[137] In some patients, a newly gained daytime activity could be used to (re-)motivate for weight loss programs to further improve OSA reduction or to stabilize to surgical result.

10.3.3 Follow-Up in Active and Passive Implants for Sleep Apnea

Special aspects need to be considered when implants have been used to stabilize the upper airway during sleep. As implants can induce foreign body reaction and extrusion over time up to 10%, a more long-term follow-up is recommended.[138,139]

In active implants such as hypoglossal nerve stimulation, several aspects make a long-term follow-up necessary.[140,141] The first 12 months require an intense monitoring as the systems are activated delayed for several weeks, a polysomnographic assessment is performed 2 months after implantation and might require an additional sleep lab visit for advanced titration, and a 6- and 12-month follow-up are recommended. At 6-month follow-up, some patients need additional palate surgery to achieve better outcome and adherence,[1,42] and repeated adjustment of installed impulses as a potential sign of prolonged subtle nerve recovery or newly discovered obstruction sites in sleep endoscopy with stimulation.[143] Even in stimulation systems using a rechargeable battery, the impulse generator needs to be exchanged over the following years, so a lifetime support is necessary.

> ### Key Points
>
> The extent of the follow-up is strongly influenced by the severity of OSA and the expected success rate in the individual case. Especially in nonminimal invasive surgery, severe OSA with high daytime sleepiness and increased cardiovascular comorbidities, the follow-up should consist of subjective and objective outcome measurements. In such cases, equal tools for OSA testing should be preferred for pre- and post-interventional evaluation. In more complex cases, patients should be scheduled for more long-term follow-ups with 12 months and more. Sleep endoscopy can help to detect persisting obstruction sites after sleep surgery and might lead to suggestion for additional approaches. In overweight patients with improved daytime sleepiness but less favorable results, weight reduction programs should be recommended. In implants, especially active implants such as hypoglossal nerve stimulation, there are follow-ups needed for lifetime in order to check the batteries.

References

[1]   Spicuzza L, Caruso D, Di Maria G. Obstructive sleep apnoea syndrome and its management. Ther Adv Chronic Dis. 2015; 6(5):273–285

[2]   Barrera JE. Skeletal surgery for obstructive sleep apnea. Otolaryngol Clin North Am. 2016; 49(6):1433–1447

[3]   Mickelson SA. Nasal surgery for obstructive sleep apnea syndrome. Otolaryngol Clin North Am. 2016; 49(6):1373–1381

[4]   Yaremchuk K. Palatal procedures for obstructive sleep apnea. Otolaryngol Clin North Am. 2016; 49(6):1383–1397

[5]   Gupta RM, Parvizi J, Hanssen AD, Gay PC. Postoperative complications in patients with obstructive sleep apnea syndrome undergoing hip or knee replacement: a case-control study. Mayo Clin Proc. 2001; 76(9):897–905

[6]   Kaw R, Chung F, Pasupuleti V, Mehta J, Gay PC, Hernandez AV. Meta-analysis of the association between obstructive sleep apnoea and postoperative outcome. Br J Anaesth. 2012; 109(6):897–906

[7]   Kaw R, Golish J, Ghamande S, Burgess R, Foldvary N, Walker E. Incremental risk of obstructive sleep apnea on cardiac surgical outcomes. J Cardiovasc Surg (Torino). 2006; 47(6):683–689

[8]   Memtsoudis S, Liu SS, Ma Y, et al. Perioperative pulmonary outcomes in patients with sleep apnea after noncardiac surgery. Anesth Analg. 2011; 112(1):113–121

[9]   Memtsoudis SG, Stundner O, Rasul R, et al. The impact of sleep apnea on postoperative utilization of resources and adverse outcomes. Anesth Analg. 2014; 118(2):407–418

[10] Mokhlesi B, Hovda MD, Vekhter B, Arora VM, Chung F, Meltzer DO. Sleep-disordered breathing and postoperative outcomes after elective surgery: analysis of the nationwide inpatient sample. Chest. 2013; 144(3):903–914

[11] Mokhlesi B, Hovda MD, Vekhter B, Arora VM, Chung F, Meltzer DO. Sleep-disordered breathing and postoperative outcomes after bariatric surgery: analysis of the nationwide inpatient sample. Obes Surg. 2013; 23(11):1842–1851

[12] Opperer M, Cozowicz C, Bugada D, et al. Does obstructive sleep apnea influence perioperative outcome? a qualitative systematic review for the Society of Anesthesia and Sleep Medicine Task Force on preoperative preparation of patients with sleep-disordered breathing. Anesth Analg. 2016; 122(5):1321–1334

[13] Vasu TS, Grewal R, Doghramji K. Obstructive sleep apnea syndrome and perioperative complications: a systematic review of the literature. J Clin Sleep Med. 2012; 8(2):199–207

[14] Abrishami A, Khajehdehi A, Chung F. A systematic review of screening questionnaires for obstructive sleep apnea. Can J Anaesth. 2010; 57(5):423–438

[15] Drager LF, Togeiro SM, Polotsky VY, Lorenzi-Filho G. Obstructive sleep apnea: a cardiometabolic risk in obesity and the metabolic syndrome. J Am Coll Cardiol. 2013; 62(7):569–576

[16] Bahammam A, Delaive K, Ronald J, Manfreda J, Roos L, Kryger MH. Health care utilization in males with obstructive sleep apnea syndrome two years after diagnosis and treatment. Sleep. 1999; 22(6):740–747

[17] McNicholas WT, Ryan S. Obstructive sleep apnoea syndrome: translating science to clinical practice. Respirology. 2006; 11(2):136–144

[18] Franklin KA, Haglund B, Axelsson S, Holmlund T, Rehnqvist N, Rosén M. Frequency of serious complications after surgery for snoring and sleep apnea. Acta Otolaryngol. 2011; 131(3):298–302

[19] Spiegel JH, Raval TH. Overnight hospital stay is not always necessary after uvulopalatopharyngoplasty. Laryngoscope. 2005; 115(1):167–171

[20] Bachar G, Feinmesser R, Shpitzer T, Yaniv E, Nageris B, Eidelman L. Laryngeal and hypopharyngeal obstruction in sleep disordered breathing patients, evaluated by sleep endoscopy. Eur Arch Otorhinolaryngol. 2008; 265(11):1397–1402

[21] Isono S, Remmers JE, Tanaka A, Sho Y, Sato J, Nishino T. Anatomy of pharynx in patients with obstructive sleep apnea and in normal subjects. J Appl Physiol (1985). 1997; 82(4):1319–1326

[22] Patil SP, Schneider H, Schwartz AR, Smith PL. Adult obstructive sleep apnea: pathophysiology and diagnosis. Chest. 2007; 132(1):325–337

[23] Sforza E, Petiau C, Weiss T, Thibault A, Krieger J. Pharyngeal critical pressure in patients with obstructive sleep apnea syndrome. Clinical implications. Am J Respir Crit Care Med. 1999; 159(1):149–157

[24] Strauss SG, Lynn AM, Bratton SL, Nespeca MK. Ventilatory response to CO_2 in children with obstructive sleep apnea from adenotonsillar hypertrophy. Anesth Analg. 1999; 89(2): 328–332

[25] Waters KA, McBrien F, Stewart P, Hinder M, Wharton S. Effects of OSA, inhalational anesthesia, and fentanyl on the airway and ventilation of children. J Appl Physiol (1985). 2002; 92(5):1987–1994

[26] Younes M. Contributions of upper airway mechanics and control mechanisms to severity of obstructive apnea. Am J Respir Crit Care Med. 2003; 168(6):645–658

[27] Esclamado RM, Glenn MG, McCulloch TM, Cummings CW. Perioperative complications and risk factors in the surgical treatment of obstructive sleep apnea syndrome. Laryngoscope. 1989; 99(11):1125–1129

[28] Gabrielczyk MR. Acute airway obstruction after uvulopalatopharyngoplasty for obstructive sleep apnea syndrome. Anesthesiology. 1988; 69(6):941–943

[29] Neill AM, Angus SM, Sajkov D, McEvoy RD. Effects of sleep posture on upper airway stability in patients with obstructive sleep apnea. Am J Respir Crit Care Med. 1997; 155(1):199–204

[30] Nagappa M, Mokhlesi B, Wong J, Wong DT, Kaw R, Chung F. The effects of continuous positive airway pressure on postoperative outcomes in obstructive sleep apnea patients undergoing surgery: a systematic review and meta-analysis. Anesth Analg. 2015; 120(5):1013–1023

[31] Chung F, Liao P, Yegneswaran B, Shapiro CM, Kang W. Postoperative changes in sleep-disordered breathing and sleep architecture in patients with obstructive sleep apnea. Anesthesiology. 2014; 120(2):287–298

[32] American Society of Anesthesiologists Task Force on Perioperative Management of Patients with Obstructive Sleep Apnea. Practice guidelines for the perioperative management of patients with obstructive sleep apnea: an updated report by the American Society of Anesthesiologists Task Force on Perioperative Management of patients with obstructive sleep apnea. Anesthesiology. 2014; 120(2):268–286

[33] Abdelsattar ZM, Hendren S, Wong SL, Campbell DA, Jr, Ramachandran SK. The impact of untreated obstructive sleep apnea on cardiopulmonary complications in general and vascular surgery: a cohort study. Sleep. 2015; 38(8):1205–1210

[34] Mutter TC, Chateau D, Moffatt M, Ramsey C, Roos LL, Kryger M. A matched cohort study of postoperative outcomes in obstructive sleep apnea: could preoperative diagnosis and treatment prevent complications? Anesthesiology. 2014; 121(4):707–718

[35] Cordovani L, Chung F, Germain G, et al. Canadian Perioperative Anesthesia Clinical Trials Group. Perioperative management of patients with obstructive sleep apnea: a survey of Canadian anesthesiologists. Can J Anaesth. 2016; 63(1):16–23

[36] Chung F, Memtsoudis SG, Ramachandran SK, et al. Society of Anesthesia and Sleep Medicine Guidelines on preoperative screening and assessment of adult patients with obstructive sleep apnea. Anesth Analg. 2016; 123(2):452–473

[37] Sullivan CE, Issa FG, Berthon-Jones M, Eves L. Reversal of obstructive sleep apnoea by continuous positive airway pressure applied through the nares. Lancet. 1981; 1(8225):862–865

[38] Gottlieb DJ, Punjabi NM, Mehra R, et al. CPAP versus oxygen in obstructive sleep apnea. N Engl J Med. 2014; 370(24):2276–2285

[39] Gay P, Weaver T, Loube D, Iber C; Positive Airway Pressure Task Force. Standards of Practice Committee. American Academy of Sleep Medicine. Evaluation of positive airway pressure treatment for sleep related breathing disorders in adults. Sleep. 2006; 29(3):381–401

[40] Giles TL, Lasserson TJ, Smith BJ, White J, Wright J, Cates CJ. Continuous positive airways pressure for obstructive sleep apnoea in adults. Cochrane Database Syst Rev. 2006; 25(1):Cd001106

[41] Jing J, Huang T, Cui W, Shen H. Effect on quality of life of continuous positive airway pressure in patients with obstructive sleep apnea syndrome: a meta-analysis. Lung. 2008; 186(3):131–144

[42] Qureshi WT, Nasir UB, Alqalyoobi S, et al. Meta-analysis of continuous positive airway pressure as a therapy of atrial fibrillation in obstructive sleep apnea. Am J Cardiol. 2015; 116(11):1767–1773

[43] Somers VK, White DP, Amin R, et al. Sleep apnea and cardiovascular disease: an American Heart Association/American College of Cardiology Foundation Scientific Statement from the American Heart Association Council for High Blood Pressure Research Professional Education Committee, Council on Clinical Cardiology, Stroke Council, and Council on Cardiovascular Nursing. J Am Coll Cardiol. 2008; 52(8):686–717

[44] Tregear S, Reston J, Schoelles K, Phillips B. Continuous positive airway pressure reduces risk of motor vehicle crash among drivers with obstructive sleep apnea: systematic review and meta-analysis. Sleep. 2010; 33(10):1373–1380

[45] McEvoy RD, Antic NA, Heeley E, et al. SAVE Investigators and Coordinators. CPAP for prevention of cardiovascular events in obstructive sleep apnea. N Engl J Med. 2016; 375(10):919–931

[46] Kindgen-Milles D, Müller E, Buhl R, et al. Nasal-continuous positive airway pressure reduces pulmonary morbidity and length of hospital stay following thoracoabdominal aortic surgery. Chest. 2005; 128(2):821–828

[47] Liao P, Yegneswaran B, Vairavanathan S, Zilberman P, Chung F. Postoperative complications in patients with obstructive sleep apnea: a retrospective matched cohort study. Can J Anaesth. 2009; 56(11):819–828

[48] Zarbock A, Mueller E, Netzer S, Gabriel A, Feindt P, Kindgen-Milles D. Prophylactic nasal continuous positive airway pressure following cardiac surgery protects from postoperative pulmonary complications: a prospective, randomized, controlled trial in 500 patients. Chest. 2009; 135(5):1252–1259

[49] Mador MJ, Goplani S, Gottumukkala VA, et al. Postoperative complications in obstructive sleep apnea. Sleep Breath. 2013; 17(2):727–734

[50] Kempfle JS, BuSaba NY, Dobrowski JM, Westover MB, Bianchi MT. A cost-effectiveness analysis of nasal surgery to increase continuous positive airway pressure adherence in sleep apnea patients with nasal obstruction. Laryngoscope. 2017; 127(4):977–983

[51] Auckley D, Bolden N. Preoperative screening and perioperative care of the patient with sleep-disordered breathing. Curr Opin Pulm Med. 2012; 18(6):588–595

[52] Ankichetty S, Wong J, Chung F. A systematic review of the effects of sedatives and anesthetics in patients with obstructive sleep apnea. J Anaesthesiol Clin Pharmacol. 2011; 27(4):447–458

[53] Adesanya AO, Lee W, Greilich NB, Joshi GP. Perioperative management of obstructive sleep apnea. Chest. 2010; 138(6):1489–1498

[54] Haytoğlu S, Arikan OK, Muluk NB, Kuran G. Relief of pain at rest and during swallowing after modified cautery-assisted uvulopalatopharyngoplasty: bupivacaine versus lidocaine. J Craniofac Surg. 2015; 26(3):e216–e223

[55] Murphy GS, Brull SJ. Residual neuromuscular block: lessons unlearned. Part I: definitions, incidence, and adverse physiologic effects of residual neuromuscular block. Anesth Analg. 2010; 111(1):120–128

[56] Ünal DY, Baran İ, Mutlu M, Ural G, Akkaya T, Özlü O. Comparison of Sugammadex versus Neostigmine costs and respiratory complications in patients with obstructive sleep apnoea. Turk J Anaesthesiol Reanim. 2015; 43(6):387–395

[57] Brousseau CA, Dobson GR, Milne AD. A retrospective analysis of airway management in patients with obstructive sleep apnea and its effects on postanesthesia care unit length of stay. Can J Respir Ther. 2014; 50(1):23–26

[58] Chung F, Yegneswaran B, Herrera F, Shenderey A, Shapiro CM. Patients with difficult intubation may need referral to sleep clinics. Anesth Analg. 2008; 107(3):915–920

[59] Corso RM, Piraccini E, Calli M, et al. Obstructive sleep apnea is a risk factor for difficult endotracheal intubation. Minerva Anestesiol. 2011; 77(1):99–100

[60] Iyer US, Koh KF, Chia NC, Macachor J, Cheng A. Perioperative risk factors in obese patients for bariatric surgery: a Singapore experience. Singapore Med J. 2011; 52(2):94–99

[61] Kheterpal S, Healy D, Aziz MF, et al. Multicenter Perioperative Outcomes Group (MPOG) Perioperative Clinical Research Committee. Incidence, predictors, and outcome of difficult mask ventilation combined with difficult laryngoscopy: a report from the multicenter perioperative outcomes group. Anesthesiology. 2013; 119(6):1360–1369

[62] Kheterpal S, Martin L, Shanks AM, Tremper KK. Prediction and outcomes of impossible mask ventilation: a review of 50,000 anesthetics. Anesthesiology. 2009; 110(4):891–897

[63] Kim JA, Lee JJ. Preoperative predictors of difficult intubation in patients with obstructive sleep apnea syndrome. Can J Anaesth. 2006; 53(4):393–397

[64] Siyam MA, Benhamou D. Difficult endotracheal intubation in patients with sleep apnea syndrome. Anesth Analg. 2002; 95(4):1098–1102

[65] Apfelbaum JL, Hagberg CA, Caplan RA, et al. American Society of Anesthesiologists Task Force on Management of the Difficult Airway. Practice guidelines for management of the difficult airway: an updated report by the American Society of Anesthesiologists Task Force on Management of the Difficult Airway. Anesthesiology. 2013; 118(2):251–270

[66] Chung F, Liao P, Elsaid H, Shapiro CM, Kang W. Factors associated with postoperative exacerbation of sleep-disordered breathing. Anesthesiology. 2014; 120(2):299–311

[67] Kaw R, Pasupuleti V, Walker E, Ramaswamy A, Foldvary-Schafer N. Postoperative complications in patients with obstructive sleep apnea. Chest. 2012; 141(2):436–441

[68] Gaucher A, Frasca D, Mimoz O, Debaene B. Accuracy of respiratory rate monitoring by capnometry using the Capnomask(R) in extubated patients receiving supplemental oxygen after surgery. Br J Anaesth. 2012; 108(2):316–320

[69] Chung F, Nagappa M, Singh M, Mokhlesi B. CPAP in the perioperative setting: evidence of support. Chest. 2016; 149(2):586–597

[70] Camacho M, Riaz M, Capasso R, et al. The effect of nasal surgery on continuous positive airway pressure device use and therapeutic treatment pressures: a systematic review and meta-analysis. Sleep. 2015; 38(2):279–286

[71] Friedman M, Maley A, Kelley K, et al. Impact of nasal obstruction on obstructive sleep apnea. Otolaryngol Head Neck Surg. 2011; 144(6):1000–1004

[72] Liu SS, Wu CL. Effect of postoperative analgesia on major postoperative complications: a systematic update of the evidence. Anesth Analg. 2007; 104(3):689–702

[73] Lam KK, Kunder S, Wong J, Doufas AG, Chung F. Obstructive sleep apnea, pain, and opioids: is the riddle solved? Curr Opin Anaesthesiol. 2016; 29(1):134–140

[74] Doufas AG, Tian L, Padrez KA, et al. Experimental pain and opioid analgesia in volunteers at high risk for obstructive sleep apnea. PLoS One. 2013; 8(1):e54807

[75] Wang D, Marshall NS, Duffin J, et al. Phenotyping interindividual variability in obstructive sleep apnoea response to temazepam using ventilatory chemoreflexes during wakefulness. J Sleep Res. 2011; 20(4):526–532

[76] Younes M. Role of respiratory control mechanisms in the pathogenesis of obstructive sleep disorders. J Appl Physiol (1985). 2008; 105(5):1389–1405

[77] Maund E, McDaid C, Rice S, Wright K, Jenkins B, Woolacott N. Paracetamol and selective and non-selective non-steroidal anti-inflammatory drugs for the reduction in morphine-related side-effects after major surgery: a systematic review. Br J Anaesth. 2011; 106(3):292–297

[78] Riggin L, Ramakrishna J, Sommer DD, Koren G. A 2013 updated systematic review & meta-analysis of 36 randomized controlled trials; no apparent effects of non steroidal anti-inflammatory

agents on the risk of bleeding after tonsillectomy. Clin Otolaryngol. 2013; 38(2):115–129

[79] Jokic R, Klimaszewski A, Crossley M, Sridhar G, Fitzpatrick MF. Positional treatment vs continuous positive airway pressure in patients with positional obstructive sleep apnea syndrome. Chest. 1999; 115(3):771–781

[80] Gali B, Whalen FX, Schroeder DR, Gay PC, Plevak DJ. Identification of patients at risk for postoperative respiratory complications using a preoperative obstructive sleep apnea screening tool and postanesthesia care assessment. Anesthesiology. 2009; 110(4):869–877

[81] Dorn M, Pirsig W, Verse T. [Postoperative management following rhinosurgery interventions in severe obstructive sleep apnea. A pilot study] HNO. 2001; 49(8):642–645

[82] Joshi GP, Ankichetty SP, Gan TJ, Chung F. Society for Ambulatory Anesthesia consensus statement on preoperative selection of adult patients with obstructive sleep apnea scheduled for ambulatory surgery. Anesth Analg. 2012; 115(5):1060–1068

[83] Stierer TL, Wright C, George A, Thompson RE, Wu CL, Collop N. Risk assessment of obstructive sleep apnea in a population of patients undergoing ambulatory surgery. J Clin Sleep Med. 2010; 6(5):467–472

[84] Kezirian EJ, Weaver EM, Yueh B, Khuri SF, Daley J, Henderson WG. Risk factors for serious complication after uvulopalatopharyngoplasty. Arch Otolaryngol Head Neck Surg. 2006; 132(10): 1091–1098

[85] Regli A, von Ungern-Sternberg BS, Strobel WM, Pargger H, Welge-Luessen A, Reber A. The impact of postoperative nasal packing on sleep-disordered breathing and nocturnal oxygen saturation in patients with obstructive sleep apnea syndrome. Anesth Analg. 2006; 102(2):615–620

[86] Malhotra A, White DP. Obstructive sleep apnoea. Lancet. 2002; 360(9328):237–245

[87] Hai F, Porhomayon J, Vermont L, Frydrych L, Jaoude P, El-Solh AA. Postoperative complications in patients with obstructive sleep apnea: a meta-analysis. J Clin Anesth. 2014; 26(8):591–600

[88] Ravesloot MJ, van Maanen JP, Hilgevoord AA, van Wagensveld BA, de Vries N. Obstructive sleep apnea is underrecognized and underdiagnosed in patients undergoing bariatric surgery. Eur Arch Otorhinolaryngol. 2012; 269(7):1865–1871

[89] de Raaff CA, Pierik AS, Coblijn UK, de Vries N, Bonjer HJ, van Wagensveld BA. Value of routine polysomnography in bariatric surgery. Surg Endosc. 2017; 31(1):245–248

[90] Epstein LJ, Kristo D, Strollo PJ, Jr, et al. Adult Obstructive Sleep Apnea Task Force of the American Academy of Sleep Medicine. Clinical guideline for the evaluation, management and long-term care of obstructive sleep apnea in adults. J Clin Sleep Med. 2009; 5(3):263–276

[91] de Raaff CAL, Gorter-Stam MAW, de Vries N, et al. Perioperative management of obstructive sleep apnea in bariatric surgery: a consensus guideline. Surg Obes Relat Dis. 2017; 13(7):1095–1109

[92] Dumitrache-Rujinski S, Calcaianu G, Zaharia D, Toma CL, Bogdan M. The role of overnight pulse-oximetry in recognition of obstructive sleep apnea syndrome in morbidly obese and non obese patients. Maedica (Buchar). 2013; 8(3):237–242

[93] Malbois M, Giusti V, Suter M, Pellaton C, Vodoz JF, Heinzer R. Oximetry alone versus portable polygraphy for sleep apnea screening before bariatric surgery. Obes Surg. 2010; 20(3): 326–331

[94] Chung F, Zhou L, Liao P. Parameters from preoperative overnight oximetry predict postoperative adverse events. Minerva Anestesiol. 2014; 80(10):1084–1095

[95] El Shayeb M, Topfer LA, Stafinski T, Pawluk L, Menon D. Diagnostic accuracy of level 3 portable sleep tests versus level 1 polysomnography for sleep-disordered breathing: a systematic review and meta-analysis. CMAJ. 2014; 186(1):E25–E51

[96] Fredheim JM, Røislien J, Hjelmesæth J. Validation of a portable monitor for the diagnosis of obstructive sleep apnea in morbidly obese patients. J Clin Sleep Med. 2014; 10(7):751–757, 757A

[97] Oliveira MG, Treptow EC, Fukuda C, et al. Diagnostic accuracy of home-based monitoring system in morbidly obese patients with high risk for sleep apnea. Obes Surg. 2015; 25(5):845–851

[98] Gan YJ, Lim L, Chong YK. Validation study of WatchPat 200 for diagnosis of OSA in an Asian cohort. Eur Arch Otorhinolaryngol. 2017; 274(3):1741–1745

[99] Nagappa M, Liao P, Wong J, et al. Validation of the STOP-Bang Questionnaire as a screening tool for obstructive sleep apnea among different populations: a systematic review and meta-analysis. PLoS One. 2015; 10(12):e0143697

[100] Rosenthal LD, Dolan DC. The Epworth sleepiness scale in the identification of obstructive sleep apnea. J Nerv Ment Dis. 2008; 196(5):429–431

[101] Chung F, Yang Y, Liao P. Predictive performance of the STOP-Bang score for identifying obstructive sleep apnea in obese patients. Obes Surg. 2013; 23(12):2050–2057

[102] Montesi SB, Bajwa EK, Malhotra A. Biomarkers of sleep apnea. Chest. 2012; 142(1):239–245

[103] Archontogeorgis K, Nena E, Papanas N, Steiropoulos P. Biomarkers to improve diagnosis and monitoring of obstructive sleep apnea syndrome: current status and future perspectives. Pulm Med. 2014; 2014:930535

[104] de Raaff CA, Bindt DM, de Vries N, van Wagensveld BA. Positional obstructive sleep apnea in bariatric surgery patients: risk factor for postoperative cardiopulmonary complications? Sleep Breath. 2016; 20(1):113–119

[105] Neligan PJ, Porter S, Max B, Malhotra G, Greenblatt EP, Ochroch EA. Obstructive sleep apnea is not a risk factor for difficult intubation in morbidly obese patients. Anesth Analg. 2009; 109(4):1182–1186

[106] Neligan PJ. Metabolic syndrome: anesthesia for morbid obesity. Curr Opin Anaesthesiol. 2010; 23(3):375–383

[107] Strauss PZ. Perianesthesia implications of obstructive sleep apnea. Crit Care Nurs Q. 2015; 38(1):97–108

[108] Mulier JP. Perioperative opioids aggravate obstructive breathing in sleep apnea syndrome: mechanisms and alternative anesthesia strategies. Curr Opin Anaesthesiol. 2016; 29(1):129–133

[109] Schug SA, Raymann A. Postoperative pain management of the obese patient. Best Pract Res Clin Anaesthesiol. 2011; 25(1):73–81

[110] Schumann R. Anaesthesia for bariatric surgery. Best Pract Res Clin Anaesthesiol. 2011; 25(1):83–93

[111] de Raaff CA, Coblijn UK, de Vries N, van Wagensveld BA. Is fear for postoperative cardiopulmonary complications after bariatric surgery in patients with obstructive sleep apnea justified? A systematic review. Am J Surg. 2016; 211(4):793–801

[112] Goucham AB, Coblijn UK, Hart-Sweet HB, de Vries N, Lagarde SM, van Wagensveld BA. Routine postoperative monitoring after bariatric surgery in morbidly obese patients with severe obstructive sleep apnea: ICU admission is not necessary. Obes Surg. 2016; 26(4):737–742

[113] Ramirez A, Lalor PF, Szomstein S, Rosenthal RJ. Continuous positive airway pressure in immediate postoperative period after laparoscopic Roux-en-Y gastric bypass: is it safe? Surg Obes Relat Dis. 2009; 5(5):544–546

[114] Huerta S, DeShields S, Shpiner R, et al. Safety and efficacy of postoperative continuous positive airway pressure to prevent pulmonary complications after Roux-en-Y gastric bypass. J Gastrointest Surg. 2002; 6(3):354–358

[115] Jensen C, Tejirian T, Lewis C, Yadegar J, Dutson E, Mehran A. Postoperative CPAP and BiPAP use can be safely omitted after laparoscopic Roux-en-Y gastric bypass. Surg Obes Relat Dis. 2008; 4(4):512–514

[116] Scheenstra RJ, Hilgevoord AA, Van Rijn PM. [Serious haemorrhage after conventional (adeno)tonsillectomy: rare and most often on the day of the procedure] Ned Tijdschr Geneeskd. 2007; 151(10):598–601

[117] Mannaerts GH, van Mil SR, Stepaniak PS, et al. Results of implementing an enhanced recovery after bariatric surgery (ERABS) protocol. Obes Surg. 2016; 26(2):303–312

[118] Dutch society of doctors for Pulmonology and Tuberculosis. Diagnosis and treatment of obstructive sleep apnea in adults: a Dutch guideline. 2009:129;172. Available at: http://www.nvalt.nl

[119] Greenburg DL, Lettieri CJ, Eliasson AH. Effects of surgical weight loss on measures of obstructive sleep apnea: a meta-analysis. Am J Med. 2009; 122(6):535–542

[120] Bae EK, Lee YJ, Yun CH, Heo Y. Effects of surgical weight loss for treating obstructive sleep apnea. Sleep Breath. 2014; 18(4):901–905

[121] Ravesloot MJ, Hilgevoord AA, van Wagensveld BA, de Vries N. Assessment of the effect of bariatric surgery on obstructive sleep apnea at two postoperative intervals. Obes Surg. 2014; 24(1):22–31

[122] de Raaff CA, Coblijn UK, Ravesloot MJ, de Vries N, de Lange-de Klerk ES, van Wagensveld BA. Persistent moderate or severe obstructive sleep apnea after laparoscopic Roux-en-Y gastric bypass: which patients? Surg Obes Relat Dis. 2016; 12(10):1866–1872

[123] Lankford DA, Proctor CD, Richard R. Continuous positive airway pressure (CPAP) changes in bariatric surgery patients undergoing rapid weight loss. Obes Surg. 2005; 15(3):336–341

[124] Collen J, Lettieri CJ, Eliasson A. Postoperative CPAP use impacts long-term weight loss following bariatric surgery. J Clin Sleep Med. 2015; 11(3):213–217

[125] Verse T, Dreher A, Heiser C, et al. ENT-specific therapy of obstructive sleep apnoea in adults: A revised version of the previously published German S2e guideline. Sleep Breath. 2016; 20(4):1301–1311

[126] Faria AC, Garcia LV, Santos AC, Eckeli AL, Garcia DM, Mello-Filho FV. Dynamic comparison of pharyngeal stability during sleep in patients with obstructive sleep apnea syndrome treated with maxillomandibular advancement. Sleep Breath. 2016

[127] Boyd SB, Walters AS, Waite P, Harding SM, Song Y. Long-term effectiveness and safety of maxillomandibular advancement for treatment of obstructive sleep apnea. J Clin Sleep Med. 2015; 11(7):699–708

[128] Franklin KA, Anttila H, Axelsson S, et al. Effects and side-effects of surgery for snoring and obstructive sleep apnea—a systematic review. Sleep. 2009; 32(1):27–36

[129] Vroegop AV, Smithuis JW, Benoist LB, Vanderveken OM, de Vries N. CPAP washout prior to reevaluation polysomnography: a sleep surgeon's perspective. Sleep Breath. 2015; 19(2):433–439

[130] Benoist LB, Verhagen M, Torensma B, van Maanen JP, de Vries N. Positional therapy in patients with residual positional obstructive sleep apnea after upper airway surgery. Sleep Breath. 2016

[131] Steffen A, Maibücher L, König IR. Supine position and REM dependence in obstructive sleep apnea. HNO. 2017; 65(1):52–58

[132] Dongol EM, Williams AJ. Residual excessive sleepiness in patients with obstructive sleep apnea on treatment with continuous positive airway pressure. Curr Opin Pulm Med. 2016; 22(6):589–594

[133] Gagnadoux F, Le Vaillant M, Goupil F, et al. IRSR Sleep Cohort Group*. Depressive symptoms before and after long-term CPAP therapy in patients with sleep apnea. Chest. 2014; 145(5):1025–1031

[134] Li S, Wu D, Shi H. Reoperation on patients with obstructive sleep apnea-hypopnea syndrome after failed uvulopalato-pharyngoplasty. Eur Arch Otorhinolaryngol. 2015; 272(2):407–412

[135] Steffen A, Frenzel H, Wollenberg B, König IR. Patient selection for upper airway stimulation: is concentric collapse in sleep endoscopy predictable? Sleep Breath. 2015; 19(4):1373–1376

[136] Blumen MB, Latournerie V, Bequignon E, Guillere L, Chabolle F. Are the obstruction sites visualized on drug-induced sleep endoscopy reliable? Sleep Breath. 2015; 19(3):1021–1026

[137] Azbay S, Bostanci A, Aysun Y, Turhan M. The influence of multi-level upper airway surgery on CPAP tolerance in non-responders to obstructive sleep apnea surgery. Eur Arch Otorhinolaryngol. 2016; 273(9):2813–2818

[138] Choi JH, Kim SN, Cho JH. Efficacy of the Pillar implant in the treatment of snoring and mild-to-moderate obstructive sleep apnea: a meta-analysis. Laryngoscope. 2013; 123(1):269–276

[139] Neruntarat C. Long-term results of palatal implants for obstructive sleep apnea. Eur Arch Otorhinolaryngol. 2011; 268(7):1077–1080

[140] Soose RJ, Gillespie MB. Upper airway stimulation therapy: a novel approach to managing obstructive sleep apnea. Laryngoscope. 2016; 126(Suppl 7):S5–S8

[141] Friedman M, Jacobowitz O, Hwang MS, et al. Targeted hypoglossal nerve stimulation for the treatment of obstructive sleep apnea: six-month results. Laryngoscope. 2016; 126(11):2618–2623

[142] Heiser C. Advanced titration to treat a floppy epiglottis in selective upper airway stimulation. Laryngoscope. 2016; 126(Suppl 7):S22–S24

[143] Heiser C, Maurer JT, Hofauer B, Sommer JU, Seitz A, Steffen A. Outcomes of upper airway stimulation for obstructive sleep apnea in a multicenter German postmarket study. Otolaryngol Head Neck Surg. 2017; 156(2):378–384

[144] D'Apuzzo MR, Browne JA. Obstructive sleep apnea as a risk factor for postoperative complications after revision joint arthroplasty. J Arthroplasty. 2012; 27(8 Suppl):95–98

[145] Flink BJ, Rivelli SK, Cox EA, et al. Obstructive sleep apnea and incidence of postoperative delirium after elective knee replacement in the nondemented elderly. Anesthesiology. 2012; 116(4):788–796

Index

Note: Page numbers set in **bold** or *italic* indicate headings or figures, respectively.